Management of Orbital and Ocular Adnexal Tumors and Inflammations

Management of Orbital and Ocular Adnexal Tumors and Inflammations

Edited by

Joseph A. Mauriello, Jr., M.D.
Director of Oculoplastics and Ophthalmic Pathology
Eye Institute of New Jersey
University of Medicine and Dentistry of New Jersey
New Jersey Medical School
Newark, New Jersey

Joseph C. Flanagan, M.D.
Director of Oculoplastics
Wills Eye Hospital
Thomas Jefferson University
Philadelphia, Pennsylvania

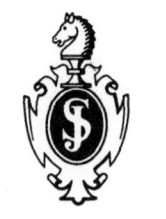 Springer-Verlag Berlin Heidelberg GmbH

Heidelberger Platz 3
1000 Berlin 33
Federal Republic of Germany

Library of Congress Catalog Card Number: 89–080876

ISBN 978-3-662-08465-6   ISBN 978-3-662-08463-2 (eBook)
DOI 10.1007/978-3-662-08463-2

Printing: 1   2   3   4   5   6   7   8   9   10

This book is dedicated to our wives, Marilyn Mauriello and Cathy Flanagan, who have allowed us to indulge ourselves in such a large undertaking in the hours after the long working day.

Contents

Plates

Contributors

Joseph C. Flanagan, M.D.
Director of Oculoplastics
Wills Eye Hospital
Thomas Jefferson University
Philadelphia, Pennsylvania

Steven E. Harms
Director of Resonance Imaging
Baylor University Medical Center
Dallas, Texas

Joseph A. Mauriello, Jr., M.D.
Director of Oculoplastics
   and Ophthalmic Pathology
Eye Institute of New Jersey
University of Medicine and Dentistry
   of New Jersey
New Jersey Medical School
Newark, New Jersey

Thaddeus Nowinski, M.D.
Oculoplastics Department
Wills Eye Hospital
Thomas Jefferson University
Philadelphia, Pennsylvania

Mark Ruchman, M.D.
Director of Oculoplastics
Waterbury Eye Associates
Waterbury, Connecticut

Mary Stefanyszyn, M.D.
Oculoplastics Department
Wills Eye Hospital
Thomas Jefferson University
Philadelphia, Pennsylvania

Preface

This book is designed to provide the busy ophthalmologist with a practical guide to the management of lid and ocular adnexal disease. The book encompasses more than tumors simply because other inflammatory conditions may mimic tumors in their presentation and vice versa. It is not meant to be an encyclopedic, definitive work on a single subject, organized around individual disease entities; instead it approaches the patient much as clinician does. It concentrates on the patient and considers various disease processes logically. Work-up, differential diagnosis, and initial treatment are discussed.

When any patient presents with an orbital or an ocular adnexal mass, the question that needs to be answered is whether the process is due to inflammation or tumor. The history and clinical features are helpful in answering this question. At times a trial of systemic antibiotics is necessary. In many cases, however, an incisional biopsy is indicated to resolve the question finally. When there are no signs of inflammation, a tumor is suspected and the initial step is incisional biopsy.

The nuances of patient management, both before and after biopsy, are considered in a logical stepwise fashion in separate chapters, covering the general approach to the patient, surgical techniques, (including pediatric orbital tumors), orbital tumors and inflammation, lacrimal gland tumors and inflammation, lacrimal sac tumors and inflammation, and lid tumors and inflammations.

This book provides the ophthalmologist with a step-by-step approach to patients with lid and orbital tumors and inflammations.

Acknowledgments

We wish to thank all the referring doctors who have allowed us to treat their patients with orbital and ocular adnexal disease and without whom a book of this type would have been impossible. We also would like to give special thanks to our teachers, Dr. Lorenz E. Zimmerman and Dr. Byron Smith.

We also thank Dr. Ian McLean, chief of ophthalmic pathology, AFIP (Washington, DC) for allowing us to use materials at the AFIP, and the various AFIP alumni who have allowed us to use their material from case presentations at the biannual meetings. Special technical assistance was received from Mr. Richard Press and Mr. David Silva, directors of photography at United Hospital (Newark, NJ) and Wills Eye Hospital (Philadelphia, PA) respectively; and from Mr. Frank Buonomo, chief CT technician, United Hospital (Newark, NJ).

Management of Orbital and Ocular Adnexal Tumors and Inflammations

1

General Approach to the Patient

Joseph A. Mauriello, Jr.
Joseph C. Flanagan

INTRODUCTION

The ophthalmologist's goal in evaluating patients with orbital and ocular adnexal disease may be simplified if he or she attempts to: (1) localize the exact site of the disease process and (2) distinguish between an inflammation and a tumor. A careful history, examination, and use of the computed tomography (CT) scan and magnetic resonance imaging (MRI) as outlined below will be instrumental in the work-up.[1]

The site of the disease process may include lacrimal gland, sac, orbit, globe, or lid. In general, inflammatory processes have a more abrupt onset, while tumors have a gradual onset and lack inflammatory signs. On the one hand, a rapidly growing tumor undergoing necrosis may result in an inflammatory-type presentation (Fig. 1-1). On the other hand, in the lacrimal gland area, for example, a gradual enlargement followed by inflammatory signs or rapid growth is classically represented by malignant change of a benign tumor such as a benign mixed tumor of the lacrimal gland.

LOCALIZING SITE OF DISEASE PROCESS

The differential diagnosis will depend on the site of the disease process at the onset of the disease. Orbital and ocular adnexal disease may originate within the lacrimal sac, lacrimal gland, orbit (intraconal, extraconal, or subperiosteal space), eyelid, the globe, or adjacent sinus or may be metastatic from elsewhere in the body.

Generally, lacrimal sac, lid, lacrimal gland, and eye tumors or inflammations confine themselves to their particular locations. However, advanced stages of some processes eventually spill over and involves other areas of the orbit.

DEFINITION OF TERMS (PSEUDOTUMOR VS. LYMPHOID INFILTRATE)

Since pseudotumors and lymphoid infiltrates are common entities that are sometimes clinically confused and may involve almost any portion of the orbit, we must thoroughly define these distinct clinicopathologic entities (Table 1-1). Chapter 2, "Orbital Inflammatory Disease," considers this subject in detail.

Classically, acute pseudotumor is characterized by an abrupt, painful onset (Fig. 1-2).[1-3] In the acute form of pseudotumor the eye is often injected, and it is important to clinically rule out a bacterial orbital cellulitis (Fig. 1-3). In many cases, a trial of intravenous antibiotics may be necessary before instituting oral steroid therapy. Patients with lymphoid infiltrates tend to have a more gradual, completely painless onset than patients with pseudotumors. Boggy chemosis of the conjunctiva may be present and a salmon-colored subconjunctival infiltrate may be apparent on examination (Fig. 1-4). An anterior orbital infiltrate may be clinically visible, while a posterior infiltrate may present with proptosis. The direction of the proptosis is determined by the location of the infiltrate.

It is crucial to understand that pseudotumor and bacterial orbital cellulitis are inflammations, while a lymphoid

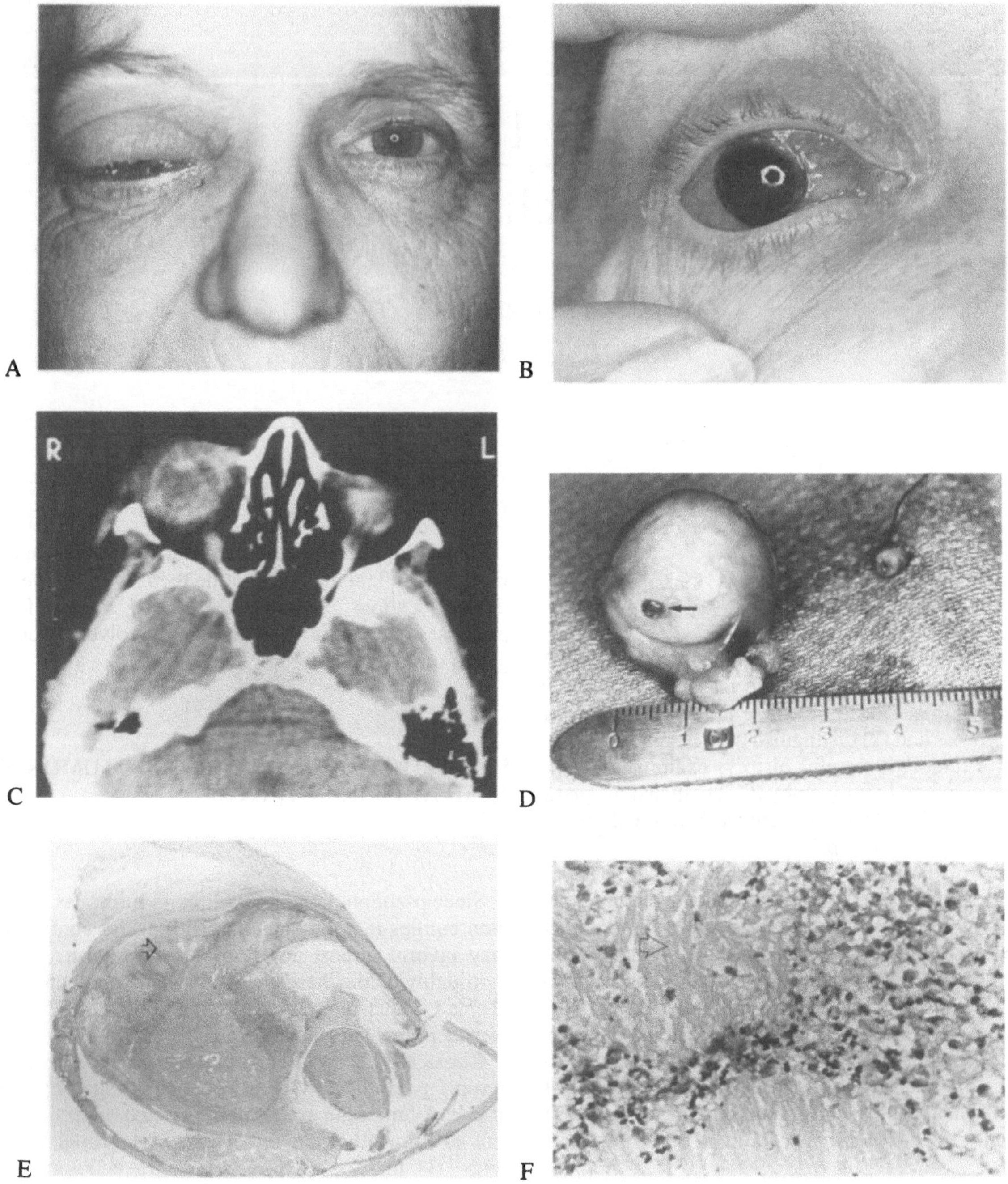

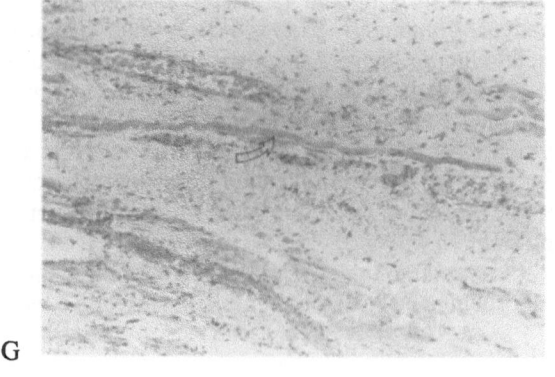

Fig. 1-1. (*A*) A 55-year-old female with 18-month history of gradual loss of vision in the right eye to no light perception (NLP) 6 month prior to presenting with an "orbital cellulitis." (*B*) Ophthalmologic examination showed a 25 percent hyphema and total vitreous opacification. (*C*) Orbital CT scan showed evidence of diffuse vitreous opacification that was compatible with intraocular hemorrhage or tumor. B scan ultrasonography showed similar findings. Because of the blind, painful eye and suspicion of an intraocular tumor, the eye was enucleated. (*D*) During the procedure, brown pigment was noted

Table 1-1
Diagnostic Signs of Pseudotumor vs. Lymphoid Infiltrate

	Pseudotumor	Lymphoid Infiltrate
History	Abrupt, painful onset	Painless onset
	Subacute and chronic forms have little if any associated pain	May be abrupt
		Usually gradual
Examination	Mimics orbital cellulitis	Salmon-colored mass
CT Scan	Centers about anterior aspect of globe or structure in orbit such as EOM, sclera tenons, optic nerve, or lacrimal gland	Diffuse, no bone destruction
	Rarely may be diffuse, "streaky" pattern in subacute or chronic pseudotumor	
Pathology	Mixed cell infiltrate	Diffuse, mostly lymphocytes and or plasma cells
		Based on cytology of individual cells classified as benign reactive, atypical, or malignant lymphoma
	Fibrosis typical	Fibrosis not found
	May be vasculitis or granuloma formation	
Systemic workup	Systemic vasculitis workup if recurrent Scd rate, ANA, Rheumatoid factor	Bone marrow, serum protein electrophoresis (SPEP), CT scan of abdomen to rule out systemic lymphoma, multiple myeloma, Waldenström's macroglobulinemia, and leukemia

infiltrate is a tumor composed of sheets of lymphocytes and plasma cells of varying degrees of cytologic maturity. The lymphoid infiltrate is considered benign reactive lymphoid hyperplasia if it is composed of sheets of cells with benign cytologic features, atypical reactive lymphoid hyperplasia if the cells have atypical cytologic

in the superonasal quadrant outside the adjacent thin sclera as well as in the cross-section of optic nerve (arrow). (E) Microscopic examination of the globe and attached superonasal orbital tissues showed a large melanoma arising from the choroid (open arrow) in the superotemporal quadrant of the right eye with massive necrosis leading to secondary intraocular and orbital hemorrhage and subacute inflammation. (F) High-power magnification of area corresponding to open arrow in E shows totally necrotic tumors cells (open arrow) with adjacent pyknotic tumor cells (black arrow). (G) High-power magnification of orbital tissues shows subacute inflammation and hemorrhage. Note striated EOM fiber (open arrow). (Patient referred by Dr. Anthony Panariello, Jersey City, NJ.)

features, or lymphoma if the infiltrate is frankly malignant. Pathologically, the classic pattern of pseudotumor is that of a mixed of inflammatory cell infiltrate (see Fig. 1-2B). At times, a nonspecific chronic granulomatous process or a vasculitis may be present and the infiltrate may be sparse. Secondary fibrosis occurs in proportion to the chronicity of the condition.

On CT scan, a lymphoid infiltrate presents as a diffuse "tumorous" mass without bone erosion (see Fig. 1-4C). On CT scan, acute pseudotumor may involve: (1) the anterior orbit, mimicking an orbital cellulitis (Fig. 1-3B) with involvement of tenons, episclera, and at times the sclera; (2) the optic nerve; (3) extraocular muscles; or (4) the lacrimal gland (Fig. 1-5). Unlike a lymphoid infiltrate, there is no definite mass to biopsy on CT scan.

In addition, it should be recognized that there are subacute and chronic forms of pseudotumor that may be clinically and pathologically confused with a lymphoid infiltrate. Patients with the latter condition have a more gradual onset of disease with minimal or no pain. Some may have a history of previous acute episodes of pseudotumor. CT scan may show a diffuse process. However, close examination of the nature of the infiltrate will show an irregular rather than homogeneous density, which is characteristic of a lymphoid infiltrate. In such cases, biopsy will not show sheets of cells typical of a lymphoid

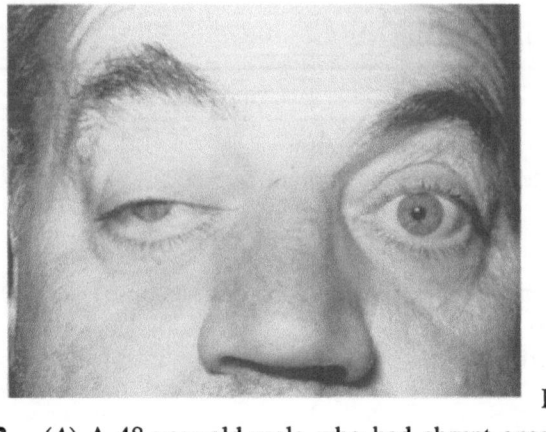
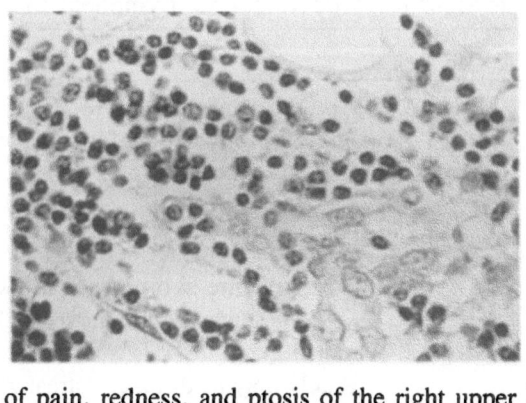

A   B

Fig. 1-2. (*A*) A 48-year-old male who had abrupt onset of pain, redness, and ptosis of the right upper lid that occurred over a 48-hour period. CT scan showed a minimal infiltrate in the superior orbit that did not erode into bone. Because of the history and CT findings consistent with pseudotumor, a trial of oral prednisone was instituted. The patient responded within a week with total resolution of his clinical signs. Steroids were gradually tapered at 10 mg/week until clinical signs of increased redness recurred at a 30-mg dose. The prednisone was more gradually tapered by 5 mg every other day without recurrence. Because of recurrence 6 months later, an orbital biopsy was obtained to rule out a systemic vasculitis such as Wegener's granulomatosis. (*B*) Biopsy showed a mixed inflammatory cell infiltrate (Armed Forces Institute of Pathology Accession AFIP ACC #67710).

infiltrate, but rather a mixed inflammatory cell infiltrate with an underlying fibrous matrix (Fig. 1-6).

Thyroid ophthalmopathy generally presents with the gradual onset of inflammation but may have an abrupt painful onset that is caused by exposure keratitis. The CT scan is often diagnostic in that there is fusiform thickening of the extraocular muscles (EOMs). Chemical workup for systemic thyroid serum abnormalities such as T3 and T4 by radioimmunoassay (RIA) are often negative (Figs. 1-7 and 1-8).

DIFFERENTIAL DIAGNOSIS

Specific orbital disease entities are summarized in Table 1-2.[4] The incidence of these entities is somewhat helpful when confronting the individual patient and is influenced by the nature of the referral institution. For example, in the Toronto series of 257 cases of proptosis, acute ethmoiditis was a more common cause of proptosis

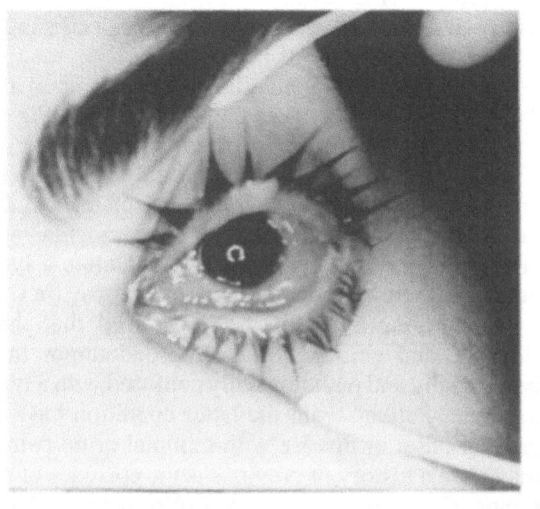
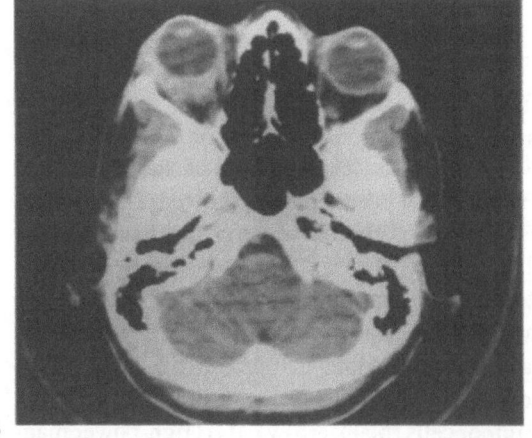

A   B

Fig. 1-3. (*A*) An 18-year-old male with purulent conjunctivitis and orbital cellulitis. Patient had a history of a penile discharge. (*B*) CT scan shows infiltrate that surrounds the globe. This CT scan pattern is consistent with orbital pseudotumor or bacterial orbital cellulitis. Gram's stain of conjunctival discharge showed gram-positive cocci and cultures grew out *Neisseria gonococcus*.

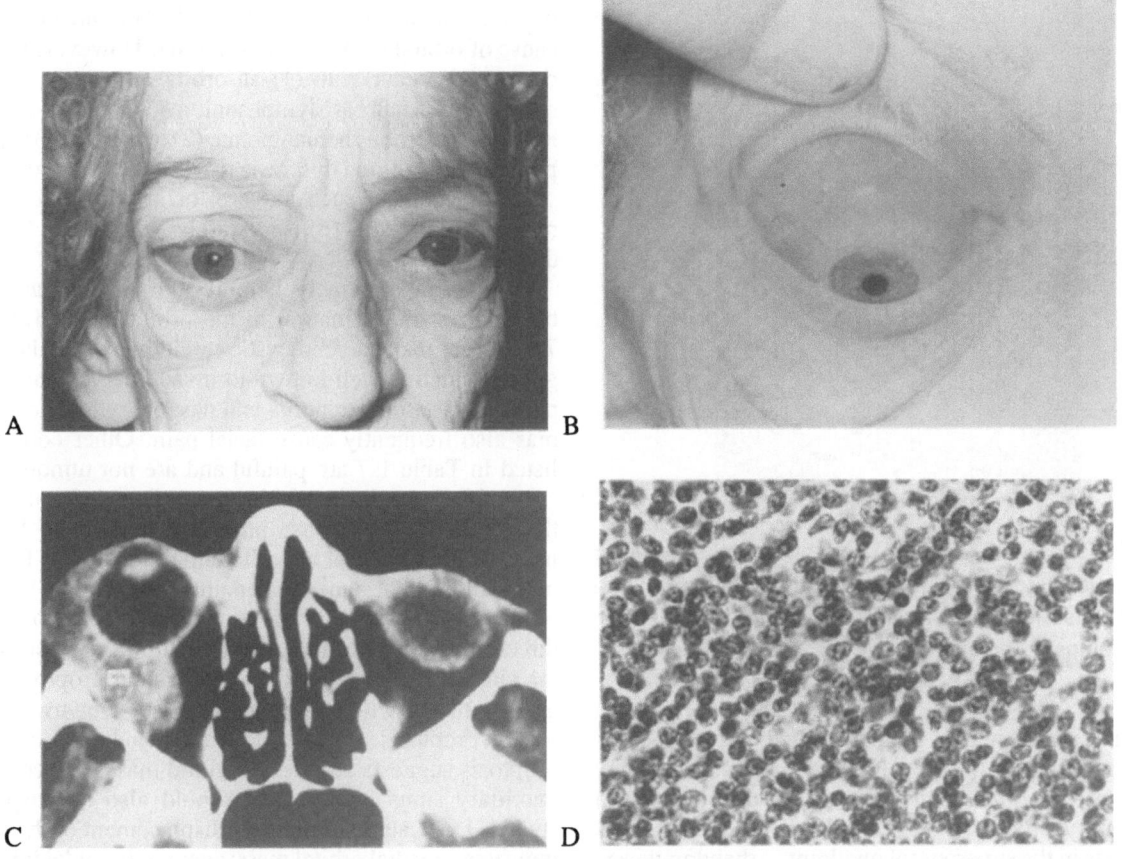

Fig. 1-4. (*A*) A 68-year-old female with gradual onset of proptosis of the right eye. (*B*) Patient had boggy swelling in the right superior orbit with a salmon-colored mass characteristic of a lymphoid infiltrate. (*C*) CT scan shows a diffuse mass without bone erosion that molds about the globe. (*D*) Biopsy shows a monotonous infiltrate of mononuclear cells with bland cytologic features consistent with a lymphoid infiltrate. Abdominal CT scan, bone marrow, and serum protein electrophoresis showed no evidence of systemic lymphoma. (Patient referred by Dr. A. Micale, Red Bank, NJ.)

than hyperthyroidism.[5] In the Children's Hospital, Washington, DC, the most common cause in 62 cases was dermoid cyst (Table 1-3).[6] Similarly, in 250 cases of orbital biopsies in children at Wills Eye Hospital, 46 percent were dermoid cysts.[7] In 214 biopsy-proven orbital tumors in children from the Armed Forces Institute of Pathology (AFIP), a tertiary referral pathology institute, rhabdomyosarcoma was the most common tumor in children.[8] Lymphoid tumors are rare in children, while granulocytic sarcoma of the orbit associated with myelogenous leukemia is more common. The most common optic nerve tumor in the Wills series was juvenile pilocytic astrocytoma.

The same bias applies to 504 consecutive cases of biopsy-proven orbital tumors from the Institute of Ophthalmology in New York (Columbia-Presbyterian) where granuloma or pseudotumor accounted for 18 percent of cases, while in the Mayo study, 31 percent had carcinoma as the most common condition.[9–11]

A list of disease entities by localized site and by presence of inflammation has been found to be helpful in approaching the individual patient (Tables 1-4 and 1-5). In addition, the patient's age at onset is extremely helpful in formulating a differential diagnosis. History, examination, and CT scan will localize the disease process. Each of the various categories will be discussed in the subsequent sections.

HISTORY

The patient's history is an important factor in determining whether the process is an inflammation or a tumor and in locating the site of onset (Figs. 1-9, 1-10). For example, an abrupt onset favors inflammation over tu-

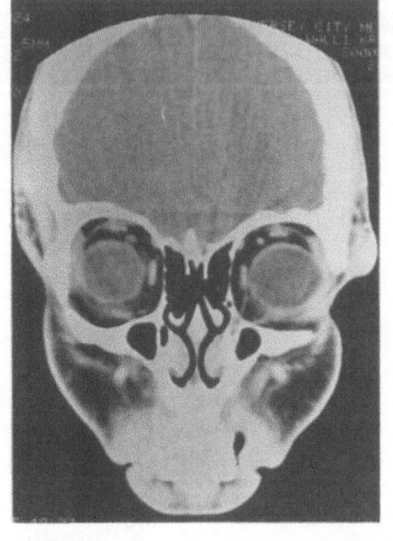

Fig. 1-5. Coronal CT scan of patient with pseudotumor involving left lateral and inferior recti. The inflammation also involves the left lacrimal gland. There is no definite mass to biopsy.

mor, while a history of a gradual growth over 2 months or longer favors a tumor. However, rapid onset may also occur with malignant tumors and may mimic an inflammatory process. For example, if a child presents with a mass in the superonasal quadrant, a rhabdomyosarcoma should always be suspected. However, a history of gradual growth over months rather than over weeks to days suggests a slowly growing tumor rather than rhabdomyosarcoma. In fact, an abrupt onset of a rhabdomyosarcoma may suggest an inflammatory process rather than a malignant tumor (Fig. 1-11). In addition to rhabdomyosarcoma, other disease processes that are inherently noninflammatory should be considered whenever there is the rapid onset of proptosis (Table 1-6).

With the exception of orbital hemorrhage, all of the conditions listed in Table 1-6 are diseases or tumors that have their onset in childhood.[12] The most common cause of orbital hemorrhage is trauma. However, hemorrhage may occur with (1) an orbital tumor that bleeds secondarily such as lymphangioma, hemangiopericytoma, or cavernous hemangioma, (2) leukemia, (3) hemophilia or other blood dyscrasia, (4) scurvy, (5) underlying vascular anomaly such as varix or arteriovenous (AV) malformation, and (6) very rarely without underlying disease (Fig. 1-12).

Pain is an extremely helpful sign in distinguishing tumor from inflammation in the orbital area (Table 1-7).[12] Other than adenoid cystic carcinoma of the lacrimal gland, which is well known to invade nerves and cause pain, metastatic carcinoma and nasopharyngeal carcinomas also frequently cause facial pain. Other conditions listed in Table 1-7 are painful and are not tumors.[12]

In addition to distinguishing tumor from inflammation, the origin of the disease process is extremely helpful in establishing a working differential diagnosis. The site of the initial enlargement will point to the original location of the disease process. In patients with proptosis, the direction of the proptosis will be helpful in determining the site of the tumor. For example, axial proptosis suggests a tumor within the muscle cone. Downward and inward proptosis suggests a lacrimal gland mass. Upward proptosis suggests an inferior orbital mass. Concomitant maxillary sinus involvement should also be suspected (Fig. 1-13). Lateral or outward displacement of the globe indicates a medial orbital mass; again, ethmoidal involvement needs to be ruled out. Downward displacement of the globe suggests a superior orbital mass. These features are usually more apparent on examination than by history.

However, during the ophthalmologic examination, the direction of proptosis will indicate the anatomic area of the orbit that is involved and will direct the ophthalmologist's investigation of the history to further pinpoint the disease process. For example, any medial orbital mass with possible sinus involvement should raise ques-

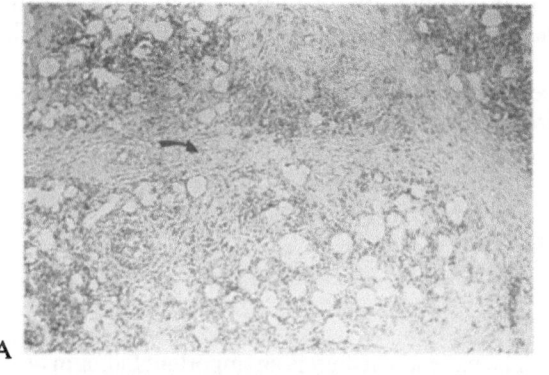
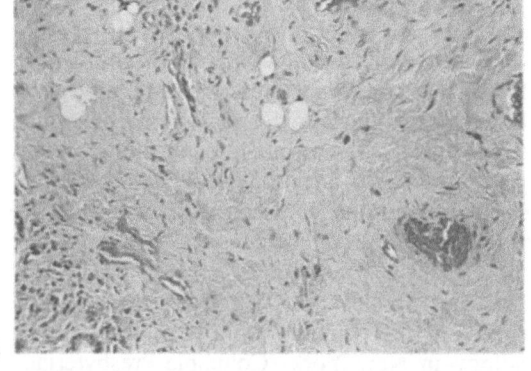

A   B

Fig. 1-6. (A) Biopsy shows bands of fibrous tissue (arrow) with islands of mature inflammatory cells including mostly lymphocytes, some plasma cells, and rare eosinophils within the orbital fat. (B) High-power magnification of another field shows marked fibrosis with scattered chronic inflammatory cells.

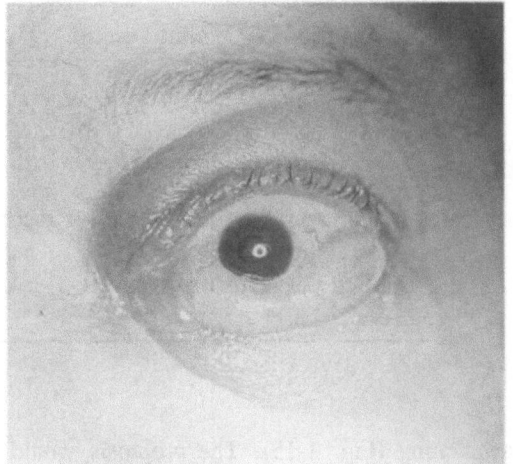

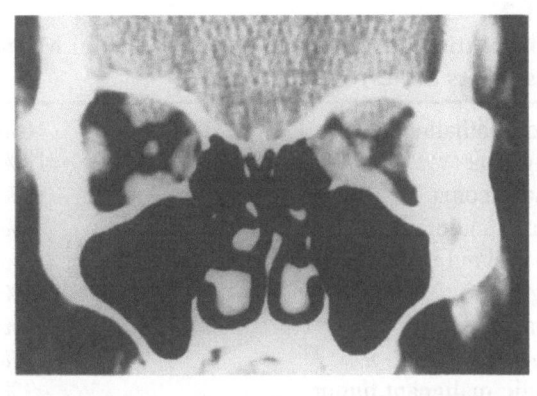

B

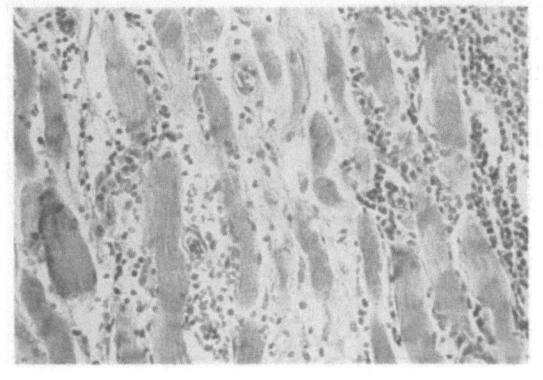

A

Fig. 1-7. (*A*) A 55-year-old female with onset of congestive thyroid ophthalmopathy left orbit over a several-week period. Coronal CT scan shows thickening of EOMs. (*B*) Axial CT scan after medial and inferior wall decompression shows fusiform thickening of the EOMs that spares the muscle tendon. C Biopsy on file at the AFIP shows a mixed inflammatory cell infiltrate within the superficial extraocular muscle (AFIP ACC #859063).

C

tions about epistaxis, nasal congestion, nasal obstruction, and previous sinus disease in the patient's history. Advanced lacrimal gland tumors may involve the entire orbit. Therefore, in any patient with an advanced orbital tumor, a malignant mixed tumor of the lacrimal gland should be suspected.

Generally, advanced lacrimal sac tumors do not extend into the orbit but invade the nose and sinus.

Eyelid tumors are usually confined to the eyelid. However, advanced basal cell carcinomas of the medial canthus are aggressive and may extend into the orbit; on occasion, rather minimal eyelid involvement may be apparent on examination, but the history will be instrumental in determining the initial site of the disease process. While advanced malignant mixed tumor of the lacrimal gland and sebaceous gland carcinoma may fill the entire orbit, the patient's history should suggest an original orbital or lid component.

The patient's history should also include the duration of proptosis. Comparison with old photographs may be helpful in determining the duration of the disease. A general medical history that includes a history of prior cancers elsewhere in the body is also necessary. For example, a history of prior breast resection for carcinoma may establish the diagnosis (Fig. 1-14). Metastatic breast carcinomas may occur years after the onset of the primary disease. History of thyroid disease, sinus disease, or trauma with a possible retained foreign body may accompany orbital inflammatory disease.

A history of intermittent or pulsating proptosis is confirmed on examination; the differential diagnosis is summarized in Table 1-8.[12] Intermittent proptosis may wax and wane; in addition, the degree of proptosis may change with body position. For example, a patient with a varix of the orbit would have increased proptosis when the head is in a dependent position or in the morning on

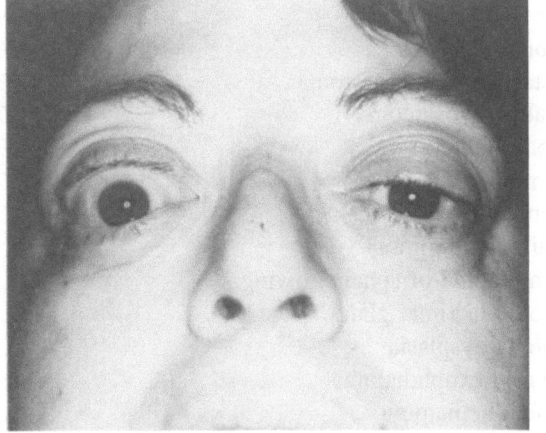

Fig. 1-8. A 48-year-old female with thyroid ophthalmopathy and marked lid retraction on downgaze. (Patient referred by Dr. Ivan Jacobs, Plainfield, NJ.)

Table 1-2
250 Consecutive Cases of Nonbiopsied Orbital Mass Lesions (Moss Series)

Thyroid ophthalmopathy	16%
Hemangioma	12%
Lymphosarcoma	10%
Chronic granuloma	8%
Lacrimal gland epithelial tumor	7%
Meningioma	5%
Lymphangioma	4%
Optic nerve glioma	3%
Metastatic malignant tumor	3%
Peripheral nerve tumor	3%
Dermoid cyst	3%
Sinusitis or mucocele	3%
Rhabdomyosarcoma	2%
Vascular aneurysm or fistula	2%
Angiosarcoma	2%
Osteoma	1%
Histiocytoma	1%
Sarcoid	1%
Other single cases	3%
Unknown cause	10%

Table 1-3
Clinical Diagnosis in 62 Cases of Suspected Orbital Tumors

Dermoid cyst	42%
Hemangioma	13%
Orbital cellulitis	10%
Metastatic neuroblastoma	9%
Rhabdomyosarcoma	3%
Sebaceous cyst	3%
Dermolipoma	3%
Pseudotumor	3%
Optic nerve glioma	1.5%
Meningioma of sphenoid wing	1.5%
Ectopic lacrimal gland	1.5%
Fibrous dysplasia	1.5%
Thyroid exophthalmos	1.5%
Orbital hematoma	1.5%
Metastatic embryonal sarcoma	1.5%
Unknown cause	4.5%

Table 1-4
Classification of Orbital Disease

1. Inflammation versus tumor
2. Site of disease
   Intraconal
   Extraconal
   Peripheral surgical space (extraconal and subperiosteal)
   Bone or sinus involvement
3. Age at onset

awakening (Fig. 1-15). The proptosis would improve when in the upright position, since gravity would serve to drain the blood from his head and orbit. Pulsating exophthalmos does not vary as much with position but is synchronous with the arterial pulse. A palpable thrill may be present. Movement of the applanation mires on slit lamp examination will demonstrate the pulsations in inconspicuous cases.

HISTORY—CAUSES OF PSEUDOPROPTOSIS

Causes of pseudoproptosis may be elicited by appropriate history. Causes of pseudoproptosis or pseudexopthalmos include craniostenosis and craniofacial dysostosis. Enlargement of the eye due to severe myopia and buphthalmos may also mimic exophthalmos. A history of amblyopia may help to support this possible diagnosis. Oculomotor palsy may result in 1–2 mm of exophthalmos.

Enophthalmos of one eye may falsely suggest exophthalmos of the other eye. Enophthalmos most commonly follows trauma, whether accidental or surgical, or may follow radiation. Asymmetry of eyelid fissures from unilateral lid retraction, ptosis, or Horner's syndrome may also mimic enophthalmos (Table 1-9).[12]

Table 1-5
Location of and Type of Disease

Orbital inflammatory disease
Adult orbital tumors
Pediatric orbital tumors
Lacrimal gland inflammations and tumors
Lacrimal sac inflammations and tumors
Eyelid tumors and inflammations

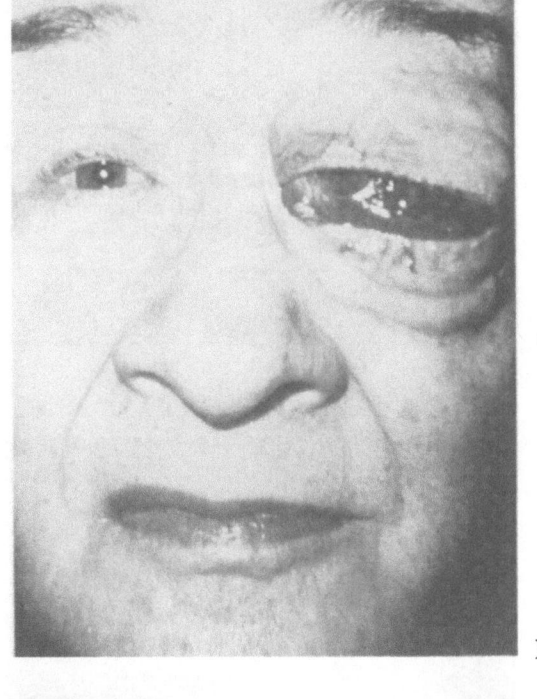

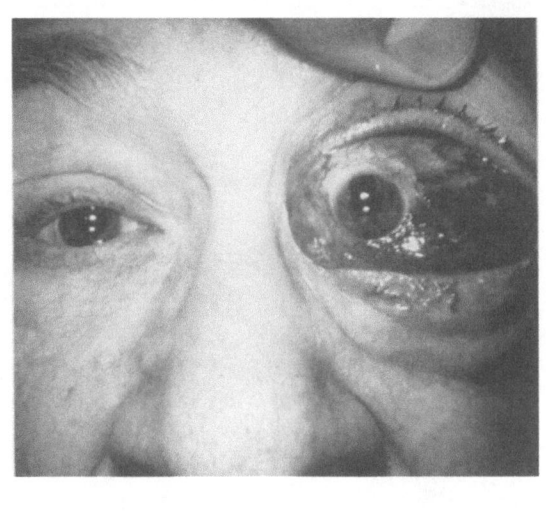

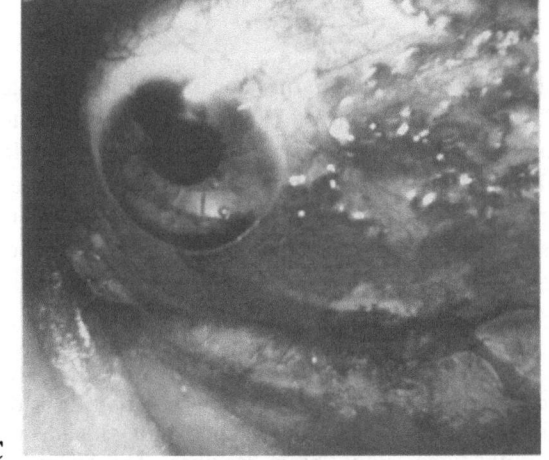

Fig. 1-9. (*A*) A 68-year-old female with spontaneous AV fistula. (*B,C*) Note arterialization of vessels to the limbus. Unlike with a varix, the proptosis does not increase with Valsalva's maneuver. The patient had a "swishing sound" in his head synchronous with the pulse. CT scan showed enlarged extraocular muscles on the left side with a markedly dilated superior ophthalmic vein (see Chapter 2.) Patient was treated expectantly with temporary tarsorrhaphy for exposure keratitis.

OPHTHALMOLOGIC EXAMINATION

Inflammation vs. Tumor

The ophthalmologic examination often confirms the history in answering two critical questions: (1) whether the process is an inflammation or a tumor, and (2) whether the site of the disease process is orbit, lacrimal gland, lacrimal sac, or eyelid. On ophthalmologic examination, inspection and palpation are extremely helpful in distinguishing inflammation from tumor. A "red hot" orbit that is tender strongly suggests an inflammatory process such as bacterial orbital cellulitis or acute pseudotumor.

During an inflammatory process, there is edema with marked tenderness on palpation. Tumors, including lymphoid infiltrates, produce boggy chemosis that is usually nontender. A salmon-colored patch may be visible in the conjunctiva. The lids should be elevated and the cul-de-sac examined (Fig. 4-*A* and *B*).

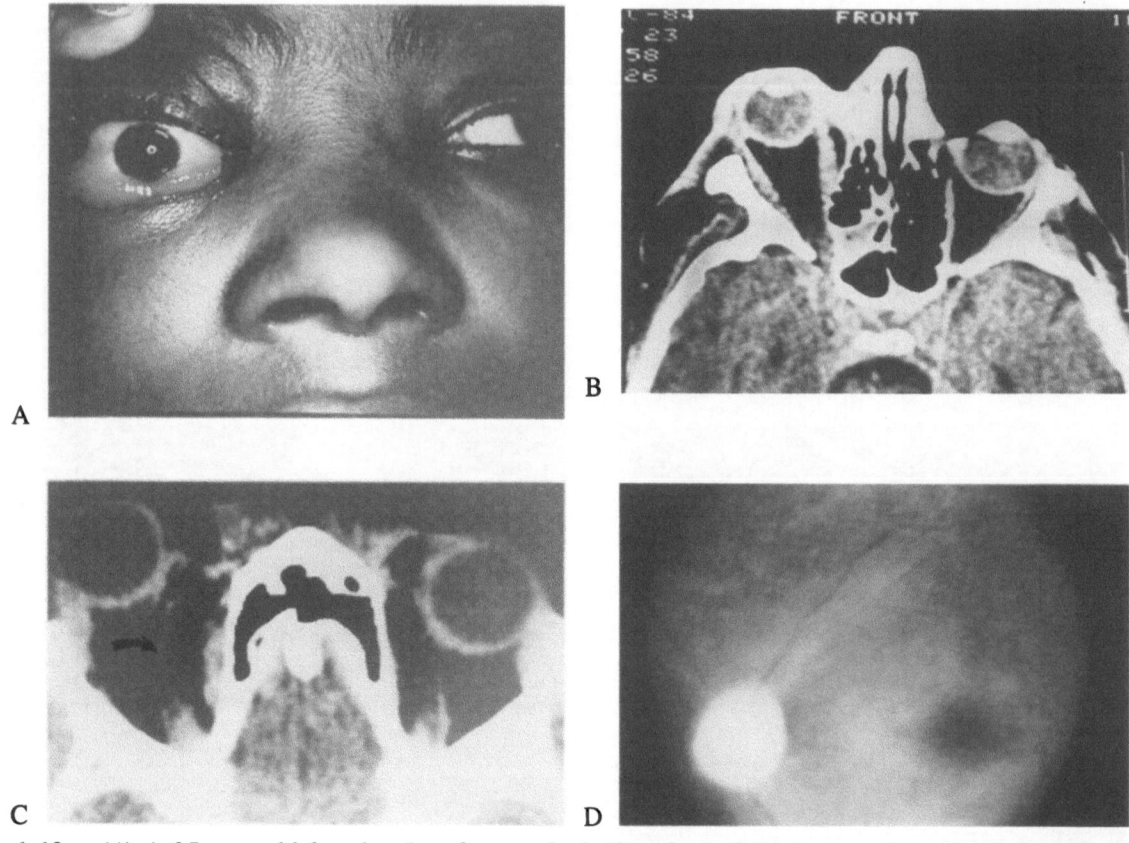

Fig. 1-10. (*A*) A 35-year-old female who after an alcoholic episode fell asleep on floor in her friend's apartment and awoke with loss of vision and congested orbit. (*B*) CT scan shows enlarged EOMs that involve the tendon. (*C*) Note lack of superior ophthalmic vein enlargement (arrow), which helps rule out an AV fistula. (*D*) Fundoscopy 3 days after the acute episode shows evidence of a central retinal artery. Later, retinal pigmentary changes from disturbance of the choroidal circulation and electroretinogram (ERG) confirmed an occlusion of the ophthalmic artery. Loss of vision is presumably due to external pressure on the globe that occurred when the patient fell asleep during the alcoholic episode.

Localizing Site of Disease Process

Proptosis may be axial or nonaxial. The history will act as a guide to the suspected location of the disease process as well as the absence or presence of inflammation.

On examination, axial proptosis suggests a retrobulbar, intraconal mass. The direction of displacement of the globe by a nonaxial mass will suggest the location of the mass. For example, displacement of the globe down and out (temporal direction) suggests a superonasal mass. In children, the downward and temporal displacement of the globe should always suggest rhabdomyosarcoma or dermoid. A less common condition is encephalocele, which, like dermoid cyst, is usually congenital. While a rapid, recent onset suggests rhabdomyosarcoma, a preexisting, slowly enlarging mass that has recently enlarged dramatically suggests a ruptured dermoid cyst. A history of trauma should be sought.

The CT-scan features of these two entities are quite distinctive. Usually a rhabdomyosarcoma is a diffuse, homogeneous, noncystic lesion that may invade adjacent orbital bone, sinus, brain, or nose. The lesion may be intra- or extraconal and enhances with contrast injection, while a dermoid is almost always extraconal due to its embryogenic association with sutures of orbital bones. The wall of the dermoid cyst appears somewhat more radioopaque than its more radiolucent, low-density central cystic keratin component. The wall or rim of the cyst enhances with intravenous contrast. A dermoid may cause fossa formation or a regular hollowing out of the adjacent bone where it is attached.

In adults, dermoid cyst and rhabdomyosarcoma are less common, but may occur. More common are frontal sinus mucoceles, which if infected present with inflammation.

Displacement of the globe down and in (inferonasal) suggests a lacrimal gland mass. A thickened lid should raise the suspicion of an eyelid mass infiltrating the orbit.

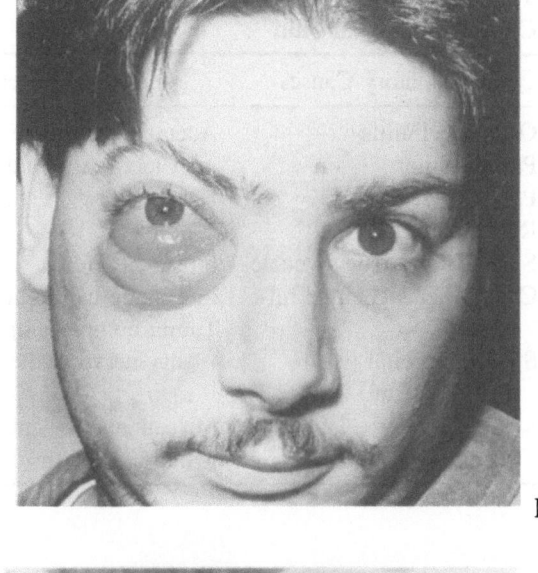

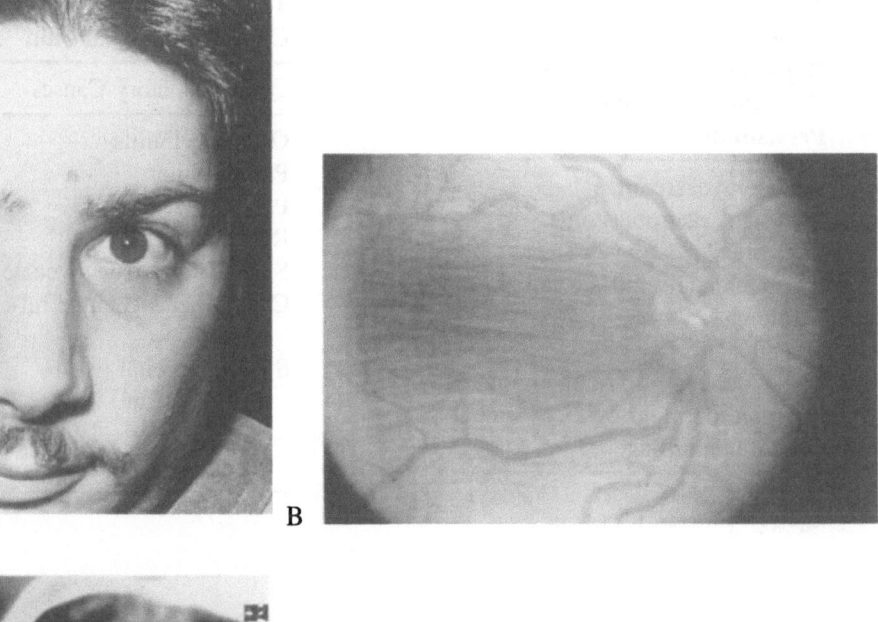

A   B

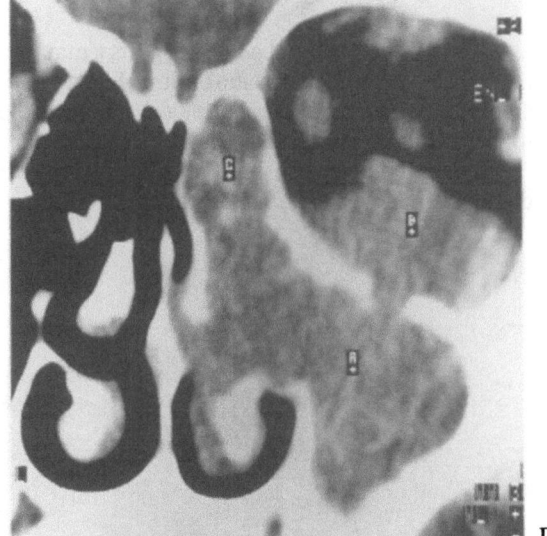

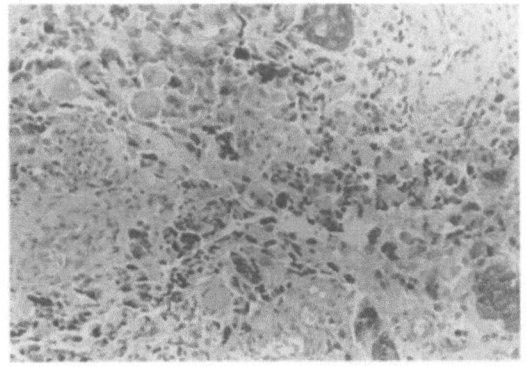

C   D

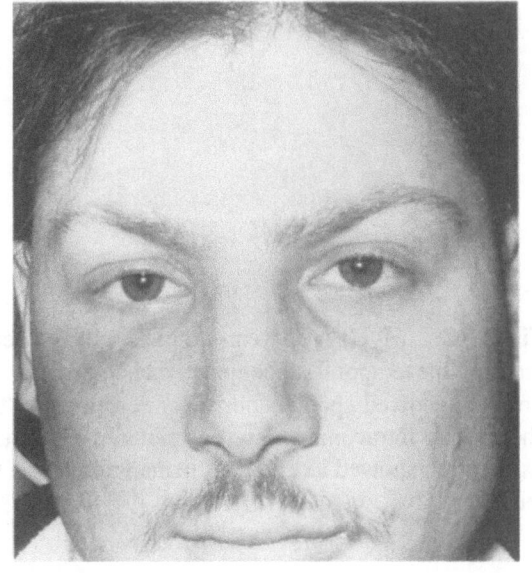

Fig. 1-11. (*A*) A 28-year-old male with history of dental abscess and ''maxillary sinusitis'' unresponsive to oral antibiotics. (*B*) Fundoscopy showed marked chorioretinal striae. (*C*) Emergency CT scan showed a soft tissue density eroding through the medial wall of the maxillary sinus and the floor of the orbit. The globe is displaced superiorly. (*D*) Biopsy showed an undifferentiated sarcoma with rhabdomyoblastic differentiation and many multinucleated giant cells (arrow) consistent with embryonal sarcoma. (*E*) Patient had an initial response to chemotherapy and local radiation to the orbit and maxillary sinus radiation. Note hair loss. Over 3-year course, patient had several recurrences that led to exenteration and death. (Patient referred by Dr. Alan Goldfedder, Newark, NJ.)

E

Table 1-6
Noninflammatory Causes of Rapid Onset Proptosis That May Have an Inflammatory-Type Presentation

Rhabdomyosarcoma
Metastatic neuroblastoma
Leukemia
Lymphoma (Burkitt's lymphoma)
Teratoma
Granulocytic sarcoma
Chocolate cyst in lymphangioma
Ruptured dermoid cyst*
Orbital hemorrhage

* Causes sudden proptosis due to granulomatous response to keratin and hair follicles.

Table 1-7
Causes of Orbital Pain

Inflammatory Causes	Tumor Causes
Orbital cellulitis	Adenoid cystic carcinoma of lacrimal gland
Pseudotumor	
Posterior scleritis	Nasopharyngeal carcinoma
Retrobulbar neuritis	
Sinusitis and mucopyocele	Sinus carcinoma
Cluster headache and migraine	Metastatic carcinoma
Superior orbital fissure (Tolosa-Hunt) syndrome	Tumor compressing a sensory nerve at the foramen
	Miscellaneous—intracranial aneurysm

Squamous cell carcinoma of the conjunctiva almost always arises at the limbus and may invade the eye or orbit.

Lateral displacement of the globe suggests a possible ethmoidal mass. Furniture makers are prone to develop adenocarcinomas of the ethmoid sinus. Mucoceles of the ethmoid sinus are not uncommon.

A superiorly displaced globe suggests a maxillary sinus mass that is extending into the orbit. A history of cigarette smoking or excessive alcohol intake might further point to a maxillary sinus carcinoma.

Bilaterality may also help to narrow the differential diagnosis (Table 1-10).[12]

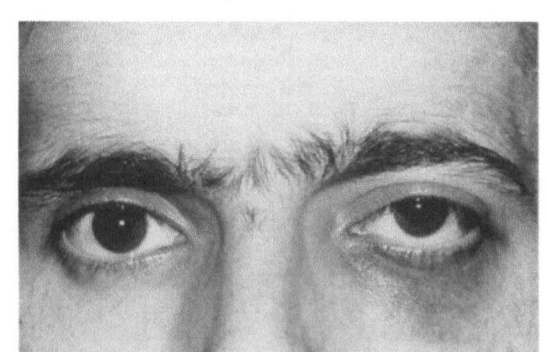

A

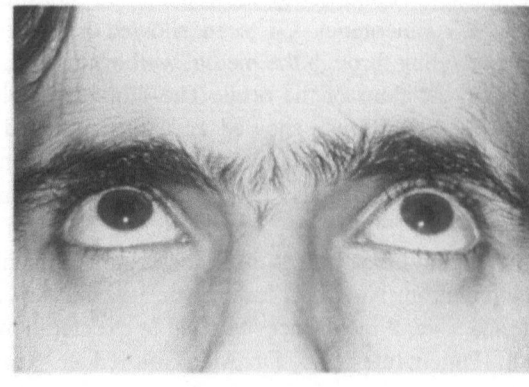

C

B

Fig. 1-12. (A–C) A 35-year-old male with sudden proptosis. Note temporal subconjunctival hemorrhage. Hemorrhage resolved spontaneously 2 weeks later. CT scan showed an intraconal mass (not pictured) and surgical exploration showed a cavernous hemangioma (see Chapter 3).

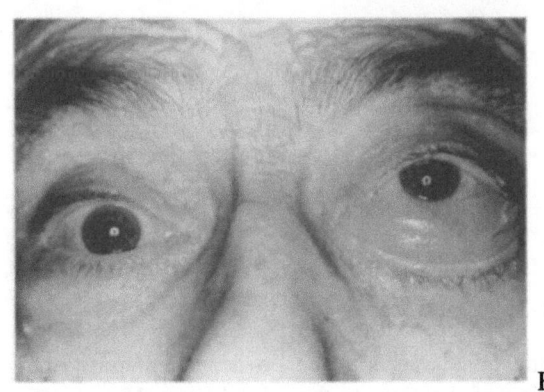
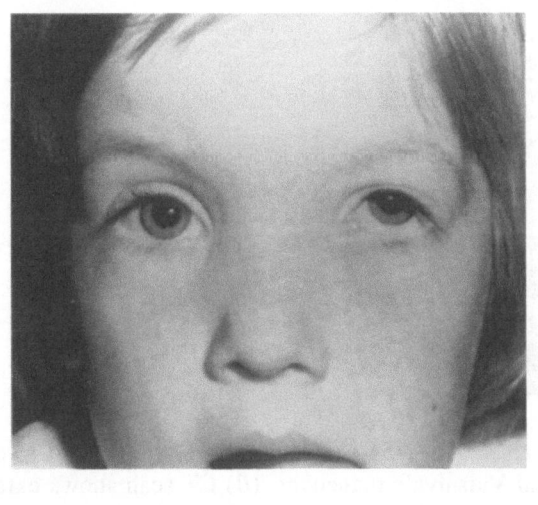

A   B

Fig. 1-13. (*A*) A 71-year-old male with gradual onset of proptosis of the left eye. CT scan showed a maxillary sinus tumor that invaded the orbital floor and inferior orbit. Initial biopsy showed an undifferentiated squamous cell carcinoma. Radical orbital exenteration with maxillectomy was performed via a Weber-Ferguson incision. (*B*) An 8-year-old female with proptosis of upward and outward displacement of left eye that was exacerbated by upper respiratory infections. CT scan showed ethmoid sinus mucocele.

Measurement of Degree of Proptosis

The degree of forward displacement of the globe is measured by an exophthalmometer. The mean normal protrusion is 16.5 mm in white males, 18.5 mm in black males, 15.4 mm in white females, and 17.8 mm in black females.[3] Upper limits of normal are 21.7 mm for white males, 24.7 mm for black males, 20.1 mm for white females, and 23 mm for black females. No normal patient has more than 2 mm of asymmetry. The normal range is 14–22 mm.[13–15]

There are several methods of measuring displacement of the globe, whether downward, lateral, medial, or forward. To measure downward displacement, a clear straight-edge is placed from medial canthus to medial canthus. Downward displacement of the eye can be measured by comparing the position of the eye with the rule and observing the relationship of the rule to the pupil of each eye. The test assumes there is no distortion of the canthi as might occur from traumatic telecanthus. Lateral or medial displacement is measured from the bridge of the nose to the nasal limbus.

Exophthalmometers are designed to measure forward displacment of the globe or proptosis. The three types of exophthalmometers include the standard Hertel, the

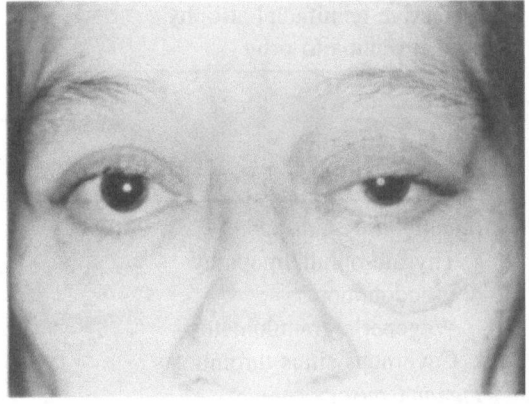

Fig. 1-14. A 63-year-old black female with mastectomy 5 years ago. Presented with recent ptosis and indurated painless mass in superior orbit. There were minimal signs of inflammation. Biopsy showed a sclerosing adenocarcinoma consistent with metastatic breast carcinoma.

Table 1-8
Intermittent or Pulsating Exophthalmos

Intermittent	Pulsating
Lymphangioma	Carotid-cavernous sinus fistula
Ruptured orbital cyst	Venous angioma
Ruptured dermoid cyst	AV malformation
	Frontal mucocele if massive
	Neurofibroma
	Meningocele
	Encephalocele
	Metastatic renal cell carcinoma

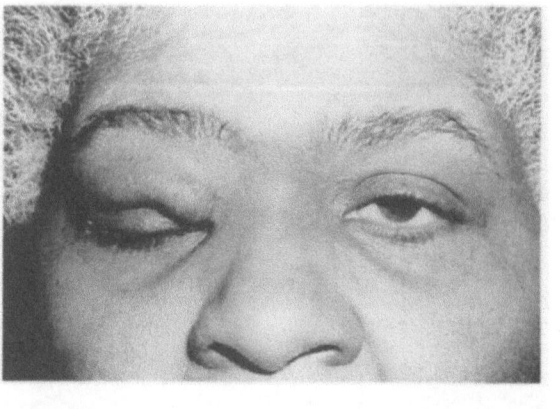
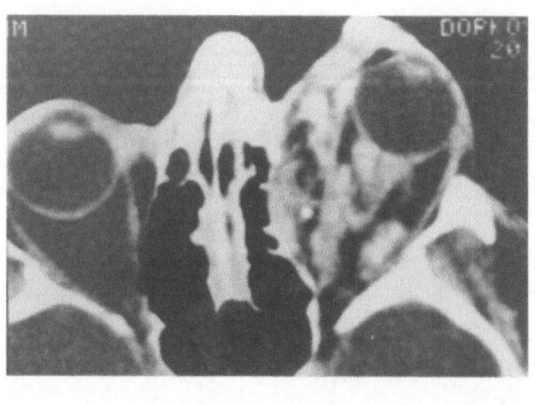

Fig. 1-15. (*A*) A 54-year-old female with eyelid swelling that is accentuated on dependent positioning of the head and Valsalva's maneuver. (*B*) CT scan shows extension of the mass to the orbital apex. Note "coke bottle" distortion of medial orbital wall.

Luedde, and the Mutch exophthalmometer (Plate 1-1). Of the three types, only the Hertel measures both eyes simultaneously with the lateral orbit rim as the reference point. The Luedde exophthalmometer can be used to measure each eye separately, also with the lateral orbital rim as the reference point. The Mutch exophthalmometer again is used to measure each eye separately with the cheek or brow as a reference point. The latter instrument is helpful when there is distortion of orbital anatomy due to surgical or accidental trauma and the lateral orbital rims cannot be used accurately as a reference point. It is calibrated to give figures comparable with the lateral orbital rim type of exophthalmometry reading.

In addition to measuring displacement of the globe, a simple method of recording ocular motility that is accurate and does not necessitate taking measurement by the alternate cover test can be employed. A rectangular potential field of binocular vision is drawn, and the particular patient's field of single binocular vision is then drawn within that field.

Other Features

All patients with orbital disease should have a complete ophthalmologic examination; the fine points of the examination are outlined below. For example, on applanation tonometry, fine degrees of pulsating exophthalmos may be evident, a finding that is consistent with an AV fistula and may be confirmed on auscultation of the orbit with a stethoscope. Bruits should be auscultated over the globe and above the eyes on both sides of the forehead. In addition, a palpable thrill will also suggest an AV fistula or a communication between the brain and orbit as in neurofibromatosis. Causes of pulsating exophthalmos, which are summarized in Table 1-8, should be distinguished from causes of intermittent proptosis that are

due to venous anomalies. In the latter conditions, such as varix of the orbit, merely asking the patient to place his or her head in a dependent position will accentuate the proptosis. Proptosis accentuated by mastication may be due to extension of a dermoid cyst into the temporal fossa (Fig. 1-16).

Table 1-9
Causes of Enophthalmos

Old blowout fracture
Radiation effect
Microophthalmos due to any cause
Neurofibromatosis
Metastatic scirrhous ca.
Parinaud's syndrome (retraction nystagmus)
Progressive hemifacial atrophy
Surgical trauma to orbit

Table 1-10
Causes of Bilateral Proptosis

Inflammatory Causes
　Thyroid ophthalmopathy
　Pseudotumor
　Wegener's granulomatosis
　Cavernous sinus thrombosis
Tumor Causes
　Metastatic neuroblastoma
　Leukemia
　Lymphoma
　Histiocytosis X
Miscellaneous cause
　Congenital orbitofacial malformation

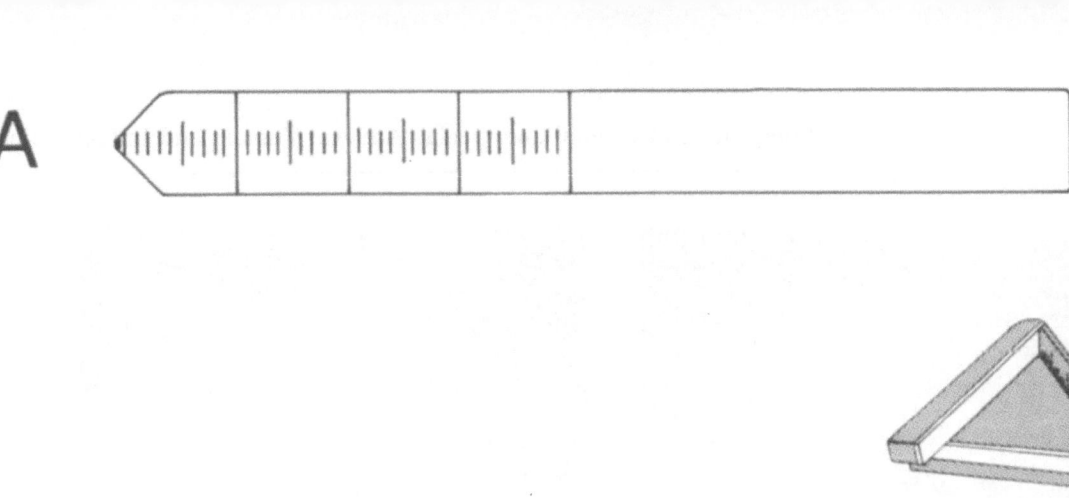

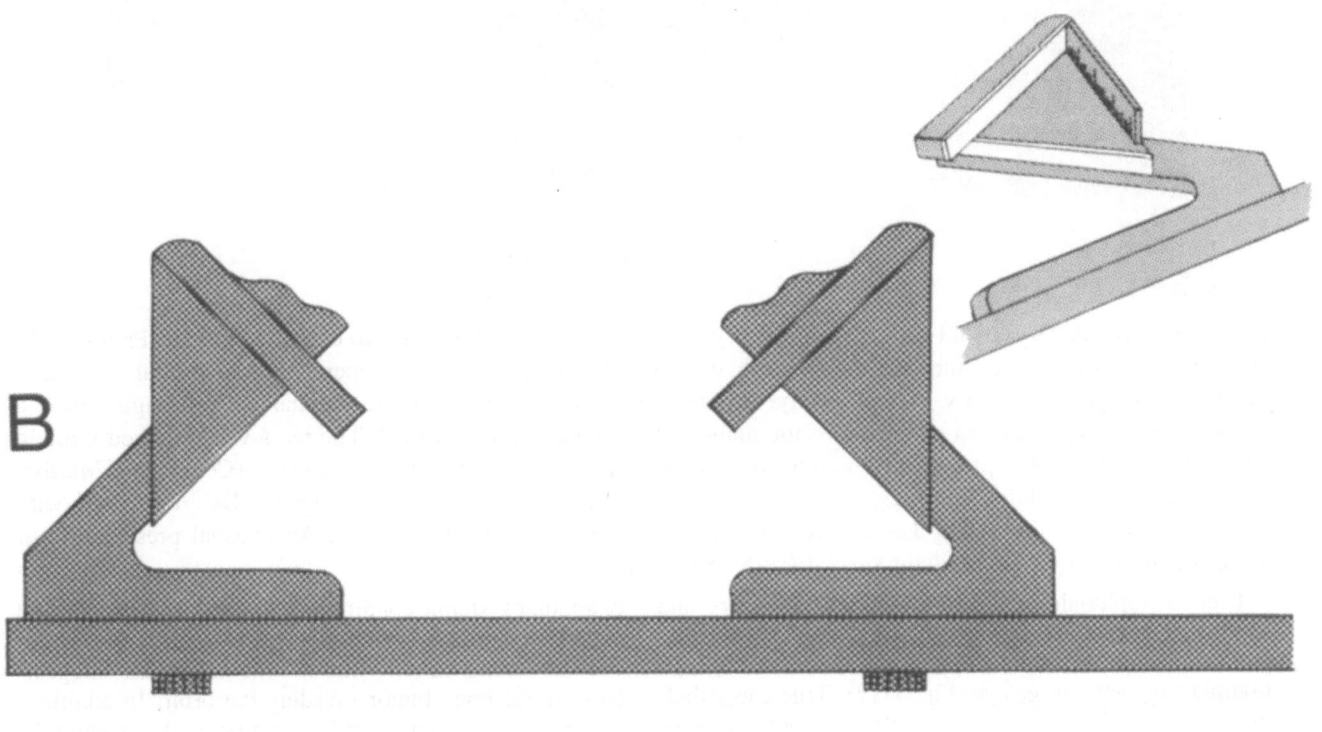

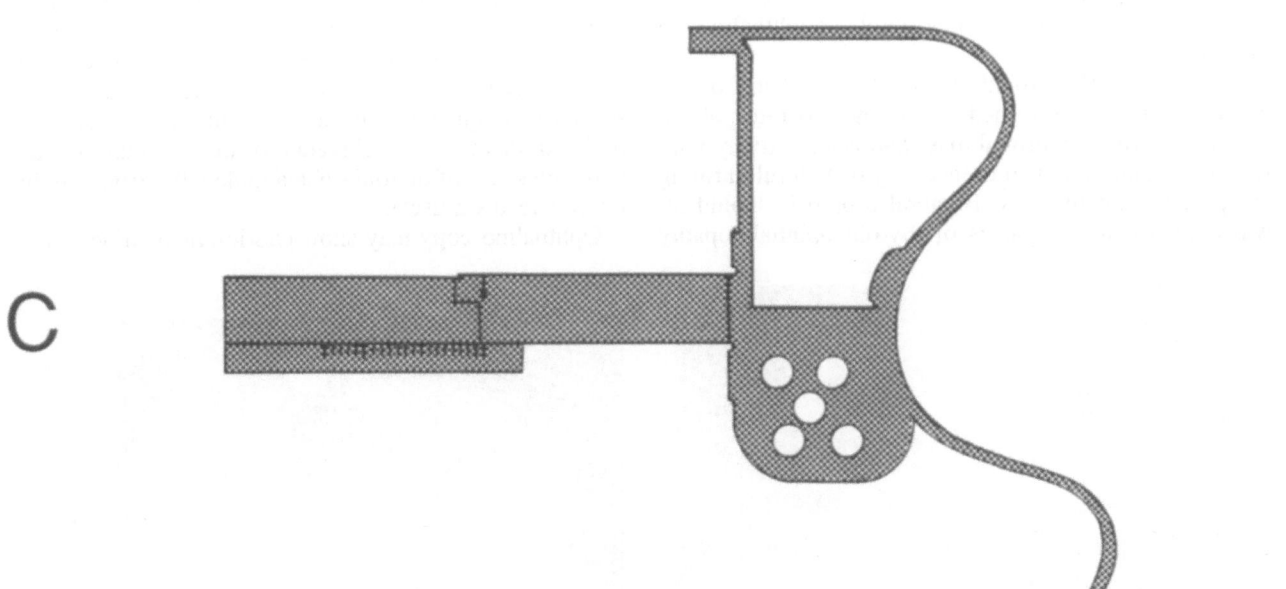

Plate 1-1. (*A*) Luedde exophthalmometer measures position of each separately with lateral orbital rim as baseline. (*B*) Hertel exophthalmometer measures two eyes simultaneously with lateral orbital rims as baseline. (*C*) Mutch exophthalmometer measures each eye separately with brow and cheek as baselines and is calibrated to give measurements comparable with other exophthalmometers. (Modified from Jones IS, Jakobiec FA, Nolan B: Patient examination and introduction to orbital disease. In Duane TD, Jaeger EA [eds] *Clinical Ophthalmology*, Volume 2 [Harper & Row, Philadelphia, 1982].)

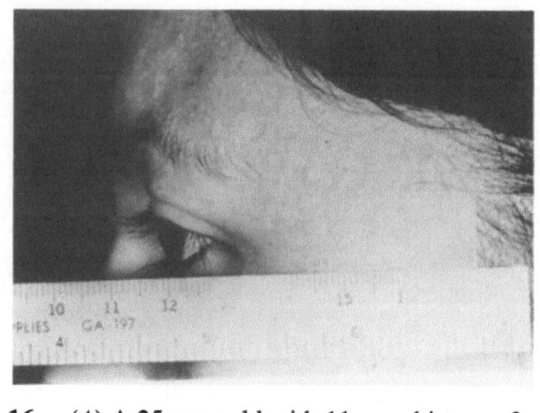
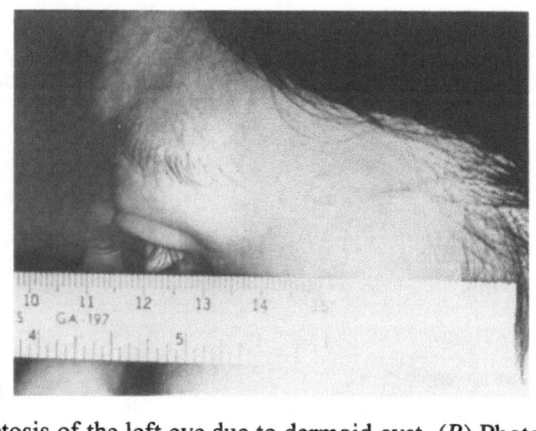

Fig. 1-16. (*A*) A 25-year-old with 11-year history of proptosis of the left eye due to dermoid cyst. (*B*) Photographs show that her eye moves forward 3 mm with chewing. CT scan showed a superotemporal orbital mass that displaced the globe medially and inferiorly. A defect was present in the lateral orbital wall through which a much smaller temporal fossa extension of the main cystic orbital mass protruded. The mass was removed through a lateral orbitotomy. The preoperative diagnosis of dermoid cyst was confirmed histologically. (Courtesy of Marilyn D. Kincaid, Ann Arbor, MI, presented at the 1985 AFIP Alumni Meeting, Washington, DC. Reprinted with permission from Whitney CE, Leone CR, Kincaid MD: Proptosis with mastication: An unusual presentation of an orbital dermal cyst *Ophthalmic Surg.* 17:295–298, 1986.)

Pseudoexophthalmos is often elicited by history and should be considered on examination. High intraocular pressure suggests buphthalmos, while unilateral high myopia suggests a large eye (Fig. 1-17). True enophthalmos on one side may falsely simulate exophthalmos of the contralateral eye. Enophthalmos is most often due to trauma and other signs of an old orbital floor fracture should be sought. Similarly, unilateral lid retraction due to thyroid ophthalmopathy may mimic enophthalmos of the other eye.

Palpation of the orbital rim and retropulsion of the globe should be performed. Resistance to retropulsion may occur with any orbital mass and is a relatively nonspecific finding, but its presence may be helpful in ruling out pseudoexophthalmos. Bilateral proptosis should always suggest the diagnosis of thyroid ophthalmopathy or another systemic condition. Adherence of a firm orbital mass to the underlying bone suggests a soft tissue orbital mass invading bone, while a bone-hard mass suggests an intrinsic bone tumor invading the orbit. In addition, the preauricular and cervical lymph nodes should be palpated for possible local metastases or signs of inflammation.

EOM rotations will be affected by the presence of a mass, and in general, there will be limited ductions in the direction of the mass. Graves' disease affects the inferior rectus most commonly and the medial rectus second in frequency. An increased intraocular pressure of 2 mm or greater on elevation of the eye may be due to the presence of thyroid ophthalmolopathy from a tight inferior rectus muscle.

Ophthalmoscopy may show chorioretinal striae in the

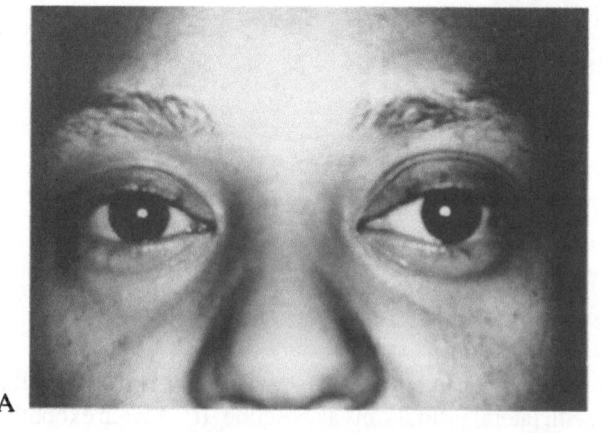
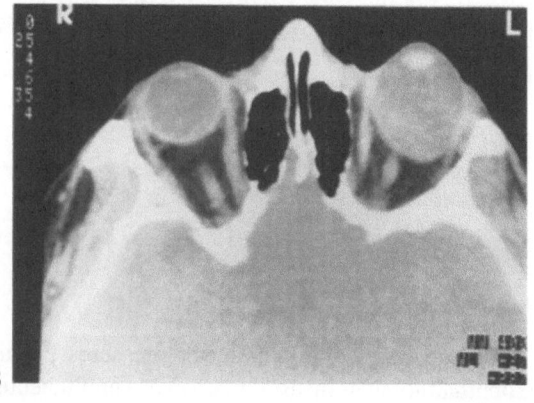

Fig. 1-17. (*A*) A 24-year-old female referred for evaluation of proptosis of the left eye. Examination showed myopia causing pseudoproptosis. (*B*) CT scan showed enlarged globe.

posterior pole. Examination of the optic nerve area may show pallor and/or opticociliary shunts as in meningioma of the optic nerve sheath, most commonly, and glioma. High myopia and a posterior staphyloma suspected in retinoscopy will be confirmed on ophthalmoscopic examination and A-scan ultrasound.

Loss of sensory cranial nerve function is common with sinus carcinoma, and sensory loss in the superotemporal eyelid may occur with infiltrating tumors of the lacrimal gland. Adenoid cystic carcinoma typically produces pain as the tumor invades the nerve.

Ancillary tests are color vision tests (Isihara color plates) for signs of optic nerve involvement and confrontation and formal visual fields. An intraocular tumor with orbital extension such as a melanoma or retinoblastoma will be elicited by history and detected on examination.

All patients should have a general medical evaluation, particularly if metastatic disease is considered. A breast or lung carcinoma may present as an orbital mass. Inflammatory conditions such as Wegener's granulomatosis or periarteritis nodosa may have other systemic findings (see Chapter 2, "Orbital Inflammatory Disease").

DIAGNOSTIC WORK-UP

Role of Radiographic Examinations and Ultrasound

The orbital CT scan will confirm the clinical suspicion of orbital disease and will localize the site of the disease. The pattern of the disease will often virtually solidify the diagnosis. Orbital ultrasound is helpful for diagnosing purely intraorbital disease and may be available immediately as an office test. It does not delineate disease of the orbital bones. Arteriography is indicated only when an arterial process such as an AV fistula is suspected. Venography is rarely necessary to diagnose a suspected varix.

The varix typically involves either the superior or inferior ophthalmic vein, both of which may have a large component in the muscle cone. CT scan with the patient's head in a dependent position may establish the diagnosis of a sausage-shaped intraorbital mass, but the mass virtually disappears or is barely visible when the CT scan is performed with the patient's head in a nondependent position. The enlarged superior ophthalmic vein and cavernous sinus are seen well on CT scan. The varix will markedly light up with intravenous contrast. Arteriography is not necessary for confirmation and shows rapid filling of the dilated superior ophthalmic vein with poor perfusion of the intracranial carotid artery branches.

The importance of the CT scan cannot be overemphasized.[1] Using the CT scan, the disease should be localized quite easily to the lacrimal gland area, intraconal space, extraconal space (between the EOMs and periorbita), and subperiosteal space. Concomitant sinus disease and/or the presence of bone erosion will be apparent. Bony windows enhance processes involving bone while soft tissue windows are helpful in analyzing soft tissue masses. Infused contrast material may be useful in demonstrating vascular tumors. The following sections will further elucidate the role of all of such CT scan parameters. When the CT scan findings are combined with those from the history and ophthalmologic examination, the disease process can usually be quite well-localized and the nature of the disease process can be defined as inflammation or tumor. A fairly specific diagnosis or narrow differential is usually determined.

A few general rules regarding the evaluation of CT scans are worth reviewing. In general, benign tumors are well-localized and if adjacent to bone may cause a minimal smooth erosion or fossa formation. Malignant tumors tend to have irregular margins and erode adjacent bone. Lymphoid infiltrates are diffuse and, therefore, do not observe normal anatomic barriers such as the EOMs. Lymphoid infiltrates tend to mold about the globe and orbital bones. They are homogeneous masses of relatively high density that mildly enhance with injection of intravenous contrast. Pseudotumors often show inflammation about a particular structure such as the EOM, lacrimal gland, episclera, or optic nerve. Typically, a halo or ring of increased density is present about the globe (sclera), fat, and EOMs.

The presence of sinus involvement coupled with clinical presentation will lead to a diagnosis of a tumor or inflammatory process. In general, inflammatory processes do not erode bone. A recent study shows that bone erosion may be present in patients with orbital pseudotumor.[16] These presentations are clearly the exception.

MANAGEMENT

Based on a careful history, ophthalmologic examination, and review of the CT scan, a management protocol may be established. Once the physician is able to localize the original site of the disease process, he or she may proceed to the various sections of this book where the particular nuances of management are outlined. In some cases, a trial of systemic antibiotics will be necessary to rule out a bacterial orbital cellulitis or dacryoadenitis before the patient is committed to (1) a trial of systemic steroids in the case of a presumed pseudotumor, or (2) an incisional biopsy in the case of an orbital tumor. The incisional biopsy will then lead to further definitive work-up and treatment.

REFERENCES

1. Mauriello JA, Flanagan JC: Management of orbital inflammatory disease. A protocol. *Surv Ophthalmol* 29(2):104–116, 1984.
2. Birch-Hirshfeld A: Krankheiten der Orbita, in Graefe-Saemisch, *Handbuch des Gesamten Augenheilk.* Band 9, Abt 1, Teil. Berlin: Springer, 1930, p 1947.
3. Jakobiec FA, Jones IS: Orbital Inflammations, in Duane TD, Jaeger EA (eds): *Clinical Ophthalmology.* Philadelphia: Harper and Row, 1982, pp 1–70.
4. Moss HM: Expanding lesions of the orbit: A clinical study of 250 consecutive cases. *Am J Ophthalmol* 54:761, 1962.
5. Crawford JS: Disease of the orbit, in Hughes WF (ed): *Toronto Hospital for Sick Children Department of Ophthalmology: The Eye in Childhood.* Chicago: Year Book, 1967, p 331.
6. Youssefi B: Orbital tumors in children: A clinical study of 62 cases. *J Pediatr Ophthalmol* 6:177, 1969.
7. Shields JA, Bakewell B, Augsburger JJ, et al: Space-occupying orbital masses in children. A review of 250 consecutive biopsies. *Ophthalmology* 93:379–384, 1986.
8. Porterfield JF: Orbital tumors in children: A report on 214 cases. *Int Ophthalmol Clin* 2:319, 1962.
9. Reese AB: Expanding lesions of the orbit. *Trans Ophthalmol Soc UK* 91:85, 1971.
10. Henderson JW, Farrow GM: *Orbital Tumors.* Philadelphia: Saunders, 1973.
11. Shields JA, Bakewell B, Augsburger JJ, et al: Classification and incidence of space-occupying lesions of the orbit. A survey of 645 biopsies. *Arch Ophthalmol* 102:1606–1611, 1984.
12. Jones IS, Jakobiec FA, Nolan BT: Patient examination and introduction to orbital disease, in Duane TD, Jaeger EA (eds): *Clinical Ophthalmology.* Philadelphia: Harper and Row, 1982, pp 1–30.
13. Duke-Elder A, MacFaul PA: The ocular adnexa, lacrimal, orbital, and paraorbital disease, in Duke-Elder A (ed): *Systems of Ophthalmology.* St. Louis: CV Mosby, 1974, pp 780–782, 785.
14. Migliori ME, Gladstone GJ: Determination of the normal range of exophthalmometric values for black and white adults. *Am J Ophthalmol* 98:438–442, 1984.
15. Musch DC, Frueh BR, Landis JR: The reliability of Hertel exophthalmometry. Observe variation between physician and lay readers. *Ophthalmology* 92:1177–1180, 1985.
16. Frohman LP, Kupersmith MJ, Lang J, et al: Intracranial extension and bone destruction in orbital pseudotumor. *Arch Ophthalmol* 104:380–384, 1986.

2

Orbital Inflammatory Disease

Joseph A. Mauriello, Jr.
Joseph C. Flanagan

INTRODUCTION

By applying the principles in Chapter 1, the physician should be reasonably assured whether he or she is dealing with an orbital inflammation or a tumor. Acute periorbital swelling with or without proptosis and pain generally accompanies an inflammatory process.

On a clinical basis, some diseases do not present with inflammatory signs, although on pathologic examination, these entities consist of mainly inflammatory cells, and are discussed in this chapter. For example, a lymphoid infiltrate defined in Chapter 1 as a "tumor" ranges from reactive lymphoid hyperplasia to malignant lymphoma. The entity classically presents as a painless mass with minimal or no inflammatory signs. When pathologically benign, the mass is composed of mostly bland lymphocytes, plasma cells, and rare eosinophils. Similarly, although sarcoid of the lids and orbit is purely an inflammatory process pathologically, the clinical presentation is usually noninflammatory. In this book, such entities are discussed under the "inflammatory" category because lymphoid infiltrate, a tumor, and pseudotumor, an inflammation, are part of the same differential diagnosis. Inflammations of the lacrimal gland, sac, or lids are considered in their respective chapters.

The following step-by-step approach to orbital inflammatory disease is extremely helpful in approaching the individual patient.

When confronted with the patient with orbital inflammatory disease, a life-threatening bacterial orbital cellulitis must initially be ruled out. Because the orbital disease presentation may be part of a systemic disease process, a good history and appropriate systemic work-up are mandatory (Fig. 2-1). If any suspicion of bacterial orbital cellulitis exists, intravenous antibiotics should be instituted.

Concurrently, orbital computed tomography (CT) scan is extremely helpful in the work-up. Specifically, three findings—the presence of an orbital mass lesion without sinus involvement or bone erosion, the presence of an orbital mass lesion with sinus involvement or bone changes, or thickened extraocular muscles (EOMs) on CT scan—lead to the differential diagnosis, decision to biopsy, and appropriate treatment.

DIFFERENTIAL DIAGNOSIS AND NOMENCLATURE

The main causes of orbital inflammation as well as some of the rare causes are listed in Table 2-1. Thyroid ophthalmopathy is the most common cause of unilateral or bilateral proptosis in adults and the most common cause of bilateral proptosis in children. Orbital cellulitis is the most common cause of unilateral proptosis in children and is often associated with an ethmoid sinusitis or upper respiratory infection.

Pseudotumor is a confusing term that may be clinically useful when its definition is sufficiently narrowed. The term *pseudotumor* means "pseudoneoplasm," although the disease actually presents as an inflammatory process. There is no mass lesion to biopsy; however, if a biopsy is performed, mature chronic inflammatory cells and varying degrees of fibrosis proportionate to the chronicity of the process are present. Pseudotumor may be defined as a nonspecific idiopathic inflammatory condition for which no local identifiable cause or systemic disease can be found (see Chapter 1).[1,2] Under this definition, local orbital causes of inflammation are not considered pseudotumor because an identifiable cause is present: ruptured dermoid cyst, ectopic lacrimal gland, retained

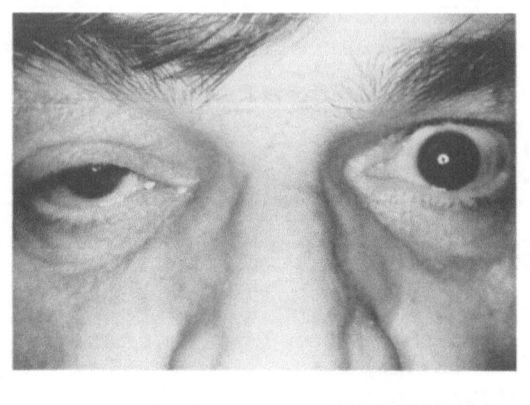

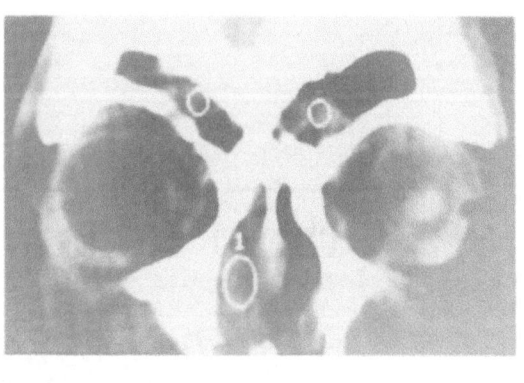

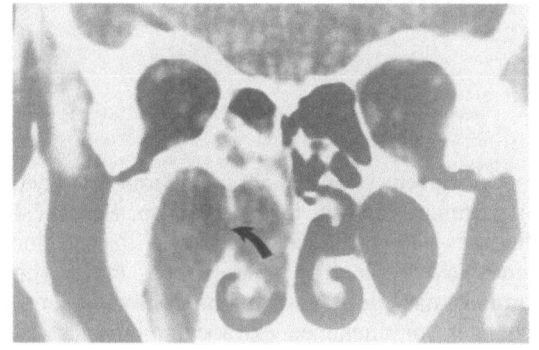

Fig. 2-1. (*A*) A 55-year-old male with incipient orbital cellulitis. CT scan shows minimal orbital inflammation but bilateral frontal (*B*), right ethmoid and right maxillary sinus opacities (*C*). Because of the evidence of bone destruction (arrow in *C*), the diagnosis of Wegener's granulomatosis was considered. The patient was admitted and after a course of intravenous antibiotics, sinus drainage, and biopsy of the maxillary sinus, mucosa showed evidence of Wegener's granulomatosis.

foreign body, sclerosing hemangioma, and infected mucoceles. Systemic causes of orbital inflammation such as Wegener's granulomatosis and sarcoidosis would not be considered a form of pseudotumor. While the latter diseases are themselves idiopathic, the orbital inflammation in such patients would be ascribed to a systemic condition and would not be considered a pseudotumor.

Orbital hemorrhage may mimic an orbital inflammatory pseudotumor because of the sudden onset of proptosis and edema. In addition, there is accompanying subacute inflammation that serves to biograde the collected blood. The possible local causes of orbital hemorrhage include trauma, hemophilia or other blood dyscrasia, scurvy, varix, arteriovenous (AV) fistula, or orbital tumor (Fig. 2-2). Systemic causes of orbital hemorrhage are hemophilia, scurvy, leukemia, and lymphoma.

A lymphoid infiltrate is a distinct clinicopathologic entity that should be distinguished from pseudotumor (see Chapter 1). While a lymphoid infiltrate that had entirely benign cytologic and morphologic features in the past has been considered a form of pseudotumor, such a classification is not clinically useful and should be abandoned.[3] Classically, acute pseudotumor has an abrupt onset with a clearly inflammatory clinical presentation, while a lymphoid infiltrate presents as a painless salmon-colored subconjunctival mass or retrobulbar mass often with a gradual onset (Figs. 2-3–2-7). The chronic form of pseudotumor has a history of recurrent episodes that result in chronic fibrosis and a frozen globe (Fig. 2-6).

Pseudotumor has several different possible CT presentations, including: (1) a diffuse anterior orbital process due to inflammation of tenons capsule and sclera (Fig. 2-3) and optic nerve involvement ("lollipop sign" on CT scan), and (2) a more localized process that appears to have a particular orbital structure such as EOM (myositis) or lacrimal gland as its target for inflammation (Fig. 2-8), and (3) a subacute or chronic form with either recurrent attacks of acute pseudotumor or chronic sclerosing pseudotumor (Fig. 2-6).[4] Rarely, pseudotumor will show bone destruction or even intracranial extension (Fig. 2-9).[5] The CT scan appearance of pseudotumor reflects these presentations and is quite distinctive from a lymphoid infiltrate, that is, a diffuse process. The lymphoid tumor is a homogeneous infiltrate that molds around the globe and orbital bones and rarely destroys bone (Fig. 2-8C). The subacute and chronic forms of pseudotumor may mimic a lymphoid infiltrate; however, the history of recurrent attacks, the nonhomogeneous streaked density in the orbit that corresponds to the fibrosis, and the sometimes frozen globe due to the fibrosis are helpful clues in the differential diagnosis. Rarely, however, both the clinical presentation and CT scan appearance may be identical; in that case only biopsy will separate the entities.

Pathologically, pseudotumor is composed of mature chronic inflammatory cells such as lymphocytes and plasma cells often within a fibrous matrix. The presence of fibrosis is extremely helpful in distinguishing pseudotumor from a lymphoid infiltrate that is composed of

Table 2-1
Differential Diagnosis of Orbital Inflammatory Disease

Thyroid ophthalmopathy
Acute orbital cellulitis (bacterial)
Idiopathic inflammatory pseudotumor
Lymphoid infiltrate
   reactive lymphoid hyperplasia
   atypical reactive lymphoid hyperplasia
   lymphoma
Leukemia
Vasculitis
   Wegener's granulomatosis
   periarteritis nodosa
   lethal midline granuloma
Sarcoid
Nonbacterial infections (fungal and parasitic)
Infected mucoceles
Local causes of inflammation
   ruptured dermoid cyst
   ectopic lacrimal gland
   retained foreign body
   sclerosing hemangioma
   infected mucocele
   orbital hemorrhage
Primary or secondary orbital tumor associated with inflammation
Unifocal or multifocal eosinophilic granuloma (formerly termed *diffuse histiocytosis*)
Varix with or without thrombophlebitis or hemorrhage
Arteriovenous fistula with or without orbital hemorrhage

sheets of cells without fibrosis, especially when the clinical and CT findings suggest a chronic diffuse process. Reactive lymphoid hyperplasia is a combination of mature lymphocytes, plasma cells, and histiocytes with follicle formation. The cytologic features are benign. In atypical reactive lymphoid hyperplasia, the cytologic features are not sufficiently worrisome to warrant the diagnosis of lymphoma. A lymphoma is a frankly malignant tumor that by definition cannot be considered a pseudotumor. We favor the diagnosis of a lymphoid infiltrate over pseudotumor when both follicles and significant fibrosis are present.

Lymphoid infiltrates may have many cells with plasma cell features. Such tumors with plasmacytic differentiation may be associated with myeloma or immunoglobulin secretion. All patients with lid, conjunctival, or orbital lymphoid or lymphoplasmacytic infiltrates should have serum protein electrophoresis studies and bone marrow biopsy.

Not only are the clinical, CT scan, and pathologic features distinctive, but the prognosis of a patient with an orbital pseudotumor as defined above is different from that of a patient with a lymphoid infiltrate. Any of the latter patients may eventually develop a systemic lymphoma, while the former patients are not at risk. In one autopsy series of 1269 patients with systemic lymphoma, only three patients presented with orbital disease and an additional 13 patients developed orbital involvement later in the course of their disease.[6] Another prognostic factor is the anatomic location of the infiltrate. In general, conjunctival lymphoid infiltrates are salmon-colored patches that are moveable over the epibulbar surface and do not cause proptosis or motility disturbances. Orbital lesions cause proptosis or displacement of the globe with consequent motility imbalance. Conjunctival lymphoid lesions are much less likely to be associated with systemic lymphomas (less than 10 percent of cases) than lid or orbital lymphoid lesions in which systemic disease is present in approximately 50 percent of the cases. This prognosis may be related to the fact that lymphoid tissue is normally present in the conjunctiva (and lacrimal gland) but not in the lid and orbit. Bilateral involvement points toward malignancy.[6-9] In general, lymphoid lesions tend to occur in the superior orbit.

Aside from pseudotumor and lymphoid infiltrate, other, more rare causes of orbital inflammation include various fungal and parasitic infections. In addition, any primary or secondary orbital tumor may be associated with inflammation, particularly if the tumor undergoes necrosis.

WORK-UP

History

Patients with orbital inflammation tend to present with pain, some degree of lid or conjunctival injection, or chemosis. Proptosis is usually present. The patient's history helps differentiate thyroid ophthalmopathy and pseudotumor. Patients with thyroid ophthalmopathy tend to have a more gradual, painless onset (unless there is exposure keratopathy) and generally do not feel sick, whereas patients with pseudotumor tend to have a more explosive, painful onset and may have general malaise. The clinical differential diagnosis is summarized in Table 2-2.

Orbital pseudotumor is uncommon in children yet has certain distinctive features in children.[10] Bilaterality is more common in children than in adults. Iritis is also seen in children and is not common in adults. Trauma may play a precipitating role in pseudotumor in children. The youngest patient documented with orbital pseudotumor is 3 months old.[11]

Thyroid ophthalmopathy is a fairly common cause of proptosis in children and appears to be a much less severe disease than when it presents in the adult. In a recent large series, optic neuropathy and corneal exposure did not occur. Motility disturbances, however, may occur. Ocular complications are more likely the older the age of the child at the onset of the disease.[12]

Like patients with acute classic orbital pseudotumor, patients with acute orbital cellulitis have an abrupt onset of disease with pain. Bacterial orbital cellulitis is rarely painless by history and even more rarely painless on palpation. The latter findings may be consistent with pseudotumor. A history of trauma, sinusitis, or a retained foreign body such as an orbital floor implant can aid in determining the cause of orbital cellulitis. Sinusitis is the most common cause of acute bacterial orbital cellulitis. Sinusitis may precede the development of mucoceles.

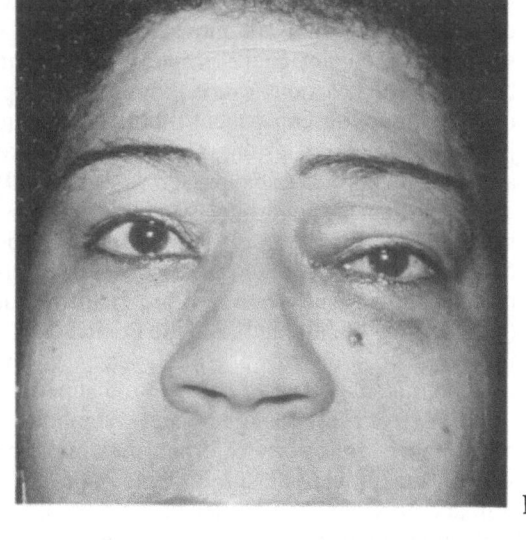

A

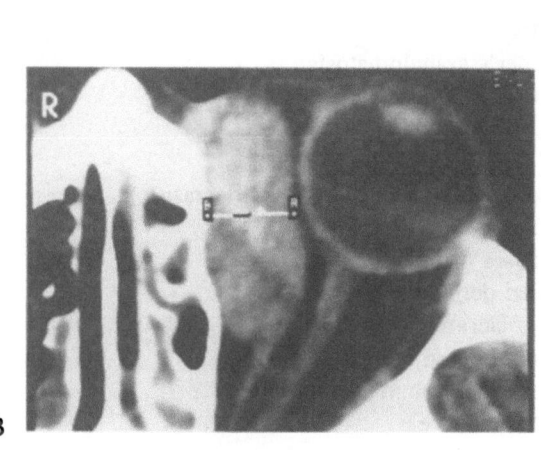

B

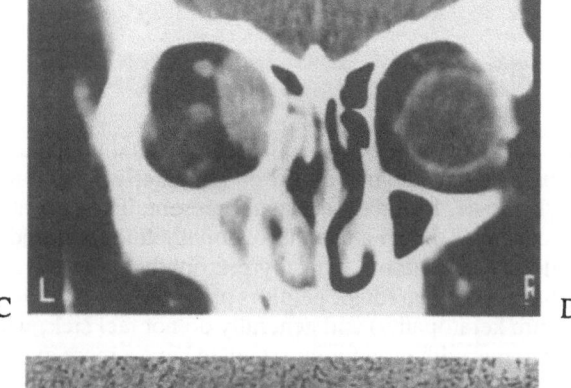

C

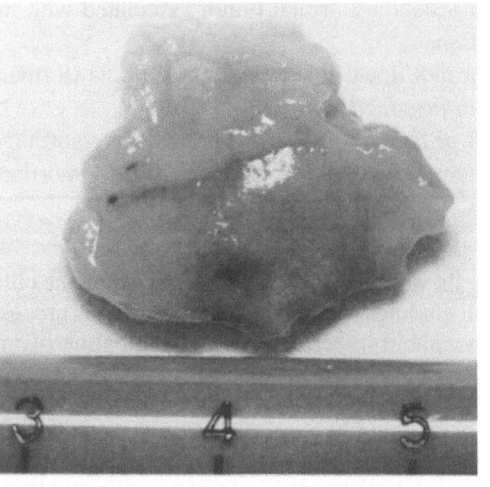

D

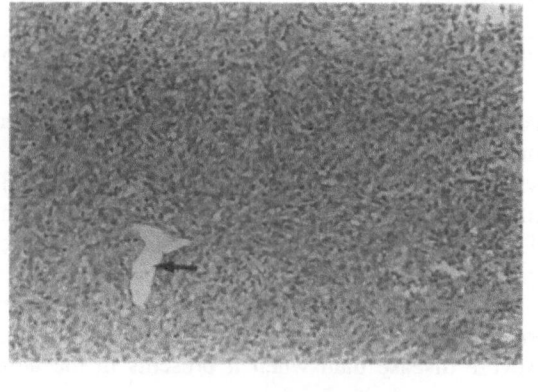

E

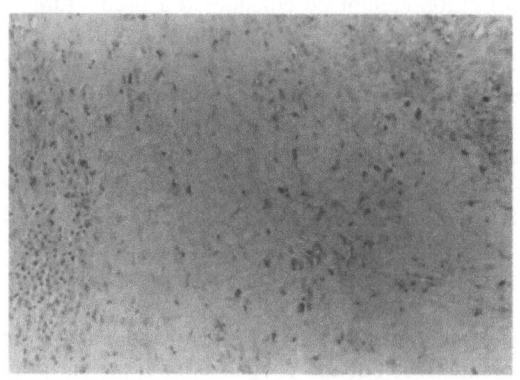

F

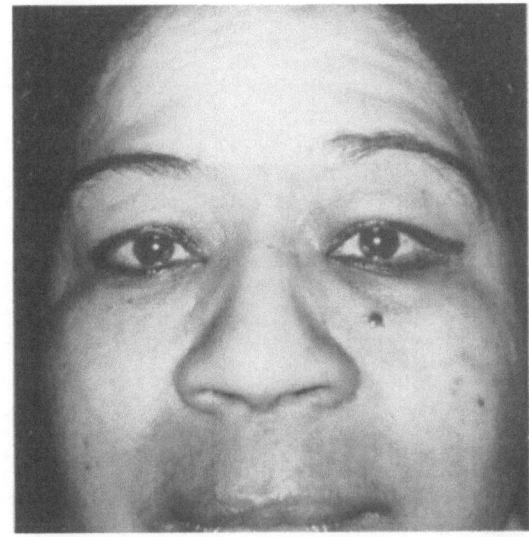

G

Fig. 2-2. (*A*) A 44-ycar-old female with episode of epigastric pain and vomiting resulting in left orbital hemorrhage. (*B-C*) Orbital CT scan shows a mass both inside and outside the muscle cone that infiltrated the medial rectus. (*D*) Gross specimen in operating room shows an irregular friable tannish-red unencapsulated mass with smooth surface. (*E*) Photomicrograph shows a cellular tumor with irregular vascular channels (arrow) that is composed of pericytes that have round-to-oval hyperchromatic nuclei. (*F*) Areas of the tumor show evidence of orbital hemorrhage with fibrosis and hemosiderin-laden macrophages. (*G*) Appearance of patient 1 month after surgery.

A dental abscess with or without dental extraction, particularly in the upper teeth, may predispose to maxillary sinusitis or orbital cellulitis.[13] Other possible foci of infection, including concurrent dacryocystitis, osteomyelitis of contiguous orbital bone, or subclinical pneumonia, should be considered.[14,15]

Patients with Wegener's granulomatosis or periartitis nodosa may have pulmonary, kidney, or skin involvement. A history of travel may suggest a parasitic or infectious origin. Metastatic cancer to the orbit may present as an inflammatory process.

OPHTHALMOLOGIC EXAMINATION AND GENERAL MEDICAL EVALUATION

The important features of ophthalmologic examination include vision, visual field, and exophthalmometry. Patients with acute bacterial orbital cellulitis show signs of acute inflammation, including pain, swelling, and erythema. Tense edema on external examination helps to differentiate patients with orbital cellulitis from patients with thyroid disease or pseudotumor. Patients with suspected acute bacterial orbital cellulitis should be observed for signs of cavernous sinus thrombosis, including decreasing vision, internal and external ophthalmoplegia, fifth nerve involvement, signs in the fellow eye, and meningeal signs.[2]

In any child with unilateral or bilateral rapidly evolving proptosis with chemosis and hemorrhage, the diagnosis of rhabdomyosarcoma should be considered. Other possible diagnoses include granulocytic sarcoma, metastatic neuroblastoma, and Ewing's sarcoma (see Chapter 4).

Patients with reactive lymphoid hyperplasia or lymphoma often have a painless salmon-colored subconjunctival mass (Fig. 2-7). Boggy chemosis, in contrast to the tense chemosis of the conjunctiva associated with bacterial infection, generally accompanies such lesions as lymphoid infiltrates. In addition, a tumor with necrosis may mimic a bacterial orbital cellulitis. Patients with idiopathic orbital inflammation (pseudotumor) may present acutely, subacutely, or chronically (Figs. 2-8 through 2-10). The acute form presents with pain and is most easily distinguished from a lymphoid infiltrate on clinical involvement. The subacute and chronic forms of pseudotumor are difficult to distinguish from a lymphoid infiltrate. The key to an understanding of the more chronic forms of pseudotumor is that fibrosis occurs, and this will give an anteriorly located palpable mass a rock-hard consistency that is not found in a lymphoid infiltrate, which has sheets of cells with little, if any, associated fibrosis (Fig. 2-11).

Eosinophilic granuloma is a histiocytic disorder of the orbit that in the past was considered part of a spectrum of entities termed *histiocytosis X*. Other diseases similarly classified included eosinophilic granuloma, Letterer-Siwe disease, and Hand-Schüller-Christian disease. All three diseases are now termed either (1) *unifocal (local) eosinophilic granuloma* or (2) *multifocal eosinophilic granuloma*. The formerly termed *diffuse histiocytoses* are pathologically indistinguishable and have the common histologic feature of an abnormal proliferation of bland mononuclear as well as binuclear histiocytes, multinucleated histiocytes, giant cells, and eosinophils in a minimally fibrotic stroma. In addition, Langerhans' cells contain characteristic Birbeck or Langerhans' granules, racquet-shaped ultrastructural intracytoplasmic bodies. Hemorrhage, frequently present within the tumor, leads to secondary pathologic features including hemosiderin-laden macrophages and sclerosis.[3]

As stated above, the processes may be unifocal (localized) or multifocal (systemic). Focal eosinophilic granuloma presents typically as a swelling in the superotempo-

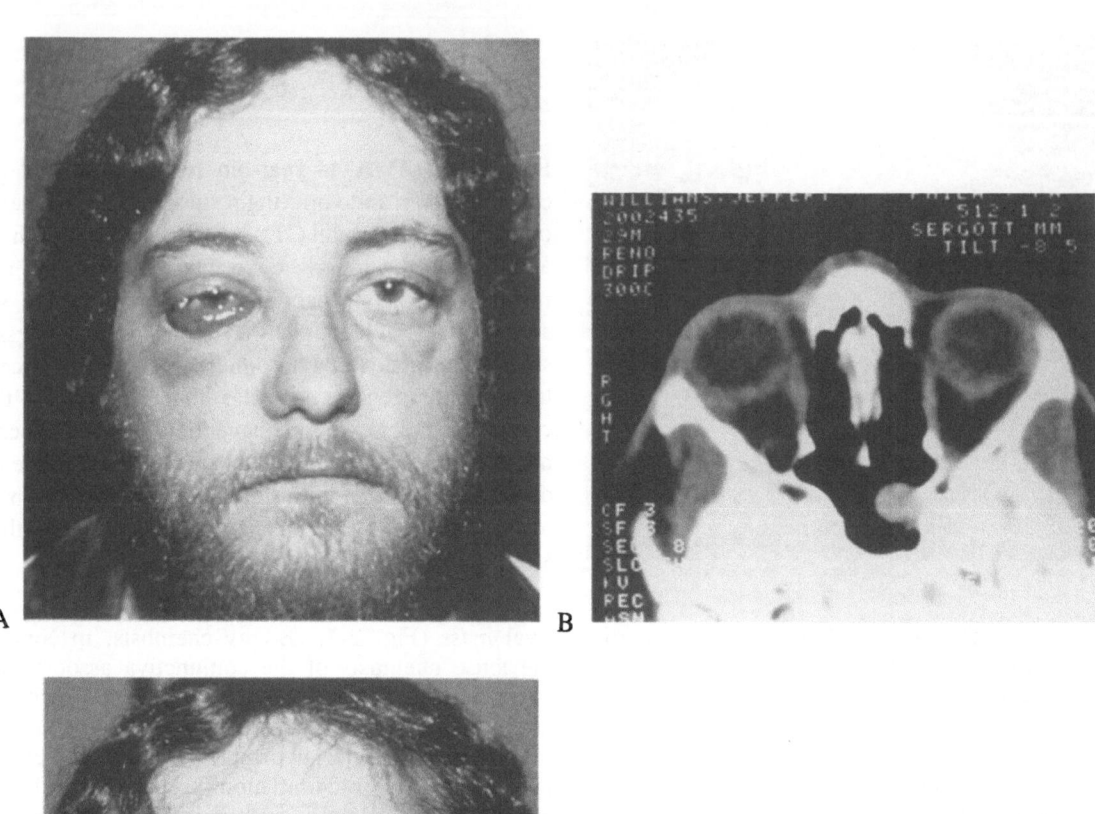

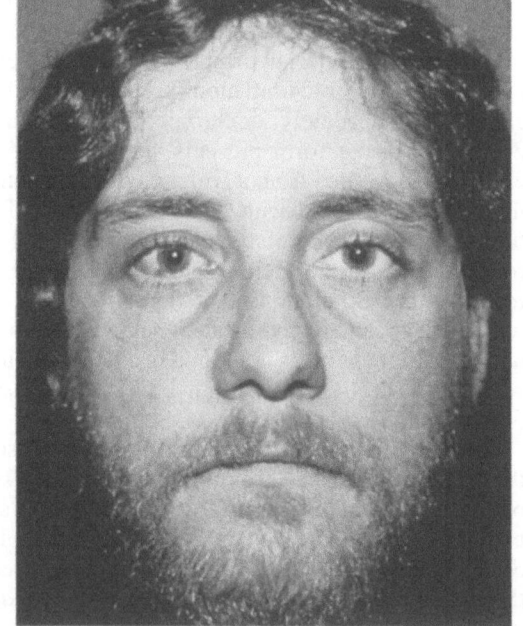

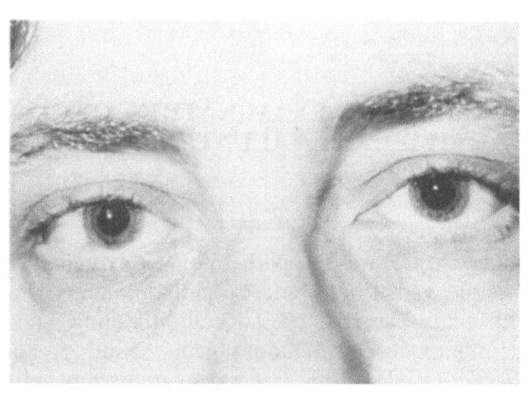

Fig. 2-3. (*A*) Patient with acute onset of pain/tenderness on right side that was unresponsive to antibiotics. (*B*) CT scan shows inflammation (sclerotenonitis pattern) that surrounds the right globe. There is no definite mass. Abrupt onset, lack of response to therapeutic antibiotic trial, and CT pattern strongly support diagnosis of presumed pseudotumor. High-dose steroids were administered. (*C–D*) 48 hours after oral prednisone, inflammation has resolved. (Courtesy of Dr. Robert Sergott, Philadelphia, PA; reprinted with permission from Mauriello JA, Flanagan JC: Recommended protocol for management of orbital inflammatory disease. *Surv Ophthalmol* 29:104–116, 1984.)

ral quadrant of the orbit adjacent to the orbital rim. Pain may or may not be present. The multifocal form of eosinophilic granuloma occurs in the first 2 years of life with cutaneous, visceral, lymph node, and rarely orbital and ocular involvement. This entity was formerly known as the Letterer-Siwe form of histiocytosis X. These patients often present with fever, wasting, hepato-splenomegaly, lymphadenopathy, anemia, and thrombo-

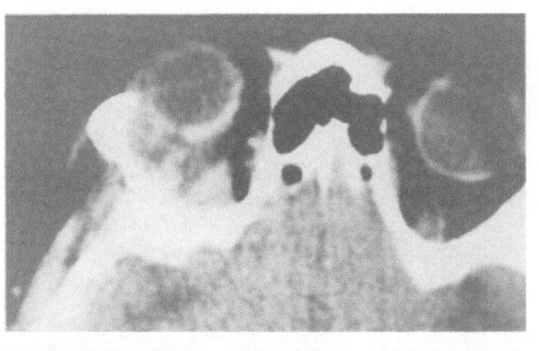

Fig. 2-4. CT scan of another patient with pseudotumor. Note that infiltrate unlike that of lymphoid infiltrate is not homogeneous but slightly granular.

cytopenia. Patients usually die within 6 months. The classic triad of multiple osteolytic lesions, diabetes insipidus, and exophthalmos, is rare. The latter disease was formerly called Hand-Schüller-Christian disease.[16]

Other histiocytic disorders of the orbit include juvenile xanthogranuloma, Erdheim-Chester disease, pseudorheumatoid nodules, necrobiotic xanthogranuloma, and sarcoidosis. The latter entities present as tumors without significant clinical evidence of inflammation and are considered in Chapters 3 and 8.

In patients with a palpable thrill or audible bruit, an AV fistula should be considered. Arterialization of the conjunctival vessels up to the limbus will often be present.

In addition to an ophthalmologic history and examination, a general medical history and physical examination are recommended to rule out primary malignancy or evidence of other systemic disease. Patients with Wegener's granulomatosis and periarteritis nodosa may have pulmonary, kidney, or skin lesions.

DIAGNOSTIC STUDIES

The main diagnostic studies include orbital CT scan, magnetic resonance imaging (MRI), and orbital ultrasound. Plain x-ray films of the orbit are not necessary. The most significant information that can be obtained from these studies are: (1) presence of an orbital mass lesion without sinus involvement or bone erosion, (2) presence of an orbital mass lesion with sinus involvement or bone changes, or (3) thickened EOMs. In our experience, determination of these features is critical to the management of patients with orbital inflammatory disease.[1] Patients with pseudotumor should have blood studies including sedimentation rate, antinuclear antibodies (ANA), and rheumatoid factor to rule out a systemic vasculitis.

It should be added that in patients with a palpable thrill or audible bruit in the orbital region, arteriography may be necessary to rule out an A-V fistula.

General medical evaluation will suggest other appropriate systemic studies.

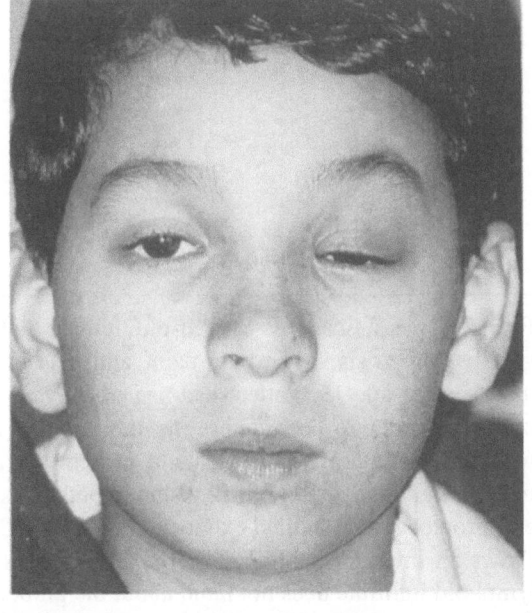
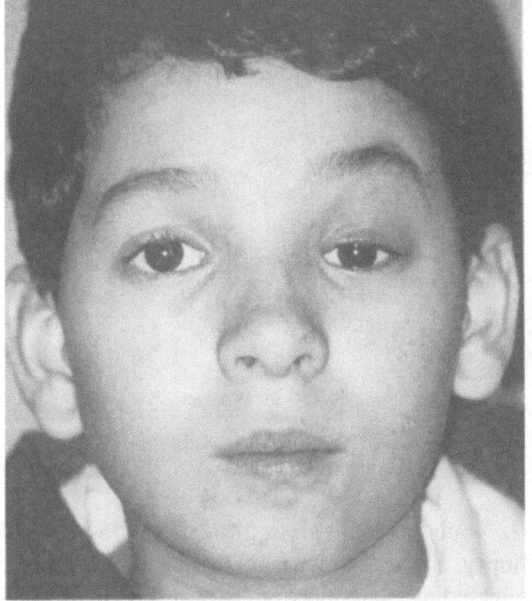

A   B

Fig. 2-5. (A) A 12-year-old child with acute onset of pain and tenderness of left orbit. There was no history of trauma, sinusitis, or dental abscess. (B) After trial of intravenous antibiotics, patient had a dramatic response to oral prednisone.

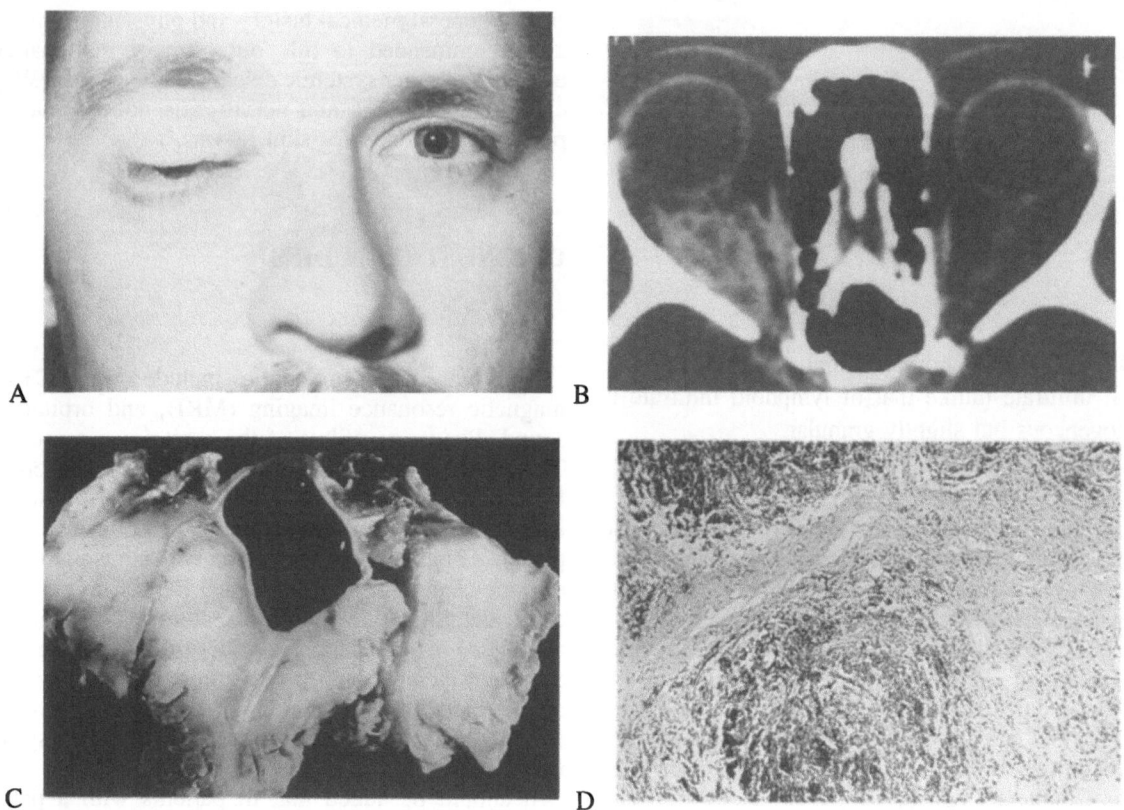

Fig. 2-6. (*A*) A 38-year-old male with 5-year history of recurrnt bouts of pseudotumor unresponsive to medical management with systemic steroids. (*B*) Orbital CT scan shows a diffuse orbital infiltrate. CT scan shows "streak" densities due to fibrosis. The lack of homogeneity of the orbital infiltrate on CT scan combined with the history are helpful in clinically differentiating pseudotumor and lymphoid infiltrate. Patient had undergone multiple orbital debulking procedures. (*C*) Orbital exenteration specimen of another patient showing fibrous replacement of orbital contents due to pseudotumor (AFIP ACC #1307043). (*D*) Biopsy (AFIP ACC #280758) shows bands of fibrous tissue that replace orbital fat and are interspersed with foci of mature chronic inflammatory cells.

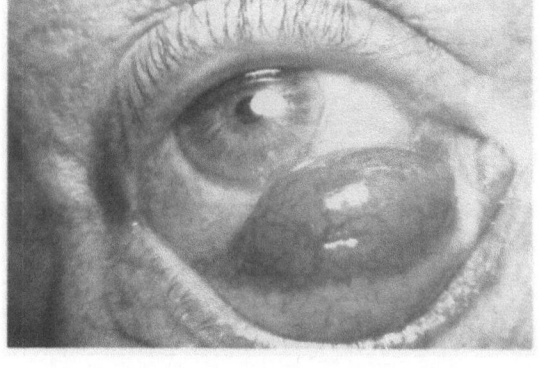

Fig. 2-7. Subconjunctival infiltrate in 55-year-old male. Biopsy showed a lymphoplasmacytic infiltrate. Work-up including bone marrow, serum protein electrophoresis, and abdominal CT scan showed evidence of systemic multiple myeloma. The patient was referred to an oncologist for treatment and further follow-up.

Fig. 2-9. CT scan of 48-year-old female with progressive proptosis, periorbital pain, and loss of vision that dates to age 19. Patient had had transfrontal craniotomy in order to decompress the left orbit at age 29 with only temporary relief. Patient presents at age 48 with no light perception (NLP) vision in both eyes, bilateral proptosis, and limited extraocular motility. CT scan shows an irregular nonhomogeneous mass that unlike a lymphoid infiltrate does not mold about the globe. There is bony destruction with extension in the right cavernous sinus and middle cranial fossa. The history of pain, "frozen globe," and CT pattern favor chronic sclerosing

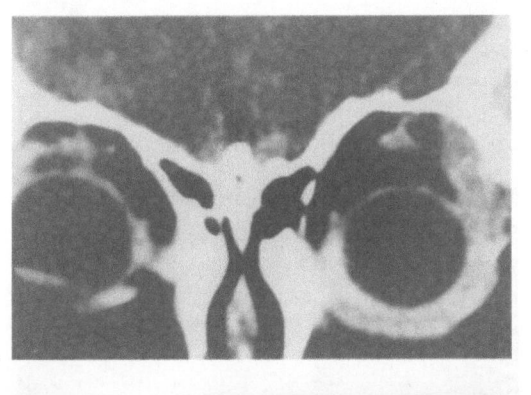

A

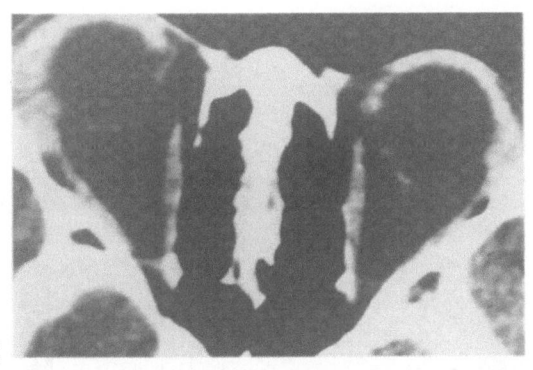

C

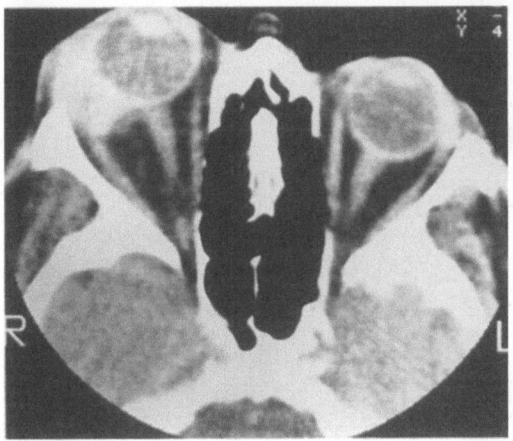

B

Fig. 2-8. (*A*) Coronal CT scan from patient with acute orbital pseudotumor involving the right orbit. (*B*) On axial CT scan, infiltrate involves lacrimal gland as well as tendon of lateral rectus muscle. Note mild lacrimal gland enlargement on left side. The infiltrate partially surrounds the eye as seen on coronal view. The latter CT scan pattern should be compared with the next pattern of a 55-year-old female with 1-month history of gradual onset of painless swelling of right orbit. (*C*) CT scan of this latter patient shows diffuse mass inside and outside the muscle cone in the lacrimal gland area. As compared with the CT pattern in *A* and *B*, in *C* there is "something to biopsy." The lymphoid infiltrate has a characteristic homogeneous pattern.

pseudotumor. This diagnosis was confirmed on biopsy. The presence of bone erosion and brain extension is extremely unusual for pseudotumor. (Reprinted with permission from Frohman LP, Kupersmith MJ, Lang J, et al: Intracranial extension and bone destruction in orbital pseudotumor. *Arch Ophthalmol* 104:380–384, 1986; courtesy of MJ Kupersmith)

Table 2-2
Clinical Differential Diagnosis of Pseudotumor and Thyroid Ophthalmopathy

Pseudotumor	Thyroid Ophthalmopathy
Equal incidence of males and females	Females predominate
Sudden onset	Gradual onset
Tends to be painful	Painless unless cornea involved
Early motility problems	Later motility problems
General malaise	Well-being
No lid-lag or retraction	Lid-lag and retraction
Usually unilateral	Usually bilateral
Steroid-sensitive	Variably responds to steroids
May have photophobia	

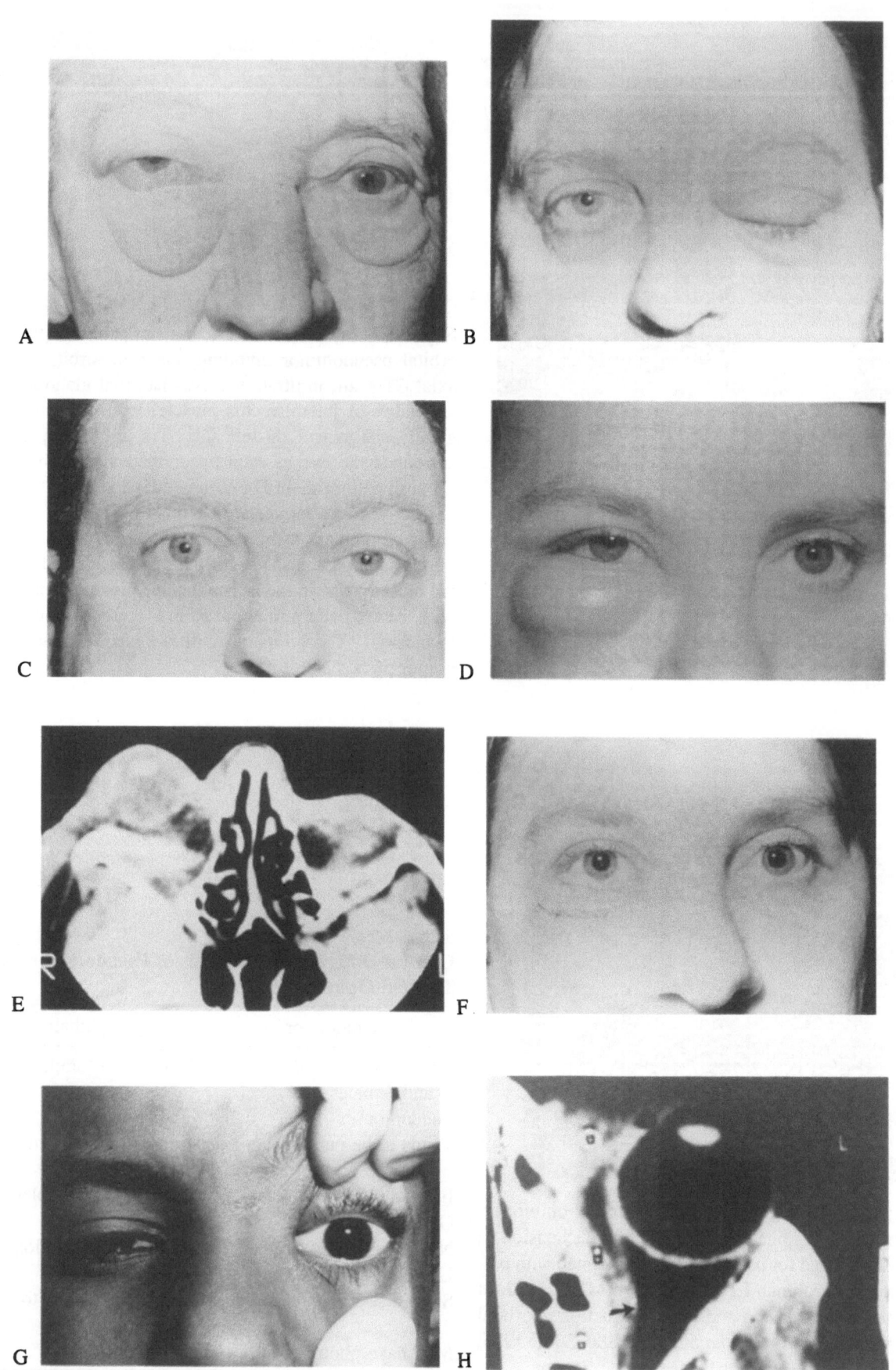

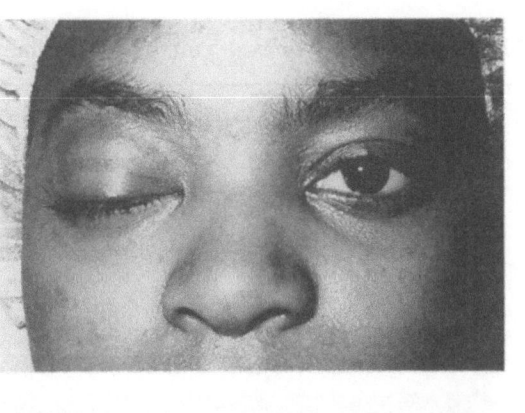

I

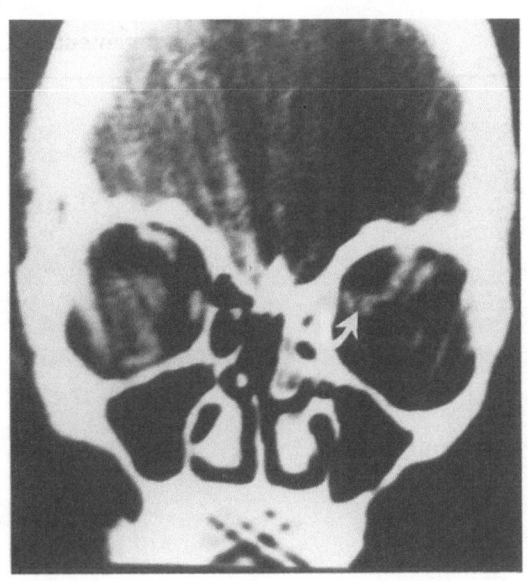

J

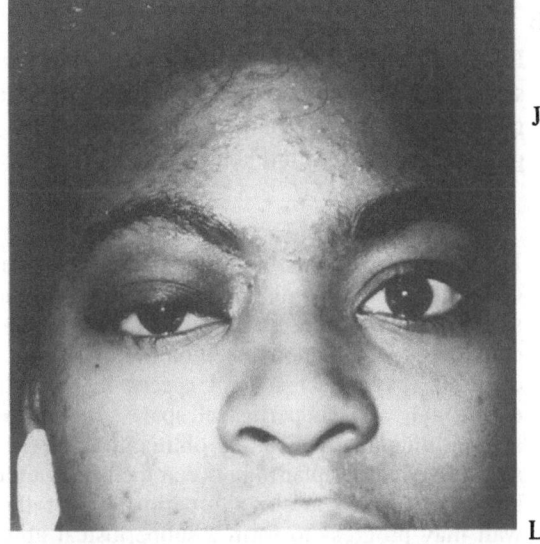

K

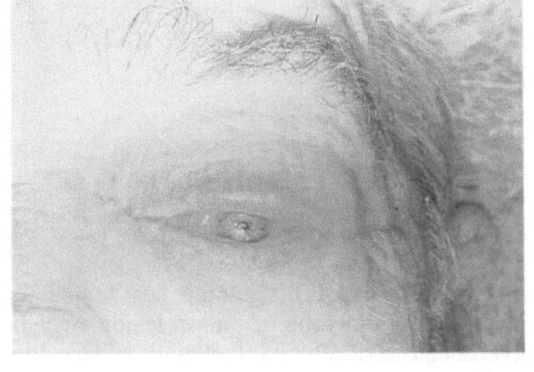

L

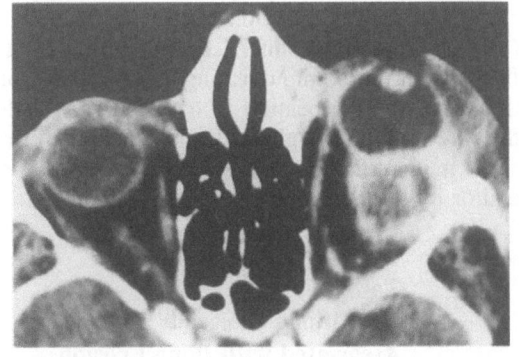

M

Fig. 2-10. (A) A 70-year-old female with gradual onset of painless proptosis with upward displacement of the globe and boggy edema of the conjunctiva inferiorly. CT scan showed a homogeneous mass in the inferior orbit. Biopsy showed a well-differentiated lymphoma. (B) A 38-year-old male with left ethmoiditis and orbital cellulitis that responded dramatically over 48 hours (C) to intravenous antibiotics. (D) Patient had a motor vehicle accident and required reconstruction with orbital floor implant 5 years previously. Two days prior to admission, he had dental work that resulted in an infected orbital floor implant. (E) CT scan shows an opacity that surrounds the implant. (F) Treatment with intravenous antibiotics for 48 hours followed by drainage of the abscess and removal of the offending foreign body implant was performed. (Reprinted with permission from Mauriello JA, Flanagan JC: Recommended protocol for management of orbital inflammatory disease. *Surv Ophthalmol* 29:104–116, 1984.) (G) A 10-year-old patient with ethmoiditis and preseptal cellulitis on the left side. The eye is white, indicating a preseptal cellulitis. (H) On CT scan, there is only a subperiosteal effusion without extension through the periorbita. (I) A 20-year-old female who had orbital cellulitis. There was no history of trauma, retained foreign body, dental extraction, or sinusitis. Patient had received a 10-day course of oral antibiotics with only partial resolution. (J) CT scan showed a well-localized superior subperiosteal abscess (arrow). (K) Three weeks after orbital drainage, there is a characteristic persistent edema that usually takes months to resolve. (L) A 68-year-old male who had had a subscapular melanoma of the skin excised 5 years ago presented with orbital inflammation unresponsive to intravenous antibiotics. (M) CT scan showed a possible intraorbital abscess or tumor abscess. Biopsy showed metastatic melanoma. (Patient referred by Martin Corwin, MD, Livingston, NJ.)

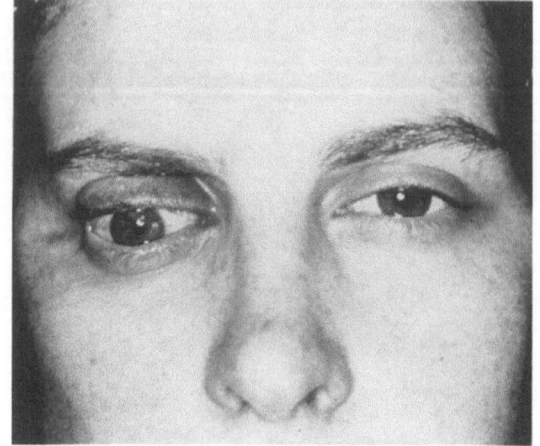

A

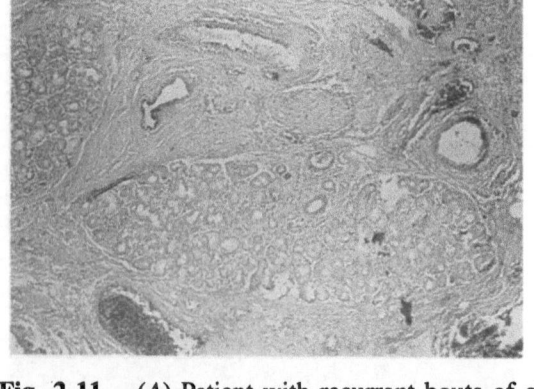

B

Fig. 2-11. (*A*) Patient with recurrent bouts of chronic sclerosing pseudotumor unresponsive to steroids and surgical debulking procedures. (*B*) Biopsy shows ectopic gland tissue amid chronic sclerosing pseudotumor matrix.

CT SCAN

Conditions Generally Not Associated with Bone Erosion or Sinus Involvement

High-resolution orbital CT scanning has supplanted plain x-ray films of the orbit. A mass lesion may be seen in diverse causes of orbital inflammation. This nonspecific finding is secondary to soft tissue edema and cellular infiltration. Causes of a mass lesion without sinus involvement or bone erosion are listed in Table 2-3. When a homogeneous mass lesion of relatively high density follows the contour of the globe and the adjacent orbital bone without causing erosion and shows mild contrast enhancement on CT scan, an orbital lymphoid infiltrate is the most likely cause; solitary plasmacytomas associated with myeloma, both of which are extremely rare in the orbit, may cause bone destruction or sinus involvement. Pseudotumors that are diffuse and fill the orbit have marked sclerosis, and therefore, there is a streak-like quality to the nonhomogeneous density (Fig. 2-6).[2] Sinus involvement is very rare with a lymphoid infiltrate.[17]

Pseudotumor most often causes enhancement confined to the anterior orbit, particularly when the patient has the classic abrupt onset with pain. CT scan may show findings consistent with a preseptal cellulitis, that is, diffuse anterior inflammation, an irregular infiltrate involving one or more EOMs (see next section), an enlarged optic nerve with a ring of scleral enhancement, "lollipop" sign, or unilateral and bilateral enlarged lacrimal glands. In all such cases, it is apparent on examining the CT scan that there is very little abnormal tissue to biopsy. There is no mass lesion except in the chronic sclerosing form with its irregular streak densities.

Orbital cellulitis can be well demonstrated on CT scan.

Eyelid edema, the first manifestation of preseptal orbital cellulitis, can not be distinguished from cellulitis on CT scan. However, preseptal versus postseptal or orbital cellulitis is well demonstrated on the axial scan. Orbital cellulitis may affect several spaces in the intraconal, extraconal, and subperiosteal space. In the intraconal space, inflammation causes obliteration of the normal soft tissue and fat planes between the optic nerve, retrobulbar fat, and muscles. A periosteitis of the orbital wall may progress to form a subperiosteal abscess that is of low tissue density; the entire mass or at least the rim of the abscess may enhance with contrast injection (Fig. 2-12). Gas produced by gas-forming bacteria or from air in the communicating sinus may be present in the abscess. The location of the abscess will determine the direction of the globe displacement. An orbital abscess is identified as an area of increased tissue density and/or by the presence of gas in the orbit.

Table 2-3
Conditions Generally Not Associated with Bone Erosion or Sinus Involvement

Pseudotumor*
Lymphoid infiltrate
Leukemia
Local causes of inflammation†
    ectopic lacrimal gland
    retained foreign body
    sclerosing hemangioma
    orbital hemorrhage

* Rarely associated with bone erosion

† If the degree of associated inflammation is severe, of long duration, and adjacent to bone, bone erosion may occur.

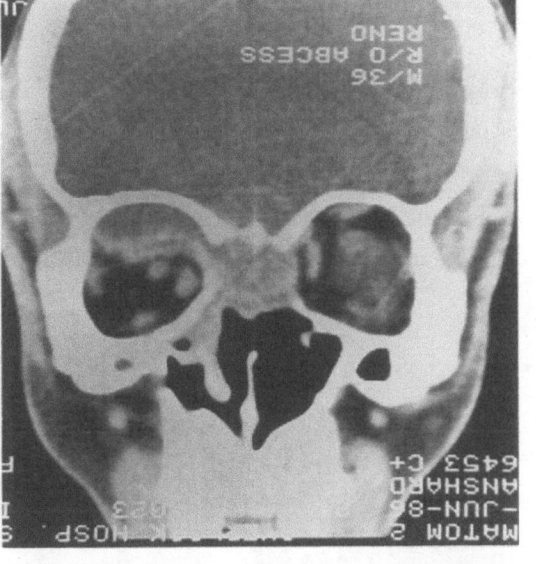

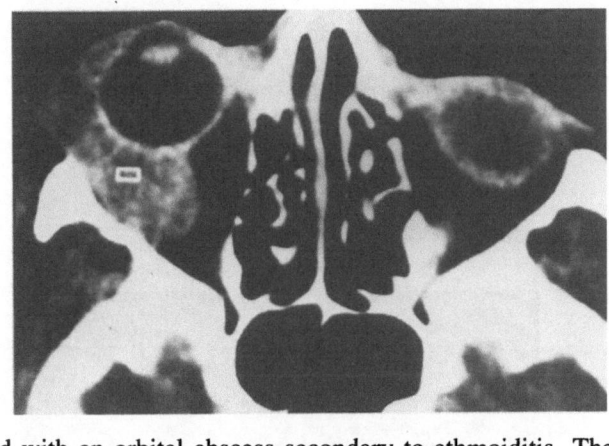

A   B

Fig. 2-12. CT scan of a 35-year-old male who presented with an orbital abscess secondary to ethmoiditis. The patient had had two prior episodes of ethmoiditis. Ethmoidectomy was performed after the second bout, which explains loss of bony wall on CT scan. There was a dramatic response to drainage of the abscess. (*B*) CT scan from a 67-year-old female with diffuse infiltrate about the lacrimal gland. Disease had gradual painless onset with no prior history suggesting pseudotumor. The lack of bone erosion and diffuse process favored the diagnosis of a lymphoid infiltrate over a primary epithelial tumor of the lacrimal gland (see Chapter 6). Biopsy showed a monotonous infiltrate of lymphoid cells.

Possible sequellae of orbital cellulitis include cavernous sinus thrombosis, meningitis, cerebral abscess, infarction, and subdural or epidural abscess, all which are well demonstrated by CT scanning. Signs of meningitis including nuchal rigidity and change in mentation should be ruled out.

The CT findings of a mass lesion that surrounds an EOM without sinus involvement or bone erosion virtually rules out thyroid ophthalmopathy. A lymphoid infiltrate is the most likely diagnosis. Pseudotumor is usually not significant enough to produce a mass unless there is sclerosis (Fig. 2-8*C* and 2-13). Myasthenia gravis has been reported to be associated with pseudotumor and thrombocytopenia and therefore should be considered in this differential diagnosis.[18]

The local causes of inflammation, including orbital hemorrhage, ectopic lacrimal gland, and retained foreign body, rarely cause bone changes. Whether such lesions produce bone erosion depends on their proximity to bone, their duration, and the degree of associated inflammation.

Conditions Associated with Sinus Involvement or Bone Erosion

Table 2-4 lists the orbital inflammatory diseases that show sinus involvement or bone changes (usually erosion). Orbital cellulitis due to ethmoiditis or maxillary sinusitis often shows clouding of the involved sinus and sometimes bone erosion (Fig. 2-1*C* and 2-10*D–K*).[19]

Primary orbital cellulitis generally does not cause bone erosion or sinus involvement. In the largest series of patients with Wegener's granulomatosis, all patients with proptosis had sinus involvement.[20–22] Sarcoidosis may also involve the paranasalsinus and rarely cause a mucopyocele (Fig. 2-14). Orbital fungal infections, including mucormycosis and sometimes aspergillosis, may be accompanied by sinus disease.

Tuberculosis of the orbit is uncommon and may involve the soft tissues, lacrimal gland, orbital bones, and sinuses. Patients may or may not have pulmonary tuberculosis. Pansinusitis may occur. In any case, acid-fast bacilli are difficult to detect in the orbital pathologic specimens. Many of the granulomatous lesions are of the sclerosing type. Aside from determining the extraorbital seeding site of the infection, a tuberculin skin test should be included in the work-up. In addition to tissue biopsy, cultures for acid fast bacilli (AFB) and fungi should be obtained.[23]

A dermoid cyst with or without rupture commonly causes bone erosion in the lacrimal fossa. The dermoid cyst has a low-density center due to the keratin content. The wall of rim of the cyst enhances with intravenous contrast. On MRI, the tumor is recognized because it yields the same signal intensity as retrobulbar fat.

Almost any primary or secondary orbital tumor with significant tumor necrosis and inflammation may be associated with sinusitis or bone erosion.

Thickening of one or more EOMs occurs most commonly in five conditions: thyroid ophthalmopathy, pseu-

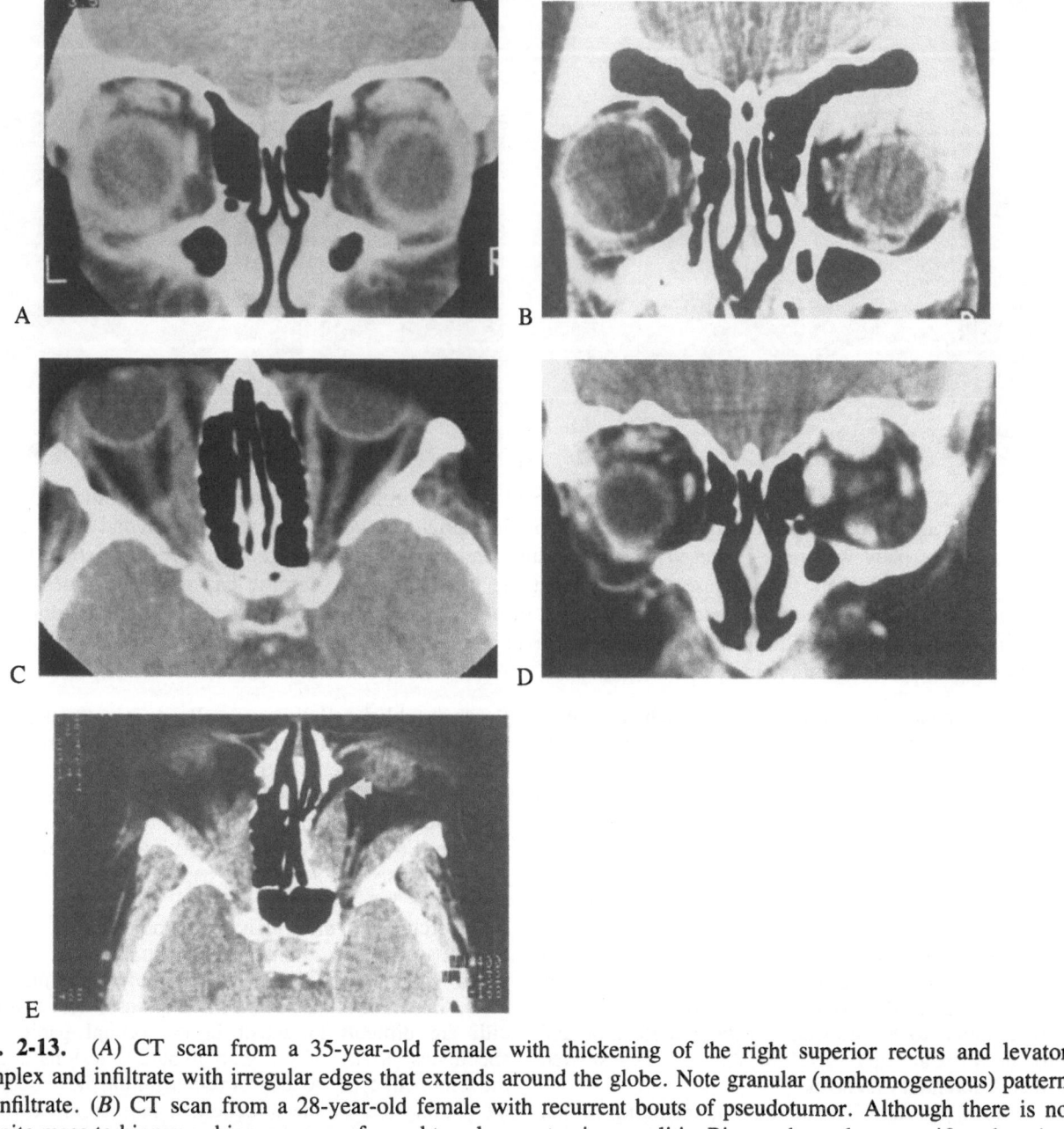

Fig. 2-13. (*A*) CT scan from a 35-year-old female with thickening of the right superior rectus and levator complex and infiltrate with irregular edges that extends around the globe. Note granular (nonhomogeneous) pattern of infiltrate. (*B*) CT scan from a 28-year-old female with recurrent bouts of pseudotumor. Although there is no definite mass to biopsy, a biopsy was performed to rule a systemic vasculitis. Biopsy showed nonspecific sclerosing pseudotumor. This myositis pattern is distinct from patients with thyroid ophthalmopathy who show fusiform thickening of the medial rectus that characteristically spares the tendon of the involved muscle on axial view (*C*) and a discrete, well-circumscribed thickening of the superior rectus and medial rectus on coronal view (*D*). Also note right lacrimal gland enlargement in *D*. (*E*) Axial CT scan of patient with thyroid ophthalmopathy who underwent left orbital decompression. Note fusiform thickening of muscle that spares the tendon (arrow).

dotumor, lymphoid infiltrate, metastatic carcinoma, and A-V fistula. Acromegaly, amyloid of the orbit, collagen vascular disease (e.g., dermatomyositis and systemic lupus erythematosis), and parasitic infections, such as trichinosis and cysticercosis, are more rare causes of EOM enlargement on CT scan (Table 2-5).

The most common differential diagnosis of thickened EOMs on CT scan is thyroid ophthalmopathy. Pseudotumor and lymphoid infiltrate are also common (Fig. 2-13*C, D, E*) Thyroid disease spares the EOM tendon.[24–28] Therefore, the pattern of muscle enlargement in thyroid disease is fusiform. The thickened EOMs have

Table 2-4
Conditions Often Associated with Sinus Involvement or Bone Erosion*

Vasculitis
 Wegener's granulomatosis
 Periarteritis nodosa
 Lethal midline granuloma
Fungal infections
 Aspergillosis
 Mucormycosis
Tuberculosis
Infected mucoceles
 Primary or secondary orbital malignancies with associated inflammation
 Unifocal or multifocal eosinophilic granuloma, diffuse malignant histiocytosis

*In any of these conditions, bone erosion or sinus involvement may not always be present.

† Primary orbital cellulitis may not show bone erosion or sinus involvement.

smooth, well-defined borders. Multiple muscles, most commonly the inferior rectus and the medial rectus, are involved and the process is usually bilateral. In contrast, pseudotumor is an infiltrative process that causes the borders of the enlarged muscles to be irregular and ill-defined. The muscle tendon is involved. Unless there is significant sclerosis, there appears to be little to biopsy on CT scan. Pseudotumor in adults is often limited to one muscle and is usually unilateral. Pseudotumor is rare in children and is more often bilateral in children than in adults. A lymphoid infiltrate most often presents as a contrast-enhancing mass (usually in the superior orbit). The mass tends to mold around the globe and may show EOM enlargement that is best seen on coronal views.[28] There is a mass that may be biopsied.

Orbital myositis is a form of pseudotumor localized to the EOM.[28] In contrast to a lymphoid infiltrate, there is little to biopsy. However, pseudotumor may affect any orbital structure including episclera, retrobulbar space, optic nerve and sheath, optic canal or superior orbital fissure (Tolosa-Hunt syndrome), and lacrimal gland. Involvement of any of the above structures combined with EOM enlargement is virtually pathognomonic of pseudotumor. Enhancement of the posterior sclera and optic nerve due to edema in the retrobulbar space and around the optic nerve gives the appearance of a thickened sclera and optic nerve on CT scan. This finding is characteristic of pseudotumor and is rarely present with thyroid disease.

A mottled retrobulbar fat pattern is typical of pseudotumor, but the pattern is also observed rarely in the CT scan of patients who have thyroid ophthalmopathy. In general, however, the radiodensity of orbital fat is normal in thyroid ophthalmopathy. In addition, swelling of the optic nerve or its sheath does not occur in thyroid ophthalmopathy.

Enlarged lacrimal glands that enhance with contrast may be found in patients with pseudotumor or thyroid disease, so this finding is of limited value in the differential diagnosis. In patients with thyroid ophthalmopathy, enlargement of the lacrimal gland correlates with the severity of the EOM enlargement and/or the congestive changes that also cause a noticeable enlargement of the superior ophthalmic vein.

In patients that show only bilateral lacrimal gland enlargement on CT scan, sarcoidosis and viral infections such as infectious mononucleosis should be considered. Serum angiotensin-converting enzyme and a chest x-ray should be obtained (see Chapter 6).

The lamina papyracea of the ethmoid bone may be displaced medially in severe thyroid ophthalmopathy to form a "wasp-waisted" or "Coca-Cola bottle" contour appearance on CT scan.

Aside from the presence of lid lag and retraction, we have found that the most helpful differential point is the chemical work-up for thyroid disease. Screening tests, including T3 and T4 by radioimmunoassay (RIA) and T3 resin uptake, may be normal while the thyroid-releasing hormone (TRH) infusion test may be abnormal and diagnostic. The differential diagnosis of any suspected pseudotumor that shows bilateral involvement includes systemic diseases, that is, thyroid ophthalmopathy, sarcoidosis, vasculitis, Waldenstöm's macroglobulinemia, and rare infectious causes such as tuberculosis and syphilis.[2]

Metastatic carcinoma usually involves one muscle, and the pattern of involvement on CT scan shows a homogeneous mass that causes irregular muscle margins similar to orbital myositis (Fig. 2-15). Typically, there is a mottled nonhomogeneous quality to the infiltrate. Bone erosion is not unusual. The process is usually extraconal. Metastatic carcinoma shows slight-to-moderate enhancement, while orbital myositis causes moderate-to-marked enhancement. Unlike orbital myositis, metastatic carcinoma may cause adjacent bone erosion. The greater wing of the sphenoid is the most common site

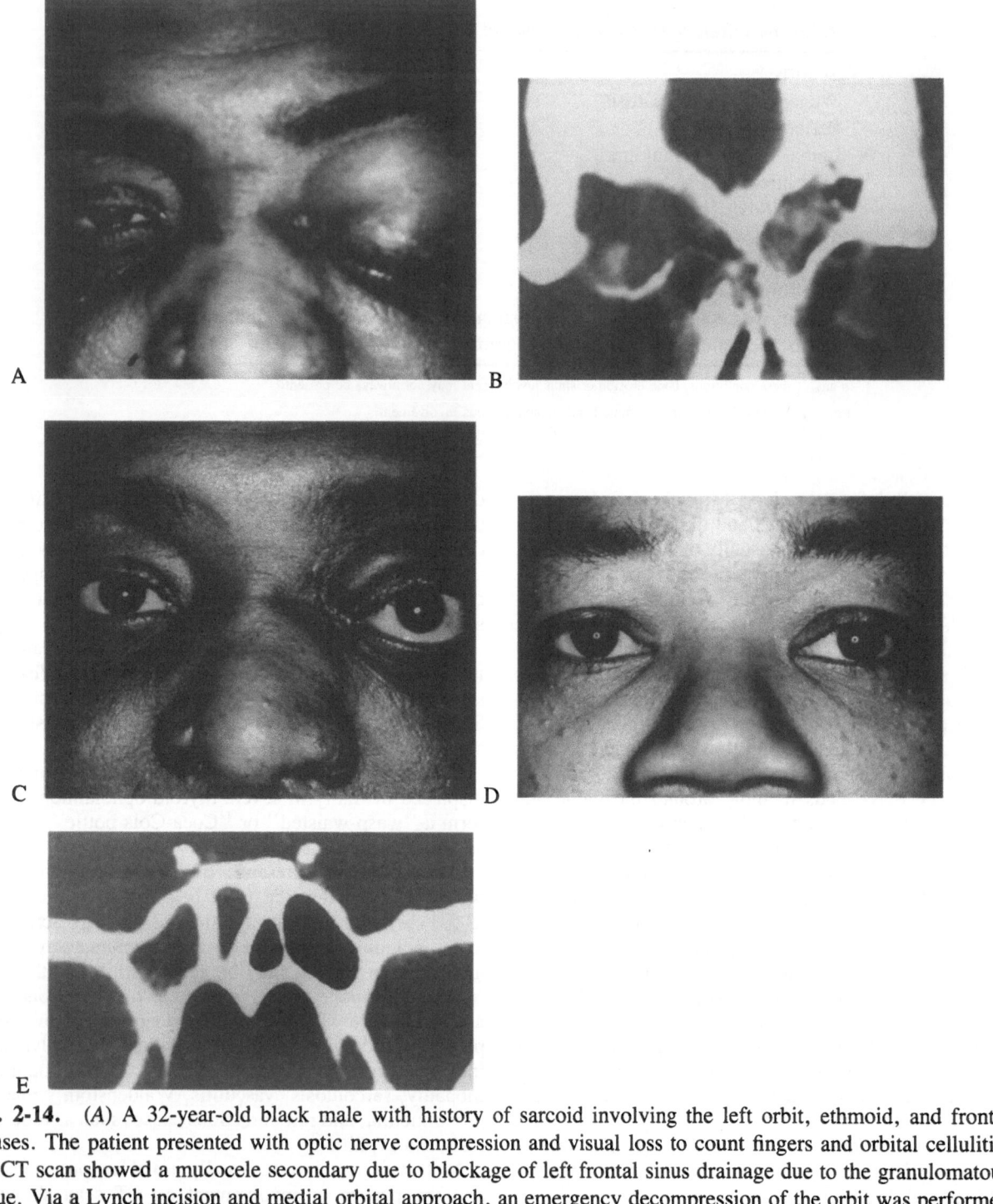

Fig. 2-14. (*A*) A 32-year-old black male with history of sarcoid involving the left orbit, ethmoid, and frontal sinuses. The patient presented with optic nerve compression and visual loss to count fingers and orbital cellulitis. (*B*) CT scan showed a mucocele secondary due to blockage of left frontal sinus drainage due to the granulomatous tissue. Via a Lynch incision and medial orbital approach, an emergency decompression of the orbit was performed with dramatic improvement of vision to the 20/30 level. (*C*) Definitive sinus surgery was performed 1 month later to allow drainage of the frontal sinus directly into the nose. (*D*) A 54-year-old female with proptosis of the right eye for 1 month with loss of vision to count fingers. (*E*) Orbital CT scan showed opacification of the right sphenoidal sinus. Biopsy of the sphenoid sinus showed granulation tissue and nonspecific chronic inflammatory cell. Cultures and special stains for microorganisms were negative. After a course of intravenous antibiotics, the patient responded dramatically to oral steroids. The patient later developed orbital myositis. Work-up for systemic vasculitis has been negative. (Patient referred by Dr. Lawrence Frohman, Newark, NJ.)

Table 2-5
Conditions Associated with EOM Enlargement*

Thyroid ophthalmopathy
Pseudotumor
Lymphoid infiltrate
Metastatic carcinoma

*Other rare causes include amyloid, acromegaly, collagen vascular disease, including systemic lupus erythematosis and dermatomyositis, and parasitic infections such as trichinosis and cysticercosis.

of bone metastasis. For this reason, bone metastases may be confused with meningioma of the greater wing of the sphenoid. Meningiomas have greater enhancement than metastases, and angiography shows middle meningeal artery supply to the meningioma. Other than metastatic disease and sphenoid ridge meningioma, myeloma should always be considered when bone erosion occurs in the orbit. A systemic work-up for myeloma is often diagnostic. In some cases, biopsy will be necessary.

A-V (carotid-cavernous) fistula usually involves all four muscles and shows enlargement of the superior ophthalmic vein and cavernous sinus on CT scan (Fig. 2-16). The diagnosis may be confirmed on arteriography in which rapid filling of the dilated superior ophthalmic vein with poor perfusion of the intracranial carotid artery branches is demonstrated. Other signs on ophthalmologic examination usually make this diagnosis apparent, including arterialization of the conjunctival and episcleral veins, presence of a bruit or thrill, and third or sixth nerve palsy.

Amyloidosis does not present clinically as an inflammatory process (Fig. 2-17). In general, lid involvement usually suggests systemic disease, while orbital and conjunctival amyloid suggests a localized process. Patients with amyloid of the lids, conjunctiva, or orbit should undergo a work-up for multiple myeloma including serum protein electrophoresis, urine for Bence Jones protein,

and possibly bone marrow examination. Patients with orbital involvement have external ophthalmoplegia. Pupillary abnormalities may also occur. On CT scan, calcifications are often present within the diffuse mass that infiltrates the lid or EOMs (Table 2-6).[29-30]

ULTRASOUND

The main advantage of orbital ultrasonography is that information can be obtained in the office quickly and economically. Its prime disadvantage is that the examiner must have considerable experience and skill with the technique. Both EOM enlargement and mass lesions can be detected by ultrasound, but bone erosion is difficult to determine. A mass with decreasing internal reflectivity suggests the presence of a cellular mass without vascular or cystic spaces and is most commonly due to bacterial cellulitis, pseudotumor, or a lymphoid infiltrate. A well-localized bacterial abscess is characterized by the presence of a focal, acoustically hollow area within a cellular mass that shows decreasing internal reflectivity. The characteristic "T sign" suggests the presence of a pseudotumor and is the ultrasonic counterpart of the thickened sclera and optic nerve on CT scan.[4,31]

INITIAL MANAGEMENT AND INDICATIONS FOR BIOPSY

On the basis of clinical presentation and CT findings, patients with orbital inflammation may be divided into four groups: group I—patients clinically suspected of having acute bacterial orbital cellulitis; group II—patients

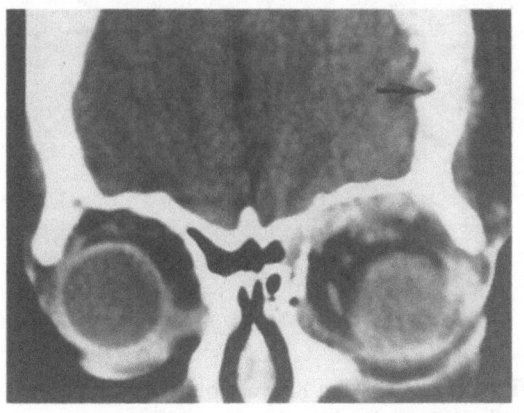
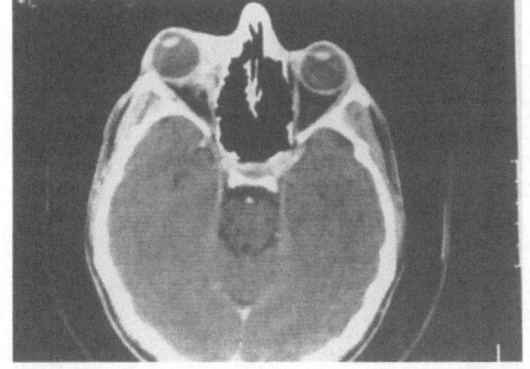

A   B

Fig. 2-15. (*A*) CT scan of patient who had undergone mastectomy for adenocarcinoma 6 years previously. Scan shows bone erosion and nonhomogeneous mass with irregular margins and granular appearance. (Patient referred by Dr. Walter Mazzanti, Roseland, NJ.) (*B*) CT scan from a 55-year-old male with granular nonhomogeneous infiltrate. Patient presented with painless, gradual proptosis. Biopsy showed metastatic carcinoma from the lung.

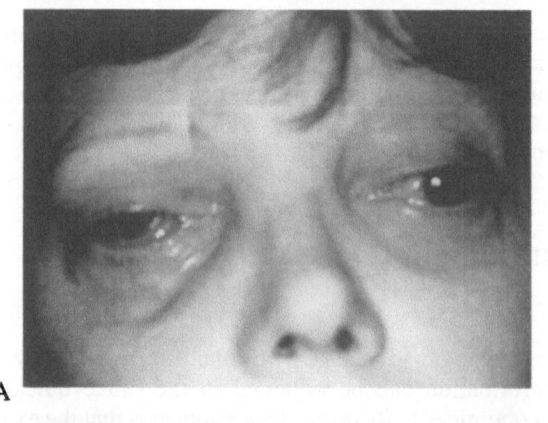

A

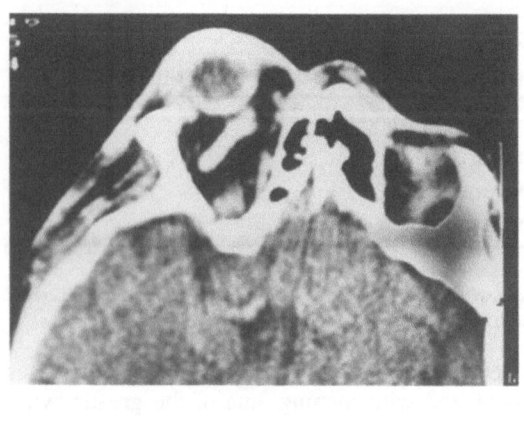

B

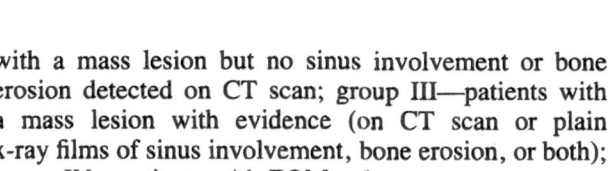

C

Fig. 2-16. (*A*) A 48-year-old female with history of head trauma secondary to a fall 2 years previously. (*B*) CT scan shows enlarged EOMs and markedly dilated superior ophthalmic vein on the right side characteristic of a carotid cavernous fistula. (*C*) Note improved proptosis and orbital congestion after closure of fistula with glue using balloon catheterization technique. (Patient referred by Dr. Louis Morrone, North Arlington, NJ.)

with a mass lesion but no sinus involvement or bone erosion detected on CT scan; group III—patients with a mass lesion with evidence (on CT scan or plain x-ray films of sinus involvement, bone erosion, or both); group IV—patients with EOM enlargement.

According to this protocol, patients who on clinical examination alone appear to have an acute bacterial orbital cellulitis (group I) should be treated before or during the diagnostic work-up (CT scan or ultrasound). Because

patients with CT findings in any of the four groups may have systemic disease, a careful history and systemic work-up are essential. Patients with Wegener's granulomatosis and periarteritis nodosa tend to have sinus and orbital involvement on CT scan.

Patients with suspected acute bacterial orbital cellulitis are hospitalized and an infectious disease consultation is obtained. Blood, throat, nose, and conjunctival cultures are taken and intravenous antibiotics that include cover-

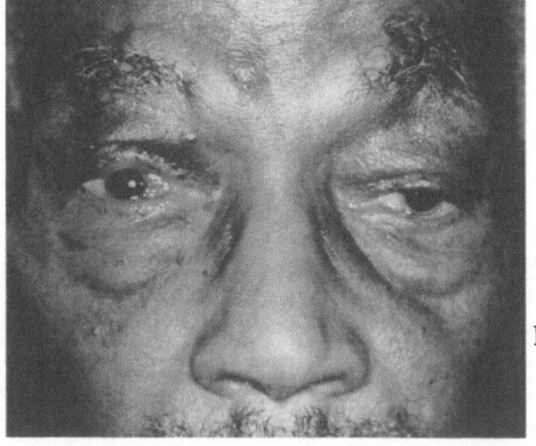

A

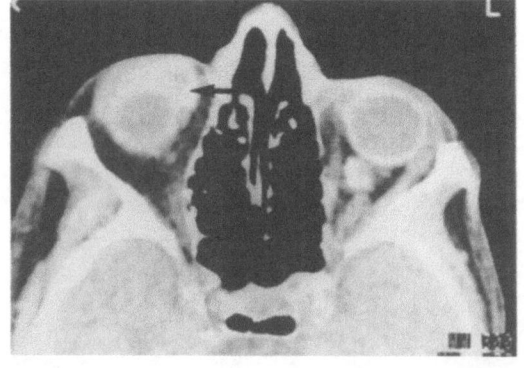

B

Fig. 2-17. (*A*) An 82-year-old male with amyloidosis of the lids and orbit with no conjunctival involvement. (*B*) CT scan shows diffuse homogeneous process with calcifications (arrow). (Patient referred by Dr. Robert Cunningham, East Orange, NJ.)

Table 2-6
Conditions Associated with Orbital Calcifications

Systemic disease
  Mönckeberg's sclerosis
  hyperparathyroidism
  hypervitaminosis D
  Paget's disease
Vascular lesions
  phlebolith
  venous angiomas
  cavernous hemangioma
  lymphangioma
  hemangiopericytoma
Fibroosseous tumors
  osteoma
  ossifying fibroma
  osteogenic sarcoma
Lacrimal fossa calcifications
  dermoid cyst
  dermolipoma
  plasmacytoma
  malignant and rarely benign epithelial lacrimal gland
    tumors
Other orbital tumors
  meningioma
  glioma
  schwannoma
Parasites
Foreign body
Amyloid
Intraocular calcifications
  retinoblastoma
  retinopathy of prematurity
  choroidal hemangioma
  phthisis bulbi
  optic nerve drusen
  choroidal osteoma
  senile hyaline plaque of sclera
  trisomy 13
  retinal angioma of von Hippel's disease
Edge of mucocele

age for *Staphylococcus aureus, Diplococcus pneumoniae, Streptococcus pyogenes,* and gram-negative organisms are administered. *Hemophilus influenzae* is a more common cause of acute cellulitis in children than in adults, especially in children under 36 months of age because of their lack of a *H. influenzae* anticapsular antibody. Typically, patients with *H. influenzae* have a sharply demarcated purple discoloration on examination that is usually only present the first few days of the cellulitis. The illness is often severe at the onset and the child is usually symptomatic for less than 24 hours

prior to admission to the hospital. A high fever, elevated white count, and positive blood culture are usually present with *H. influenzae*.

In all cases of orbital cellulitis, meningitis-level doses of antibiotics are recommended. Antibiotic coverage is adjusted based on culture results.

Unfortunately, in some patients with orbital cellulitis a drop in vision may be precipitous and despite heroic measures described above, the process may be irreversible. The intraocular pressure must be monitored in all patients, especially those that present with decreased vision. Harris reported a patient who presented with arterial pulsations and an amaurotic pupil.[32] A subperiosteal abscess had formed. There are several possible mechanisms of loss of vision in these patients: (1) external compression on the globe and optic nerve, (2) increased intraorbital pressure, (3) elongation and stretching of the optic nerve that leads to ischemia, and (4) septic emboli and optic neuritis.

In any patient who shows only partial resolution of an orbital cellulitis, orbital or subperiosteal abscess should be suspected and may be diagnosed on repeat ultrasound or CT scan.[33] Such patients may require biopsy and surgical drainage with intraoperative insertion of a drain that is advanced a few centimeters a day postoperatively until drainage cases. An ear, nose, and throat surgeon may also need to drain the paranasal sinuses in patients who do not respond to maximal medical therapy. In patients who show progression of neurologic signs or involvement of the other eye, cavernous sinus thrombosis must be considered. In addition, any patient with persistent inflammation, abscess, fistula formation, or chronic osteomyelitis should be suspected of a retained foreign body. In a case report, a 12-year-old white female had a chronic 8-year course that resulted in osteomyelitis due to a retained wood foreign body from when she had fallen off a horse into a tree branch.[34] We often administer a trial of intravenous antibiotics to patients in group II (patients with a mass lesion without evidence of sinus involvement) in whom a clinical diagnosis of bacterial orbital cellulitis is suspected (Fig. 2-10). In most cases, however, the suspected diagnosis is pseudotumor. The absence of pain is helpful in distinguishing a lymphoid infiltrate from orbital cellulitis, which is almost always painful. Unless the history and clinical findings are absolutely classic for pseudotumor, a confirmatory biopsy might be appropriate before instituting a trial of steroids for patients in group II.

Low-dose radiation (1500 rad) is an acceptable alternative to steroids for those elderly patients who cannot tolerate steroids. Because of the long-term complications of radiation, including secondary tumors, cataracts, and dry eyes, radiation might be reserved for such elderly patients.

Virtually all patients with EOM enlargement and an orbital mass have a lymphoid infiltrate; pseudotumor as defined in this text is much less likely. The absence of clinical features typical of pseudotumor including sudden onset of pain would also favor the diagnosis of a lymphoid infiltrate. A metastatic cancer may have a similar orbital CT scan presentation.

Group III patients have inflammatory orbital disease and radiographic evidence of sinus or bone erosion. Patients with sinus involvement are treated with antibiotics, which are effective against bacteria that are found in both the sinus and the orbit. Infectious disease consultation is recommended. Patients who do not respond to trial of the appropriate antibiotics should receive an internal medicine consultation to rule out Wegener's granulomatosis, lethal midline granuloma and periarteritis nodosa (PA). Mucormycosis should also be considered in the appropriate clinical setting. Rarely, pseudotumor of the orbit and an adjacent sinus has been reported.[17]

The presence of sinus and orbit involvement with bone erosion also suggests the possibility of a malignant tumor. Classically, unifocal eosinophilic granuloma causes clearly punched-out lesions of the frontal bones without sclerosis. Typically, multifocal eosinophilic granuloma does not present in the orbit.

Certain points are helpful in the clinical differential diagnosis of Wegener's granulomatosis, lethal midline granuloma, and periarteritis nodosa (PAN). Patients with Wegener's granulomatosis with orbital involvement tend to have concomitant sinus involvement.[35–38] In its limited form, Wegener's granulomatosis affects the lung and spares the kidney. In its systemic form, death results from renal failure. Chronic low-dose cyclophosphamide (Cytoxan), an antimetabolite, and steroids or a combination of these may be life-saving.

Idiopathic midline destructive disease (formerly termed *lethal midline granuloma*) is a local disease. Like Wegener's, it characteristically involves the sinuses, but unlike Wegener's, it may cause erosion through the palate or through the sinus and skin of the face. Even with radiation, the treatment of choice, this disease is uniformly fatal due to inanition and secondary infection. As in Wegener's granulomatosis, orbital involvement in periarteritis nodosa may be accompanied by adjacent sinus involvement. Periarteritis nodosa is a systemic vasculitis that tends to involve the kidney. Skin lesions may be striking. Unlike Wegener's granulomatosis, periarteritis nodosa tends to spare the lung. Systemic steroids are the treatment of choice. In Wegener's, lethal midline granuloma, and periarteritis, both biopsy and clinical findings are necessary for diagnosis and treatment.

Group IV consists of patients with EOM enlargement. If the chemical work-up for thyroid disease, including a TRH infusion test, is negative, a trial of steroids, 80–120 mg by mouth for at least 5 days, may be warranted. In most patients with pseudotumor, the response to steroids within the 5-day period is shown by improved vision on color-plate testing and decreased exophthalmos and orbital congestion. Thyroid patients usually take longer to respond. The management of compressive thyroid ophthalmopathy will be discussed in Chapter 5. Patients with suspected pseudotumor who respond to

steroids should be maintained on high-dose steroids for 1–2 weeks and the dosage should be tapered 10 mg each week.[1]

Children with idiopathic orbital myositis typically respond to oral steroids, but this condition is subject to recurrence. Patients not responding to treatment may require biopsy. Some patients may show a combination of features and require individual management according to the basic principles we have outlined (Fig. 2-8).

BIOPSY AND MANAGEMENT

Assuming there has been an adequate trial of systemic antibiotics, diagnostic orbital biopsy may be appropriate. Where there is sinus involvement, a Caldwell-Luc or other ear, nose, and throat (ENT) surgical approach may be more desirable than exploration of an inflamed orbit. The management of patients with acute bacterial orbital cellulitis was considered above in the discussion of group I. The various possible biopsy results and management of the other three groups are outlined below.

Possible Biopsy Results for Group II Patients

A general note about the pathology of lymphoid infiltrates and pseudotumor is necessary before considering specific biopsy findings. Lymphoid infiltrates are characterized by diffuse sheets of cells that are predominantly lymphocytes. The morphologic features of the infiltrate and the individual cells determine whether the infiltrate is classified by the pathologist as a benign reactive lym-

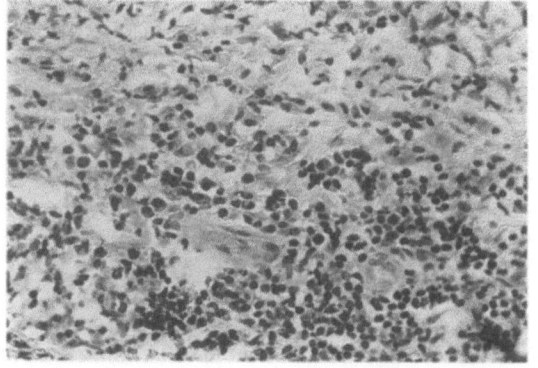

Fig. 2-18. Biopsy shows mixed inflammatory cell infiltrate consisting mainly of lymphocytes and some plasma cells. Fibrous tissue between inflammatory cells favors diagnosis of pseudotumor over lymphoid infiltrate, which is characterized classically by sheets of cells without fibrosis. Diagnosis cannot be rendered on basis of this field alone.

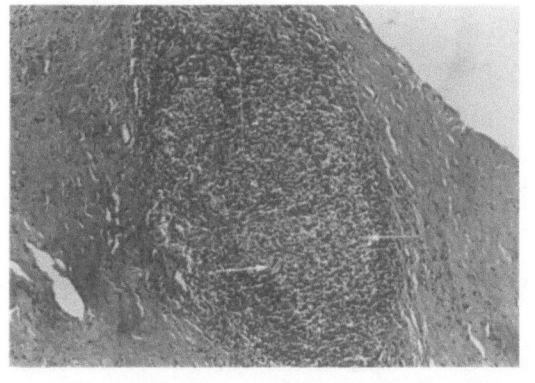
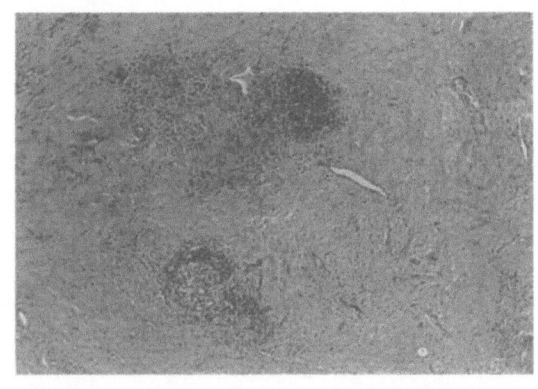

A   B

Fig. 2-19. (*A*) Biopsy shows background of sclerosis with lymphoid follicle present in field. (*B*) A pale germinal center (arrows) is present. Presence of follicles favors diagnosis of lymphoid infiltrate (benign reactive) over sclerosing pseudotumor.

phoid hyperplasia, atypical reactive lymphoid hyperplasia, or a malignant lymphoma.

Pseudotumor is by definition an "idiopathic" inflammation in that no identifiable systemic or local cause is found.[3] Therefore, noncaseating granuloma in the lid or orbit that is accompanied by other systemic findings of sarcoid that fulfill the diagnostic criteria for the diagnosis of sarcoid would not be classified a "pseudotumor." Similarly, a ruptured dermoid cyst that incites inflammation is not a pseudotumor. However, noncaseating granuloma without other signs of systemic disease such as sarcoid would be diagnostic of pseudotumor and not a lymphoid infiltrate. Similarly, a vasculitis in the orbit without other stigmata of a known systemic vasculitis would favor the diagnosis of pseudotumor and not lymphoid infiltrate for two reasons: (1) there is no known local or systemic identifiable cause, and (2) the nature of the pathologic component is consistent with pseudotumor and not lymphoid infiltrate.

As pseudotumor becomes chronic, there will be a sclerosing or fibrosing component. In fact, while the presence of follicles with germinal centers favors the diagnosis of a lymphoid infiltrate over pseudotumor, concomitant fibrosis strongly favors the diagnosis of pseudotumor. The fibrosis is responsible for the streak densities seen on CT scan. In cases of lymphoid infiltrates, germinal centers strongly favor a benign reactive lymphoid hyperplasia over an atypical or malignant infiltrate. The prognosis of a pseudotumor is quite different from a lymphoid infiltrate in that systemic lymphoma may develop in the latter while lymphoma does not develop in patients with pseudotumor. Pseudotumor, in general, does not lead to permanent sequellae; however, in a small percentage of patients, a frozen sclerosed globe will result.

Case Study 1. Biopsy shows chronic nongranulomatous inflammation (Fig. 2-18). Because this biopsy is nonspecific, such patients should be followed clinically and reevaluated with the subsequent possible diagnoses in mind: (1) pseudotumor or lymphoid infiltrate, (2) re-

tained foreign body, (3) ectopic lacrimal gland tissue, and (4) underlying orbital tumor. Depending on the clinical findings, a working diagnosis of pseudotumor is appropriate and a steroid trial may be warranted. The ophthalmologists should suspect an underlying orbital tumor if the inflammatory condition persists. Follow-up CT scans are recommended. It is appropriate to request that the pathologist cut deeper sections from the block when follow-up clinical data or later CT scans suggest one of the above four conditions.

Case Study 2. Biopsy shows reactive lymphoid hyperplasia with follicles containing germinal centers (Fig. 2-19). All such patients should have a systemic oncologic work-up for lymphoma. Steroids or low-dose radiation of 1500–2000 rad over 10 days are possible therapeutic alternatives. All patients should be followed because a small percentage of patients in this group may develop fatal systemic lymphoma at a later time.[7]

In patients with a classic pseudotumor presentation both clinically and on CT scan, including inflammation involving tenons capsule and scleral *sclerotenonitis*, diffuse streaking inflammation anterior to the equator, or thickening of the EOMs with irregular edges, biopsy is not necessary and is not recommended because it will only worsen the inflammation. Only in those patients who do not respond to steroids should biopsy be performed. Patients with presumed pseudotumor who respond to a trial of steroids should have the steroids tapered 5–10 mg per week. If there is recurrence of disease, the previous dose at which response was attained should be reinstituted and tapering should be done at a slower level, perhaps 2.5 mg per week.

In patients who do not respond to steroids, a biopsy should be performed. If the diagnosis of pseudotumor is confirmed, the alternatives include (1) high-dose oral prednisone, 150 mg, or (2) trial of intravenous steroid (4 mg dexamethasone) IV every 4 hours until there is a clinical response followed by oral prednisone. Patients unresponsive to steroids may be candidates for radiation.

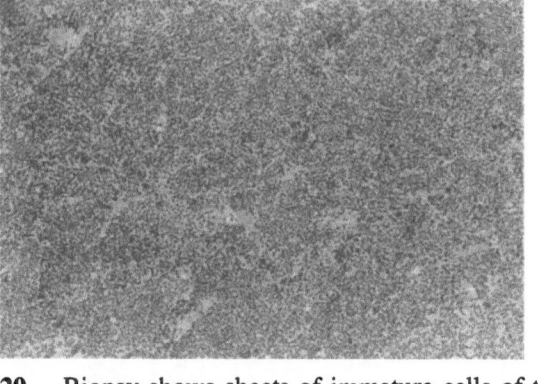
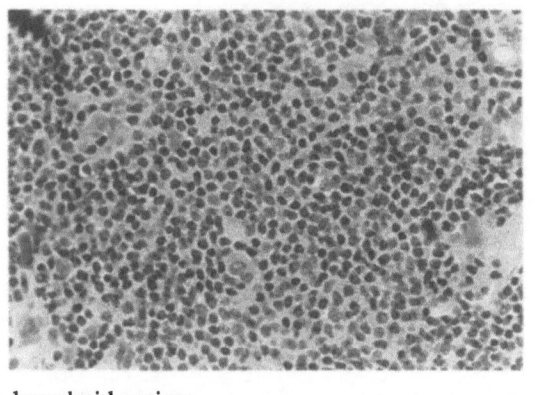

Fig. 2-20. Biopsy shows sheets of immature cells of the lymphoid series.

A sufficient dose may be 1000 rad. In some cases, 3000 rad in fractional doses may be necessary.[39–41] In one series, a patient received 4300 rad and developed a frozen globe with count-fingers vision. Clearly, some patients will have this result no matter what treatment protocol is adopted. Long-term cyclophosphamide, 200 mg/day, may be necessary in some patients refractory to steroids and radiation. Such patients must be followed by a hematologist for adverse effects to the hemopoetic system with periodic blood counts, platelet counts, and observation for hematuria and melena.

Recently, intralesional corticosteroids for inflammatory lesions of the orbit have been proposed for use in patients with orbital pseudotumor and sarcoid who have significant side effects from systemic corticosteroids and in patients in whom radiation therapy is contraindicated. In a case report of a 13-year-old girl with sarcoidosis who had repeated exacerbations in the lacrimal gland area after withdrawal of systemic steroids, a mixture of 40 mg triamcinolone and 6 mg betamethasone was injected into the lacrimal glands. There was a dramatic response within three days.[42]

Case Study 3. Biopsy shows atypical reactive lymphoid hyperplasia (ARLH). A larger percentage of patients with atypical RLH develop systemic lymphoma than do those with RLH.[7] Immunoperoxidase staining of the paraffin sections may help the pathologist differentiate typical RLH from a well-differentiated lymphoma. Concomitant choroidal involvement should always be considered.[43]

Case Study 4. Biopsy shows malignant lymphoma (Fig. 2-20). The Rappaport modified classification has been often used by ophthalmic pathologists (Table 2-7).[44] The pattern is diffuse or nodular. Histologically, a lymphoma is diagnosed on the basis of cytologic atypia. Immature cells are characterized as round (noncleaved) or indented nuclei. In general small cells are less mitotically active and less malignant than large-cleaved or noncleaved cells.

Again, these patients should be examined by an oncologist to rule out systemic disease. If there is no evidence of systemic disease, radiotherapy (approximately 3500 rad) and oncologic follow-up are recommended. If systemic disease is present, local radiotherapy and chemotherapy are appropriate. If malignant lymphoma is diagnosed in a child, the ophthalmologist should alert the pathologist to the possibility of granulocytic sarcoma. Orbital lymphoma is very uncommon in children. Burkitt's lymphoma is extremely rare in the United States, and Hodgkin's disease rarely involves the orbit except in its late stages.[45,46] Burkitt's lymphoma is always a systemic disease and is characterized by a blastic proliferation of immature lymphocytes with interspersed pale-staining histiocytes that provide a low-power microscopic "starry sky" appearance. Zimmerman and Font described 33 patients with granulocytic sarcoma, a form of leukemia.[47] The Leder stain for cytoplasmic granules of esterase is diagnostic. A pediatric oncologist should be consulted.

Case Study 5. Biopsy shows a well-differentiated lymphocytic lymphoma in an adult. Again, a systemic oncologic work-up is recommended. A hematologist should be consulted to rule out chronic lymphocytic leukemia that may be pathologically confused with a lymphoma. (Reprinted with permission from Mauriello JA, Flanagan, JC: Recommended protocol for management of orbital inflammatory disease. *Surv Ophthalmol* 29:104–116, 1984.)

Case Study 6. Biopsy shows a lymphoplasmacytic infiltrate with PAS-positive intranuclear inclusions of immunoglobulins (Dutcher bodies) (Fig. 2-21). An oncologist or hematologist should be consulted to rule out an immunoglobulin-producing tumor such as multiple myeloma, Waldenström's macroglobulinemia, or a lymphoplasmacytic lymphoma. Amyloid may rarely be found in the orbital lesions associated with myeloma. A methyl green pyronine stain for cytoplasmic RNA characteristically found in plasma cells may be helpful in distinguishing a poorly differentiated myeloma from an undifferentiated carcinoma.

In patients with a lymphoplasmacytic infiltrate, a serum protein electrophoresis, bone marrow biopsy, and CT

Table 2-7
Non-Hodgkin's Lymphoma: International Formulation (Modified Rappaport Classification)

Low-Grade
    small lymphocytic (well-differentiated lymphocytic)
      with/without chronic lymphocytic leukemia
      with/without plasmacytoid features
    follicular, small-cleaved cell (nodular, poorly differentiated
      lymphocytic)
    follicular, mixed small-cleaved and large-cell
Intermediate-Grade
    follicular large cell
    diffuse, small-cleaved cell
    diffuse, mixed small- and large-cell
    diffuse, large-cell
High-Grade
    immunoblastic-plasmacytoid, clear-cell, polymorphous types
    lymphoblastic-convoluted and nonconvoluted cell types
    small noncleaved-cell Burkitt's
Miscellaneous
    mycosis fungoides
    hairy-cell leukemia
    malignant histiocytosis
    unclassified

scan of the abdomen is indicated. In patients with a malignant plasma cell tumor, multiple myeloma should be ruled out and a skeletal survey should also be preformed. A localized extramedullary plasmacytoma, a malignant tumor, cannot be distinguished from well-differentiated multiple myeloma on histologic or immunohistologic grounds alone. An orbital plasmacytoma is

treated with radiotherapy. Persistent or recurrent local orbital tumors or systemic involvement may require chemotherapy.

Immunoperoxidase staining for monoclonal or polyclonal patterns is somewhat disappointing in predicting patients who will develop systemic disease. Polyclonality

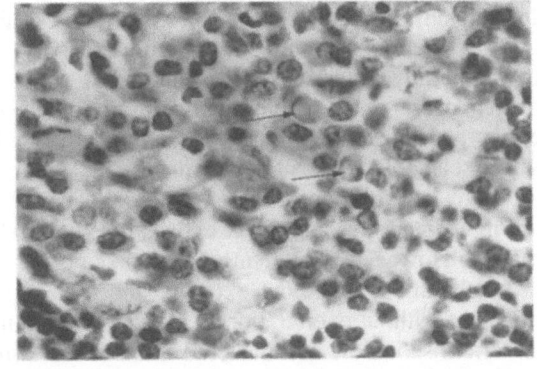

Fig. 2-21. Biopsy shows lymphoplasmacytic cell infiltrate with PAS-positive intranuclear inclusions (arrows). (Reprinted with permission from Mauriello JA, Flanagan, JC: Recommended protocol for management of orbital inflammatory disease. *Surv Ophthalmol* 29:104–116, 1984.)

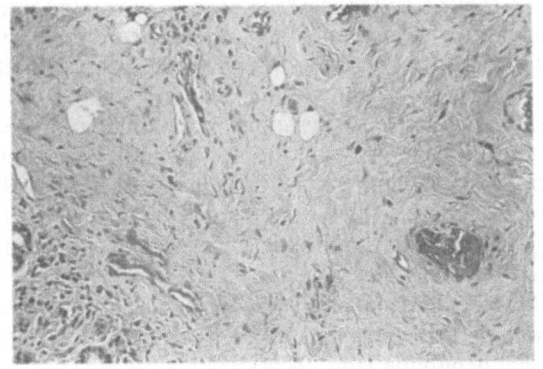

Fig. 2-22. Biopsy shows inflammatory cells in the orbital fat with resultant fat necrosis and a lipogranulomatous reaction with foreign body giant cells (arrows). (Reprinted with permission from Mauriello JA, Flanagan, JC: Recommended protocol for management of orbital inflammatory disease. *Surv Ophthalmol* 29:104–116, 1984.)

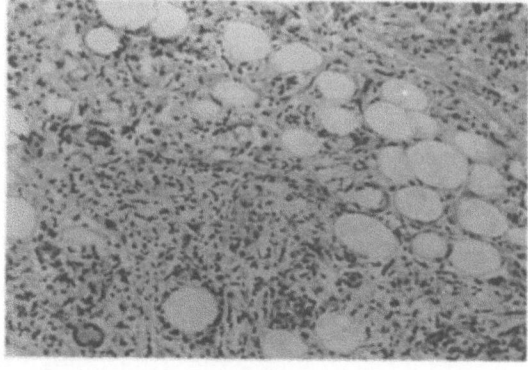

Fig. 2-23. Biopsy shows sclerosing pseudotumor. Note minimal number of inflammatory cells.

is generally associated with benignity, and monclonality with malignancy. For example, 11 specimens from patients with uveal lymphoplasmacytic infiltrates were all found to have a monoclonal-staining pattern and yet only two patients developed systemic disease.[48,49]

Case Study 7. Biopsy shows chronic sclerosing lipogranulomatous inflammation (Fig. 2-22). Any cause of fat necrosis in the orbit results in a lipogranulomatous inflammation. The differential diagnosis includes ectopic lacrimal gland, ruptured dermoid cyst, sclerosing hemangioma, trauma, retained foreign body, and Weber-Christian disease. The pathologist should be alerted to cut deep sections to look for hair follicles and keratin in the case of a ruptured dermoid cyst (Fig. 2-23). A dermoid cyst with or without rupture commonly causes bone erosion in the lacrimal gland fossa. Fat necrosis may also simply be the result of inflammation that accompanies a pseudotumor or lymphoid infiltrate. Sclerosing pseudotumors may be associated with systemic fibrosclerosis particularly in the retroperitoneal area.[50–51]

Regardless of the cause of the lipogranulomatous reaction, a trial of systemic prednisone is warranted unless the underlying cause such as a retained foreign body is treated. Most importantly, foreign body giant cells adjacent to fat (as a result of fat necrosis) should not be considered a sign of systemic granulomatous disease whereby a systemic work-up for sarcoid, Wegener's, tuberculosis, and other conditions is instituted. The slide should be polarized by the pathologist to rule out a foreign body, and special stains for acid-fast organisms and fungi should be obtained.

Chronic sclerosing pseudotumors are usually refractory to steroids and will only respond partially, if at all, to surgical debulking (Fig. 2-24).

Possible Biopsy Results for Group III Patients

The following biopsy results may be found in group III patients.

Case Study 8. Biopsy shows necrotizing granulomas involving the small blood vessels (Fig. 2-25). This biopsy suggests Wegener's granulomatosis. Internal medicine consultation may be obtained to determine whether the kidneys or lungs are involved. Chronic low-dose cyclophosphamide, systemic steroids, or a combination may be life-saving. Wegener's granulomatosis may also affect children. All patients require follow-up systemic evaluation, even if the disease is initially limited to the orbit.

Case Study 9. Biopsy shows lymphocytes and granulation tissue. Focal granulomatous vasculitis associated with fibrinoid necrosis may be present as well as central facial lymphomas, the latter having been referred to as polymorphic reticulosis or lymphomatoid granulomatosis. If the patient has other clinical findings consistent with the diagnosis of idiopathic midline destructive disease (polymorphic recitulosis, lethal midline granuloma) including erosion of the face and palate, the biopsy result strongly supports the clinical diagnosis. Other diseases that produce destruction of the central face include chronic syphilis, tuberculosis, blastomycosis, histoplasmosis, and coccidioidomycosis. Systemic oncologic work-up is appropriate since patients may develop systemic lymphoma.[50] Local radiation of approximately 5000 rad, is presently the treatment of choice.

Case Study 10. Biopsy shows vasculitis with fibrinoid necrosis of the small- and medium-sized muscular arteries. This biopsy suggests periarteritis nodosa. Consultation from an internist for possible systemic steroid therapy is appropriate.

Case Study 11. Biopsy shows thrombosis of orbital vessels with secondary ischemic necrosis. Large, nonseptate hyphae are present. This biopsy in a diabetic or immunosuppressed patient is consistent with the rhinoorbitocerebral syndrome or mucormycosis. Although the infection may originate in the palate or nose, multiple sinuses are often involved.

Mucormycosis may be cured by radical surgery that includes exenteration combined with sinus surgery and antibiotic therapy. Infectious disease and ENT consultations are necessary. When ischemic infarction of the optic nerve occurs due to the organism's affinity for blood vessels, vision is markedly decreased. In these cases, there is extensive necrosis, and radical surgery including exenteration and sinus extirpation is a viable alternative. However, in patients with good vision and intense inflammation without extensive necrosis, local debridement without exerteration is indicated. Systemic amphotericin should be administered in all cases. Since infarction of the blood vessels hampers delivery of the drug, local daily amphotericin packs including the orbit and sinuses may be effectively combined with surgical management.[52]

Case Study 12. Biopsy shows chronic granulomatous inflammation. Special stains show branching hyphae with

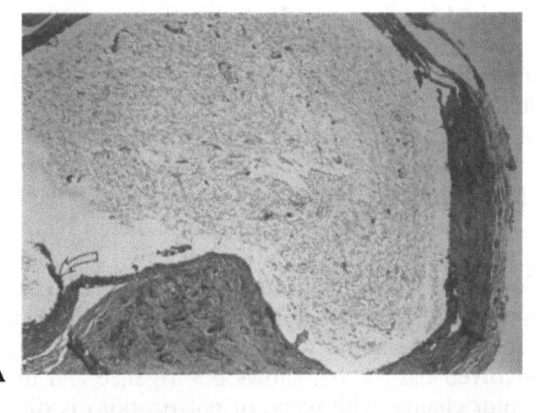

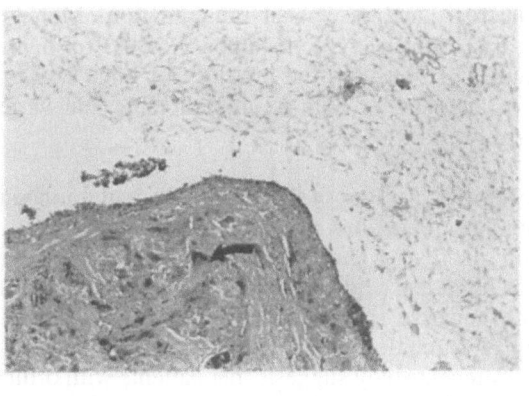

A   B

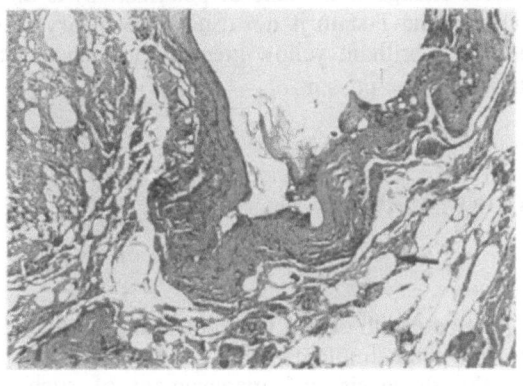

C

Fig. 2-24. (*A*) Biopsy shows dermoid cyst lined by stratified squamous keratinizing epithelium. (*B*) Cyst wall shows granulomatous reaction to keratin secondary to rupture of cyst. (*C*) Note fibrosis in surrounding orbital fat. (Reprinted with permission from Mauriello JA, Flanagan JC: Recommended protocol for management of orbital inflammatory disease. *Surv Ophthalmol* 29:104–116, 1984.)

septation. The biopsy result suggests the *Aspergillus* organism, although cultures are absolutely diagnostic. The fungus *Aspergillus* often starts as a sinus infection and involves the orbit secondarily. In some cases, the orbit alone may be involved. Infectious disease consultation is suggested, although surgical drainage alone may be curative.

Fig. 2-25. Biopsy shows chronic granulomatous inflammation with giant cell reaction. The inflammation involves the small blood vessels. Biopsy is consistent with Wegener's granulomatosis. (Reprinted with permission from Mauriello JA, Flanagan JC: Recommended protocol for management of orbital inflammatory disease. *Surv Ophthalmol* 29:104–116, 1984.)

Case Study 13. Biopsy shows eosinophils and bland typical histiocytes. Birbeck's and Langerhans' granules are present in the cytoplasm of the histiocytes on electron microscopy. This biopsy is consistent with eosinophilic granuloma, especially in a child. The disease does not involve the sinuses but typically causes solitary or multiple cystic defects of bone superotemporally in the orbit. Work-up for evidence of a histiocytic disorder includes a skeletal survey that is more sensitive than a bone scan. Chest x-ray, dental evaluation, and liver function tests should be performed. The prognosis for localized or unifocal eosinophilic granuloma is excellent with greater than 90 percent survival. Management includes biopsy with surgical curettage. Radiation may be necessary in persistent cases. Spontaneous healing with incisional biopsy alone has been reported.[53] Rarely, systemic steroids may be helpful.[3]

Besides eosinophilic granuloma, the pathologic differential diagnosis of an orbital lesion in a child with eosinophils should include granulocytic sarcoma, fungal and parasitic diseases, and pseudotumor. The Leder stain is helpful in demonstrating granules in the malignant cells that accompany the eosinophils. Special stains will help rule out fungal and parasitic diseases. Pseudotumor in children may have eosinophils but also has lymphocytes and fibroblasts rather than histiocytes and clinically does not show bone erosion.

Case Study 14. Any primary or metastatic malignant orbital tumor may cause bone erosion if there is sufficient tumor necrosis and associated inflammation. Management is based on the type of tumor. For the following case studies, 15 and 16, the presence of bone erosion, sinus involvement, or both is unpredictable and varies from case to case.

Case Study 15. Biopsy shows chronic granulomatous inflammation. Tubercles are present that show central caseation necrosis. The pathologist performs special stains for fungi and acid-fast bacilli. Noncaseating tubercles with negative special stains for fungi suggest the work-up of sarcoid. On CT stain, bone erosion is not present. A recent study suggests that patients with orbital sarcoid will often be found to have evidence of systemic sarcoidosis.[54] Therefore, an internal medicine consultation for appropriate treatment of the underlying disease is warranted.

Case Study 16. Biopsy shows chronic granulomatous inflammation with prominent eosinophils. Bone erosion may not be present on radiographic studies of the orbit. The pathologist should examine all tissues at multiple levels to search for a possible parasites. Parasites in the orbit are most likely a hydatid cyst due to *Echinococcus granulosus* and cysticercus due to *Taenia solium*. Other parasites include microfilaria, *Ascaris*, and *Schistosoma*. Treatment depends on the organism.

Case Study 17. Biopsy shows chronic sclerosing lipogranulomatous inflammation. Refer to biopsy for group II, Case Study 7.

POSSIBLE BIOPSY RESULTS FOR GROUP IV PATIENTS

In our experience, group IV patients rarely come to biopsy because their disease process responds to a therapeutic trial of steroids. Occasionally metastatic carcinoma causes thickening of one or more EOMs, and biopsy is

required for diagnosis. In such patients, oncologic work-up is necessary; local radiotherapy is combined with appropriate chemotherapy. Patients with suspected amyloidosis of the orbital tissues should be biopsied. Biopsy shows pale, eosinophilic homogeneous hyaline material subepithelial and typically surrounding blood vessels (Fig. 2-26). The lumen and endothelium of the involved blood vessels is typically intact. Scattered lymphocytes, plasma cells, foreign body giant cells, and, less often, eosinophils and calcification may be present. Metachromasia with crystal violet is classic, but this stain may fade in old paraffin sections. Congo-red staining of the involved tissues that shows birefrigence and dichroism (color change with plane of polarization) is diagnostic. Thioflavine T-stain is not usually necessary. This stain shows a brilliant yellow-green fluorescence. Calcifications may be present.

CONCLUSION

Patients with orbital inflammation present a challenge to the ophthalmologist. Our protocol has been helpful in the diagnosis and management of such patients. Ophthalmologists must initially be convinced that they are not dealing with a life-threatening bacterial orbital cellulitis. If bacterial orbital cellulitis cannot be ruled out, a trial of intravenous antibiotics should be administered. Concurrently, a general medical examination is helpful in determining possible systemic disease. CT scanning helps to determine whether bone changes, sinus disease, or both are present (Table 2-8). The most common causes of a mass lesion in the orbit without bone erosion or sinus involvement include pseudotumor, lymphoid infiltrate, or underlying tumor with inflammation. Such conditions probably warrant a biopsy before instituting steroid therapy unless the clinical presentation is absolutely classic for pseudotumor. Patients with pre-

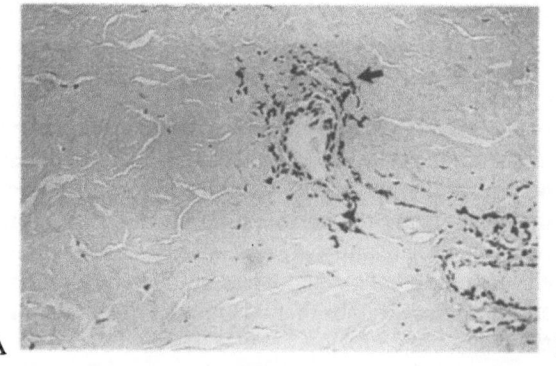
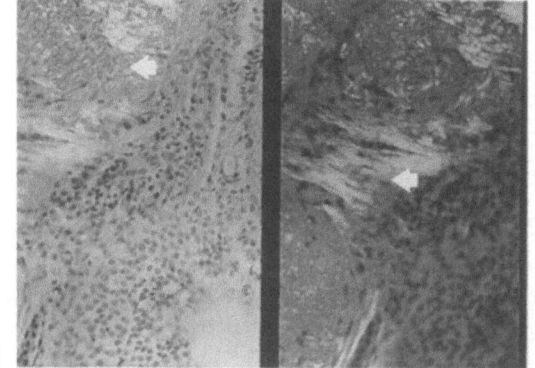

Fig. 2-26. (*A*) Biopsy shows pale eosinophilic homogeneous material that is dichroic and birefringent (*B*, arrows) and stains with congo-red stain (AFIP ACC #1404851).

Table 2-8
Summary of Differential Diagnosis and Management of Orbital Inflammatory Disease

Group I (Patient appears toxic with signs of acute inflammation)

Rule out acute bacterial orbital cellulitis

Immediate admission blood cultures, and intravenous antibiotics, infectious disease consult

Rule out sinusitis, retained orbital foreign body, and history of dental abscess

Concurrent with treatment, obtain orbital CT scan and medical consult to rule out systemic disease

If minimal response to antibiotics, rule out intraorbital or subperiosteal abscess that may require surgical drainage

Group II (CT scan shows mass lesion without bone erosion or sinus involvement)

Rule out pseudotumor

Biopsy to rule out the following conditions and refer to appropriate specialist: (1) pseudotumor, (2) lymphoid infiltrate, or leukemia, (3) local causes of inflammation, orbital hemorrhage, ectopic lacrimal gland, retained foreign body, sclerosing hemangioma

Group III (CT scan shows orbital sinus involvement or bone erosion)

Trial of antibiotics and if no response, biopsy to rule out the following conditions: (1) vasculitis, including Wegener's granulomatosis, periarteritis nodosa, and lethal midline granuloma; (2) fungal including *Aspergillosis* and mucormycosis infections; (3) infected mucocele, which usually responds to antibiotics, surgical drainage, and curettage; (4) primary or secondary orbital malignancies associated with inflammation; (5) eosinophilic granuloma; and (6) ruptured dermoid cyst.

Group IV (CT scan shows enlarged EOMs)

Rule out the following conditions: (1) thyroid disease (obtain chemical work-up including TRH infusion test), (2) pseudotumor (idiopathic myositis) (perform steroid trial), (3) A-V fistula (obtain neurosurgical consultation), and (4) metastatic carcinoma (obtain oncology consultation and prescribe possible local radiation)

---

sumed bacterial orbital cellulitis who do not respond to antibiotics and who have sinus involvement or bone erosion on CT scan may have a systemic vasculitis such as Wegener's granulomatosis, periarteritis nodosa, lethal midline granuloma, or a malignant tumor.

EOM enlargement on CT scan is most commonly found in thyroid ophthalmopathy and pseudotumor (idiopathic myositis), although metastatic carcinomas and AV fistula have to be considered. EOM enlargement along with the presence of a mass lesion strongly suggests the diagnosis of pseudotumor. An incisional biopsy, however, is probably warranted before systemic steroids or local radiation are instituted. The various biopsy results lead to refinement of the differential diagnosis and appropriate management.

REFERENCES

1. Mauriello JA, Flanagan JC: Management of orbital inflammatory disease. *Surv Ophthalmol* 29:104–116, 1984.

2. Jakobiec FA, Jones IS: Orbital Inflammations, in Duane TD, Jaeger EA (eds): *Clinical Ophthalmology*, vol 2. Philadelphia: Harper and Row, 1982, pp 1–75.

3. Jakobiec FA, Font RL: Orbit, in Spencer WH (ed): *Ophthalmic Pathology: An Atlas and Textbook*, vol 3. Philadelphia: WB Saunders, 1986, pp 2459–2860.

4. Keeney AH, Hafner JN: Ultrasonic evidence of inflammatory thickening and fluid collection within the retrobulbar fascia: The T sign. *Ann Ophthalmol* 9:1557–1563.

5. Frohman LP, Kupersmith MJ, Lang J: Intracranial extension and bone destruction in orbital pseudotumor. *Arch Ophthalmol* 104:380–384, 1986.

6. Rosenbery SA, Diamond HD, Jaslowitz B, Craver LF: Lymphosarcoma: A review of 1269 cases. *Medicine* 40:41–84, 1961.

7. Jakobiec FA, McLean I, Font R: Clinicopathologic characteristics of orbital lymphoid hyperplasia. *Ophthalmology* 86:948–966, 1979.

8. Sigelman J, Jakobiec FA: Lymphoid lesions of the conjunctiva: Relation of histopathology to clinical outcome. *Ophthalmology* 85:818–843, 1978.

9. Jakobiec FA, Gibralter RA, Knowles DM, Iwamoto T: Lymphoid tumor of the lid. *Ophthalmology* 87:1058–1064, 1980.

10. Mottow LS, Jakobiec FA: Idiopathic inflammatory orbital pseudotumor in childhood. *Arch Ophthalmol* 96:410–417, 1978.

11. Levine MR: Pseudotumor in 3 month old child. Paper presented at the Spring meeting, American Society of Ophthalmic Plastic and Reconstructive Surgery, 1984.

12. Uretsky SH, Kennerdell JS, Gutai J: Graves' ophthalmopathy in childhood and adolescence. *Arch Ophthalmol* 98:1963–1964, 1980.

13. Watters EC, Waller PH, Hiles DA, Michaels RA: Acute orbital cellulitis. *Arch Ophthalmol* 94:786–788, 1976.

14. Weiss IS: Pseudomonas orbital cellulitis. *Am J Ophthalmol* 87:368–370, 1975.

15. Londer L, Nelson DL: Orbital cellulitis due to *Hemophilus influenzae*. *Arch Ophthalmol* 91:89–91, 1974.

16. Jakobiec FA, Font RL: Noninfectious orbital inflammations, in Spencer WH (ed): *Ophthalmic Pathology: An Atlas and Textbook*. Philadelphia: WB Saunders, 1986, pp 2716–2725.

17. Esphagian J, Anderson RL: Sinus involvement in inflammatory orbital pseudotumor. *Arch Ophthalmol* 99:627–630, 1981.

18. Blodi FC: Orbital Pseudotumor mit Thrombozytopenic und Myasthenie. *Klin Monatsbl Augenheilkd* 170:397–400, 1977.

19. Jarret WH, Gutman FA: Ocular complications of infection in the paranasal sinuses. *Arch Ophthalmol* 81:683–688, 1969.

20. Haynes BF, Fishman ML, Fauci AS, Wolff SM: The ocular manifestations of Wegener's granulomatosis. *Am J Med* 63:131–141, 1977.
21. Haynes BF: Treatment of granulomatous vasculitides, in Fauci AS (moderator): The spectrum of vasculitis. Clinical, pathologic, immunologic, and therapeutic considerations. *Ann Intern Med* 89:660–676, 1978.
22. Bullen CL, Liesegang TJ, McDonald TJ, DeRemmee RA: Ocular complications of Wegener's granulomatosis. *Ophthalmology* 90:279–290, 1983.
23. Khalil M, Lindley S, Matouk E: Tuberculosis of the orbit: *Ophthalmology* 92:1624–1627, 1985.
24. Grimson BS, Simmons KB: Orbital inflammation, myositis, and systemic lupus erythematosis. *Arch Ophthalmol* 101:736–738, 1983.
25. Dal Pozzo G, Boschi MC: Extraocular muscle enlargement in acromegaly. *J Comp Assist Tomog* 6:706–707, 1982.
26. Slavin ML, Glaser JS: Idiopathic orbital myositis. *Arch Ophthalmol* 100:1261–1265, 1982.
27. Blodi FC, Gass JDM: Inflammatory pseudotumor of the orbit. *Trans Am Acad Ophthalmol Otolaryngol* 71:303–323, 1917.
28. Trokel SL, Jakobiec FA: Correlation of CT scanning and pathologic features of ophthalmic Graves' disease. *Ophthalmology* 88:553–564, 1981.
29. Smith ME, Zimmerman LE: Amyloidosis of the eyelid and conjunctiva. *Arch Ophthalmol* 75:42–50, 1966.
30. Levine MR, Buckman G: Primary localized orbital amyloidosis. *Ann Ophthalmol* 18:165–167, 1986.
31. Coleman DJ, Jack RL, Jones IS, Fransen LA: High resolution B-scan ultrasound of the orbit: VI pseudotumors. *Arch Ophthalmol* 88:472–489, 1972.
32. Harris GJ: Subperiosteal abscess of the orbit. *Arch Ophthalmol* 101:751–757, 1983.
33. Krohel GB, Krauss HR, Christensen RE, Minckler D: Orbital abscess. *Arch Ophthalmol* 98:274–278, 1980.
34. Townsend DJ, Beyer-Machule CK, Fabian RL: Osteomyelitis of the orbit. *Ophthalmol Plast Reconstruc Surg* 2:15–19, 1986.
35. Char DH, Ablin A, Beckstead J: Histiocytic disorders of the orbit. *Ann Ophthalmol* 16:867–872, 1984.
36. Fauci AS, Johnson RE, Wolff SM: Radiation therapy of midline granuloma. *Ann Intern Med* 84:140–147, 1976.
37. Harcourt RB: Orbital granulomata associated with widespread angiitis. *Br J Ophthalmol* 49:673–677, 1964.
38. Van Wein S, Merz EH: Exophthalmos secondary to periarteritis nodosa. *Am J Ophthalmol* 56:204–207, 1963.
39. Sergott RC, Glaser JS: Graves' ophthalmopathy. A clinical and immunologic review. *Surv Ophthalmol* 26:1–21, 1981.
40. Sergott RC, Glaser JS, Komanduri C: Radiotherapy for idiopathic inflammatory orbital pseudotumor. *Arch Ophthalmol* 99:853–856, 1981.
41. Leone CR, Lloyd WC: Treatment protocol for orbital inflammatory disease. *Ophthalmology* 92:1325–1331, 1985.
42. Krohel GB, Carr EM, Webb RM: Intralesional corticosteroids for inflammatory lesions of the orbit. *Am J Ophthalmol* 101:121–123, 1986.
43. Ryan S, Zimmerman LE, King FM: Reactive lymphoid hyperplasia: An unusual form of intraocular pseudotumor. *Trans Am Acad Ophthalmol Otolaryngol* 76:652–671, 1972.
44. Rosenberg S: National Cancer Institute-sponsored study of classification of non-Hodgkin's lymphomas. Summary and description of a working formulation for clinical usage. *Cancer* 49:2112–2135, 1982.
45. Fratkin JD, Shammas HF, Miller SD: Disseminated Hodgkin's disease with bilateral orbital involvement. *Arch Ophthalmol* 96:102–104, 1978.
46. Arseneau JC, Canellos GP, Banks PM, et al: American Burkitt's lymphoma: A clinicopathologic study of 30 cases. 1. Clinical factors relating to prolonged survival. *Am J Med* 58:314–321, 1975.
47. Zimmerman LE, Font RL: Ophthalmologic manifestations of granulocytic sarcoma (myeloid sarcoma or chloroma). A clinicopathologic study of 33 cases. *Am J Ophthalmol* 80:975–990, 1975.
48. Mauriello JA, Langloss JM, Weiner J, Zimmerman LE: A clinicopathologic and immunohistologic study of lymphoproliferative lesions of the uveal tract. ARVO Abstracts. *Invest Ophthalmol Vis Sci* 22(suppl):172, 1982.
49. Jakobiec FA, Iwamoto T, Patell M, Knowles DM: Ocular adnexal monoclonal lymphoid tumors with a favorable prognosis. *Ophthalmology* 93:1547–1557, 1986.
50. Richards AS, Skalka HW, Roberts FJ: Pseudotumor of the orbit and retroperitoneal fibrosis: A form of multifocal fibrosclerosis. *Arch Ophthalmol* 98:1617–1620, 1980.
51. Fauci AS, Haynes BF, Costa J, et al: Lymphomatoid granulomatosis: Prospective clinical and therapeutic experience over 10 years. *N Engl J Med* 306:68–74, 1982.
52. Kohn R, Hepler R: Management of limited rhino-orbital mucormycosis without exenteration. *Ophthalmology* 92:1440–1444, 1985.
53. Glover AT, Grove AS: Eosinophilic granuloma with spontaneous healing. *Ophthalmology* 94:1008–1012, 1987.
54. Collison JM, Miller NR, Green WR: Involvement of orbital tissues by sarcoid. *Am J Ophthalmol* 102:302–307, 1986.

3

Orbital Tumors

Joseph A. Mauriello, Jr.
Joseph C. Flanagan
*Steven E. Harms**

As outlined in Chapter 1, the physician should determine whether the disease process is an inflammation or a tumor. Next, the disease process should be localized to the orbit, lacrimal gland, lacrimal sac, or eyelids. Tumors in the orbit may be further localized to the intraconal, peripheral (between the muscle cone but within the periorbita), and subperiosteal surgical spaces. Orbital tumors may arise secondarily from the adjacent brain and meninges, the sinus, surrounding orbital bones, lacrimal gland, lacrimal sac, surface of the globe, lid, or an intraocular tumor. Recognition of such possible origins will enhance the physician's determination of the appropriate clinical differential diagnosis.

This chapter considers orbital tumors exclusive of those that originate in the lacrimal gland and lacrimal sac. Adult orbital tumors will be considered separately from pediatric tumors since age is often a helpful criterion for differential diagnosis. Optic nerve meningioma and glioma are considered in this chapter since the clinical presentation and computed tomography (CT) scan and magnetic resonance imaging (MRI) pattern may be confused.

A step-by-step approach consisting of differential diagnosis, work-up, initial management, and management after biopsy will be considered.

Table 3-1 lists all orbital tumors, both pediatric and adult, and includes some inflammatory processes that may mimic a tumor as well. The classification is based on CT appearance. Any given tumor will most likely present as outlined in the table, but in many cases, the pattern suggested in the table is not always that of the given tumor. In addition, many tumors have more than one type of presentation. For example, a rhabdomyosarcoma often presents as a peripheral tumor, but sinus involvement may occur, as may extensive bone destruction. All such possible presentations should be kept in mind; otherwise, this important diagnosis may be clinically missed. For this reason, as many CT presentations that may be practically included within the limits of a table are listed in Table 3-1.

The CT classifications outlined in Table 3-1 will serve as the framework for the differential diagnosis and discussion of the various orbital tumors.

INTRACONAL TUMORS—OPTIC NERVE TUMORS

Differential Diagnosis—Glioma vs. Meningioma

The main differential diagnosis of an enlarged optic nerve that has a noninflammatory-type presentation includes optic nerve glioma (juvenile pilocytic astrocytic harmatoma) and optic nerve sheath meningioma. Gliomas are considered hamartomas and are composed of astrocytes with hair-like (pilocytic) cytoplasmic processes. Optic nerve glioma is generally a disease of children with a median age of 6 years, and optic nerve sheath meningioma is a disease of middle-aged females. The two conditions may be clinically confused.[1,2] A detailed differential diagnosis of optic nerve lesions is listed in Table 3-2.

Anatomic Site of Origin

Both optic nerve glioma and meningioma may cause minimal proptosis of usually not more than 2 mm with

* Author of MRI section.

Table 3-1
Differential Diagnosis of Orbital Tumors and Some Inflammations—Adults and Children

EOM Involvement (see Chapter 2)
   Thyroid ophthalmopathy
   Pseudotumor
   Lymphoid infiltrate
   Metastatic carcinoma
Intraconal Tumors
   Intrinsic optic nerve tumors
      glioma
      meningioma
      giant drusen (astrocytoma) of tuberous sclerosis
      optic nerve sheath cyst—colobomatous arachnoid cyst
      melanocytoma
      blue nevus
   Juxtaneural tumors
      metastatic
      hemangioblastoma (von Hippel's disease)
      juvenile xanthogranuloma
      leukemia
      cellular blue nevus
Inflammatory Optic Nerve Conditions That May Mimic Tumor
   Pseudotumor involving optic nerve
   Optic neuritis
   Thyroid ophthalmopathy
   Sarcoid
Miscellaneous Causes of Optic Nerve Enlargement
   Traumatic hematoma involving nerve sheath and nerve
   Optic nerve drusen
Localized Intraconal Tumors
   Cavernous hemangioma
   Hemangiopericytoma
   Schwannoma
   Neurofibroma—may be localized and unencapsuled
   Intravascular papillary endothelial hyperplasia
   Leiomyoma
Focal Intraconal or Extraconal (Noncystic)
   Benign vascular tumors
   Fibroma
   Nodular fasciitis
   Rhabdomyoma
   Leiomyoma
   Chondroma
   Spindle cell lipoma
   Myxoma
   Metastatic carcinoma
   Neuroblastoma[*]
   Ewing's sarcoma[*]
   Juvenile xanthogranuloma[*] or xanthogranuloma in adults
   Teratoma[*]
   Leiomyoma
   Kaposi's sarcoma

Varix
Granular cell myoblastoma
Lipoma
Juvenile fibromatosis—extraconal, with lid component[*]

Diffuse (Intraconal and Extraconal) (Noncystic)
Lymphoid infiltrate (see Chapter 2)
Pseudotumor (sclerosing)
Orbital hemorrhage
Amyloid deposition
Leukemia
Sinus histiocytosis (may be bilateral) (see Chapter 4)
Rare spindle cell tumors
  fibrous histiocytoma
  hemangiopericytoma
  Erdheim-Chester disease
  fibromatosis
  fibrosarcoma
  leiomyosarcoma
  malignant schwannoma
  neurofibroma
  malignant neurofibroma
  chondrosarcoma
  liposarcoma
  myxosarcoma
  angiosarcoma
  postradiation sarcoma
  undifferentiated sarcoma

Diffuse (predominantly children) (see Chapter 4)
Rhabdomyosarcoma[*†]
Granulocytic sarcoma[*†]
Metastatic neuroblastoma[*†]
Metastatic Ewing's sarcoma[*†]
Alveolar soft part sarcoma—involves EOMs and may be well-localized[†‡]
Sinus histiocytosis
Endodermal sinus tumor
Heterotopic brain tissue
Capillary hemangioma—may have prominent lid component
Undifferentiated sarcoma

Diffuse (cystic)[*]
Microphthalmos with cyst[*]
Congenital cystic eyeball[*]
Lymphangioma[*]
Teratoma[*†]

Focal (Cystic) with Bone Involvement[*]
Dermoid cyst[§]
Epidermal inclusion cyst[§]
Encephalocele[‖]
Meningocele[‖]
Mucocele (most often frontal and ethmoid sinus)

Peripheral Tumors (Soft Tissue Mass) (may be extraconal or subperiosteal)
Orbital or subperiosteal hemorrhage
Hematic cyst

Cholesteatoma
Arteriovenous malformation
Venous malformation
Vascular malformation

Sinus and/or Bone Involvement
Osseous and other tumors that primarily involve bone
  osteoma
  osteogenic sarcoma
  fibrous dysplasia*
  ossifying fibroma*
  cavernous hemangioma of bone
  intradiploic meningioma of orbital roof
  chordoma
  aneurysmal bone cyst*
  Paget's disease (a metabolic disease)
  metastatic neuroblastoma
  lipoma of frontal bone
  giant cell tumor (osteoclastoma)*
  osteoblastoma*
  reparative granuloma*
  infantile cortical hyperostosis (Caffey's syndrome)*
  brown tumor
  melanoma

Soft Tissue Tumors That Secondarily Involve Bone (predominantly in children)
Angiofibroma*
Unifocal (local) and multifocal (systemic) eosinophilic granuloma or Langerhans
  cell histiocytosis (formerly termed *histiocytoses X*)*#
  Letterer-Siwe
  eosinophilic granuloma
  Hand-Schüller-Christian Syndrome
Erdheim-Chester disease
Necrobiotic xanthogranuloma
Granulocytic sarcoma*#
Melanotic ectodermal tumor of infancy (retinal anlage tumor)*
Metastatic neuroblastoma*
Teratoma* involves maxillary sinus
Rhabdomyosarcoma—usually not of sinus origin
Mesenchymal chondrosarcoma
Angiofibroma
Alveolar soft part sarcoma
Endodermal sinus tumor
Esthesioneuroblastoma

Nonosseous Tumors Originating in Sinus, Nose, and Oropharynx
Tumors of epithelial sinus origin
  squamous cell carcinoma
  sarcomatoid carcinoma
  inverted papilloma (arises from sinus epithelium, especially ethmoid or nasal
    mucosa)
  mucoepidermoid carcinoma
  inverted papilloma
Adenocarcinoma

Adenocystic carcinoma
    malignant mixed tumor
    mucoepidermoid carcinoma
    inverted papilloma
Angiofibroma (oropharyngeal tumor)
Lymphoepithelioma
Esthesioneuroblastoma
Cholesteatoma
Rhabdomyosarcoma
Fibrosarcoma (see "Adult Orbital Tumors")
Melanoma
Mesoectodermal leiomyosarcoma
Alveolar soft part sarcoma (see "pediatric orbital tumors")
Metastatic Ewing's sarcoma
Mucocele secondary to sinus tumor

Intraocular Tumors with Orbital Extension
Malignant melanoma of the choroid
Retinoblastoma
Medulloepithelioma
Carcinoma of the nonpigmented ciliary epithelium
Granulocytic sarcoma
Lymphoma of uvea
Leukemia—unilateral or bilateral mainly of choroid

Orbital Tumors with Intraocular Invasion
Optic nerve glioma
Optic nerve meningioma
Adenoid cystic carcinoma of the lacrimal gland

Lid Tumors with Orbital Extension (see Chapter 8)
Basal cell carcinoma (BCC)
Squamous cell carcinoma (SCC)
Sebaceous gland carcinoma
Adnexal carcinomas other than sebaceous
Melanoma

Conjunctival Tumors with Orbital Extension
Squamous cell carcinoma (SCC)
Mucoepidermoid carcinoma
Melanoma

Lacrimal Sac Tumors with Orbital Extension (see Chapter 7)
Papilloma—Exophytic and endophytic
Squamous cell carcinoma (SCC)
Lymphoma
Melanoma

Cranial Tumors with Orbital Extension
Sphenoid ridge meningioma—most common
Chordomas
Esthesioneuroblastoma—of olfactory origin

---

* involving children, see Chapter 4

† may have adjacent bone invasion

‡ may extend from paranasal sinus into orbit

§ are localized at suture line, usually superotemporal with focal erosion of bone (fossa formation)

‖ at suture lines between maxillary, lacrimal, ethmoid, and frontal bones

6 of 33 in largest series involved orbital or adjacent sinus

Table 3-2
Differential Diagnosis of Optic Nerve Tumors and Inflammations

Intrinsic Tumors
   glioma
   meningioma
   giant drusen (astrocytoma) of tuberous sclerosis
   optic nerve sheath colobomatous (arachnoid) cyst
   melanocytoma
   blue nevus
Juxtaneural
   metastatic
   hemangioblastoma (von Hippel's disease)
   JXG
   leukemia
   cellular blue nevus
Secondary Optic Nerve Tumors
   malignant melanoma of choroid (very rare)
   retinoblastoma
   metastatic disease (often associated with intraocular
     metastases)
Inflammations of optic nerve that mimic tumor
   pseudotumor
   optic neuritis
   thyroid ophthalmopathy
   sarcoid
Miscellaneous causes of optic nerve enlargement
   traumatic hematoma
   optic nerve drusen

significant visual loss.[3,4] Glioma causes an earlier loss of vision than meningioma because glioma involves the substance of the nerve, while meningioma arises in the meninges that surround the nerve. Unfortunately, children with gliomas will often present with profound visual loss. In cases in which a meningioma arises within the confines of the optic canal, vision is affected extremely early due to optic nerve compression. In general, meningiomas of the optic nerve are more aggressive than gliomas, especially when they arise in children. Therefore, the diagnosis of meningioma should always be considered in a child with an optic nerve tumor.[5,6]

Optic glioma or juvenile pilocytic astrocytoma and grehamartomas may be conceptually thought of as involving or originating from the following possible sites: (1) the optic nerve proper, (2) the chiasm, or (3) structures adjacent to the chiasm such as the hypothalamus and third ventricle. In the latter group, the optic chiasm is thought to be secondarily invaded by tumor. When the optic nerve alone is involved, visual loss and proptosis are the predominant signs, and overall prognosis for survival is excellent. Pure chiasmal involvement will result in loss of vision and an overall favorable prognosis for survival.[7-12]

Gliomas are considered benign hamartomas and tend to have a self-limited growth pattern. They do not extend beyond the dura. However, gliomas that originate in structures adjacent to the chiasm have a much worse prognosis for survival than those that arise in the optic nerve or chiasm. Seizures, hydrocephalus, abnormalities of gait, headache, nystagmus, and hypothalamic and pituitary dysfunction may lead to death in such patients.

A rare, fatal type of malignant optic glioma of adulthood that arises intracranially and is composed of malignant astrocytes has been reported. Unilateral visual loss progresses to bilateral blindness within a few months. The disease is uniformly fatal in less than 1 year.[9] When originally reported, the disease was thought to affect elderly males predominantly, but a more recent report shows that this rare form of glioma affects males and females aged 22–79 years.[8,9]

Meningiomas may originate from several possible sites. They may arise primarily from the meningothelial cells (arachnoidal cap cells) that surround the intraorbital or intracanalicular portion of the optic nerve, or they may arise ectopically and extradurally in the orbit, presumably from embryonic rests of arachnoidal cells of ciliary nerves or within the orbital bones.[13-15] Meningiomas may also arise within the intracranial portion of the central nervous system, and in these cases, the tumor has a tendency to arise where the dura fuses to bone. This fact helps to explain why meningiomas arise at the apex of the orbit at the annulus of Zinn. Because meningiomas tend to invade the dura, local bone erosion occurs as well as hyperostosis. Gliomas do not extend beyond the dura, and, therefore, optic canal enlargement occurs without significant bone erosion or hyperostosis.

Patients with meningiomas and gliomas should always be clinically suspected of having systemic neurofibromatosis (Fig. 3-1). Meningiomas may be multicentric, especially in patients with neurofibromatosis. "Bilateral" meningiomas may not reflect multifocality but may represent spread of a meningioma from one optic nerve via the chiasm to the other optic nerve, and in these cases neurofibromatosis will not be present. Bilateral gliomas almost always suggest multifocality, and, therefore, such patients will have neurofibromatosis.[16] Gliomas are rarely aggressive enough to spread from one optic nerve to the other.

Patients with gliomas that have neurofibromatosis may have a more benign course than other patients with gliomas. In addition, optic nerve gliomas in patients with neurofibromatosis tend to have more of a perineural tumor component than a parenchymal optic nerve component.[17] All patients with gliomas should be examined for neurofibromatosis. In general, about 15 percent of patients with neurofibromatosis have optic gliomas.[18] Seventy-five percent of tumors become symptomatic in the first decade of life, and 90 percent in the first two decades. All cases of bilateral glioma appear to be related to neurofibromatosis.

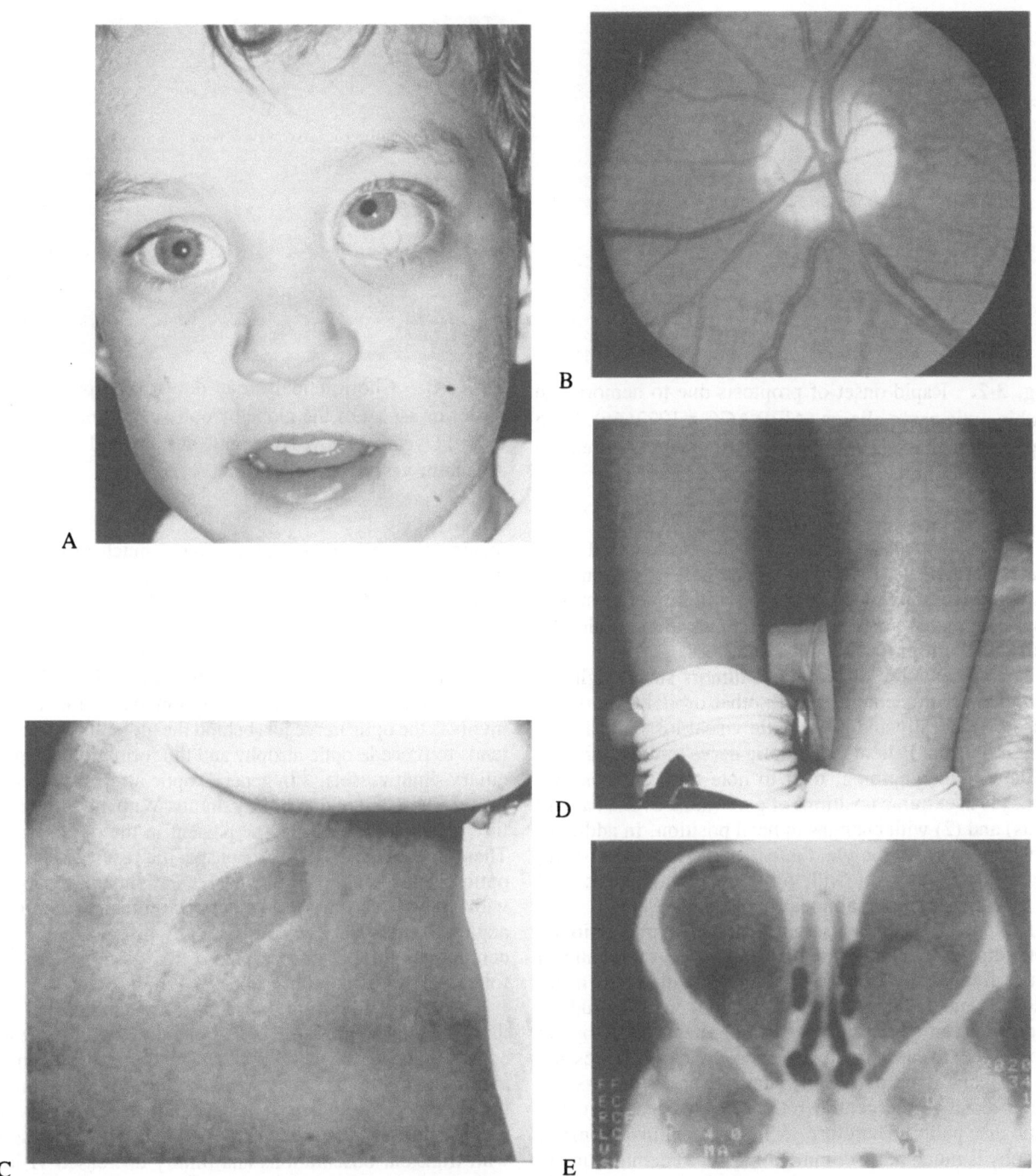

Fig. 3-1. (*A*) A 4-year-old female who presented with nonaxial proptosis of the left eye. Fundoscopy showed severe optic atrophy on the left side (*B*) with minimal optic atrophy on the right. On physical examination, there are multiple café-au-lait spots involving the trunk (*C*) and extremities (*D*). (*E*) Orbital CT scan shows bilateral optic nerve glioma. Diagnosis of neurofibromatosis was made.

History and Ophthalmologic Examination—Optic Nerve Glioma vs. Meningioma

As stated above, optic nerve tumors cause a mild degree of proptosis with a significant gradual loss of vision. Visual loss tends to be particularly profound with a glioma because of its involvement of the nerve substance.[19,20] While in general proptosis develops slowly, rapidly evolving proptosis may occur in patients with optic nerve gliomas due to the accumulation of mucinous or hemorrhage material within the tumor (Fig.

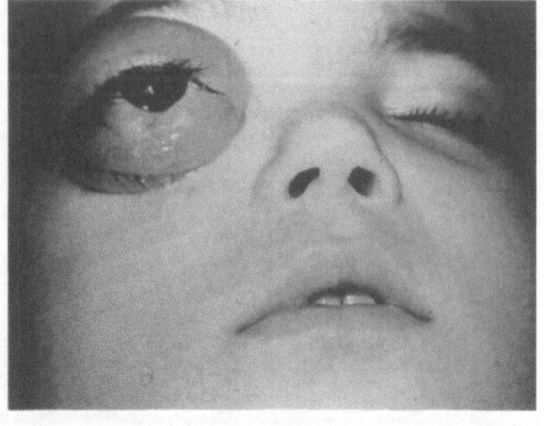

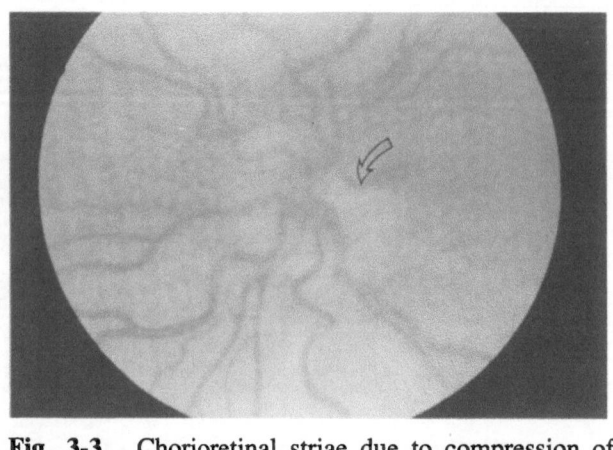

Fig. 3-2. Rapid onset of proptosis due to hemorrhage within optic nerve glioma (AFIP ACC #1222666). Such rapid enlargement may also occur after mucoid degeneration of an optic nerve glioma.

Fig. 3-3. Chorioretinal striae due to compression of posterior aspect of the globe by optic nerve meningioma in an 11-year-old boy. Note optic atrophy and opticociliary shunt vessel (arrow).

3-2).[21] Rarely, visual acuity may be excellent and color plates normal, yet optic disc edema will be present and an extensive anterior optic glioma will be demonstrated on CT scan. A meningioma that extends extradurally will give both proptosis and visual loss.

The presentation of intradural tumors such as glioma and meningioma contrasts with other orbital tumors that arise extradurally and cause little visual loss and significant proptosis. Patients with optic nerve tumors, whether glioma or meningioma, tend to note transient obscurations (1) in extreme positions of gaze (gaze-evoked amaurosis) and (2) with changes in head position. In addition, with movement of the eye, there is an increase in pressure, especially in upgaze, with optic nerve tumors as well as with thyroid ophthalmopathy.

In general, in patients with glioma or meningioma, optic disc edema and optic disc pallor occur with almost equal frequency. Rarely, in patients with optic nerve gliomas and meningiomas, visual loss may be sudden and mimic an optic neuritis. Tumors near the globe are more likely to cause optic disc edema due to compression of the central retinal vein. Tumors that compress the nerve distal to the central retinal vessels tend to cause optic disc pallor. Therefore, with chiasmal involvement, atrophy is much more common than disc edema. Tumors in the optic canal cause early loss of vision with optic atrophy that may mimic a retrobulbar neuritis and few if any radiographic signs of tumor. Improvement of vision with steroids does not confirm the diagnosis of retrobulbar neuritis. Progressive visual loss suggests a tumor.

On occasion with glioma, an enlarged optic nerve may be observed ophthalmoscopically. An enlarged optic nerve may occur in other conditions such as congenital glaucoma, megalopapillae, and congenital disc anomalies including optic pits, colobomas, and morning glory syndrome.[22,23]

Optociliary shunt vessels may be present with either meningioma or glioma but are found much more commonly with meningioma of the optic nerve (Fig. 3-3). Other conditions associated with optociliary shunt vessels include optic disc drusen, chronic atrophic papilledema, glaucoma, arachnoidal cyst, central retinal vein occlusions, or as a congenital anomaly. Optociliary shunts, like papilledema, are more common when the tumor involves the optic nerve just behind the globe. Disc edema tends to precede optic atrophy and the formation of optociliary shunt vessels.[24] In general, optic atrophy precedes the development of optociliary shunts. With meningioma, tiny refractile bodies may be present in the optic nerve. These bodies are probably a nonspecific result of chronic optic disc edema due to any cause. Patients may present with venous stasis, iris neovascularization, and secondary angle-closure glaucoma. As with any orbital tumor that compresses the posterior aspect of the globe, choroidal folds and circumpapillary folds may be present.

On visual field testing, the most consistent and earliest finding with meningioma is peripheral constriction with enlargement of the blind spot.[13] Centrocecal scotomas are not common. The peripheral constriction may sometimes respect the horizontal meridian. Other causes of unilateral optic disc edema with an enlarged blind spot with transient obscurations and mildly decreased vision include papillophlebitis (big blind-spot syndrome), optic disc vasculitis, ischemic optic neuropathy, diabetic papillopathy, thyroid optic neuropathy, optic perineuritis, and asymmetric papilledema.[10]

In patients with small optic nerve meningiomas, the visual fields, color plates, pupils, and CT of the head may be normal. Proptosis may be minimal. Orbital CT scan in some of these patients may reveal a tumor. Therefore, any patient with visual loss and normal testing should be followed with repeat clinical testing and orbital scans or MRI scans every 3 to 6 months depending on the degree of clinical suspicion. Intracanalicular tumors,

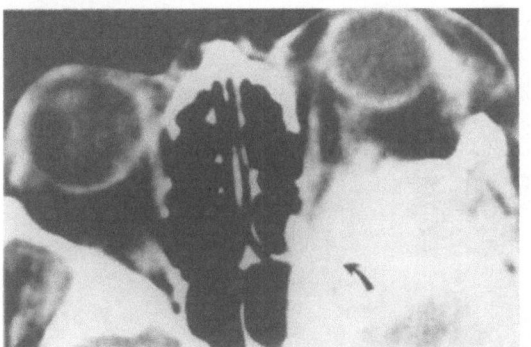

Fig. 3-4. CT scan from 60-year-old female with gradual onset of proptosis and loss of vision to the light perception level over a 10-year period. The patient had refused surgery for several years. The patient underwent a combined frontal craniotomy and surgical decompression of the orbit. Note interface between bone and soft tissue (arrow).

especially meningiomas, may be difficult to detect radiologically and yet visual loss may occur. Meningioma should always be suspected in a young female with slowly progressive uniocular loss of vision. Headache may occur with intraorbital or intracranial meningiomas. Intracranial sphenoidal ridge tumors have varying clinical features depending on their location (Fig. 3-4). In general, tumors involving the inner one-third of the sphenoid ridge affect vision early and cause unilateral optic atrophy. Cranial nerves III through VI may be involved. When orbital invasion occurs, proptosis may result. Gustatory hallucinations and convulsions may occur. In tumors of the middle third of the sphenoid ridge, bilateral papilledema is often present. Meningiomas of the lateral one-third of the sphenoidal ridge may present as a mass in the temporal fossa, may cause elevated intracranial pressure, and may affect vision late. Diploic meningiomas of the orbital roof have also been reported (peripheral orbital

tumors section, Chapter 3). Meningiomas may show acceleration of growth during pregnancy and after head trauma.

Visual field testing is often difficult to perform on patients with gliomas because of their age and often profound visual loss. In most cases of optic nerve gliomas, arcuate, altitudinal, or central defects are found. Chiasmal gliomas will often cause a bitemporal defect, although the field defects may be nonspecific. Homonymous defects or blindness in one eye and contralateral temporal field loss also occur.

CT Scan—Differential Diagnosis of Optic Nerve Glioma and Meningioma

On CT scan, patients with optic nerve gliomas often show a markedly thickened optic nerve with a fusiform pattern with clear-cut margins (Table 3-3 and Fig. 3-5). The margins are well-delineated because the tumor is almost universally confined within the dura. Kinking and buckling of the optic nerve occur due to infarction cysts that contain mucopolysaccharides. Gliomas normally have a high mucopolysaccharide content.

On CT scan, the density pattern of optic glioma is homogeneous and close to the density pattern of the normal optic nerve; there is no clear separation between the tumor and nerve on CT or ultrasonography. Enhancement of optic gliomas after contrast injection varies from imperceptible to moderate, but is generally less intense than that of a meningioma, neurofibroma, metastatic lesion, or other lesion that may mimic an optic glioma (Fig. 3-6). Calcifications are only occasionally seen and are much more likely to be found in meningiomas. Metrizamide cisternography may aid in detecting subtle gliomas. Metrizamide enters the optic nerve sheath during cisternography and is used to delineate the sheath's subarachnoid space. Uniform enlargement and contrast en-

Table 3-3
CT Scan Differential Diagnosis of Optic Nerve Glioma and Meningioma

Glioma	Meningioma
Fusiform thickening of nerve	Narrow thickening
Thickening of same density as optic nerve	Thickening of somewhat greater density than optic nerve
With kinking of nerve	With railroad tracking (lucent center optic nerve surrounded by radiopaque tumor—"tramtrack sign")
Smooth edges	Irregular edges of extradural spread
May be posterior in orbit	Fusiform globular perioptic masses often posterior
Optic canal enlarged	Optic canal not often enlarged
No bone erosion or hyperostosis	Bone erosion, hyperostosis likely
Calcifications rare	Calcifications may be seen

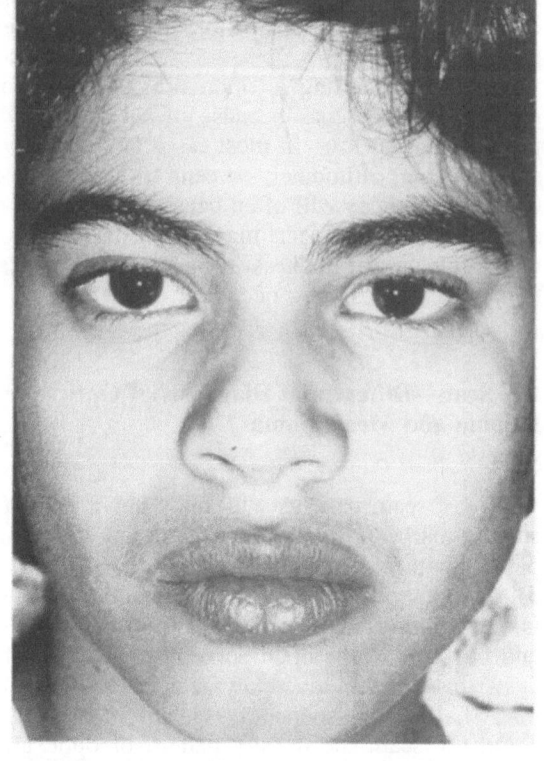

A

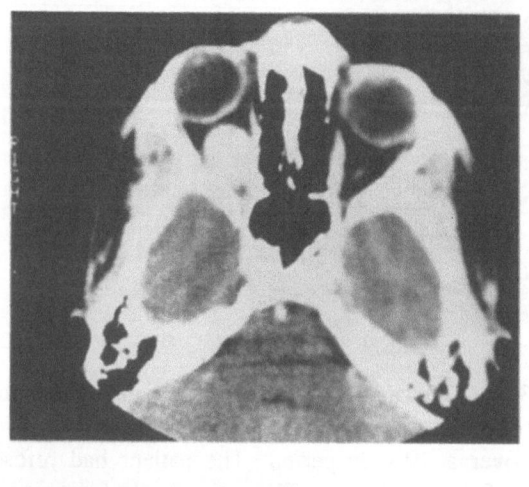

B

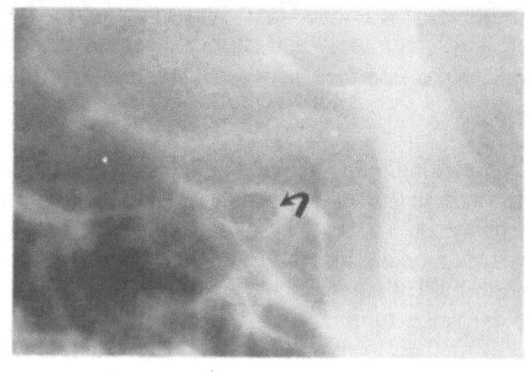

D

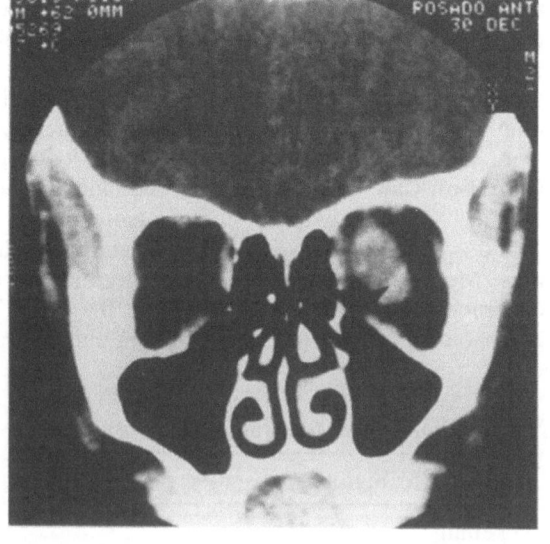

C

Fig. 3-5. (*A*) An 11-year-old male with loss of vision in the right eye. Orbital CT shows a tumor that involves the optic nerve. (*B*) Axial view of the tumor suggests an intraconal tumor while the (*C*) coronal view definitely shows an enlarged intrinsic optic nerve tumor with calcifications (arrow). Note the smooth margins of the tumor and that the thickening of the nerve is of the same density as the optic nerve. (*D*) Enlargement of optic foramen (arrow) due to optic nerve glioma. Note lack of erosion or hyperostosis, which is more common with meningioma.

hancement of the optic nerve is also seen with optic papillitis and retrobulbar neuritis.

Unlike gliomas, meningiomas are usually more dense than the normal optic nerve on CT scan (Fig. 3-7). These findings are confirmed with MRI; with MRI, optic nerve gliomas show intensity characteristics similar to the normal optic nerve, while optic nerve sheath meningiomas yield a slightly stronger signal. Meningiomas of the optic nerve cause a ligneous and leathery thickening of the optic nerve that does not allow for kinks. Most com-

monly, meningiomas tend to cause narrow, diffuse enlargement of the nerve with localized expansions either at the orbital apex or behind the globe. Expansions at the apex are most common. On high-resolution CT scanning, a less radiopaque shadow centrally is due to the compressed atrophic radiolucent optic nerve creating the so-called "railroad track sign" or "tram track sign" (Fig. 3-8). The "donut" sign is seen on coronal views. This sign is rarely present in other conditions including optic perineuritis, perineural hematoma, and perineural

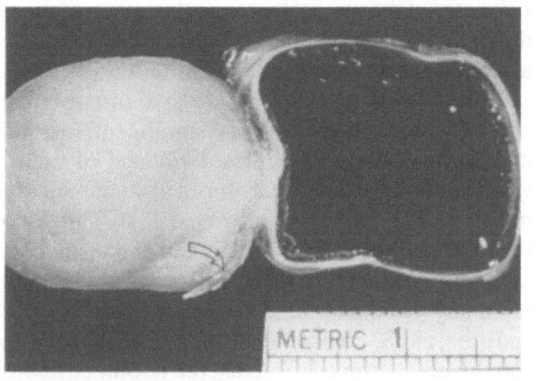
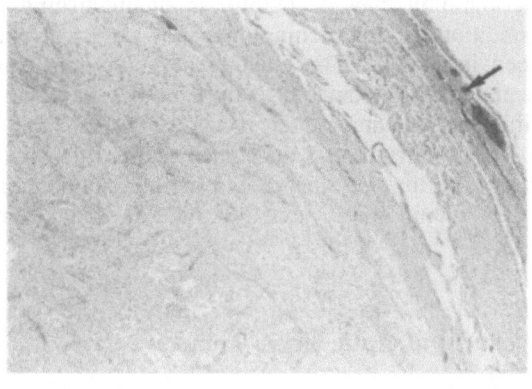

Fig. 3-6. (*A*) Specimen of eyeball with attached optic nerve glioma totally within the dura (arrow) explains CT pattern. (Courtesy of Robert Folberg, MD, Iowa City, IA.) (*B*) Biopsy shows increased number of astrocytic cells within the optic nerve. Tumor is confined within dura (arrow).

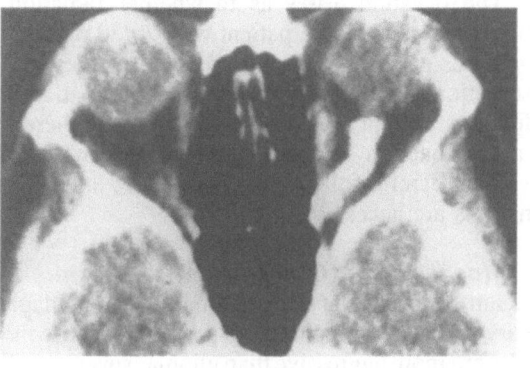
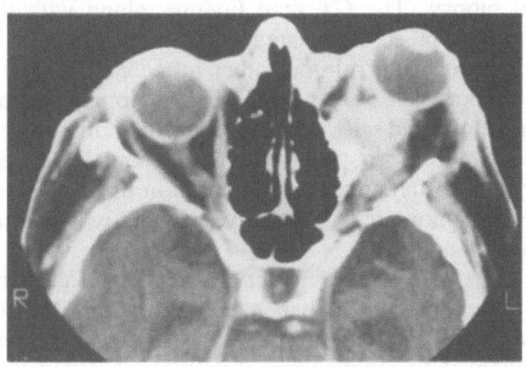

Fig. 3-7. (*A*) Axial orbital CT scan of optic nerve meningioma from 55-year-old female with history of decreased vision to NLP over 3 years. Note totally calcified optic nerve meninges. (*B*) Axial CT scan from 82-year-old female with blind painful eye due to proptosis after third recurrence of meningioma. Patient underwent exenteration. Compare density of tumor to less dense normal right optic nerve. (Patient referred by Drs. Rodger and Nicki Silverstein, Passaic, NJ.)

metastasis. Due to the extradural spread of tumor, globular enlargements of the optic nerve may occur. These irregular excrescences are often in an apical posterior location.[19,25]

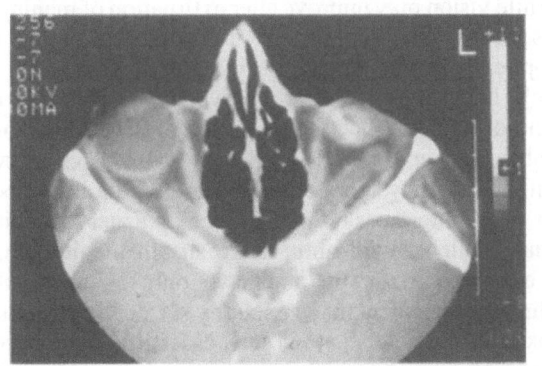

Fig. 3-8. Presumed bilateral optic nerve meningioma with ''railroad sign'' most evident on left side. (Courtesy of Dr. M. Kuppersmith, New York City, NY.)

Psammoma bodies are calcified, laminated bodies composed of whorls of degenerated meningothelial cells; they may be seen on CT scan but calcifications are generally not seen early in the course of the disease. A ring-like pattern of calcification is rare but specific for optic nerve sheath meningioma. Calcospherites seen histologically within gliomas are rarely seen on CT scan. A more posterior location in the orbit favors meningioma over glioma because of meningioma's tendency to grow where the dura fuses to bone. Because the optic nerve is diffusely and narrowly thickened on CT scan, other uncommon lesions may mimic meningioma (Table 3-1).

As stated above, meningiomas tend to be slightly hyperdense and often enhance after injection of contrast media. Unlike gliomas that almost always cause enlargement of the optic foramen, optic nerve sheath meningiomas show minimal or no enlargement of the optic canal. Erosion or hyperostosis of the adjacent bone is typical of meningioma and less common with glioma.

Ultrasonography may be helpful in differentiating these tumors in children.

Arteriography may be helpful in distinguishing the two conditions in that meningioma shows a tumor blush not seen in glioma. The change in tumor density on CT-scan contrast enhancement may be of little value in the differential diagnosis.

On MRI, both gliomas and meningiomas are similar in intensity to the optic nerve and brain. Calcifications, typical of meningioma, are seen on CT scan but not MRI.

Management of Optic Nerve Tumors

The management of optic nerve meningioma and glioma is controversial and is dependent on how firm a clinical diagnosis can be made. In general, diagnosis of an optic nerve tumor can be made on clinical grounds without biopsy. The CT scan findings along with the low-grade proptosis associated with significant loss of visual function help rule out other intraconal, nonoptic nerve tumors such as cavernous hemangioma, hemangiopericytoma, and schwannoma. The latter tumors affect vision late. CT scan, ultrasonography, and MRI may further help differentiate these tumors in difficult cases (see "Ultrasonography"). Rarely, patients will require diagnostic biopsy.

While the management is not clear-cut, the following general guidelines for management are offered. A well-localized optic nerve tumor that does not show growth in a patient with good vision should be observed.[19,26] Progression can be monitored by color plates, visual field every 3 to 6 months, and CT scans when other clinical data suggest change.

Management of Gliomas. Surgical indications for the evaluation and treatment of presumed optic glioma are controversial and depend on the tumor location.

Optic gliomas that involve the chiasm and adjacent structures are treated by the neurosurgeon and are not generally considered resectable.[27] Neurosurgeons often recommend biopsy of even chiasmal lesions because of clinical confusion with craniopharyngioma or other tumors. Radiation of gliomas in the chiasmal area is possibly effective and may serve to stabilize or even improve vision. The morbidity and mortality of neurosurgical biopsy must be evaluated in each individual case.

Gliomas confined to the intraorbital optic nerve are probably better left alone unless there is high-grade proptosis, significant loss of vision (less than 20/400), or fear of extension to the chiasm.[7,27] Incisional biopsy has yielded equivocal results, mainly because marked arachnoidal hyperplasia associated with an underlying glioma of the nerve may be confused pathologically with a meningioma. For the same reason, needle biopsy may not be helpful in distinguishing the two tumors. A biopsy taken from the edges of the lesion is more likely to show arachnoidal hyperplasia than a biopsy taken at the epicenter of the tumor, that is, at the center of the fusiform thickening.[28,29] Arachnoidal hyperplasia associated with a glioma rarely extends beyond the dura.

If there is evidence of progressive tumor enlargement or significant proptosis with significant loss of vision and no radiologic or clinical evidence of chiasmal involvement, a frontal neurosurgical approach is recommended. The chiasm is inspected first, and if no tumor is found, the optic canal is unroofed and the nerve excised at the posterior aspect of the glioma. Tumors have recurred many years later (one case report was 48 years later), and, therefore, complete excision utilizing this approach should be attempted.[30] A lateral Krönlein approach allows for only partial excision of the tumor unless the tumor is well-localized.

The routine use of radiation for optic nerve glioma has been advocated.[31] The effectiveness of radiation alone has not been well-established.

The question arises as to whether radiation should be recommended to a patient with 20/70 or better vision who has not been biopsied. The alternatives include observation or radiotherapy. If the clinical and radiologic findings strongly support a glioma, radiotherapy is the option that can be used in order to attempt to stabilize vision. Careful follow-up clinical, CT, and MRI examinations are necessary.[32]

Management of Optic Nerve Meningioma. The physician confronts the same dilemma when managing optic nerve sheath meningioma. In general, because meningiomas are more aggressive than glioma, surgical indications are less stringent. A presumed optic nerve meningioma with vision of 20/50 or better should be observed. If the vision is 20/100 or less or if there is evidence of growth, a transcranial neurosurgical approach is warranted. Certainly, a patient with no light perception should have a surgical extirpation of the entire optic nerve. Radical exenteration may not be necessary. The risk of intracranial spread of the presumed meningioma that may occur with observation must be weighed against the loss of vision that almost invariably accompanies complete surgical extirpation.

While vision may improve after extirpation of meningiomas have been reported, the intimate association of the optic nerve meningioma with the delicate pial blood vessels that supply the optic nerve makes removal of the tumor without affecting the vision difficult. It is conceivable that reports of surgical removal of optic nerve meningiomas may represent ectopic extradural components of meningiomas rather than true optic nerve meningiomas. Patients with optic nerve sheath meningiomas that extend extradurally and have only a small subarachnoid component may benefit by surgically stripping the extradural component. In such cases, the optic nerve is decompressed and vision is improved without affecting the optic nerve blood supply. The use of microsurgical techniques is strongly suggested when performing such surgery.[33]

Long-term follow-up of patients who undergo surgery is necessary before becoming too enthusiastic about surgery early in the course of the disease. We believe that in patients with advanced disease, excision of the optic nerve together with the meningioma should be performed.[34] Apical tumors should be removed through a frontal rather than a lateral Krönlein approach. Incision of the dura may lead to orbital recurrence.

As with optic nerve glioma, the role of radiotherapy is unclear in the management of meningioma.

Management Based on Biopsy

Case Study 1. Biopsy shows masses of syncytial cells with ill-defined cytoplasmic boundaries and pale, round, often empty nuclei and concentrically laminated calcified areas that represent psammoma bodies (Fig. 3-9).[4,35] Rarely, mucoprotein intracytoplasmic inclusions are present.[36] In some areas, lipid-laden xanthoma cells are present. The tumor cells extend outside the dura. The optic nerve is atrophic. This biopsy is consistent with optic nerve sheath meningioma extending through the dura. No further treatment is necessary if the lesion is completely excised.

Serial CT scans are helpful in ruling out recurrence.

Case Study 2. Biopsy shows typical meningothelial cells all contained within the dura (Fig. 3-10). Arachnoidal hyperplasia confined to the subarachnoid space is present.

Because arachnoidal hyperplasia indistinguishable from meningioma may occur with gliomas, the pathologist should obtain cross-sections through the entire nerve to rule out a glioma.

Case Study 3. Biopsy is consistent with glioma but the preponderance of tumor is present in the subarachnoid space rather than within the optic nerve substance (Fig. 3-11). Arachnoidal thickening from proliferating astrocytic neoplastic cells suggest that a clinical diagnosis of neurofibromatosis should be ruled out. Rapid enlargement of gliomas may occur due to hemorrhage or mucoid degeneration within the tumor. Proliferation of the astrocytes and pial septal columns will also cause enlargement.

Case Study 4. Biopsy shows meningioma with anaplastic cells and many mitoses per high-power field. Malignant features of optic nerve tumors include presence of many mitotic figures, dense cellularity, marked pleomorphism, necrosis, and vascular proliferation.

Malignant meningiomas of the optic nerve are rare, while malignant gliomas of the optic nerve are even more rare. A malignant glioma that is thought to have

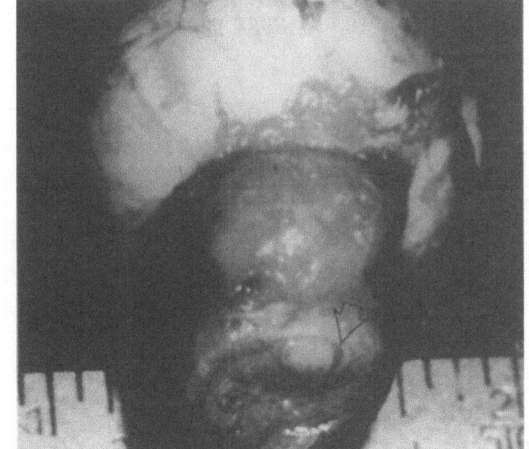

A

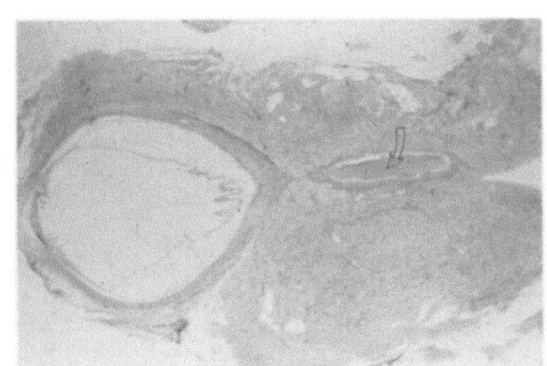

B

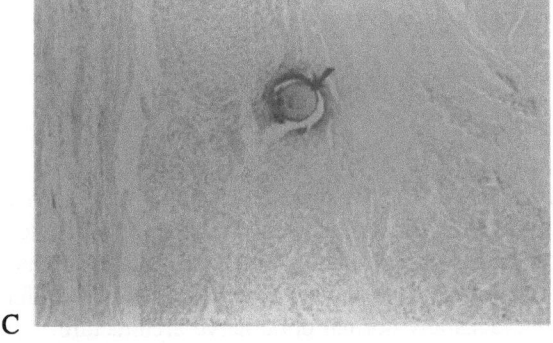

C

Fig. 3-9. (*A*) Note irregular enlargement of nerve outside the dura (arrow) in meningioma (AFIP ACC #806033). (*B*) Low-power photomicrograph shows extradural meningioma with atrophic nerve (arrow) (AFIP ACC #1527563). (*C*) High-power photomicrograph shows meningioma extending through dura. Normal optic nerve is on the right. Psammoma body (arrow) is adjacent to dura (AFIP ACC #1351072).

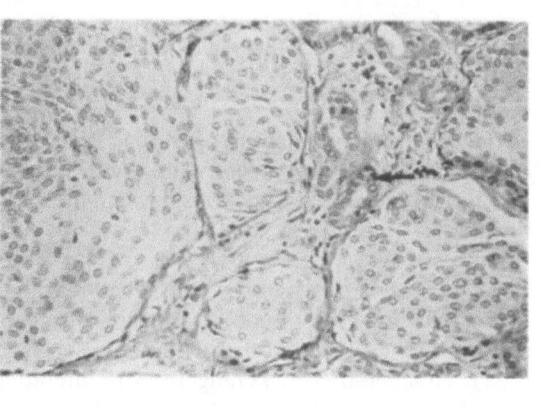

Fig. 3-10. Biopsy shows whorls of meningothelial cells that form a syncytium and are separated by fine fibrovascular septae. Note apparent ductules of lacrimal gland within tumor (arrow).

arisen in the optic nerve may have actually originated subclinically in the chiasm.

INTRACONAL TUMORS—ENCAPSULATED TUMORS

History and Ophthalmologic Examination

Unlike optic glioma and meningioma, which intrinsically involve the optic nerve or its sheath, encapsulated tumors such as cavernous hemangioma, schwannoma, and hemangiopericytoma are not intrinsic to the nerve

and therefore are less likely to compress the nerve and affect vision.[37-39] These tumors occur with such regularity that they should always be considered in the differential diagnosis. Of these three tumors, cavernous hemangioma is by far the most common. Cavernous hemangiomas occur more frequently in females, while hemangiopericytoma occurs more frequently in males.[39] Other less common encapsulated intraconal tumors include benign papillary endothelial hyperplasia, leiomyoma, and cellular blue nevus. Any of these tumors may be located anywhere in the lid or orbit (Table 3-4).

Intraconal extraneural tumors have a gradual onset over months and cause axial proptosis because of their intraconal location. Eventually, retinal striae and hyperopia will occur. A very rare tumor of blood vessel endothelium known as benign papillary endothelial hyper-

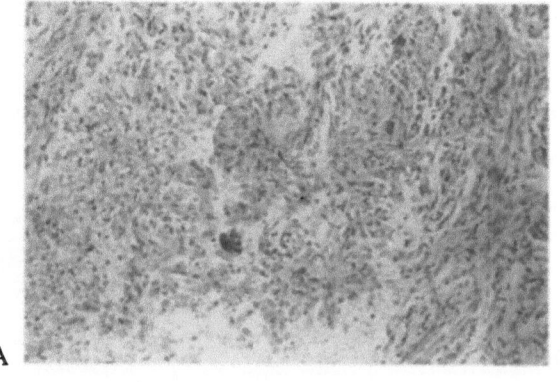

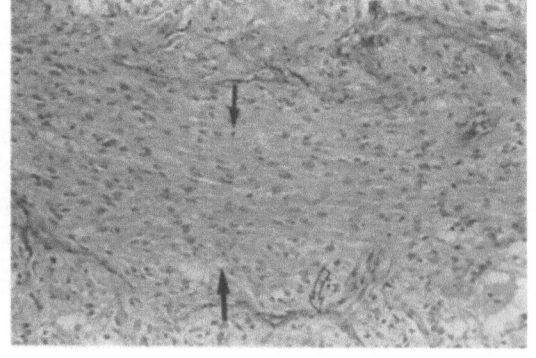

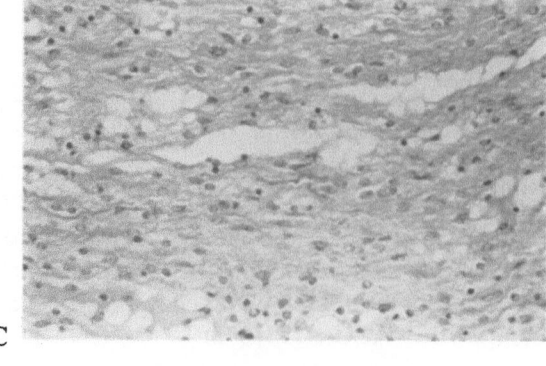

Fig. 3-11. (*A*) Meningothelial hyperplasia adjacent to glioma. (*B*) Band of increased number of astrocytes (two dark arrows) adjacent to normal pial septal columns (open arrow). (*C*) Note another area of astrocytic proliferation that lacks any normal optic nerve architecture.

Table 3-4
**Intraconal Localized Tumors That Do Not Involve
the Optic Nerve**

Cavernous hemangioma
Hemangiopericytoma[*]
Schwannoma
Benign papillary endothelial hyperplasia[†]
Leiomyoma[†]

[*] may involve meninges

[†] much less common causes

plasia does not usually induce retinal striae or hyperopia.[37] The tumor may also present in the eyelid as a localized, reddish purple mass and may be associated with a hemangioma, hematoma, arteriovenous malformation, and rarely lymphangioma.

Cavernous hemangiomas may grow during pregnancy.[38] Pain is usually not a feature of cavernous hemangioma but may occur with schwannoma and in about 20 percent of hemangiopericytomas.[39–42] Cavernous hemangiomas tend to have a more gradual onset than hemangiopericytoma. Orbital and conjunctival vascular congestion with proptosis and decreased vision may accompany either tumor. In general, the orbit and lid have greater time to adjust to the slow growth of a cavernous hemangioma than to the more rapidly growing hemangiopericytoma.

Schwannomas may be confused with neurofibromas; Table 3-5 is helpful in distinguishing the two entities.[43–46]

On ophthalmoscopic examination, chorioretinal striae are often present. Longstanding tumors may eventually cause optic disc edema. Optociliary shunt vessels do not occur.

CT Scan Appearance of Encapsulated Intraconal Tumors

There are several problems encountered in determining the nature of an intraconal mass. First, virtually any tumor may present as an intraconal mass. Second, very

Table 3-5
Neurofibromas vs. Schwannomas

Neurofibroma	Schwannoma
Diffuse	Encapsulated
Tend to be painless	May be painful
Malignant degeneration possible	Malignant change rare
Often associated with neurofibromatosis	May be associated with neurofibromatosis

often it is difficult to determine on CT scan whether the tumor involves the nerve or is, in fact, extraneural. High-resolution coronal CT scans and/or MRI are extremely helpful. In addition, as stated above, intrinsic nerve tumors generally affect vision much earlier and cause proportionately less proptosis than extrinsic nerve tumors.

The CT scan pattern of an encapsulated intraconal mass may take one of three basic patterns: (1) intraconal mass with no apical extension, (2) intraconal mass with apical extension, and (3) multiple intraconal masses. Typically, schwannoma has an apical extension, while cavernous hemangioma and hemangiopericytoma do not. (Figs. 3-12 and 3-13). Similarly, cavernous hemangioma and schwannoma may be multiple. Cavernous hemangioma is by far the most common tumor. Calcifications may be present in all three tumors but are much less common with hemangiopericytoma and are shown on CT but not MRI scan. Focal bone erosion may be present with all three tumors, but is less common with schwannoma.[38] All three tumors are well-encapsulated and enhance with contrast injection.

A case report describes a hemangiopericytoma that involved the meninges of the optic nerve. Interestingly, the patient did have significant loss of vision.[47]

The CT as well as the ultrasonic features of all three tumors may be indistinguishable.[48] Cavernous hemangiomas and schwannomas are usually rounded, well-outlined masses, while hemangiopericytomas may be bosselated and more lobulated (Fig. 3-14). Cavernous hemangiomas are slightly hyperdense with respect to the optic nerve and extraocular muscles (EOMs). Variable degrees of enhancement occur due to the very slow intratumoral circulation. The tumor is frequently seen in the intraconal space lateral to the optic nerve (Fig. 3-15).

Hemangiopericytoma, like cavernous hemangiomas, are usually of greater density than the optic nerve and rectus muscles. Hemangiopericytomas and schwannomas tend to be more homogeneous than cavernous hemangiomas because of the latter's multiple large blood-filled spaces; on ultrasonography, sound transmission may be better with hemangiopericytoma and schwannoma. There is less internal reflectivity with schwannoma and hemangiopericytoma than with cavernous hemangioma.

Arteriography should not be performed and is not indicated as part of the routine work-up unless a bruit or palpable thrill that suggests an arteriovenous (AV) fistula is present.

On MRI, schwannomas and cavernous hemangioma are hypointense on T-1 weighted and bright on T-2 weighted MRI scans.

Neurofibromas may be diffuse, plexiform, or localized. In the latter form, such tumors may be part of the differential diagnosis of a well-localized intraconal mass. Intraconal localized "isolated" neurofibromas are extremely rare in that 7 of 9 in the largest series were in the superior orbit. The tumors were circumscribed unencapsulated lesions that occurred in the third to fifth decade of life.

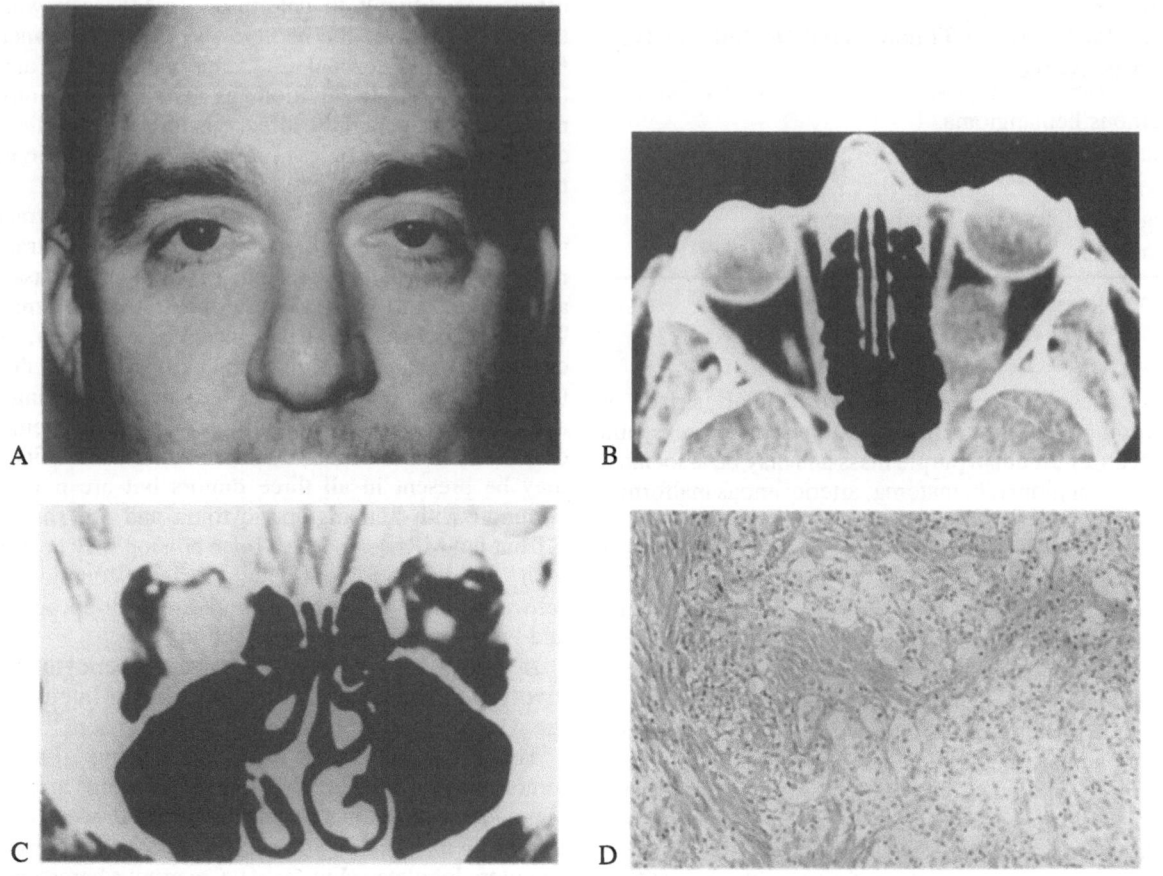

Fig. 3-12. (*A*) A 45-year-old male with gradual onset of ptosis and proptosis, left side. (*B,C*) CT scan shows intraconal mass with apical extension. (*D*) Through a lateral orbitotomy, excisional biopsy showed an encapsulated tumor composed of spindle cells with an adjacent area of lipid-laden macrophages consistent with schwannoma. (Patient referred by Dr. Roberta Strauchler, West Caldwell, NJ.)

Pain, hypesthesia, or anesthesia occur due to involvement of the trigeminal nerve. CT scan shows a well-localized mass. Ultrasonography shows rapid attenuation of the echoes within the lesion due to the cellular nature of the neurofibroma.[50,51]

Another such rare tumor is granular cell tumor that is localized and may be intra- or extraconal. Biopsy shows an unencapsulated tumor composed of rounded masses of cells with abundant granular acidophilic cytoplasmic granules and paracentral or eccentric nuclei. No mitotic activity or necrosis is present.[52,53] The granules are PAS-positive. The findings are consistent with granular cell tumor or granular cell myoblastoma.

The origin of granular cell tumor is unknown. The entity may represent a metabolic derangement, reactive process, or abnormal storage disease related to muscle degeneration rather than a primary neoplastic process. In the lid, the tumor may be associated with pseudoepitheliomatous hyperplasia.

Management of Intraconal Tumors

Treatment of an intraconal mass requires an excisional biopsy. A small mass that is causing minimal proptosis may be followed, but because the diagnosis cannot be established without a biopsy, the biopsy should eventually be performed, particularly if growth is demonstrated.

In general, biopsy necessitates an excisional biopsy, removal of the entire mass, through a Krönlein or lateral approach. This approach affords enough space to remove the mass. Posterior apical tumors, particularly schwannomas with their apical extension, may require a combined neurosurgical (frontal craniotomy) approach. Schwannomas may be firmly adherent at the orbital apex.

While cavernous hemangiomas are entirely benign, hemangiopericytomas may metastasize in 15 percent of cases, and aggressive treatment is therefore necessary.[39–41] Orbital recurrence occurred in 30 percent of

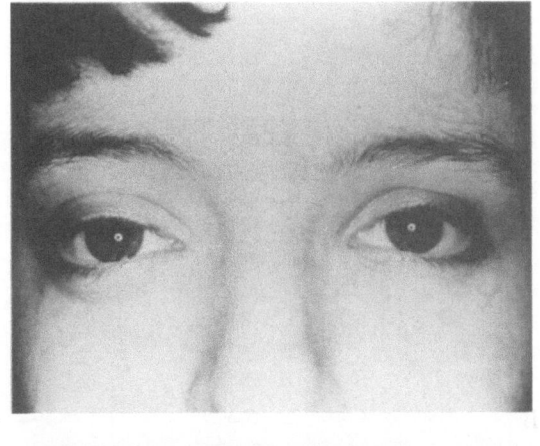

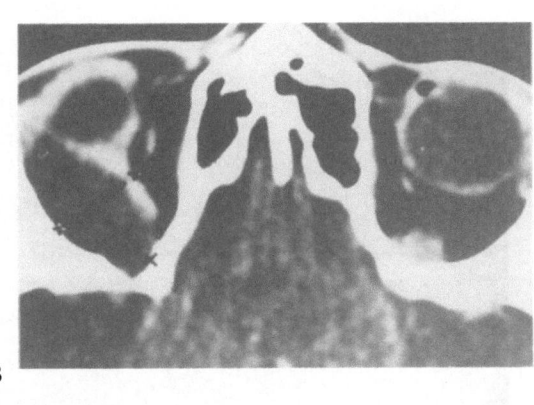

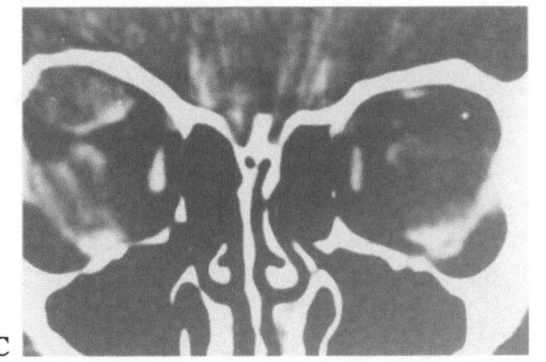

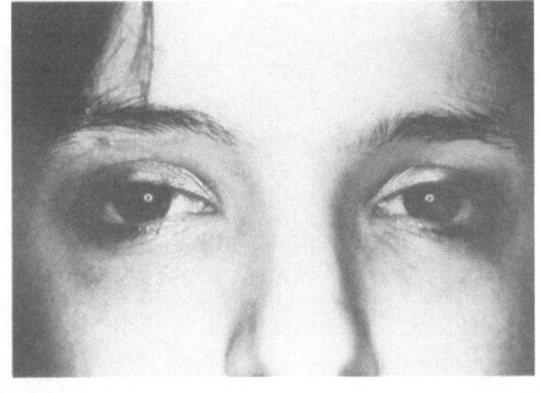

Fig. 3-13. (*A*) A 28-year-old female with 1-year history of diplopia on upgaze and right frontal headache. (*B,C*) CT scan shows encapsulated extraconal mass that extends into orbital apex. Biopsy was consistent with schwannoma. (*D*) Appearance of patient 1 month after surgery. All three extraoptic nerve intraconal tumors, cavernous hemangioma, schwannoma, and hemangiopericytoma may present as extraconal encapsulated masses. (Patient referred by Dr. William DiGiacomo, Union, NJ.)

the patients (eight patients) at a median interval of 2.9 years in the largest series reported.[39] In one patient, local intraconal extension was treated with frontal craniotomy and the patient is alive without recurrence after 10 years.

Malignant degeneration of a schwannoma is rare but may occur; therefore, excisional biopsy is imperative. The diagnosis of neurofibromatosis should be considered in all patients with a schwannoma.

The tumors discussed above are the most likely intraconal tumors to be encountered. Other tumors may occur.

Cavernous Hemangioma

Cavernous hemangioma is a reddish blue to purple, well-encapsulated tumor that on sectioning displays a honeycomb pattern corresponding to the endothelial-lined, large, "cavernous," dilated, blood-filled spaces. Cavernous hemangiomas should not be confused with capillary hemangiomas that are congenital or develop during the first year of life and start to involute after

the first year of life. Cavernous hemangiomas do not involute and may have smooth muscle in their wall surrounding the endothelial-lined channels (Fig. 3-15).

Hemangiopericytoma

Hemangiopericytomas are tannish in color and may have irregular bosselations. The tumor is often friable because the capsule is thin in certain areas. The cells are arranged about vascular channels that are often collapsed and that have elongated cleft-like lumen. The proliferating cells may surround vascular channels like ribbons or may compress the vascular spaces in a palisading pattern. A storiform or cartwheel pattern suggests the diagnosis of fibrous histiocytoma (see "Unencapsulated Diffuse Tumors").

Each cell of the hemangiopericytoma is invested by reticulin fibers and the tumor cells are outside the reticulin sheath of the blood vessels. The tumor is composed of spindle-shaped cells with minimal nuclear atypia and oval nuclei. In general, pathologic features cannot be

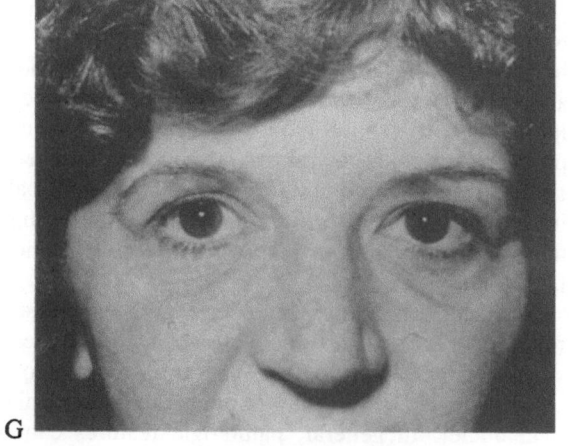

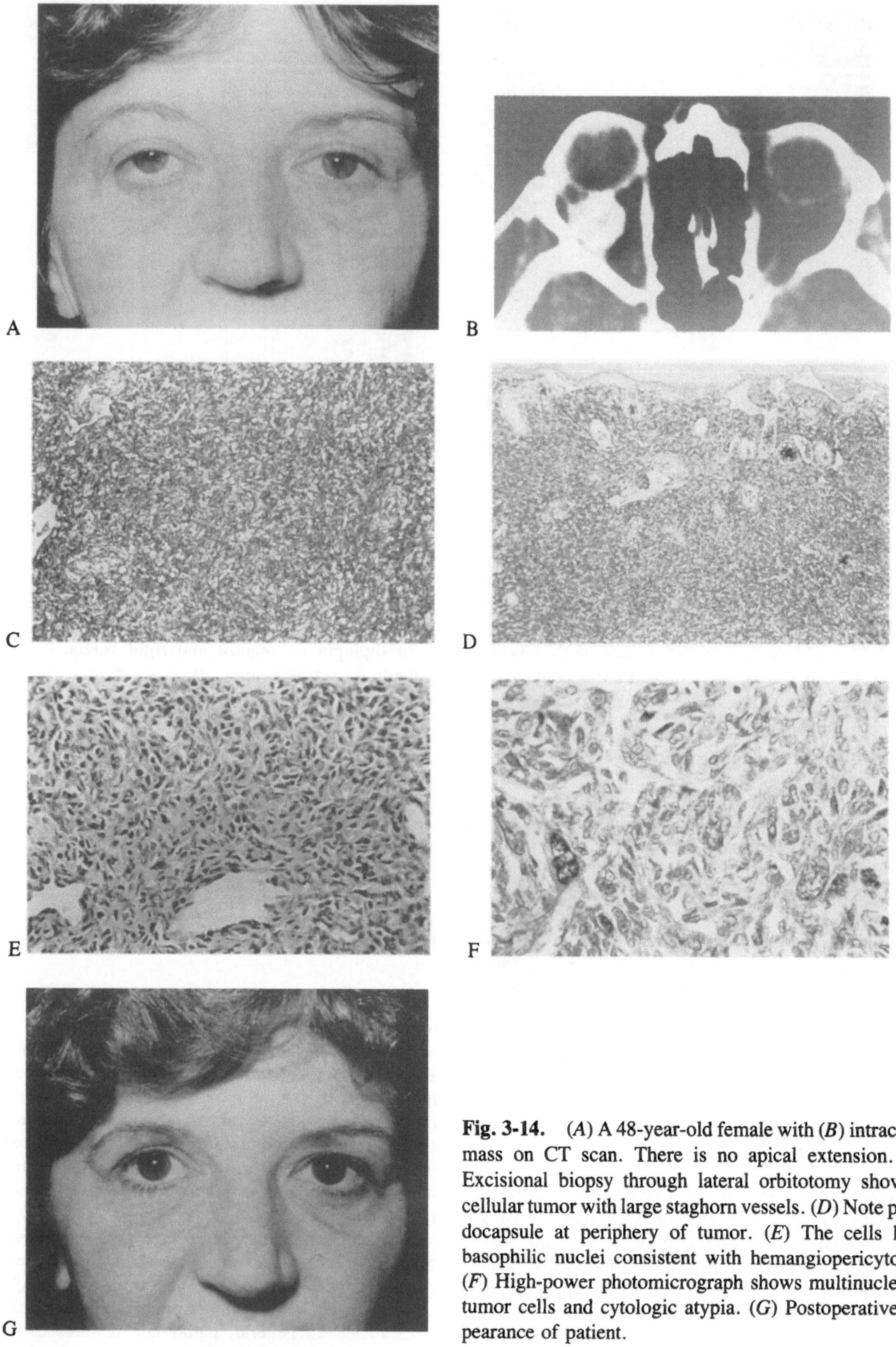

Fig. 3-14. (*A*) A 48-year-old female with (*B*) intraconal mass on CT scan. There is no apical extension. (*C*) Excisional biopsy through lateral orbitotomy shows a cellular tumor with large staghorn vessels. (*D*) Note pseudocapsule at periphery of tumor. (*E*) The cells have basophilic nuclei consistent with hemangiopericytoma. (*F*) High-power photomicrograph shows multinucleated tumor cells and cytologic atypia. (*G*) Postoperative appearance of patient.

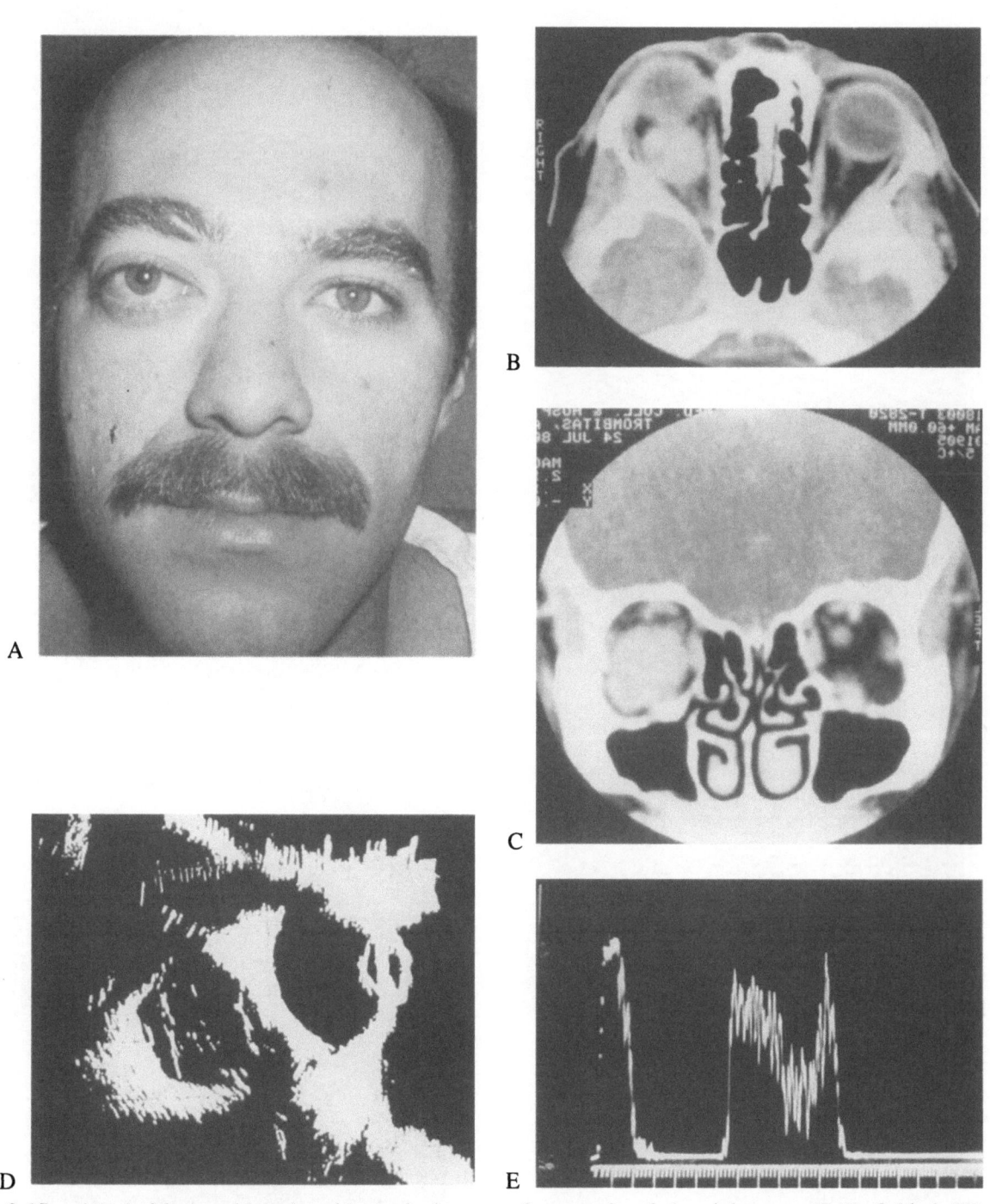

Fig. 3-15. (*A*) A 36-year-old male with gradual onset of proptosis of the right eye. (*B,C*) Orbital CT scan shows an intraconal mass that enhances with contrast. (*D*) B scan shows a well-demarcated intraconal tumor while (*E*) A scan shows a heterogeneous echo pattern with high-amplitude internal echoes and minimal attenuation due to the various fibrous septae within the tumor. (*F*) Tumor was removed with a cryoprobe through a lateral orbitotomy. (*G,H*) Intraoperatively, an encapsulated tumor that showed many fibrous septae between the vascular spaces was found. (*I,J*) Microscopic examination shows a tumor composed of "cavernous"-sized blood-filled spaces separated by fibrous septae and lined by endothelium. (*K*) Postoperative appearance of patient showing resolution of proptosis.

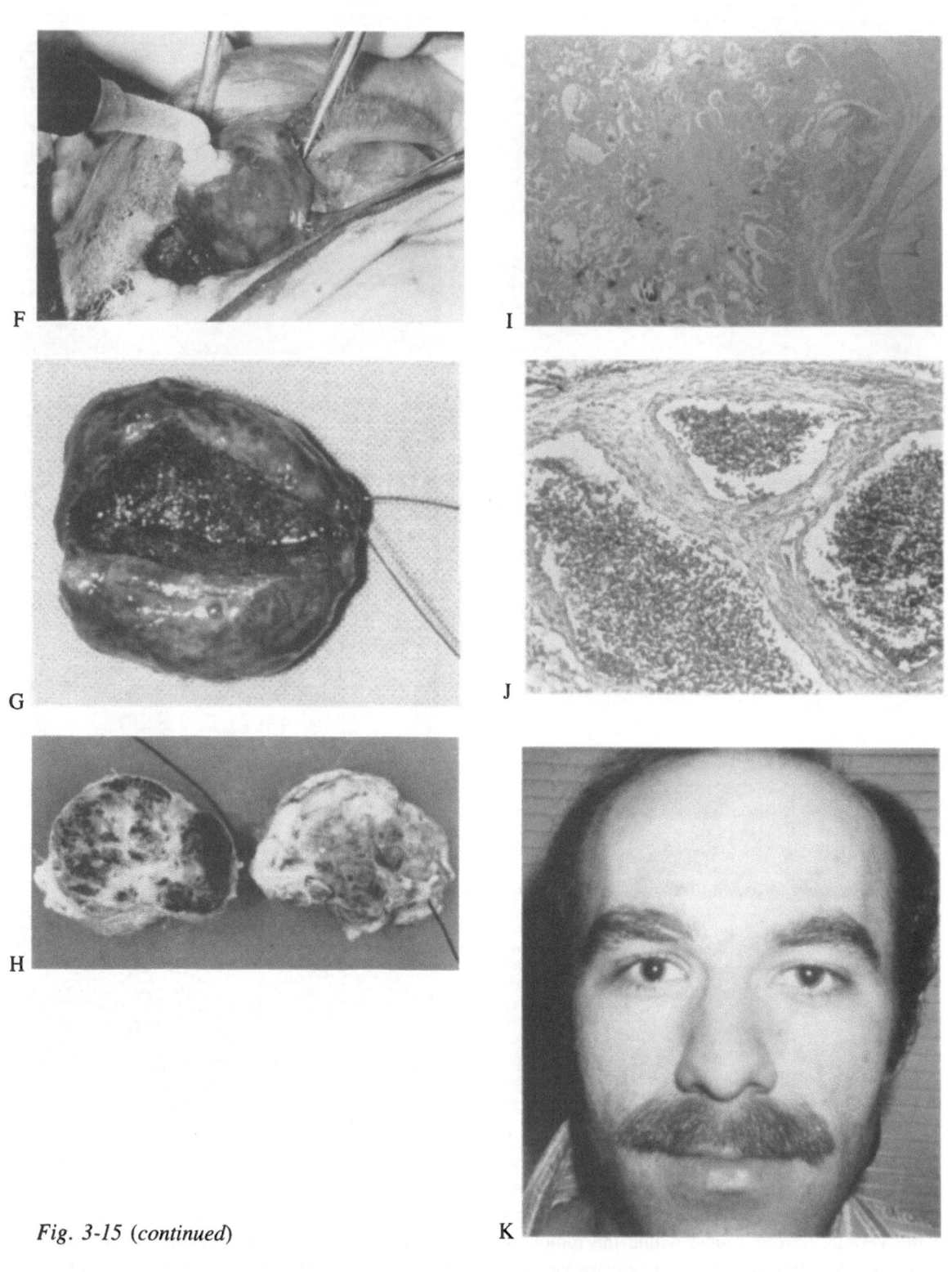

Fig. 3-15 (continued)

correlated with clinical and biologic behavior (Fig. 3-14). While the tumors appear encapsulated on CT scan, pathologically a pseudocapsule of compressed orbital tissue is present.

The pathologic differential diagnosis of orbital heman-

giopericytoma includes angioblastic meningioma and fibrous histiocytoma. The former tumor presents as an intracranial mass attached to the dura. Electron microscopy may be helpful.

Schwannoma

Schwannoma may also have a tannish capsule and if incised, the yellow "slimy" mustard-like contents are evident. Schwannomas are encapsulated with solid and cystic areas corresponding to mucinous degeneration or thrombosis with hemorrhagic areas containing xanthoma cells and hemosiderin-laden macrophages. Solid cellular areas are Antoni A. Tightly arranged cellular areas may contain Verocay bodies that have polarized palisading nuclei. Hyalinized areas surrounded by palisading cells may give the impression of pacinian (tactile) corpuscles. Antoni B areas contain stellate cells loosely arranged in a myxomatous or mucinous matrix that is alcian-blue negative, while such areas are alcian-blue positive in neurofibromas. Hyalinization, calcification, and necrosis may be present. The number of mitotic figures influences prognosis (Fig. 3-12).

Schwannoma and optic nerve glioma may have an indistinguishable cellular pattern. In these instances, the clinical location of the tumor is helpful in the differential diagnosis. Optic gliomas are intradural, while schwannomas are outside the central nervous system (CNS) and involve peripheral nerves. Vision is affected quite early in glioma. The presence of arachnoidal tissue or Rosenthal fibers (hyalinized lipocytic degenerated glioma cells that appear brightly eosinophilic) is typical of glioma. Electron microscopy (EM) may be helpful.[38,49–51]

Isolated Neurofibroma

Biopsy for isolated neurofibromas has been described elsewhere. The tumor is unencapsulated. At the time of surgery, the tumor is found attached to a peripheral nerve. The localized neurofibromas are discrete orbital masses that are often multiple and because of their association with sensory orbital nerves often present with anesthesia or mild pain. When completely excised, they do not recur, unlike diffuse or plexiform neurofibromas.

Intravascular Papillary Endothelial Hyperplasia (IPEH) (Benign Papillary Endothelial Hyperplasia)

Benign papillary endothelial hyperplasia appears red in color. The tumor is intimately attached to a vessel wall that contains the endothelial cells from which it arises. The tumor is composed of multiple layers of endothelial cells that have collagenous cores. An associated hemangioma, hematoma, arteriovenous malformation, or lymphangioma may be present. These tumors may be pathologically confused with angiosarcoma. They are difficult to resect.

FOCAL TUMORS

Clinical Features and CT Appearance

Focal tumors that grow inside or outside the muscle cone (intraconal or extraconal) are a nonspecific group of benign tumors that include the intraconal tumors described above and a number of other benign tumors (see Table 3-6). Many of the latter tumors are benign spindle cell tumors including fibroma, nodular fasciitis (see Chapter 8), rhabdomyoma, leiomyoma, chondroma, and spindle cell lipoma. The benign spindle cell tumors have malignant counterparts that are diffuse and described in a separate chapter.

On CT scan, all such tumors appear solid except for the spindle cell lipoma, which may appear as a radiolucent orbital "cyst." Any of the malignant counterparts of the spindle cell tumors may be localized, although they are more often diffuse.

Biopsy Results

Fibroma, Nodular Fasciitis, Rhabdomyoma, Leiomyoma, Myxoma, Chondroma, Spindle Cell Lipoma (See also Chapter 8). A myxoma is an extremely rare form of fibroblastic proliferation consisting of stellate spindle cells that are widely separated by a mucinous matrix of hyaluronic acid. Normal fibroblasts have the

Table 3-6
Focal Intraconal or Extraconal (Noncystic)

Benign vascular tumors
Fibroma
Nodular fasciitis
Rhabdomyoma
Leiomyoma
Chondroma
Spindle cell lipoma
Myxoma
Metastatic carcinoma
Metastatic neuroblastoma
Ewing's sarcoma
JXG or xanthogranuloma in adults
Teratoma
Leiomyoma
Kaposi's sarcoma
Varix
Granular cell myoblastoma
Lipoma
Juvenile fibromatosis—extraconal with lid component

potential to produce collagen and hyaluronic acid as in this rare tumor (also see "malignant cells").[53]

Spindle Cell Lipoma. Biopsy shows a circumscribed but unencapsulated mass composed of mature adult lipocytes (spindle) cells and many capillaries. The spindle cells are uniform without pleomorphism, atypia, or mitotic figures. No necrosis is present. The biopsy is consistent with spindle cell lipoma, a tumor first described by Enzinger in 1975 in the neck and shoulders of men aged 45 to 65 years.[53–56] Grossly, the tumor appears variegated with yellow areas of fat and gray-white areas of spindle cells.

FOCAL (CYSTIC) WITH BONE INVOLVEMENT

Dermoid cyst, epidermal inclusion cyst, encephalocele, meningocele, and mucocele. See Chapters 2 and 4.

DIFFUSE (INTRACONAL AND EXTRACONAL) NONCYSTIC ORBITAL TUMORS

Clinical Features and CT Appearance

Certain tumors will present as a mass lesion generally with minimal or no inflammatory signs (Tables 3-7 and 3-8). Some conditions listed in the table are discussed more appropriately in other chapters. Aside from fibrous histiocytoma and rhabdomyosarcoma, other mesenchymal tumors of the orbit are distinctly rare and include (1) malignant fibrosarcoma, (2) leiomyosarcoma, (3) liposarcoma, (4) chondrosarcoma and extraskeletal mesenchymal chondrosarcoma, (5) angiosarcoma, and (6) postradiation sarcoma.

Fibrous histiocytoma is the most common primary mesenchymal orbital tumor of adults. The tumor may be entirely benign, locally aggressive, or frankly malignant. When benign, the lesion may be predominantly intraconal or extraconal; however, when locally aggressive or malignant, the entire orbit and/or adjacent paranasal sinus may be involved (Fig. 3-16). Bone destruction may accompany malignant tumors. In the largest series of 150 cases of orbital fibrous histiocytoma, in four patients the entire orbit was involved and in nine cases, the adjacent sinus was involved.[57] The tumor has a definite predilection for the superior nasal orbit. There is moderate-to-marked enhancement on contrast injection.

Fibromatoses are to be distinguished from fibrous histiocytoma and from fibrosis that occurs as a sequella of

Table 3-7
Diffuse (Intraconal and Extraconal) Noncystic Tumors

Lymphoid infiltrate (see Chapter 2)
Pseudotumor (sclerosing)
Orbital hemorrhage (see "Peripheral Tumors")
Amyloid
Leukemia
Sinus histiocytosis (may be bilateral)[†]
Spindle cell tumors
   fibrous histiocytoma
   hemangiopericytoma
   Erdheim-Chester disease (if bilateral)
   fibromatosis (myofibromatosis) may be congenital
   fibrosarcoma
   leiomyosarcoma
   malignant schwannoma
   neurofibroma
   malignant neurofibroma
   malignant chondrosarcoma (medial orbit)[*]
   liposarcoma
   myxosarcoma
   angiosarcoma
   postradiation sarcoma
   undifferentiated sarcoma

[*] may have adjacent bone invasion
[†] see pediatric section

inflammation. Clinical and pathologic correlations are helpful in this regard. For example, nodular fasciitis is a reactive localized fibrous proliferation that often follows trauma.[58] In addition, a sclerosing process may result from (1) orbital or peritoneal hemorrhage, (2) a sclerosing pseudotumor or other idiopathic inflammation, (3) fibro-

Table 3-8
Diffuse Tumors of Predominantly Children

Rhabdomyosarcoma[*†]
Granulocytic sarcoma[*†]
Metastatic neuroblastoma[†]
Metastatic Ewing's sarcoma[*§]
Alveolar soft part sarcoma (young adults) involve EOM, may be localized[*§]
Sinus histiocytosis
Endodermal sinus tumor
Heterotopic brain tissue
Capillary hemangioma—may be predominantly lid
Undifferentiated sarcoma

[*] may have adjacent bone invasion
[†] see pediatric section
[§] one known case of primary Ewing's of orbital roof

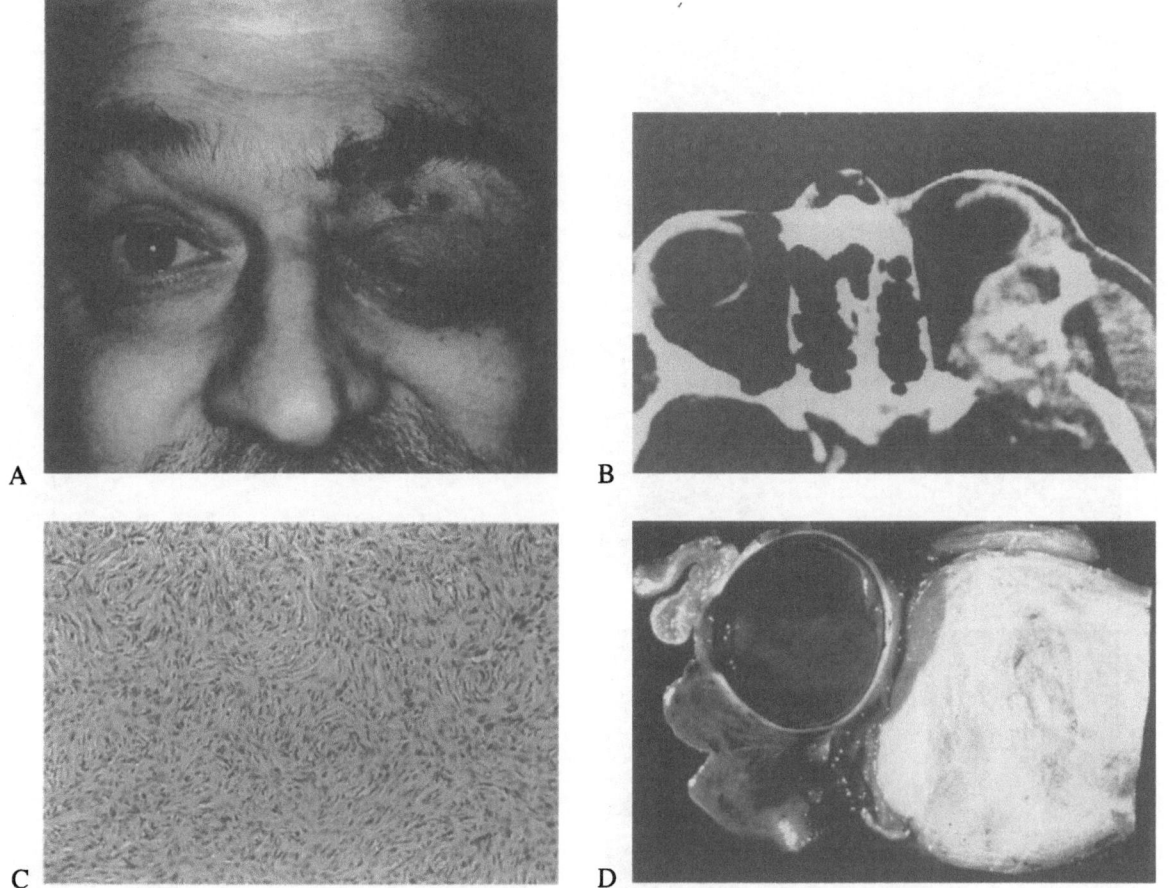

Fig. 3-16. (*A*) A 66-year-old male with rapid onset of proptosis with downward displacement of the left globe and ptosis over a 4-month period. (*B*) CT scan shows diffuse orbital tumor extending from lateral aspect of orbit through lateral orbital wall with destruction of bone. (*C*) Biopsy showed a markedly cellular tumor composed of spindle cells arranged in a storiform or cartwheel pattern (AFIP ACC #1186030). On high-power magnification (not shown), there was significant cytologic typia with several mitotic figures per high-power field. Some cells had plump nuclei with prominent nucleoli and ample cytoplasm and resembled "histiocytes." (*D*) Exenteration specimen shows solid nature of tumor (AFIP ACC #1207030).

sis of a tumor such as a ruptured dermoid cyst or sclerosing hemangioma, or (4) fibrosis about a retained foreign body. The presence of hemosiderin will suggest a previous hemorrhage. Polarization of a slide will help rule out a retained foreign body.

Neural tumors such as malignant schwannoma and benign or malignant neurofibroma may occur as diffuse tumors of the orbit. Therefore, in all patients with diffuse orbital tumors, a history and general physical examination should be performed to rule out systemic neurofibromatosis (Fig. 3-17). Five or six café-au-lait spots establish the diagnosis of neurofibromatosis. Multiple pedunculated neurofibromas may be present. Most neurofibromas of the orbit are plexiform or diffuse, while localized neurofibromas are uncommon. The latter type tend to be multiple and occur in middle-aged adults. Approximately 12 percent of localized cases are associated with systemic neurofibromatosis.[51]

Liposarcomas tend to have an indolent course with proptosis occurring slowly over years. Mesenchymal chondrosarcoma tends to occur in the bones but also may affect the soft tissues of the orbit. The tumor affects females in early adulthood aged 19 to 34; metastases to the lung has occurred years after the onset of proptosis.

Role of Radiation in Treatment of Diffuse Orbital Tumors

In all patients with a diffuse tumor, a history of radiation therapy should be obtained. Patients with inherited retinoblastoma tend to develop secondary soft tissue sarcomas especially osteogenic sarcoma of the femur. The incidence of second tumors is probably not related to prior radiation but appears to be associated with the

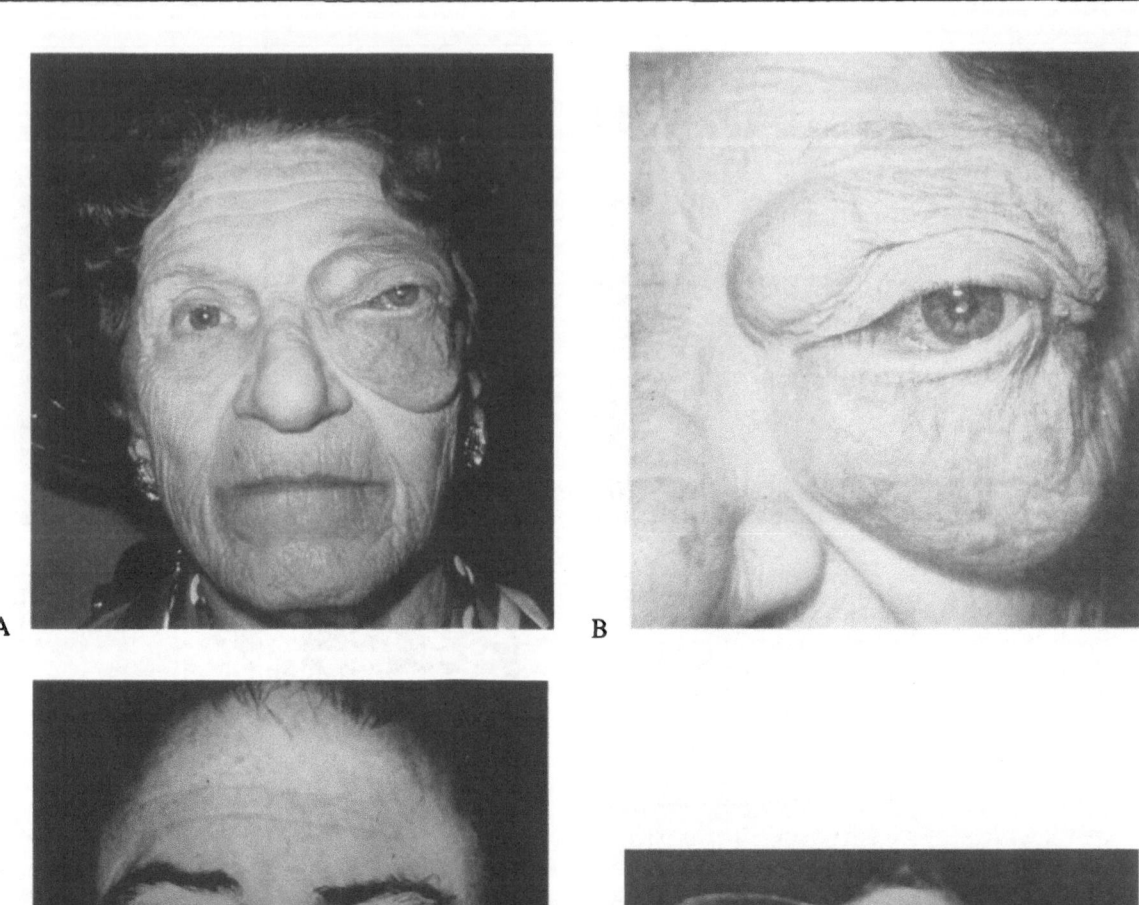

Fig. 3-17. (*A,B*) A 72-year-old female with longstanding history of neurofibromatosis involving left orbit. (*C*) A 54-year-old patient with gradual onset of proptosis of the right eye. (*D*) CT scan showed a diffuse homogeneous orbital tumor with extension into the ethmoid sinus. Biopsy of tumor showed a diffuse spindle cell tumor consistent with neurofibroma. Patient had other stigmata of neurofibromatosis.

retinoblastoma (RB) gene, which, in turn, is associated with the inherited form of retinoblastoma.[59] Inherited RB is manifest in several ways: (1) bilateral RB, (2) multifocal unilateral RB, (3) unilateral RB with a family history of RB, and rarely (d) unilateral RB without a family history with an early age of onset of 2.4 months rather than 24 months associated with the uninherited form of the disease. The chance of developing a second tumor increases from 10 percent at 10 years of age to 30 percent at 20 years of age. The types of tumors include most commonly osteogenic sarcoma, fibrosarcoma, leiomyosarcoma, and other soft tissue sarcomas (Fig. 3-18).

Fibrosarcoma of the orbit may spread from the orbit to an adjacent sinus or from the sinus to the orbit. Rapid onset of proptosis due to leiomyosarcoma of the orbit occurred after radiation for bilateral RB in two patients aged 25 and 30 years.[60–61]

It is interesting to note that leukemias, relatively common in the general population, are distinctly rare after radiation. Epithelial neoplasms may also occur. Rarely, basal cell carcinoma, squamous cell carcinoma, and sebaceous gland carcinoma have been reported. Patients with craniofacial dysostoses treated with radiotherapy may also develop secondary sarcomas.

Secondary tumors including lid melanoma and orbital

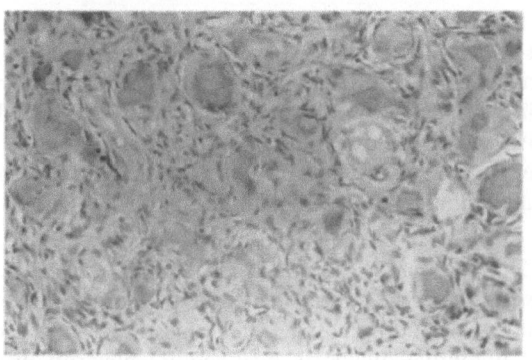

Fig. 3-18. Osteogenic sarcoma in femur of patient with history of bilateral retinoblastoma (AFIP ACC #1427982).

malignant fibrous histiocytoma have been reported after radiation therapy for rhabdomyosarcoma.[62] While tumors after RB may occur later in life, tumors that are secondary to radiation of the head and neck unrelated to the RB gene tend to occur in the first two decades of life.

Liposarcomas have not been reported after radiation for RB and have a more indolent course of proptosis. CT scan shows a radiolucency.[55]

Other mesenchymal tumors including angiosarcoma and mesenchymal chondrosarcoma, both of which have not been reported after radiation in the orbital area tend to occur in the first four decades of life.[63–64] A review of the literature regarding orbital angiosarcoma showed that the median age at the time of diagnosis was 11 years. Two reported cases of mesenchymal chondrosarcoma have been females aged 19–34 years. This tumor may occur in the bones or soft tissues of the orbit. Metastases have occurred to the lung after a long clinical course.

Diffuse Tumors Originating from the Adjacent Ocular Adnexal Structures

Sebaceous gland carcinoma of the lid or caruncle, malignant mixed tumor of the lacrimal gland, and adenoid cystic carcinoma of the lacrimal gland may have an explosive onset with diffuse orbital involvement (see Chapters 6 and 8). Such tumors of the lacrimal gland should always be considered when the process is advanced and fills the lateral portion of the orbit and extends both inside and outside the muscle cone. The location of the tumor at its onset is helpful in the differential diagnosis. For example, sebaceous gland carcinoma will originate in the lids or caruncle, while malignant mixed tumor and adenoid cystic carcinoma will originate in the lacrimal gland. Malignant mixed tumor often arises from a preexisting pleomorphic adenoma (benign mixed tumor), while adenoid cystic carcinoma arises de novo. In addition, a basal cell carcinoma or squamous cell carcinoma of the

lid or the limbus may fill the orbit. In the latter cases, there is generally a fairly long history of growth over years for basal cell carcinoma and several months to years for squamous cell carcinoma.

CT Features of Diffuse Orbital Tumors

CT scan will show both an intraconal and extraconal involvement. The most common lesion to present in this way is a lymphoid infiltrate and presents as a homogeneous mass that molds around the globe and does not cause bone destruction (see Chapter 2). On CT scan, rhabdomyosarcomas are also homogeneous lesions but unlike lymphoid infiltrates, rhabdomyosarcomas are quite aggressive and may extend into the paranasal sinuses, nasopharynx, and brain. Extensive bone destruction may occur. Moderate enchancement occurs after contrast injection (see Chapter 4).

The malignant counterparts of fibroma, leiomyoma, lipoma, chondroma, and the extremely rare myxoma are more likely to be diffuse on CT scan and have few, if any, differentiating CT features. Lipomas and liposarcomas tend to have a low density (fat density) similar to that of dermoids. Chondrosarcomas may invade the orbit secondarily from the adjacent ethmoid sinus, while mesenchymal chondrosarcomas tend to involve the orbital bones. Chondrosarcomas show foci of calcification on CT scan. The advantage of CT scan over MRI in showing calcifications is significant. The benign variants are almost without exception well-localized either intraconally or extraconally.

Erdheim-Chester disease is a systemic lipoid granulomatosis that involves the orbit, bones, lung, heart, and retroperitoneum. Ophthalmic complications include optic neuropathy and lid lesions that are more indurated than the garden variety xanthelasma. The condition often affects both orbits. The serum lipids are generally not abnormal, although the histiocytes show the presence of cytoplasmic cholesterol.

Amyloidosis. Amyloid depositions may occur in the extraocular muscles, levator, subconjunctival space, or as diffuse depositions in the orbit that may be calcified on CT scan. The conjunctival form is generally not associated with systemic disease, although a recent report of lymphoma in the scapula in an amyloid stroma was associated with a large asymptomatic amyloid nodule.[65,66]

Diffuse Orbital Tumors—Management

A diffuse orbital tumor warrants a histologic permanent section diagnosis before definitive therapy is recommended. Incisional biopsy is performed and often may be performed under local anesthesia through the eyelid.

Diffuse Orbital Tumors—Management Based on Biopsy

Fibrous Histiocytoma and Hemangiopericytoma. Biopsy shows spindle-shaped fibroblast-like cells and plump histiocytic-like cells arranged in a storiform (cartwheel or whorled) pattern. Foamy xanthoma cells, multinucleated benign giant cells, and anaplastic bizarre giant cells are also present. Number of mitoses, degree of nuclear pleomorphism, hypercellularity, and the overall lack of circumscribed pattern favor a malignant over a benign fibrous histiocytoma. Histologic parameters are correlated with prognosis.

Pathologically, fibrous histiocytoma may be confused with nodular fasciitis.[57] The latter condition is a benign reactive nodular proliferation of connective tissue that is rapidly growing and has also been confused with fibrosarcoma because of its often alarming cytologic features. Inflammation often accompanies the lesion. This lesion has an abrupt, often painful onset and rapid growth phase that may follow trauma. It is a localized growth that usually occurs in subcutaneous and fascial tissues such as the lid and eyebrow and rarely the orbit.

Complete surgical excision of fibrous histiocytoma usually requires exenteration in advanced cases. Local radiation offers limited if any value.

Incompletely excised benign tumors may be observed. Incompletely excised malignant tumors probably require more radical excision or exenteration.

The pathologic description of hemangiopericytoma has been described above. Diffuse recurrent tumors may be treated with reexcision. Radiotherapy may be of benefit for multiple recurrences. The threat of metastases, although low, must be weighed in the treatment of any recurrent hemangiopericytoma. The CO_2 laser is helpful in eradicating bleeding diffuse hemangiopercytomas.

Erdheim-Chester Disease. Biposy shows sheet of xanthomatous histiocytic cells including Touton giant cells; interspersed lymphocytes and plasma cells are present with marked sclerosis. This systemic histiocytic disorder involves the viscera (lungs, hearts, and kidneys) and metaphyses of long tubular bones. A medical consult is recommended; oral prednisone results in partial response (Fig. 3-19).[67]

Neurofibroma. Biopsy shows interwoven bundles of Schwann's cells, peripheral nerve axons, and endoneural fibroblasts. Plexiform neurofibromas are considered pathognomic of neurofibromatosis and unlike diffuse neurofibromas, the proliferation of cellular elements occurs within a distinct perineural sheath. The nuclei of neural tumors are eel-like and wavy unlike the spindle-shaped nuclei of fibroblastic tumors that have sharp tips or the cigar-shaped nuclei that arise from smooth muscle tumors such as leiomyoma.[68]

The treatment of neurofibromatosis is relatively simple

in the case of localized neurofibromas that, although not encapsulated, may be surgically shelled out without recurrence. The diffuse forms tend to be more vascular than the localized forms and often recur. The CO_2 laser is helpful in the treatment of such tumors.

Malignant neurofibromas are extremely rare and are treated similarly to malignant fibrous histiocytomas.

Angiosarcoma, Fibrosarcoma, Leiomyosarcoma, Liposarcoma, and Chondrosarcoma. Many spindle cell tumors are undifferentiated and are so rare in the orbit that definitive diagnosis may require electron microscopy. These EM features are beyond the scope of this book.[63–64]

Angiosarcoma. Biopsy shows small, dilated, blood-filled anastomosing vascular channels lined by hyperchromatic endothelial cells. In some areas, the endothelial cells form intraluminal buds and papillary projections. There is often a spindle cell component that does not form vascular channels. The spindle cells are arranged in compact bundles and have indistinct cell outlines and small nucleoli. Undifferentiated areas consist of pleomorphic polygonal cells with frequent mitoses. The endothelial nature of the tumors is confirmed on EM where typical Weibel Palade bodies are found. FVIIIRA, a component of factor VIII (antihemophiliac factor) synthesized by endothelial cells or UEAI, a lectin which is a plant or animal protein that has a marked affinity for endothelial cell membranes, may be demonstrated immunohistochemically.[63]

Fibrosarcoma. Biopsy shows spindle cells in a dense cellular herring-bone pattern. The tips of the nuclei are tapered to a point unlike the nuclei of leiomyosarcoma, which are blunt, rounded, and cigar-shaped. Mitotic figures suggest malignancy. Fibrosarcomas that are radiation-induced as in all soft tissue radiation-induced sarcomas show marked nuclear pleomorphism and tumor giant cells.

Fibromas are less cellular with no atypia or mitoses. Intercellular collagen is abundant. Fibromatosis describes a group of tumors that are more aggressive than fibromas yet less aggressive than fibrosarcomas (see Chapter 7). Again, while fibromatoses are cellular and locally infiltrating, they lack the anaplasia or mitotic activity of fibrosarcoma. An excellent review of this subject has been recently published.[69]

Leiomyosarcoma, Liposarcoma, and Chondrosarcoma. Smooth muscle tumors typically have cigar-shaped blunt ended nuclei.[68] The cells form fascicles with palisading of the nuclei. A perinuclear halo can be seen in some tumor cells cut in cross-section due to separation of the myofilaments from the nucleus. The PAS stain may show intracytoplasmic glycogen. The tumor may have significant collagen. A prominent vascu-

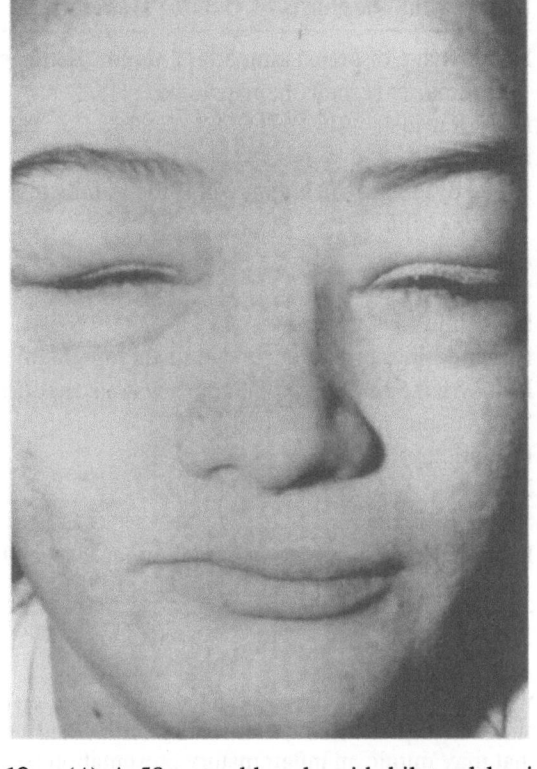

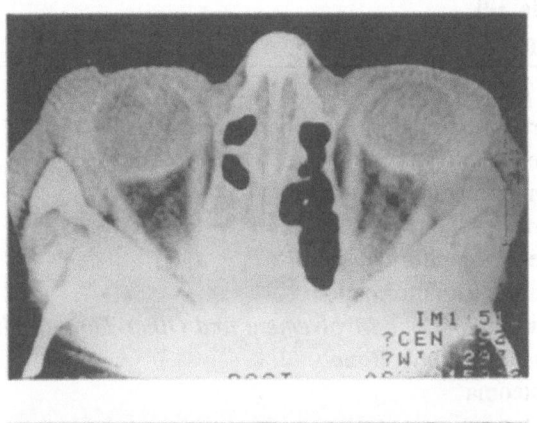

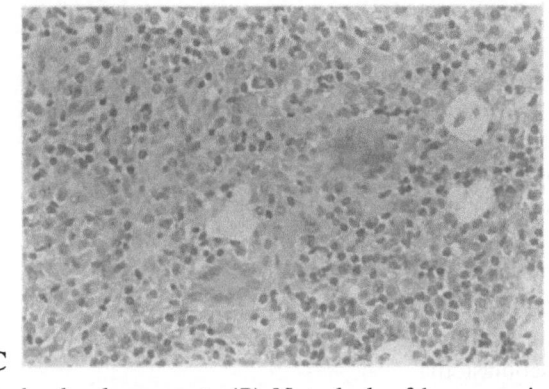

Fig. 3-19. (*A*) A 58-year-old male with bilateral lacrimal gland enlargement. (*B*) Note lack of bone erosion on CT scan. (*C*) Biopsy showed sheets of histiocytic cells containing lipid. Diagnosis of Erdheim-Chester disease was confirmed, but there was no visceral or bone involvement. The patient was treated with oral prednisone with only a partial response.

lar pattern resembling hemangiopericytoma is characteristic.

Both liposarcoma and chondrosarcomas may occur. Both tumors have a prominent vascular pattern. Cartilaginous differentiation will be present in the latter tumor, while in the former, a myxoid pattern with prominent plexiform capillary pattern is present. Hyaluronic acid is present in the myxoid areas.

Mesenchymal chondrosarcoma contain islands of cartilage and primitive mesenchymal cells in the stroma that mimic hemangiopericytoma.[64]

Amyloid

Biopsy shows large accumulations of homogeneous pink subepithelial material stained with congo-red and showing apple-green birefringence with polarized light. Conjunctival amyloidosis is generally not a sign of systemic disease and is most often found after inflammatory local conditions such as trachoma and more rarely chronic recurring uveitis, rheumatoid arthritis, and Churg-Strauss syndrome (allergic granulomatosis and angiitis). Recently, conjunctival amyloid has been reported to be associated with an extranodal lymphoma. The association of primary amyloidosis that involves the lids and multiple myeloma is well known (see Chapter 8).[65–66]

DIFFUSE CYSTIC TUMORS

Microphthalmos with cyst, congenital cystic eyeball, lymphangioma, and kratoma. Also see Chapter 4.

PERIPHERAL TUMORS

Peripheral tumors may be in the peripheral surgical space or subperiosteal and adjacent to bone. Because of their adjacency to bone, secondary bone erosion may occur and is better visualized on CT than MR scan. In addition, tumors of the bone are also considered in this chapter. While the tumors and disease processes listed

Table 3-9
Peripheral Tumors

Soft Tissue
    Orbital or subperiosteal hemorrhage
    Hematic cyst
    Cholesteatoma
    Arteriovenous malformation
    Venous malformation
    Vascular malformation
Sinus and/or Bone Involvement and Other Tumors That
Primarily Involve Bone
    Osteoma
    Osteogenic sarcoma
    Fibrous dysplasia
    Ossifying fibroma
    Cavernous hemangioma of bone
    Meningioma of orbital roof
    Chordoma
    Aneurysmal bone cyst
    Paget's disease
    Metastatic neuroblastoma
    Lipoma of frontal bone
    Giant cell tumor (osteoclastoma)
    Osteoblastoma
    Reparative granuloma
    Infantile cortical hyperostosis (Caffey's syndrome)
    Brown tumor
    Melanoma

Table 3-10
Differential Diagnosis of Orbital Hemorrhage

Hemorrhage of preexisting orbital tumor (hemangiopericytoma, cavernous hemangioma)
Hypertension
Labor
Blood dyscrasias including von Willebrand's disease and hemophilia
Anemia
Scurvy
Leukemia
Ruptured intraorbital aneursym of the ophthalmic artery
Hemorrhage of preexisting arteriovenous malformation or venous malformation
Hematic cyst
Malaria
Sickle cell anemia
Hemorrhage of preexisting orbital tumor, especially neuroblastoma, often bilateral

in Table 3-9 tend to occur in peripheral locations within the orbit, many may occur anywhere within the orbit. Tumors that originate in the adjacent sinuses and invade the peripheral orbit will be analyzed in a separate section.

Many of the entities that present in the peripheral orbit have clinical features that are more easily understood in conjunction with the CT findings. For this reason, both the CT findings and clinical features will be discussed in the following section. Soft tissue peripheral tumors will be analyzed before intrinsic osseous tumors. The management of such tumors is also considered.

Clinical Features and CT Scan Findings

CT scan shows a soft tissue mass adjacent to bone without significant bone involvement.

Orbital Hemorrhage.   The differential diagnosis of orbital hemorrhage is listed in Table 3-10.

Of the soft tissue tumors that may occur in the peripheral orbit, many are of vascular origin and may present with orbital hemorrhage. Such patients will often develop sudden proptosis, conjunctival injection, and chemosis that may mimic an inflammatory presentation (see Chapter 2). Often the patient has sudden pain and vomiting. The onset may be more gradual (Fig. 3-20). A preliminary diagnosis of orbital cellulitis or malignant orbital tumor is often made.[70] Any malformation with an arterial component will have an accompanying bruit or palpable thrill.[71] Similarly, a venous malformation characteristically enlarges on dependent positioning.[72]

An orbital varix or venous malformation may present with orbital hemorrhage (Fig. 3-21). Patients develop proptosis that is intermittent and positional. Bloody tears may also accompany an orbital varix. Should the varix thrombose, an indurated mass may be palpable and the proptosis may not increase on Valsalva's maneuver. In addition, thrombosis may lead to an inflammatory-type presentation. Secondary orbital hemorrhage may also occur.

Pulsating exophthalmos may be present with an arterial venous malformation. Strictly venous malformations such as varix do not have pulsations. *Dynamic proptosis* is a term that may be substituted for pulsating exophthalmos; it may be a better term because in some patients, these are not pulsations.[73] Dynamic proptosis can be defined as exophthalmos that occurs when a variable force is applied to the orbital contents under certain pathologic conditions such as orbital varix (see Chapter 1). In the case of varix, the dynamic proptosis is induced by head position, jugular compression, Valsalva's maneuver, or mastication. The direction of the proptosis is dependent on the location of the hemorrhage. Subperiosteal orbital hemorrhage may occur rarely and is most common in children or young adults after trauma.

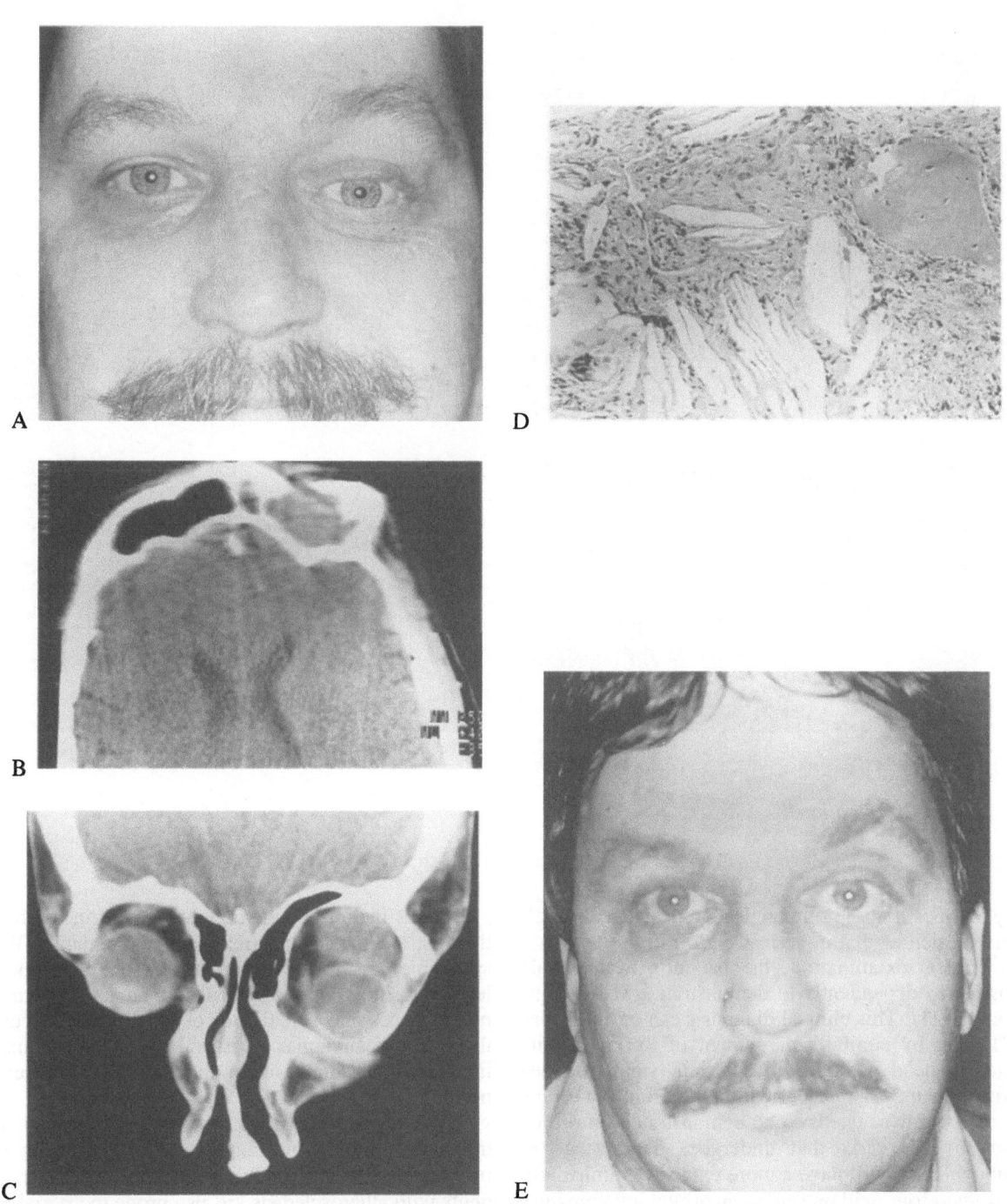

Fig. 3-20. (*A*) A 36-year-old male who developed gradual proptosis and downward displacement of the left eye. (*B,C*) Orbital CT scan showed a left frontal sinus density that eroded through the bone of the frontal sinus and extended into the left superior orbit. Patient underwent superior orbitotomy with evacuation of sinus contents and removal of orbital component. (*D*) Biopsy showed evidence of hemorrhage with hemosiderin-laden macrophages and cholesterol clefts. The patient had had a history of an auto accident 2 years ago that probably caused a frontal sinus fracture and hemorrhage. Subsequent organization of the hemorrhage occurred and led to proptosis. (*E*) Postoperative appearance 1 month after surgery. (Patient referred by Dr. Robert Serniuk, Newton, NJ.) (*F*) A 72-year-old female who presented with nausea, vomiting, and sudden proptosis. (*G,H*) CT scan shows intraconal mass. (*I*) A dark blue mass was excised through a lateral Krönlein approach and found to be a ruptured varix.

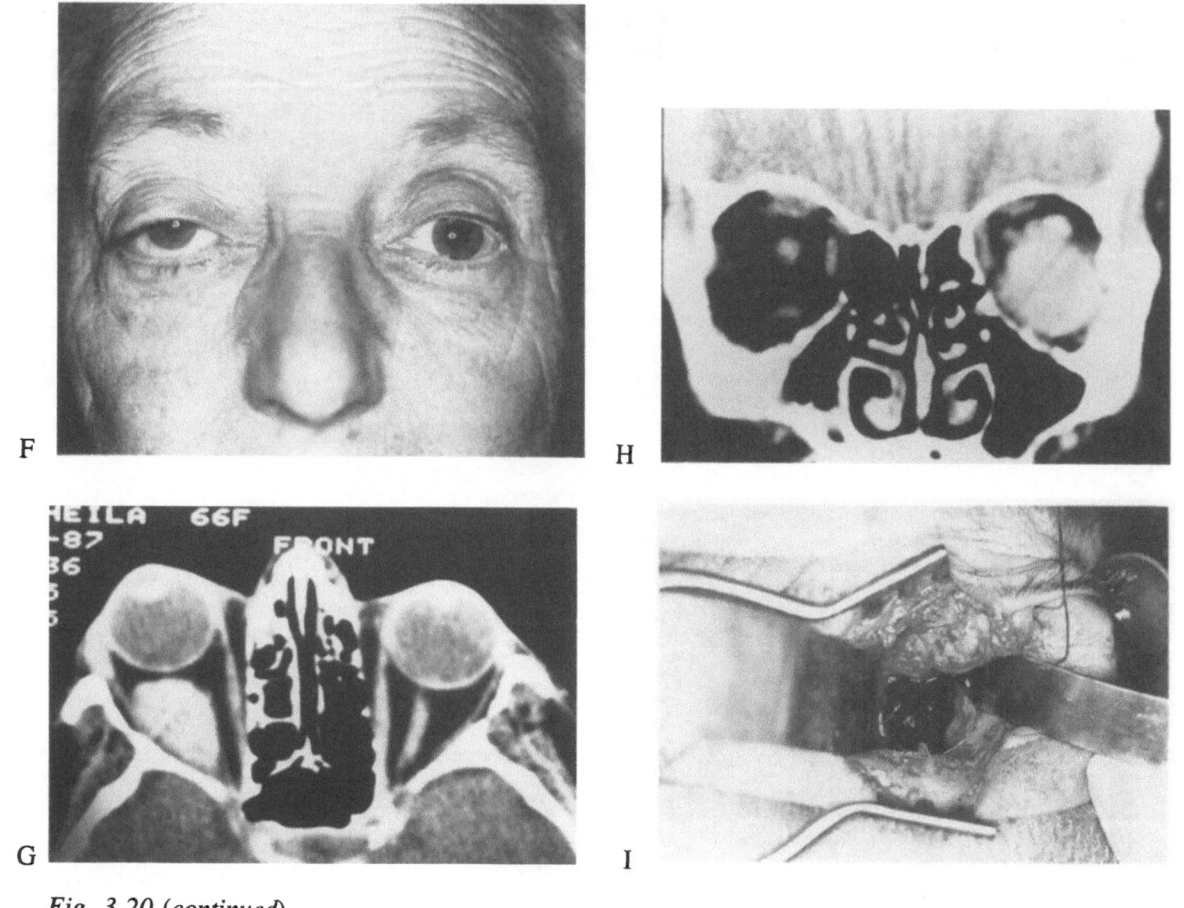

Fig. 3-20 (continued)

It may also occur after prolonged and repeated Valsalva's maneuver such as that done in weight lifting.[74]

On clinical examination, the patient's head should be positioned dependently to demonstrate a varix (Figs. 3-22 and 3-23). This clinical diagnosis can be confirmed on CT scan by similar enlargement of the mass with changes in head position. In addition, small rounded calcifications may be present within the orbit. An orbital varix rarely if ever needs to be demonstrated on orbital venography. A varix that undergoes hemorrhage or thrombophlebitis will have a more explosive clinical onset and, therefore, will present as an orbital inflammatory process. After thrombosis has occurred, the proptosis may no longer be "dynamic." Unlike varix and capillary hemangioma, lymphangiomas do not enlarge with Valsalva's maneuver.

If pulsatile exophthalmos is present or if a thrill is palpable or a bruit audible, noninvasive arterial studies are necessary to rule out an arterial component. The possibility of a carotid cavernous fistula should be considered (Fig. 3-24). Glaucoma may result from increased episcleral pressure. On examination, venous abnormalities are most common on the buccal mucosa, extremities, or chest wall (Fig. 3-25).

Venous malformations may be present in the fornix, the lids, and the canthal area. Klippel-Trenaunay-Weber syndrome consists of orbital venous malformation and leg varicosities, cutaneous hemangioma, and hypertrophy of the bones and soft tissues of the limbs that contain the venous angiomas. Visceral involvement including nephroblastomatosis of the kidneys has been reported.[75–77]

In the largest series of patients with spontaneous, nontraumatic orbital hemorrhages, venous anomalies were responsible for most of the hemorrhages.[70] Elderly patients with atherosclerosis are also prone to arterial hemorrhages.

All patients with spontaneous orbital hemorrhage should have a medical work-up for a blood dyscrasia including von Willebrand's disease, anemia, and hypertension. Other less common predisposing conditions include scurvy, hemophilia, leukemia, and intraorbital aneurysm of the ophthalmic artery. Straining such as that undergone in labor may cause orbital hemorrhage.

In any patient with orbital hemorrhage, optic nerve compression is the most important immediate consideration in the management of the patient. Any compromise of vision should lead to immediate emergency medical

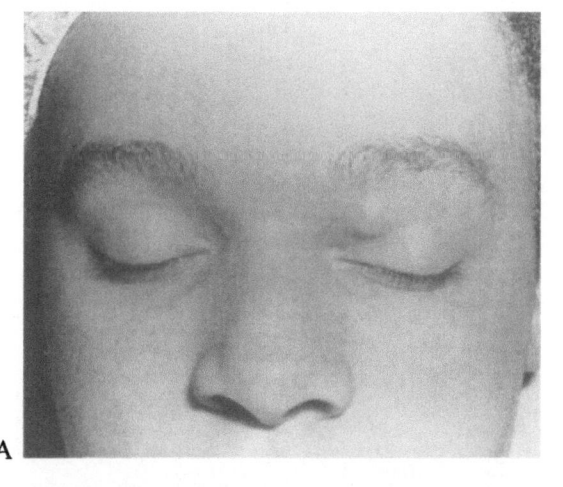

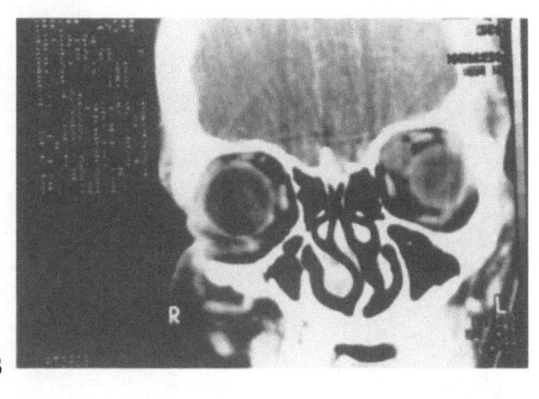

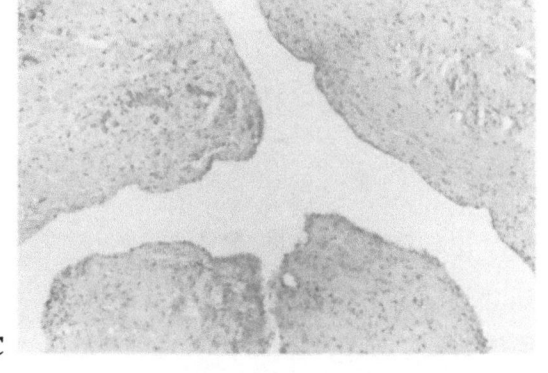

Fig. 3-21. (A) An 18-year-old male without history of trauma who developed left bluish colored mass in superomedial anterior extraconal space. On Valsalva's maneuver, there is no expansion of the mass. (B) CT scan shows an irregular density. (C) Biopsy showed an endothelial-lined vascular space with secondary fibrosis consistent with a fibrosed varix. (Patient referred by Dr. John Norris, South Orange, NJ.)

treatment. Intravenous mannitol, systemic acetazolamide, and topical beta blockers are concomitantly administered. Surgical decompression of the orbit may be necessary. A drain should be left in place at least 48 hours.

CT scan will define the process as subperiosteal or in the peripheral surgical space. An underlying tumor should be apparent on CT scan. If there is any question of an underlying tumor, the scan should be repeated when the hemorrhage resorbs. For example, on CT scan, a diffuse mass with cystic spaces should raise the suspicion of any underlying lymphangioma. A varix or venous malformation should also be suspected. Orbital calcifica-

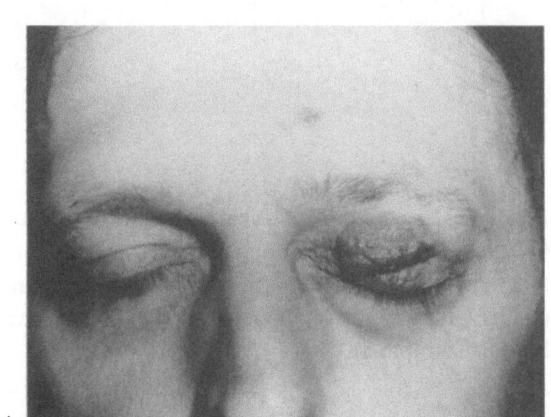

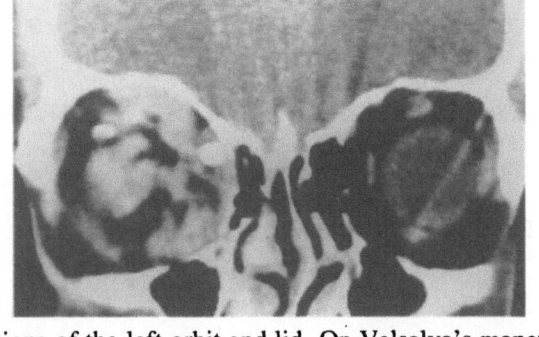

Fig. 3-22. (A) A 34-year-old male with vascular malformations of the left orbit and lid. On Valsalva's maneuver, the mass enlarges. There was no palpable or audible bruit. (B) Orbital CT scan shows multiple large vessels consistent with a varix.

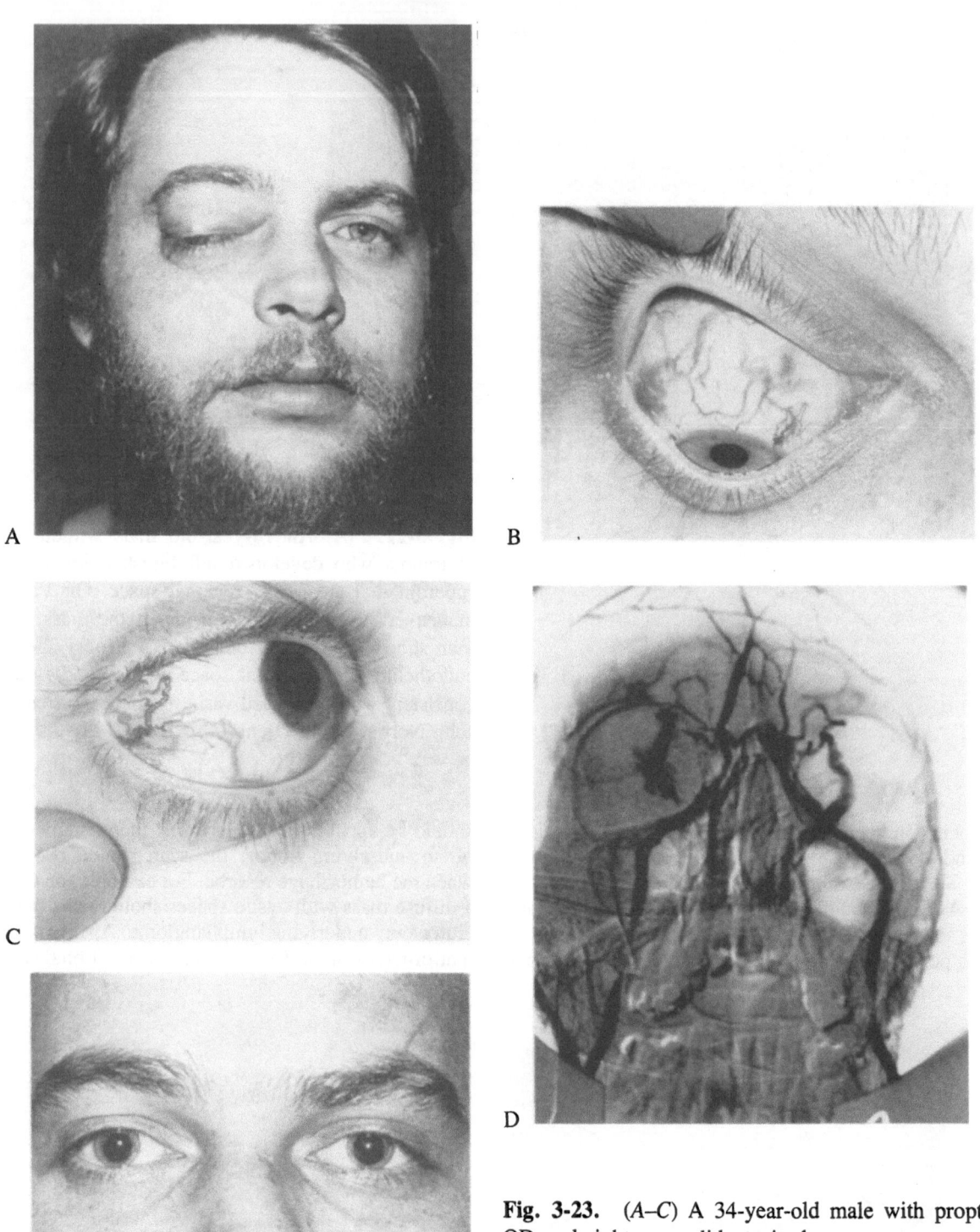

Fig. 3-23. (*A–C*) A 34-year-old male with proptosis OD and right upper lid ptosis due to venous anomaly noted on conjunctival surface and confirmed on venogram (*D*). (*E*) Postoperative appearance of patient shows resolution of proptosis.

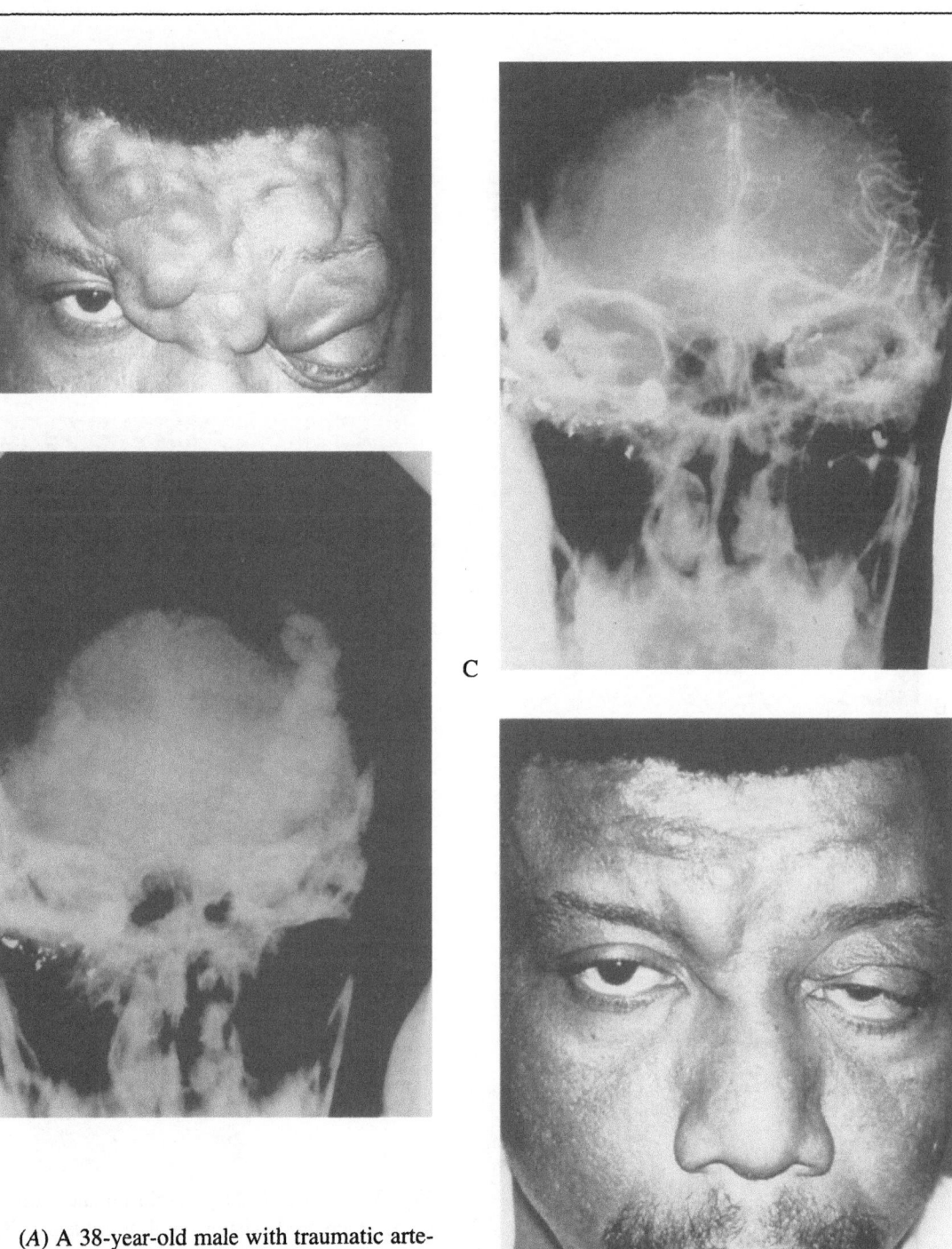

Fig. 3-24. (*A*) A 38-year-old male with traumatic arteriovenous fistula. Patient had bilateral optic atrophy. (*B*) Note dilated ophthalmic artery on carotid arteriography. (*C*) Postembolization angiogram shows marked improvement. (*D*) Clinically improved appearance after treatment.

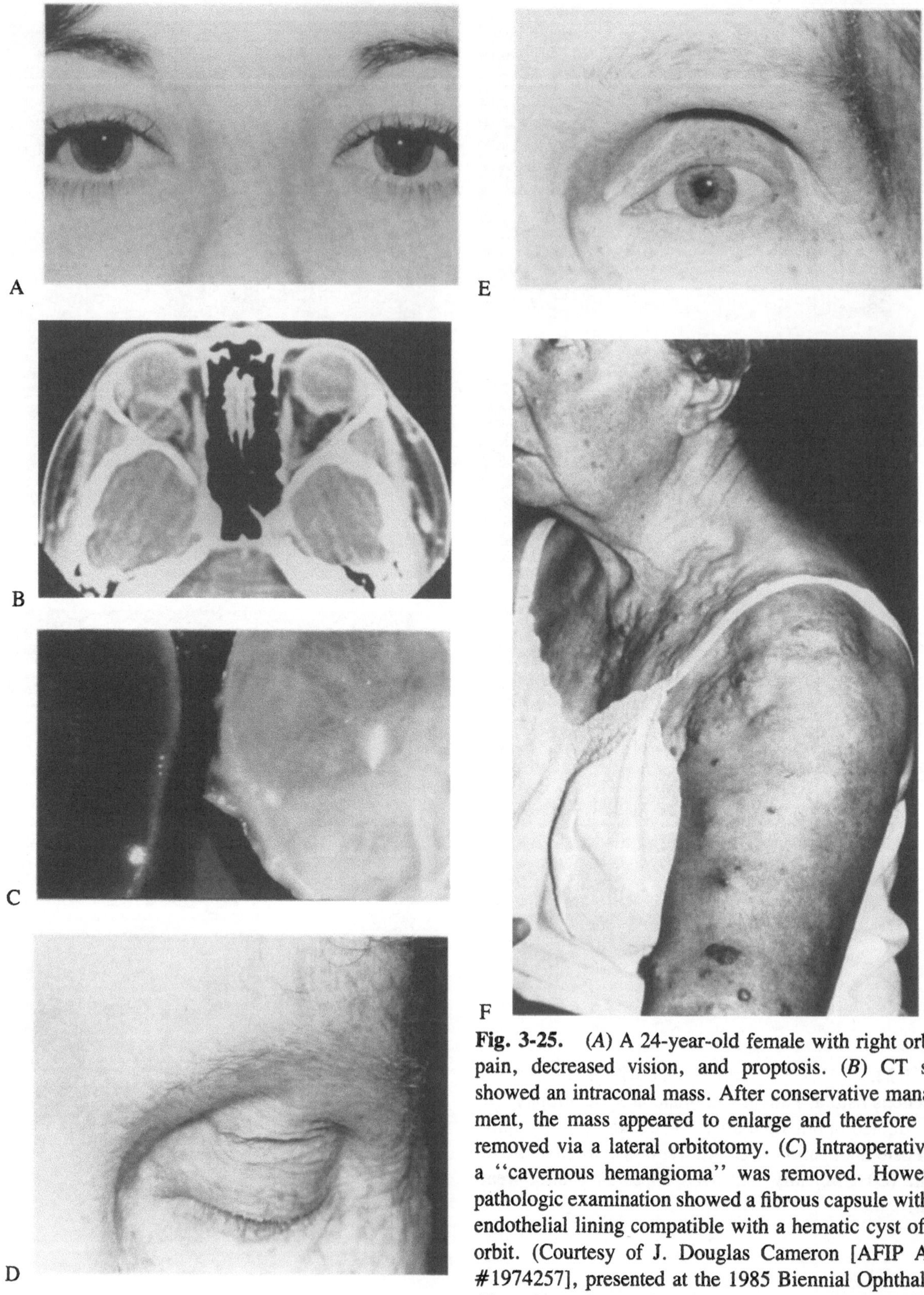

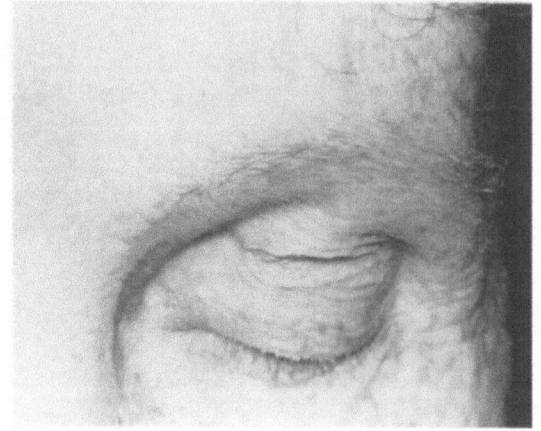

Fig. 3-25. (*A*) A 24-year-old female with right orbital pain, decreased vision, and proptosis. (*B*) CT scan showed an intraconal mass. After conservative management, the mass appeared to enlarge and therefore was removed via a lateral orbitotomy. (*C*) Intraoperatively, a "cavernous hemangioma" was removed. However, pathologic examination showed a fibrous capsule without endothelial lining compatible with a hematic cyst of the orbit. (Courtesy of J. Douglas Cameron [AFIP ACC #1974257], presented at the 1985 Biennial Ophthalmic Alumni meeting at the AFIP). (*D–F*) A 70-year-old female with vascular anomalies of lid and similar vascular anomalies involving shoulders and extremities.

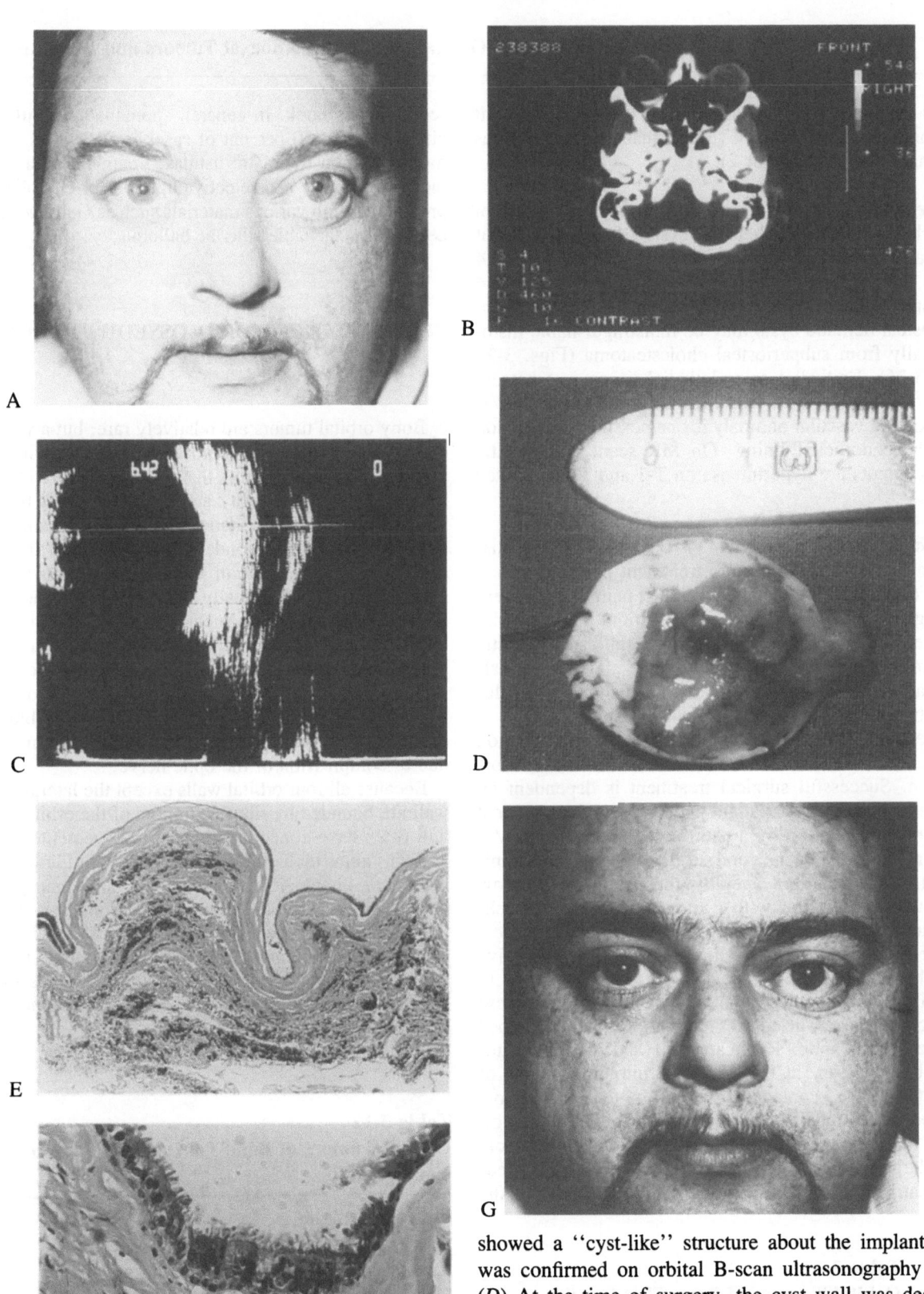

Fig. 3-26. (*A*) A 32-year-old male had undergone orbital floor exploration on the left side for an orbital floor fracture 16 years previously. At that time, the left orbital floor was reconstructed with a Teflon implant. He presented with gradual proptosis on the left side after mild trauma to the orbit 4 months prior. (*B*) Orbital CT scan showed a "cyst-like" structure about the implant that was confirmed on orbital B-scan ultrasonography (*C*). (*D*) At the time of surgery, the cyst wall was decompressed and the Teflon implant was removed. The cyst contents were blood breakdown products and (*E*) the cyst wall was fibrous tissue lined by (*F*) ciliated respiratory epithelium presumably of maxillary sinus origin. Note hemorrhage within the fibrous capsule. (*G*) The patient has had no recurrence of proptosis 3 years after removal of the implant. (Reprinted with permission from Mauriello JA, Flanagan JC, Peyster R: An unusual late complication of orbital floor fracture repair. *Ophthalmology* 91:245–248, 1984.)

tions may accompany many vascular lesions of the orbit and are best visualized on CT rather than MR scan (Tables 3-7 and 3-8; see Chapter 2).

Hematic Cyst. An orbital hemorrhage that does not resorb will result in a hematic cyst. Of the 14 cases of orbital hematic cyst described histologically, 11 of 14 were extraconal, of which 7 were subperiosteal and 4 juxtaperiosteal in the peripheral surgical space.[78–80] Subperiosteal hematic cysts may be indistinguishable histologically from subperiosteal cholesteatoma (Figs. 3-25 and 3-26). Epithelial or endothelial lining was present in 3 of 14 cases. The origin of the lining is unclear. A preexisting vascular anomaly is one possible explanation for the endothelial lining. On MR scan, the hematic cyst contents are hyperintense on T-1 and T-2 weighted scans.

Management of Orbital Varix. We believe that orbital varices do not require treatment unless there are (1) recurrent orbital hemorrhages, (2) pain that is severe enough to interfere with daily function, (3) diplopia, (4) secondary glaucoma, or (5) a significant cosmetic deformity. Patients with orbital varices and venous malformations with cutaneous involvement should be evaluated by an internist for visceral involvement.

Treatment consists of orbital exploration with plication of the feeder vessels and excision of the varix or malformation. Successful surgical treatment is dependent on proper diagnosis. Any patient with an arterial component requires consultation by a neurovascular specialist. Venous anomalies demand good surgical exposure and minimization of bleeding. Generally, these lesions are a brow or lower lid incision with a transperiorbital approach. A transeptal lid incision may also be utilized. Surgical silver clips of small or medium size with hypotensive anesthesia are helpful. The varices are cut anterior to the clip. Suture ligatures may also be utilized, but these may come loose. The varices may also need to be clipped at the orbital apex. Replication of a dehisced levator may be necessary at the time of orbitotomy.[81] Use of the CO_2 or YAG contact laser is helpful to excise tumors composed of small vessels such as a capillary hemangioma, but they are not helpful when approaching tumors with large vessels. Such feeder vessels must be ligated.

Treatment of arterial venous fistulas are beyond the scope of this book. In general, spontaneous fistulas occlude in about 50 percent of cases in 2–3 years. In the more common traumatic fistulas, treatment alternatives include complete and selective ligations or embolization procedures with various materials such as Gelfoam, glass beads, or detachable silicone balloons.

PERIPHERAL TUMORS—OSSEOUS TUMORS

Bony orbital tumors are relatively rare, but a working diagnosis is helpful in approaching patients with such tumors. In general, tumors that involve the orbital bones may affect ocular motility and cause proptosis by their mass effect. When the bones of the optic foramen and canal are involved, secondary compression of the optic nerve may occur. Certain tumors rarely affect vision since they characteristically do not involve the bones of optic foramen. These include meningioma of the orbital roof, aneurysmal cyst, hemangioma of the skull, brown tumor, and reparative granuloma (Table 3-11).

In addition, in Paget's disease, vision may decrease from lack of perfusion of the optic nerve as blood is shunted away from the nerve to supply the tumor and due to compression of the optic nerve.

Because all four orbital walls except the lateral orbital wall are bounded by sinuses, tumors of the orbital bones will often have concomitant sinus involvement.

Each tumor including clinical features, radiologic appearance, histologic considerations, and management will be discussed in the following section. Bone tumors that affect children will be discussed in this section. In all patients with bone tumors, the radiographic features must be correlated with the pathologic features (Table 3-12). Pediatric tumors of orbital bones will be considered before adult tumors.

Table 3-11
Orbital Tumors of Bone That Rarely Affect Vision

Intradiploic meningioma of orbital roof
Aneurysmal bone cyst
Hemangioma of skull
Reparative granuloma
Brown tumor

Table 3-12
Orbital Tumors of Bone That Affect Children and Young Adults

Fibrous dysplasia
Ossifying fibroma
Aneurysmal bone cyst
Giant cell tumor (benign osteoclastoma)
Reparative granuloma
Intradiploic meningioma of orbital roof*
Osteoblastoma
Osteogenic sarcoma
Infantile cortical hyperostosis (Caffey's syndrome)

---
* One case involved a 40-year-old. Note: ectopic meningioma may involve sinuses independent of orbital roof.

PEDIATRIC AND ADOLESCENT ORBITAL TUMORS OF BONE

Ossifying Fibroma

Nomenclature and Clinical Features. The classification of ossifying fibroma is controversial. Some authorities have written that the tumor in the head region is a variant of fibrous dysplasia and not a separate entity.[82] We believe that ossifying fibroma should be separated from fibrous dysplasia because ossifying fibromas tend to be more aggressive and more likely to recur. In the 1960s, some researchers classified ossifying fibroma as an osteoblastoma, yet today the histopathologic features have been more clearly outlined and no longer allow for such confusion.[83–86] The term *juvenile ossifying fibromas* has been discouraged since the lesion can occur in adults. Recently, the term *psammomatoid ossifying fibroma* was suggested.[87]

Often fibrous dysplasia and psammomatoid ossifying fibroma are confused clinically and pathologically. The clinical features of fibrous dysplasia and ossifying fibroma are outlined in Table 3-13. The most common clinical presentation is proptosis, but decreased vision, ptosis, headaches, and nasal obstruction may also occur. Fibrous dysplasia may be polyostotic and associated with Albright's syndrome (cutaneous pigmentation and precocious puberty). Both entities are more common in males than females.

Radiographic Signs. Fibrous dysplasia causes bony sclerosis in a more diffuse fashion than ossifying fibroma, which is well-defined and localized. Typically, ossifying fibroma arises from either the orbital plate of the frontal bone or the ethmoid sinus. The tumor of the frontal bone has a characteristic radiologic appearance: a reduced internal density surrounded by an incomplete bony plate. The tumor appears to expand the bone as if it were a balloon. In the ethmoid bone, the pattern is variable and only sometimes resembles the frontal bone pattern. Usually, the large mottled radiodense mass does not enhance with contrast. Radiolucent areas often correspond to psammomatoid ossicles or cystic degeneration.

Biopsy. Ossifying fibroma has a fibrous stroma with many fibroblasts and is, therefore, predominantly a fibrous lesion with variable amounts of woven and lamellar trabeculae that may appear connected and resemble psammoma bodies. Osteoblasts rim the trabeculae. The tumor may be mistaken for meningioma.

The pathologic pattern can be distinguished from fibrous dysplasia in which the bony spicules are immature woven bone, not lamellar bone. As stated above, osteoblasts are present in ossifying fibroma and not in fibrous dysplasia. Unlike fibrous dysplasia, ossifying fibroma has all of the elements of bone development. Therefore, ossifying fibroma can be considered an aberrant form of bone maturation, while fibrous dysplasia may be considered an arrested form of bone development at the woven bone stage before osteoid is laid down by mesenchymal cells and osteoblasts complete the transition from woven into lamellar bone.[83–86] The shell that often surrounds the tumor is composed of woven bone that is formed nonspecifically in a number of pathologic conditions in which new bone is deposited rapidly.

Management. Treatment is surgical, but recurrence is more likely than with fibrous dysplasia. Complete removal of the lesion is indicated.

Table 3-13
Ossifying Fibroma vs. Fibrous Dysplasia

	Ossifying Fibroma	Fibrous Dysplasia
Clinical Features	7 to 28 years of age	First decade
	Slow progressive proptosis	Painless facial asymmetry with proptosis
Radiographic Findings	Well-defined margins, round or ovoid, localized expansion of involved bone, may be eggshell-thin, expands bone-like balloon	Diffuse, sclerotic, poorly defined borders, involves whole bone length
	Monostotic	Often polyostotic
Pathologic Features	Variable fibrous stroma with many fibroblasts	Variable immature woven bone without lamellar bone or osteoblasts
	Isolated spicules of bone resembling psammoma body, spicules rimmed by osteoid and osteoblasts	
	True neoplasm	Arrest in maturation of bone

Fibrous Dysplasia

Clinical Features. The presenting clinical features of fibrous dysplasia and ossifying fibroma are similar and have been outlined above. It is important to emphasize that ossifying fibroma is more locally aggressive than fibrous dysplasia, yet neither tumor has any associated mortality. Fibrous dysplasia may be both monostotic or polyostotic and may rarely be associated with McCune-Albright syndrome, a systemic disease characterized by ipsilateral cutaneous pigment abnormalities and preco-cious puberty with early menstruation (as early as the second day of life). The skin pigmentation may have a "coast of Maine" irregular configuration that may be contrasted with the café-au-lait spots in neurofibromatosis that have a smooth "coast of California" contour. The actual triad is quite rare. The disorder is more common in males than females.[87–91]

Radiologic Appearance. The frontal, ethmoid, and sphenoid bones may be involved, with the frontal bone being most commonly involved. The bones are affected

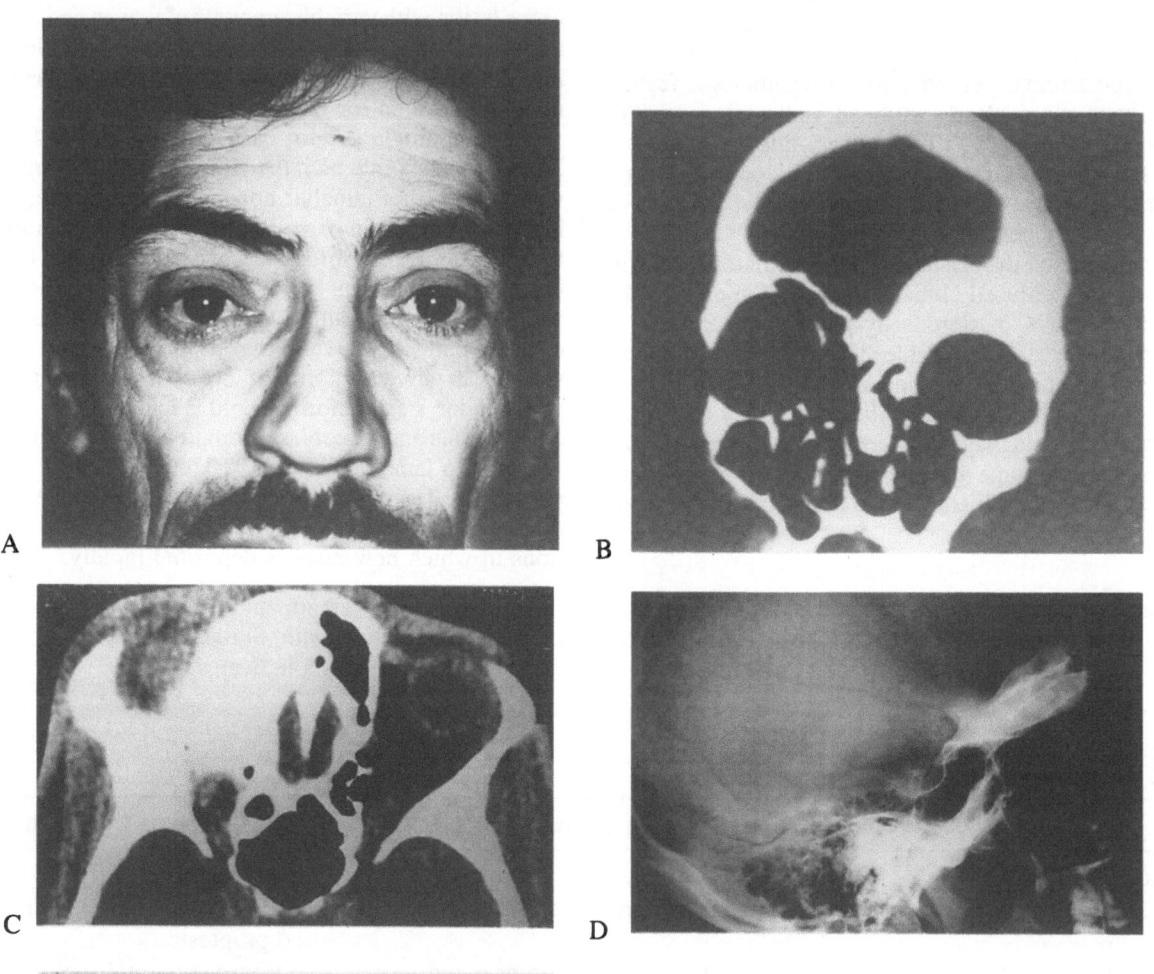

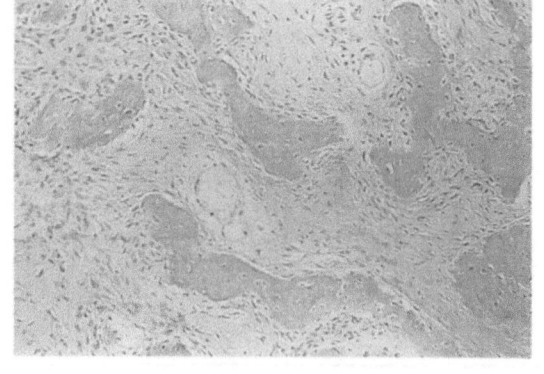

Fig. 3-27. (*A*) A 42-year-old male with downward displacement of the right eye. (*B,C*) CT scan shows marked diffuse thickening of the orbital bones on the right side. The abnormal thickened bone is well seen on plain films of the orbit (*D*). (*E*) Combined orbital and neurosurgical approaches showed a tumor on pathologic examination consistent with fibrous dysplasia.

diffusely, that is, along their entire length. Orbital roof involvement causes proptosis and downward displacement of the globe (Figs. 3-27 and 3-28). Much less common maxillary bone involvement causes upward displacement of the globe. Optic atrophy may occur from sphenoidal bone narrowing of the optic canal. Overall the most common bones involved in fibrous dysplasia are not the skull bones but the femur, tibia, and ribs.

The lesions are most often sclerotic, but rarely the lesions may appear lytic. Obliteration of medullary canals and thinning of the overlying cortex result in a homogeneous ground-glass appearance with an imperceptible blending into normal cortical bone. Tangential views show a more sclerotic appearance. The lesion may be mistaken for Paget's disease, meningioma en plaque, a unicameral bone cyst, or eosinophilic granuloma.

Biopsy. Biopsy shows spindle-appearing cells with trabeculae of curvilinear, coarse-woven bone without the fine cement lines of lamellar bone that appear unconnected in a single section. The lesion may be confused with ossifying fibroma, which is a predominantly fibrous lesion with variable amounts of woven and lamellar bone trabeculae that appear interconnected in a single section. Unlike fibrous dysplasia, where osteoblasts are usually absent except near the area of transition to normal bone, osteoblasts in ossifying fibroma usually rim the trabeculae.

Management. Treatment of fibrous dysplasia is symptomatic. Unlike Paget's disease where hemorrhage and recurrence often mitigate against surgery, excellent surgical results can be achieved with fibrous dysplasia. Radiotherapy of the bone lesions is probably not indicated because of the development of secondary tumors in the field of radiation. Treatment is indicated if there is a significant cosmetic deformity or a risk of developing optic nerve compression. Rarely, malignant transformation has occurred either spontaneously or following radiotherapy.

Aneurysmal Bone Cyst

Clinical Features. First described in 1942 by Jaffee and Lichtenstein, aneurysmal bone cyst primarily affects adolescent and young adults and is more common in males than females.[92] The nonneoplastic cyst usually involves the metaphyses of long bones and vertebra. Typically, the child or adolescent patient has a fracture or an enlarging mass. Rarely, the skull and orbit are involved and most commonly the orbit roof. Typically, vision is spared. Patients may present with slowly progressive or rapidly progressive proptosis. In the latter instance, the tumor has been mistaken clinically for rhabdomyosarcoma. Therefore, the necessity for CT scan prior to biopsy of any rapidly progressive tumor

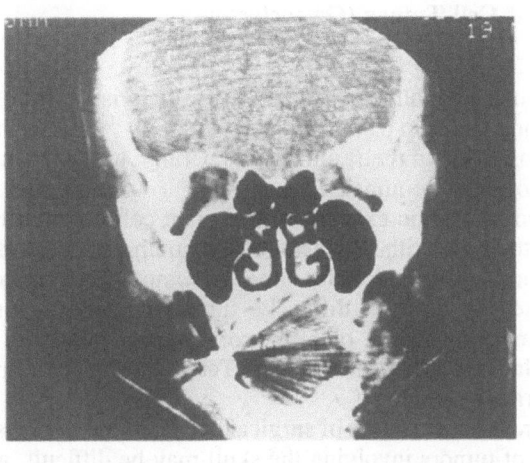

Fig. 3-28. CT scan of a 35-year-old female with fibrous dysplasia. Patient had a pressure feeling in the right orbit. Patient refused neurosurgical intervention; lateral orbitotomy with removal of the lateral orbital wall afforded relief. (Patient referred by Dr. Matthew Marano, Roseland, NJ.)

cannot be overemphasized. In addition to painless proptosis, the distinctive feature is accompanying hemorrhage.[93–96]

Radiographic Features. While the radiographic appearance of cysts in the long bones and spine is of an expansile "blown out" nature, orbital involvement is less specific and shows expansion and destruction of bone; opacification of the paranasal sinuses may occur. Aneurysmal cysts may, in fact, represent a local intraosseous vascular disturbance rather than a true neoplasm. Therefore, the findings of a cystic intraosseous lesion should be examined carefully to rule out an underlying tumor. For example, a giant cell tumor or even an osteogenic sarcoma may present as a cystic mass both radiographically and even pathologically. In addition, a subperiosteal hemorrhage or arteriovenous malformation may lead to cystic lesion as well.

Biopsy. Biopsy shows a fibrous matrix with spindle cells in which large and small endothelial-lined, blood-filled channels are present. Osteoblasts and osteoclasts may be present as well as giant cells with hemosiderin-laden macrophages. The possibility of an underlying tumor should always be considered.

Management. Surgical curretting and reconstruction with bone chips is the treatment of choice. Radiotherapy has been successful but the possibility of radiation-induced sarcoma exists.

Giant Cell Tumor (Osteoclastoma)

Giant cell tumors characteristically arise at the end of long bones in patients under age 20.[97-101] When these tumors arise in the skull, they generally arise in a sinus. Vision may be affected.

On radiologic examination of giant cell tumors, there is osteolysis with expansion and thinning of the cortex.

Biopsy shows that the tumor is composed of multinucleated giant cells diffusely spread within a cellular stroma of fusiform, plump, stromal cells with ovoid vesicular orthochromatic nuclei (Table 3-14). The tumors are rarely malignant.

Treatment consists of surgical excision, but total resection of tumors involving the skull may be difficult, and, therefore, ancillary radiation may be helpful.

Reparative Granuloma

Reparative granuloma is a reactive process that may follow trauma or infection in patients under age 20. The radiographic appearance is nonspecific.[53]

Pathologically, there is an irregular distribution of giant cells and zones of new and old hemorrhage. The zonal location of the giant cells in this lesion helps to differentiate reparative granuloma from giant cell tumor, where the giant cells are present throughout the tumor. Osteoid formation and spicules of new bone may be present.

Brown tumor is considered under the next section, "Adult Orbital Tumors of Bone."

Benign Osteoblastoma

Benign osteoblastoma of the orbit is a rare tumor that predominantly involves children and young adults. Adjacent sinus involvement may be present and also occurs in osteomas (discussed below) and giant cell tumor.[98] In the case of osteoblastoma reported by Fu and Perzin, the tumor arose in the ethmoid sinus of a 12-year-old girl. Osteoid osteoma is similar histologically to osteoblastoma. However, it is a static lesion that if untreated

Table 3-14
Pathologic Differential Diagnosis of Tumors of Orbital Bones That Contain Giant Cells

Aneurysmal bone cyst
Giant cell tumor (osteoclastoma)
Reparative granuloma
Brown tumor

is usually less than 1 cm in diameter, while osteoblastoma, if untreated, tends to grow progressively.[97]

Radiographically, the tumor is well circumscribed. It has a dense cortical margin that corresponds to dense sclerotic bone on histologic examination and a radiolucent osteolytic expanding central zone that corresponds to edematous fibrovascular tissue with irregular trabeculae of new bone and varying degree of calcification. MR, unlike CT scan, does not show calcifications.

Biopsy. Biopsy shows spicules consisting of fiber bone, osteoid, and mineralization. Osteoblasts form irregular trabeculae of osteoid with occasional multinucleated giant cells.

Management. The single orbital tumor was curetted and did not recur. Usually only curettage is possible, yet recurrence rates are approximately 10–15%.

Osteogenic Sarcoma

Clinical Features. Primary osteogenic sarcoma of the orbital bones, sinuses, and skull is extremely rare. Postradiation sarcomas are much more common. In any patient with a head and neck tumor, a history of a previous tumor such as a retinoblastoma and radiation exposure should be obtained. As discussed above, the hereditary form of retinoblastoma has a significant incidence of associated secondary soft tissue malignancies that occur with or without radiation.[102-103] Also, in approximately 2.3 percent of patients with bilateral retinoblastoma, an intracranial neuroblastic tumor occurs in the pineal region. To date no survivors have been reported despite neurosurgery, radiotherapy, and chemotherapy. In addition, fibrous dysplasia after radiotherapy may undergo sarcomatous degeneration.

Osteogenic sarcoma of the skull and jaw tend to develop in the third decade, while those of the long bones predominate in the second decade. Clinical signs include facial edema with or without pain, epistaxis, poor wound healing after loose tooth extraction, proptosis, and numbness of the upper lip.

On radiographic examination, a poorly defined mass with increased bone density is often found; clouding of the sinuses, especially the maxillary sinus may be present.

Biopsy. Biopsy shows hyperchromatic nuclei within anaplastic malignant spindle cells with tumor osteoid and neoplastic bone formation. Electron microscopy may be necessary to differentiate from chondrosarcoma in certain cases in which the extracellular matrix is not clearly that of bone or cartilage.

Management. Oncologic consultation should be sought. Surgical treatment may result in local recurrence. Pulmonary metastases may develop shortly after surgery.

Radiotherapy and chemotherapy do not appear to halt the disease.

Infantile Cortical Hyperostosis (Caffey's Syndrome)

This disease is a periosteitis of the mandible that may present with lid edema and proptosis and thereby mimic a bacterial orbital cellulitis during the first year of life. The proptosis is due to concomitant involvement of the orbital bones.

CT scan shows periosteal reaction and sclerosis of the mandible and orbital bones.

Knowledge of this disease may relieve anxiety about a possible orbital malignancy. The infants are quite irritable and there is no definitive treatment. Patients recover uneventfully in weeks to months. Bacterial infection should be ruled out.[104]

ADULT ORBITAL TUMORS OF BONE

Brown Tumor

A brown "tumor," synonymous with von Recklinghausen's disease of bone, is not a true tumor but a reactive process secondary to the changes of calcium metabolism that are a direct result of hyperparathyroidism. The tumor is so named because of the accompanying hemorrhage and resultant hemosiderin-laden macrophages that give the lesion a brown discoloration. Underlying causes include parathyroid carcinoma, adenoma, or hyperplasia of the parathyroid gland due to secondary hyperparathyroidism.

Clinically, proptosis and pain with nasal obstruction may be the presenting sign. Vision is generally not affected. The tumor affects patients aged 22 to 48 (Table 3-15). One patient reported 70 years of age. Typically, the maxillary bone, ethmoid, and frontal bone are involved.[105–107]

Radiologically, the osteolytic appearance may resemble those of giant cell tumor, giant cell reparative granuloma, and aneurysmal bone cyst. However, generalized decreased bone mineralization secondary to the disease process may be present.

Biopsy shows findings that are identical to that of reparative granuloma.

Management should include endocrine consultation. Serum calcium, phosphorus, and alkaline phosphatase should be obtained in all patients with lytic orbital bone lesions in order to rule out this diagnosis and thereby obviate the need for biopsy.

Table 3-15
Adult Orbital Tumors of Bones

Brown tumor
Intradiploic meningioma of the orbital roof
Osteoma
Benign hemangioma of the skull
Paget's disease
Lipoma of the frontal bone

Intradiploic Meningioma of the Orbital Roof

Origin of the Tumor. Ectopic meningiomas arise from arachnoidal cell nests entrapped in extradural tissue during embryonal development or after head trauma with fracture or dural tear. They may also originate ectopically from mucosa of the frontal sinus or other paranasal sinuses.[108–110]

Clinical Features. In a review of five previously reported patients, all five patients presented with proptosis and downward displacement of the eye. Vision was not affected. Four of the five patients were male.

Radiographically, in four of five cases, a "plum-like" well-delineated, calcified opacity with hyperdense borders was present. This finding may be pathognomonic. In the fifth case, a split in the orbital roof was present.

Histologically, the tumor is identical to a meningioma elsewhere in the body.

Management. These tumors should be removed by a neurosurgeon. Removal represents little surgical difficulty in that the tumors are contained in a bony shell, and the orbit is therefore protected from surgical trauma. The tumor can be removed en bloc. The entire orbital roof should be removed to prevent recurrence and the orbital roof reconstituted in some fashion such as with a wire mesh. An extradural surgical approach is indicated.

Osteomas

Osteomas are the most common tumor of bone to encroach on the orbit, and like all osteomas of the skull, they are typically slow-growing.[111] In the skull, they arise from the mandible and paranasal sinuses. Most originate in the frontal and ethmoid sinuses, but they may arise much less commonly from the maxillary sinus and least commonly from the sphenoid sinus. In the latter location, optic atrophy and visual loss with proptosis are most common. Possible symptoms include unilateral headache, hemifacial, paranasal sinus pain, ptosis, extraocular muscle imbalance, and nasal discharge (Fig. 3-29).

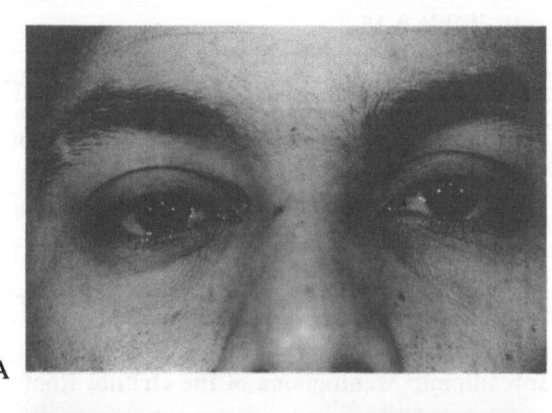

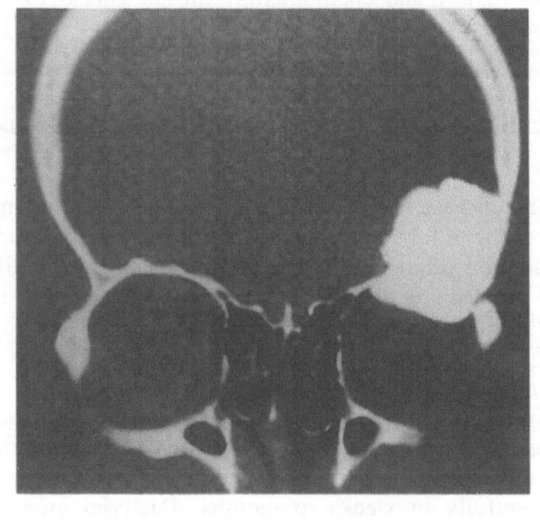

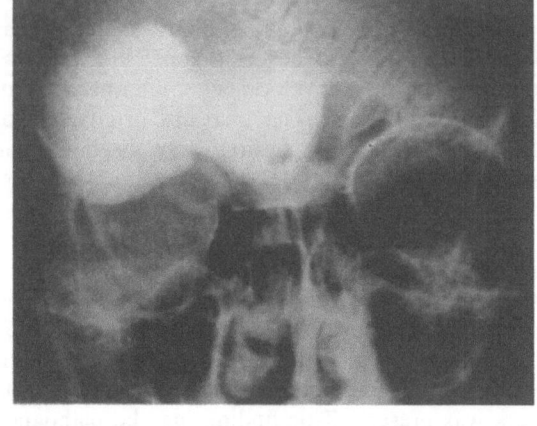

Fig. 3-29. (*A*) A 28-year-old male with gradual onset of proptosis and downward displacement of the right eye. (*B*) Orbital CT scan shows a localized thickening of the right superolateral orbital rim. The tumor was well-demonstrated on plain films (*C*). Combined orbital and neurosurgical approaches showed an osteoma.

The average age of presentation is 29 to 45 years. Most studies show a male predominance. Rarely, these tumors may grow rapidly and present with signs of chronic sinusitis and orbital cellulitis.[112]

Radiographic Findings. Osteomas are radiopaque, well-outlined, and homogeneously calcified.

Biopsy. Biopsy shows three types: ivory (eburnated), compact, and spongiose. The ivory osteoma, the most common form of osteoma to involve the orbit, consists of solid bone without haversian canals. The compact form is similar to the ivory osteoma except that the interior has haversian canals with concentric lamellae of bone formation. The spongiose type is primarily connective tissue with large areas of new bone formation. The various types may occur in any given patient.

Management. Surgical removal is recommended for symptomatic orbital osteomas. Patients with multiple osteomas of the bony skeleton should be suspected of having Gardner's syndrome, and autosomal, dominantly inherited disorder characterized by intestinal polyposis in which the risk of developing colonic adenocarcinoma approaches 100 percent. Total colectomy has been suggested as a prophylactic measure. Other eye-related findings associated with Gardner's syndrome include angioid streaks, epidermal inclusion cysts of the lids, and multiple patches of congenital hypertrophy of the retinal pigment

epithelium. The latter finding may indicate those patients who are at risk later in life of developing other phenotypic evidence of Gardner's syndrome.

Benign Hemangioma of the Skull

Clinical Features. Unlike ossifying fibroma, fibrous dysplasia, and aneurysmal bone cyst, hemangioma of the skull bones is more common in females. Seventy-five percent of patients are females and 25% are males. Like other bone tumors, symptoms are dependent on location. These tumors occur in the 31–40-year age group and rarely before age 30. Hemangioma of the orbital bones is extremely rare in that there have been only two reported cases, one of which involved the zygoma and the other involved the latter aspect of the inferior orbital rim.[113–114]

Radiographic Findings. Characteristic findings include a rounded area of rarefaction with a diagnostic honeycomb appearance. There is rarely evidence of sclerosis. A sunray appearance produced by bony trabeculae that radiate from a common center may be evident on tangential view.

Biopsy. Biopsy shows cavernous endothelial-lined space, although the spaces may be capillary in size. No smooth muscle or elastic tissue is present.

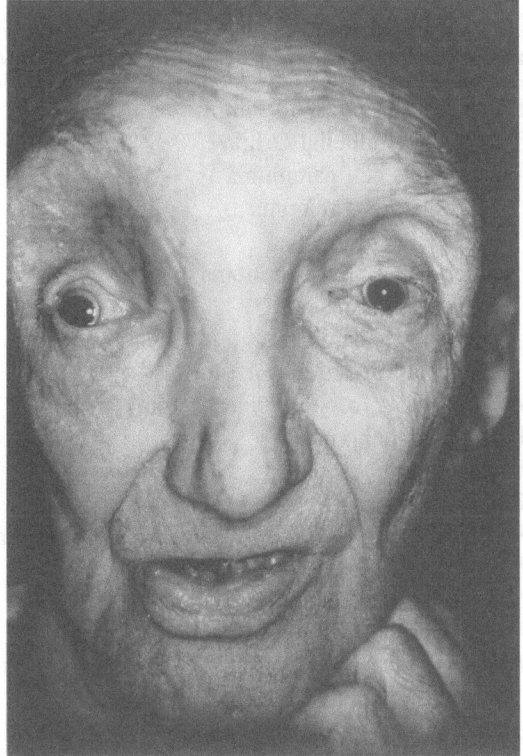

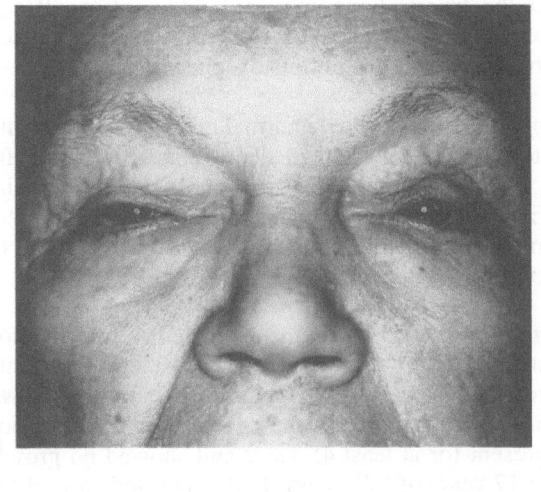

A

B

Fig. 3-30. (*A*) A 74-year-old male with lid retraction due to Paget's disease. (*B*) A 68-year-old with Paget's disease and right-sided hemifacial spasm due to bony compression of the root of the seventh nerve.

Management. Management includes surgical excision and reconstruction with bone grafts or alloplastic materials.

Paget's Disease

Clinical Features. Visual field tests including color plates are necessary to rule out optic nerve compression when any bone tumor is noted on CT scan. In addition, ocular motility should be followed. Patients with Paget's disease may have associated neurologic findings including deafness, vertigo, trigeminal neuralgia, vertebrobasilar insufficiency, seventh nerve palsy with hemifacial spasm, nystagmus, and headache.[115–117] Hemifacial spasm may also occur (Fig. 3-30).

Radiographic Findings. These changes are due to bone resorption and chaotic bone formation; the former produces osteolytic lesions, while the latter gives a characteristic "cotton-wool" appearance.

Rapid bone turnover increases serum alkaline phosphatase and may result in an abnormal bone scan even before symptoms or changes in plain skull x-rays occur.

Biopsy. Biopsy shows coarsely fibered bone with prominent cement lines. The bone is laid down as disorga-

nized wide trabeculae. The cement lines are a mosaic, rather than ordered in their appearance.

Management. Most patients with Paget's disease are free of optic neuropathy. The incidence of optic neuropathy correlates with headache, hearing loss, and skull involvement on x-ray.

In some patients treatment with calcitonin may be effective. Calcitonin decreases the bone mass and the vascularity of the pathologic bones and thereby decreases the "stealing" of blood from the surrounding neural structures. Surgical decompression may be fruitless in that the pathologic bone may reform and the surgical procedure may be significantly hampered by poor hemostasis in the operative field.

Because patients with Paget's disease may rarely develop secondary tumors such as osteosarcoma, chondrosarcoma, fibrosarcoma, and giant cell tumor, such tumors should be considered in patients with Paget's disease who develop proptosis.

Lipoma of the Frontal Bone

Clinical Features. Ptosis with downward displacement of the globe was present in the one case reported.[118] On plain films, there was no bone destruction but thickening of the frontal bone and obliteration of the lateral portion of the frontal sinus were present. The lesion may be confused with fibrous dysplasia.

Biopsy. Biopsy shows normal cancellous bone with an interior irregular shell of dense bone containing fat cells, myxoid ground substance, and scattered fibrillar material. Focal areas of bone metaplasia are present within the tumor. The tumor is located in the diploe of the bone.

Management. Management includes observation and surgical extirpation if a severe cosmetic deformity or threat to vision exists. The tumor is extremely slow-growing; for example, in the case reported, the lesion was present for at least 45 years and showed no growth during 17 years of follow-up. In the reported case, diagnosis was based on autopsy findings.

NONOSSEOUS SINUS, OROPHARYNGEAL, AND NASAL TUMORS THAT EXTEND SECONDARILY INTO THE ORBIT

Many tumors may cause initial sinus involvement followed by secondary orbital extension (Table 3-16). The need for otolaryngologic consultation cannot be overemphasized. At times, the origin of the tumor, whether primary orbit or primary sinus, will not be clear. Symptoms that relate to the teeth, nose, and sinuses and antedate ocular symptoms are helpful in this determination. In most instances, the epicenter of the mass, in the orbit or sinus, is evident on CT scan.

This section will discuss the more common clinical features of sinus tumors in general before each entity is considered in more detail.

Clinical Signs and Symptoms of Sinus Tumors Extending into the Orbit

The clinical features of sinus tumors that invade the orbit secondarily are fairly similar. Patients are generally in their 40s and 50s. Males are affected twice as commonly as females. Patients with sinus and orbital masses often present with proptosis and/or lid edema with ptosis, visual loss, tearing, and signs and symptoms relating to the sinus or nose such as nasal obstruction, discharge, epistaxis, nasal mass, facial pain, and/or edema.

Patients often have a history of chronic sinusitis that is on an allergic or infectious basis. Many patients have a history of smoking. In addition, a history of polyps is not unusual. Development of trismus reflects extension into the pterygoid fossa.[119]

Table 3-16

Nonosseous Tumors Originating in the Sinus, Nose, and Oropharynx That Extend Secondarily into Orbit

Mucocele secondary to tumor
Tumors of Epithelial Origin
   squamous cell carcinoma
   sarcomatoid carcinoma
   inverted papilloma
   mucoepidermoid carcinoma
   adenocarcinoma
   adenocystic carcinoma
   malignant mixed tumor
Angiofibroma (oropharyngeal tumor)
Lymphoepithelioma
Esthesioneuroblastoma
Cholesteatoma
Rhabdomyosarcoma (see "Pediatric Orbital Tumors")
Fibrosarcoma (see "Adult Orbital Tumors")
Melanoma of the sinus
Mesectodermal leiomyosarcoma
Alveolar soft part sarcoma (see "Pediatric Orbital Tumors")
Ewing's sarcoma metastatic to the orbit
Ameloblastoma

Maxillary sinus tumors are the most common sinus tumors to invade the orbit secondarily. The frontal sinus and nose are the primary site less frequently. Ethmoid sinus tumors more often invade the nose than the orbit, and basilar skull invasion also occurs (Fig. 3-31).[119]

With maxillary sinus tumors that extend into the orbit, upward displacement of the eye occurs; with ethmoid tumors, lateral displacement of the globe is the rule (Fig. 3-32). Concomitant involvement of the maxillary and ethmoid sinus is rare except in advanced tumors. Primary frontal and sphenoidal sinus tumors are rare and often are due to secondary spread from the ethmoid and maxillary sinus. Because of the adjacency to the pituitary gland and optic chiasm, vision may be affected. Overall, the most common type of tumor of the sinuses and nose is squamous cell carcinoma.

Perineural invasion occurs with all carcinomas, especially adenoid cystic carcinoma, and results in pain.[120] The infraorbital nerve is commonly involved in antral carcinomas. Adenoid cystic carcinomas tend to cause less sclerosis and frozen globes than squamous cell carcinoma or adenocarcinoma. Typically, inverted papillomas do not produce pain.

A history of chronic sinusitis, whether infectious or allergic and with or without polyp formation, does not rule out a tumor. Seventh and eighth nerve palsies occur with involvement of the base of the brain. Patients with tumors of the mouth and hypopharynx develop cranial

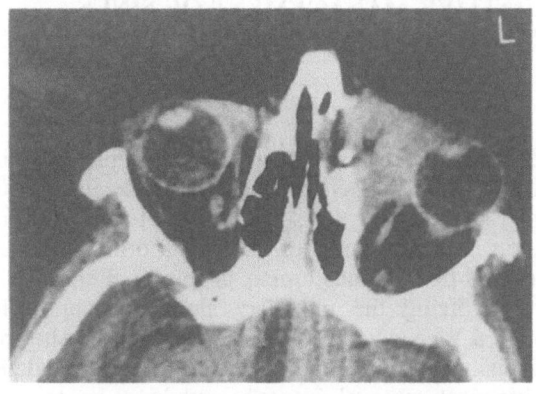

Fig. 3-31. CT scan from 70-year-old female with history of lateral displacement of left globe due to ethmoid sinus tumor that eroded through wall of ethmoid sinus into medial orbit. Initial biopsy showed squamous cell carcinoma arising from ethmoid sinus. Radical debulking procedure followed by radiation was performed rather than exenteration, which was refused by patient.

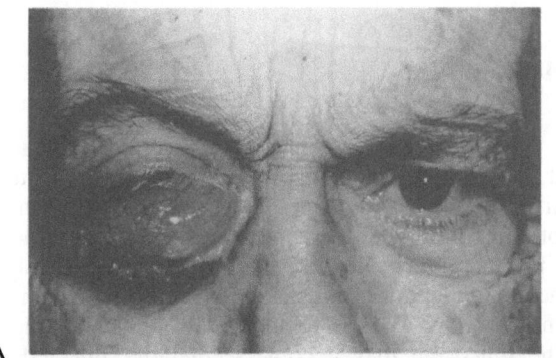

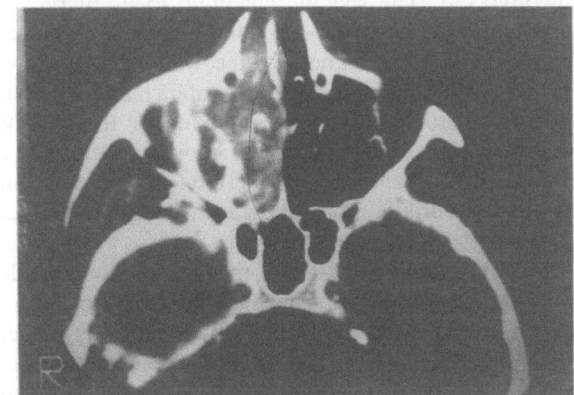

Fig. 3-32. (*A*) A 72-year-old male with maxillary sinus carcinoma causing upward displacement of right eye and nasal congestion. Preoperative CT scan shows maxillary sinus and nasal mass. (*B*). Patient underwent combined exenteration and maxillectomy through a Weber-Ferguson incision.

nerve complications more frequently than patients with sinus carcinomas.

Lymphoepithelioma is an extremely aggressive tumor that involves the oropharynx and may have only a small primary, yet metastases to the local lymph nodes occur in 70 percent of patients. Fourth, fifth, and sixth nerve palsies may be present.[119,121]

In most cases, the interval between the onset of sinus disease and orbital presentation is less than 1 year. Patients with maxillary carcinomas generally do not seek medical attention because of symptoms for 6 months or more after the onset of their disease when the disease is advanced. The patient's median survival from the time of diagnosis of orbital involvement is approximately 6 months. In one series, survival beyond 21 months is a good prognostic sign.[119]

CT Scan Findings—Sinus Tumors with Secondary Orbital Involvement

CT scan shows orbital mass with adjacent sinus, nasal, nasopharyngeal, or oropharyngeal mass. Bone erosion suggests malignancy. In approximately 70 percent of sinus tumors invading the orbit, bone destruction is present. CT scans should include views of all sinuses as well as the base of the skull.

Initial Management and Biopsy Results

All patients should have an incisional biopsy at a location where the tumor is most readily biopsied. In many patients, a biopsy through the skin may be performed under local anesthesia. In other patients, a biopsy of the mass through the nasal mucosa is more direct. In any case, the site of biopsy should later be included in the radical excision or in the radiation site.

Maxillary Sinus Carcinoma. Biopsy shows many squamous cells that are poorly keratinized and moderately-to-poorly differentiated. Ciliated columnar respiratory epithelium, a normal lining of the sinus, is not present and has presumably undergone squamous metaplasia. Peripherally placed columnar cells are present and belie a sinus origin of the tumor rather than a surface epithelial origin.

Lymphoepithelioma (Schmincke Tumor). Biopsy shows a tumor composed of poorly differentiated squamous cells with large vesicular nuclei. The tumor cells are nonkeratinizing and occur in a lymphoid stroma. Lymphoepithelioma (Schmincke tumor) has two histologic variants. In both types, nonkeratinizing squamous cells are present. In the Regaud type, the cells are arranged in nests, cords, and islands, while the Schmincke shows isolated cells scattered diffusely throughout the lymphoid stroma. Both types are variants of squamous cell carcinoma and have a similarly poor prognosis.

Sarcomatoid Carcinoma. Biopsy shows a spindle cell neoplasm with features of squamous cell carcinoma as outlined above. The sarcomatoid pattern often occurs in patients after radiation therapy.

Adenocarcinoma, Adenoid Cystic Carcinoma, and Malignant Mixed Tumor. The histologies of adenocarcinoma, adenoid cystic carcinoma, and malignant mixed tumor are identical to the lacrimal gland counterparts (see Chapter 6). All three entities in the case of a sinus origin presumably arise from the minor salivary glands of the sinus submucosa. Any adenocarcinoma should arouse suspicion of a metastatic carcinoma, and a systemic work-up should be undertaken in order to determine if the tumor is primary in the sinus and a systemic work-up should be undertaken before assuming that the tumor is primary in the sinus. Primary adenocarcinomas occur more commonly in the ethmoid sinus than the other sinuses. Mucus-producing carcinomas may also occur in the sinuses. In these cases, nests and lobules of tumor cells float in a sea of mucin.[122]

Mucoepidermoid Carcinoma. Biopsy shows features suggestive of squamous cell carcinoma. In addition, there are mucus-producing malignant cells dispersed within the tumor. Alcian-blue and colloidal iron stains demonstrate mucin within the cytoplasm of the malignant tumor cells.[121]

Ameloblastoma. This rare epithelial odontogenic tumor arises from the teeth and spreads to the sinus and the orbit.[55] Biopsy shows islands of cells with an outer layer of tall columnar cells and central portion of epithelial cells showing squamous metaplasia.

Mesectodermal Leiomyoma. Only one of these tumors has been reported. It arose from the maxillary sinus and involved the inferior orbit.

Biopsy shows a smooth muscle tumor that has a distinctly neural appearance and somewhat resembles a schwannoma. EM will confirm the smooth muscle origin of the tumor. The term *mesectodermal* refers to regions of the head that contain cells of the neural crest that contribute to the formation of bone, cartilage, connective tissue, and smooth muscle.[123]

Melanoma. Scattered melanocytes in the sinus epithelium may cause rare sinus melanomas that extend into the orbit.[54]

DEFINITIVE MANAGEMENT OF SINUS TUMORS THAT INVOLVE THE ORBIT

Most entities are best treated with complete surgical excision with an ENT colleague. The details of such surgery are beyond the scope of this book. A Lynch incision in small tumors of the medial orbit, nose, ethmoid, and frontal sinus tumors is helpful. Extensive tumors involving the maxillary sinus are approached through a Weber-Ferguson incision. The tract site from the incisional biopsy should be excised when the definitive surgical removal is performed in order to avoid seeding of the tumor along the incisional biopsy site. Preservation of the lacrimal system should be of secondary concern. The lacrimal system, especially in advanced cases, may be reconstructed at a later date if necessary. At times, maxillectomy is combined with an orbital exenteration.

Radiation may be helpful in those patients in whom the tumor has not been completely excised. A radiation therapy consultation should be obtained in such patients. Other distinct clinical entities are discussed below.

Mucocele

Clinical Features. A mucocele is an outpouching of the paranasal sinus that presumably results from obstruction of the ostium of the sinus due to chronic sinusitis (primary mucocele) or tumor (secondary mucocele). In a primary mucocele, the sinus expands as a result of the accumulation of mucus produced by the glands that line the sinus. There is no tumor causing the obstruction. The mucocele may become secondarily infected as a mucopyocele. The specific anatomic locus of pressure atrophy of the bone is dependent on the individual's anatomy and the thickness of the wall. The sinus will expand in the direction of least resistance and will cause gradual erosion of the adjacent bone of the involved paranasal sinus. Mucoceles are most common in the frontal sinus because the sinus drains dependently, and, therefore, debris is more likely to accumulate and clog the ostium.

The signs and symptoms of mucoceles are dependent on both the area of presentation and the presence or absence of secondary infection. If infection is present, a mucopyocele results. The patient presents with inflammatory signs, including pain that mimics an orbital cellulitis. Erosion of the anterior wall of the frontal sinus from a mucocele may present as a tender fluctuant mass beneath the periosteum of the frontal bone known as Pott's puffy tumor. Erosion of the posterior wall of the frontal sinus may result in an epidural, subdural, or brain abscess (Fig. 3-33).

If there is no infection, the signs and symptoms of

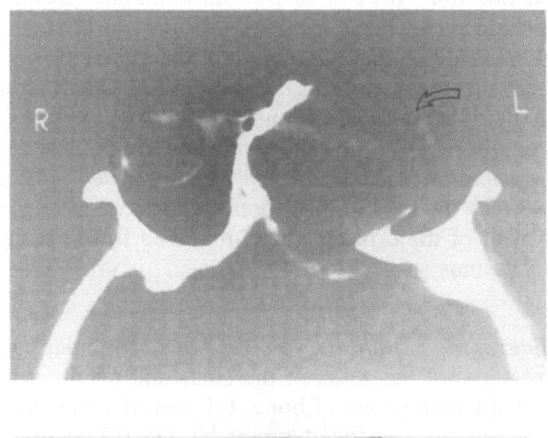

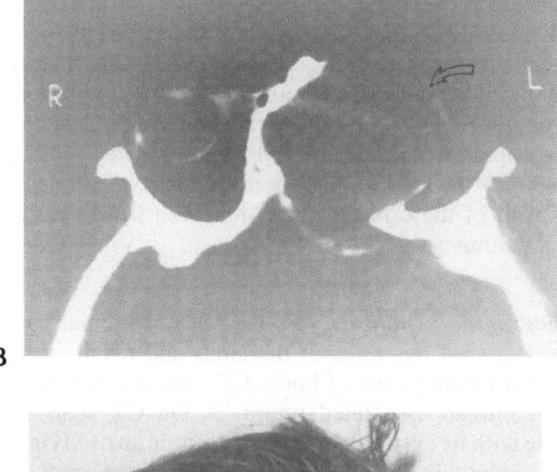

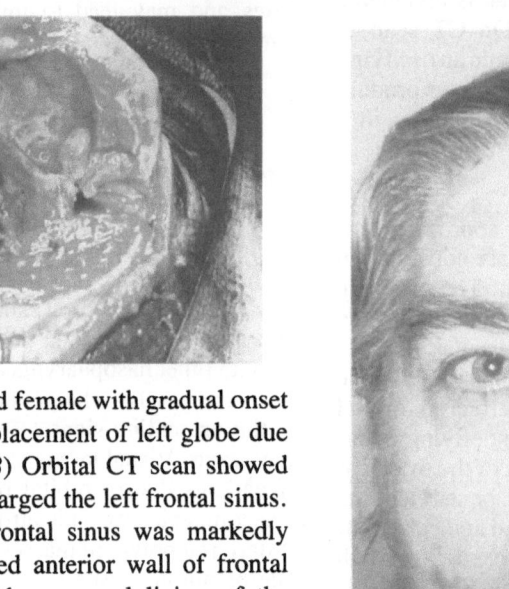

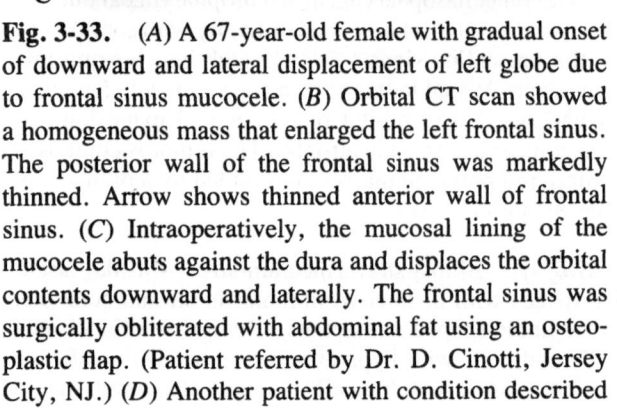

Fig. 3-33. (*A*) A 67-year-old female with gradual onset of downward and lateral displacement of left globe due to frontal sinus mucocele. (*B*) Orbital CT scan showed a homogeneous mass that enlarged the left frontal sinus. The posterior wall of the frontal sinus was markedly thinned. Arrow shows thinned anterior wall of frontal sinus. (*C*) Intraoperatively, the mucosal lining of the mucocele abuts against the dura and displaces the orbital contents downward and laterally. The frontal sinus was surgically obliterated with abdominal fat using an osteoplastic flap. (Patient referred by Dr. D. Cinotti, Jersey City, NJ.) (*D*) Another patient with condition described in (*A*).

the mucocele will be similar to those of intrinsic fibroosseous tumors of the orbital bone in which headache, proptosis, and EOM abnormalities with diplopia are common. With mucoceles, vision is rarely affected unless the sphenoid sinus is involved.

Maxillary sinus mucoceles are relatively uncommon because the ostium is located superiorly and is, therefore, less likely to become clogged. However, the prevalence is much greater in Japan. Therefore, chronic sinusitis of the antrum may lead to its contraction and secondary enophthalmos, but globe elevation and proptosis also may occur. Globe and lower lid distortion, tethering of extraocular muscles, ptosis, and rarely optic nerve compression have been reported.[124] Other findings include pain, erosion of the inferior orbital rim including the

infraorbital nerve, and epiphora due to obliteration of the nasolacrimal duct. The presence of an inner canthal mass may mimic a lacrimal sac tumor or inflammation. The mass is typically inferior and lateral to the sac. Anterior ethmoidal mucoceles may rarely compress the lacrimal sac or nasolacrimal duct and result in tearing.

Ethmoid sinus mucoceles take a long time to form because each of 20 air cells must individually become infected before the wall of sinus expands laterally toward the orbit. A sphenoid sinus mucocele may threaten vision because of possible secondary optic nerve compression. A sinus tumor that obstructs the drainage of the sinus must be ruled out.

Mucoceles are uncommon in children. However, children with cystic fibrosis may develop ethmoidal sinus mucoceles since these are the first sinuses to aerate. In a child, one must always suspect an ethmoidal meningoencephaloceles when considering the diagnosis of ethmoidal mucocele. Other predisposing causes include previous sinus or intranasal surgery, polyps, deviated nasal septum that occludes the sinus, trauma, and allergy. Occasionally massive ethmoidal sinus polyposis may result in proptosis. In this unusual circumstance, polyps prolapse into the orbit either spontaneously or after the medial wall of the orbit has been removed for previous ethmoidal sinus surgery.[125–132]

Radiographic Findings. As the mucocele enlarges, it presses against the walls of the sinus and results in a thin-walled leading edge of bone. CT scan is invaluable in ruling out an associated tumor.[130] On CT scan, a mucocele with its cystic character may mimic an ossifying fibroma except that the latter is diffuse and shows production of bony tumor rather than the bone-thinning in a mucocele.

Management. If infection is present, appropriate antibiotic therapy guided by infectious disease consultation is necessary prior to surgical intervention. The principle of surgical treatment is to reestablish drainage into the nose or nasofrontal duct in the case of frontal sinus or frontal ethmoidal sinus mucoceles. An incision is made just below the brow down to the superonasal orbital rim. The periosteum is freed from the underlying bone. Care is taken to allow for reestablishment of the trochlear anatomy. The thin-walled mucocele is penetrated, its contents expressed, and the lining removed and curretted. Irregular edges of bone are rongeured to create a smooth surface. A catheter that drains the sinus and extends through the nose is left in place for 2–3 weeks. The catheter is either sutured to the nasal septum or kept in place with packing. Initial placement of the catheter is facilitated by advancing a hemostat through the nose into the sinus. For large or bilateral mucoceles, all the sinus mucosa is excised and the bare bone burred with a drill to ensure removal of epithelium. An osteoplastic flap procedure with adipose obliteration of the sinus should be performed with an otolaryngologist. The periosteum may be closed with 4–0 chromic sutures. The skin is closed with 5–0 and 6–0 sutures.

Inverted Papilloma

Clinical and CT Scan Features. Inverted papillomas typically arise from the mucosa of the nasal cavity and paranasal sinus (schneiderian membrane). The absence of pain may be helpful in distinguishing this benign lesion from other malignant tumors arising in the sinus and nose. Some patients may have had a previous poly-

pectomy without histologic confirmation years earlier.[133–138] Due to mucinous degeneration, the lesion may have a cystic appearance on CT scan (Fig. 3-34).

A cyst-like structure may be encountered on surgical exploration.

Pathologic Features. Grossly, the specimen may be mistaken for a dermoid or epidermoid cyst. The lack of a keratin core favors the diagnosis of inverted papilloma. The tumor appears gelatinous and gray in color. A small biopsy might not be representative. Multiple sections need to be reviewed in order to rule out a carcinoma originating in an inverted papilloma. Malignant transformation occurs in approximately 5–10 percent of cases and may lead to intracranial extension or local lymph node metastases as well as lung metastases.

Angiofibroma

Clinical Signs. Angiofibroma is a vascular tumor of the oropharynx that occurs in adolescent males and may erode into the orbit, sinuses, and intracranial extension into the base of the skull in 10–20 percent of cases. As with other nasopharyngeal and oropharyngeal tumors, epistaxis, nasal discharge, and difficulty with speech may be the presenting signs.[139–141] In addition, hearing loss may occur. Visual loss occurs in approximately 5 percent of patients due to orbital or intracranial extension and is accompanied by optic atrophy. The tumor is composed of dark red polypoid masses surrounded by a pseudocapsule of fibrous tissue.[126]

Biopsy. Biopsy shows medium-sized, slit-like vascular spaces with distinctive fibroblastic stroma cells that are spindle-shaped or stellate. Benign multinucleated cells and cells with hyperchromatic nuclei may also be present. While cytologically benign, the tumor has a propensity for aggressive local growth.

Management. Complete surgical excision is the treatment of choice as with other tumors in this area, but recurrences occur in about 50 percent of cases; bleeding may be severe and may prove fatal. The CO_2 or contact YAG laser may be helpful. Adjunctive hormonal (estrogen) therapy may be helpful in that tumors often regress as sexually immature males reach maturity.

Esthesioneuroblastomas

Clinical Features. Esthesioneuroblastoma is more descriptively termed *olfactory neuroblastoma* since it

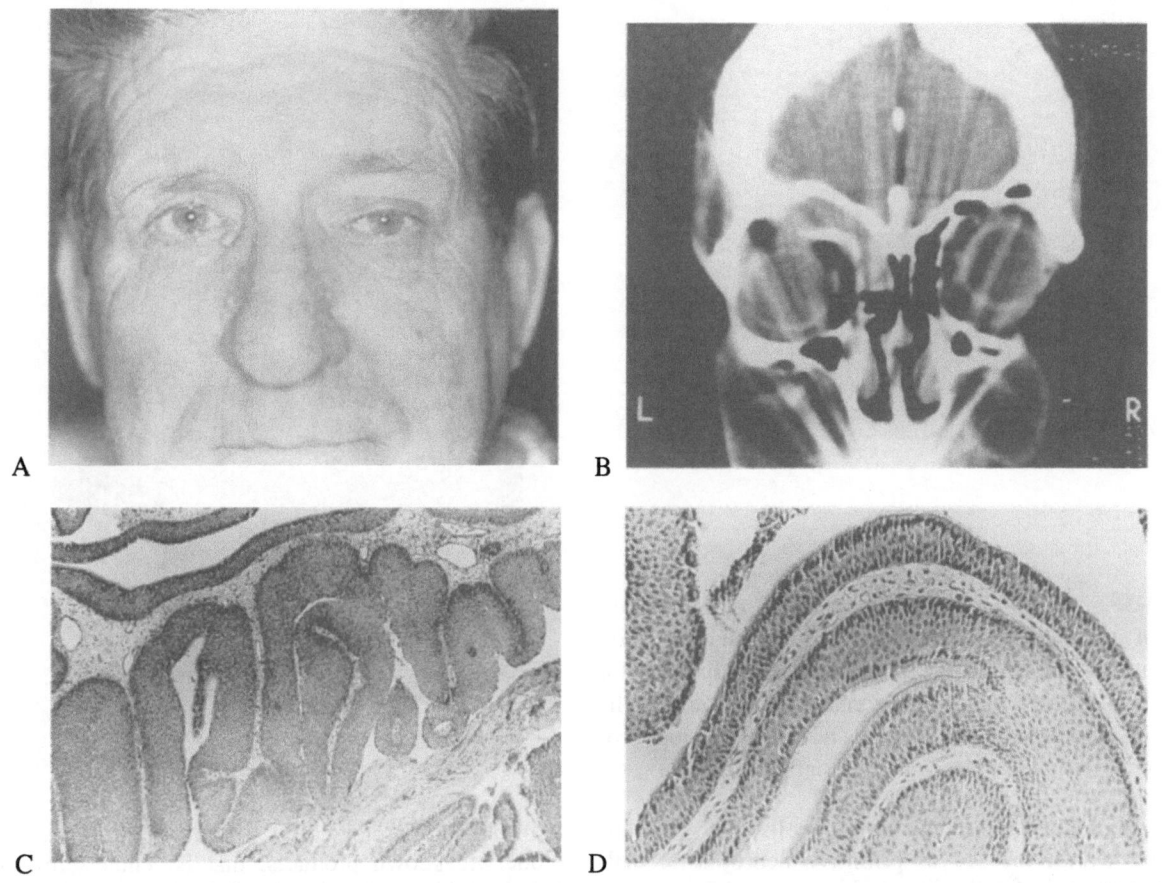

Fig. 3-34. (*A*) A 64-year-old male with proptosis and downward displacement of left globe. (*B*) CT scan showed bone erosion through the frontal sinus into the right orbit. While expansion of the entire frontal sinus as in Figure 3-33 favors a mucocele, focal erosion as present in this case may occur with a mucocele or a tumor. (*C*, *D*) In this case, an inverted papilloma arising from the ciliated respiratory epithelium of the frontal sinus was diagnosed. (Patient referred by Dr. Anthony Panariello, Jersey City, NJ.)

arises from the olfactory sensory epithelium in the roof of the nasal fossa.

Like other neuroblastic tumors and angiofibromas, the tumor primarily affects young patients in the second and third decades of life. However, the tumor is unlike other neuroblastic tumors in that middle-aged and older patients may also be affected. Males are generally more commonly affected than females. Nasal obstruction and bleeding from the nose are the most common presenting symptoms. The most common ocular symptoms include perioorbital pain, increased lacrimation, blurred vision, and diplopia. Other distinctive features include anosmia and cerebrospinal rhinorrhea. The presence of ocular and nasal symptoms should always arouse clinical suspicion of this tumor. As expected, ocular symptoms tend to occur later in the course of the disease than nasal symptoms, although the patient may seek attention ultimately because of ocular symptoms.[142–143]

CT Scan Findings. Esthesioneuroblastomas will show CT evidence of ethmoid sinus or orbital involvement. Bone erosion is present (Fig. 3-35).

Biopsy. Biopsy shows a soft-to-firm poorly circumscribed pink-to-gray tumor composed almost entirely of primitive neuroblastic cells. The tumor tends to bleed readily in the surgical field. The tumor cells are small cells with ovoid, hyperchomatic nuclei, scanty cytoplasm, and indistinct cell membrane. The tumor is indistinguishable from sympathetic neuroblastoma on light microscopy alone. Unlike sympathetic neuroblastomas, esthesioneuroblastomas do not produce catecholamines. Homer-Wright rosettes composed of cells forming central tangles of cell processes without a lumen may be present. Homer-Wright rosettes are to be distinguished from the Flexner-Wintersteiner rosettes of retinoblastoma that contain lumen formed by primitive tumor cells. In addition to esthesioneuroblastoma, there are two other subtypes of olfactory neural tumors: esthesioneurocytomas and esthesioneuroepithelioma. Esthesioneurocytomas have cells with more ample cytoplasm and more differentiated cellular processes than esthesioneuroblastoma. Esthesioneurocytomas are also more likely to have other well-differentiated features such as Homer-Wright rosettes than esthesioneuroblastomas. Esthesioneuroepitheliomas

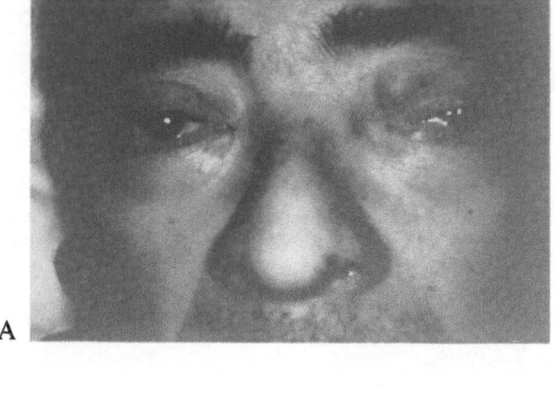

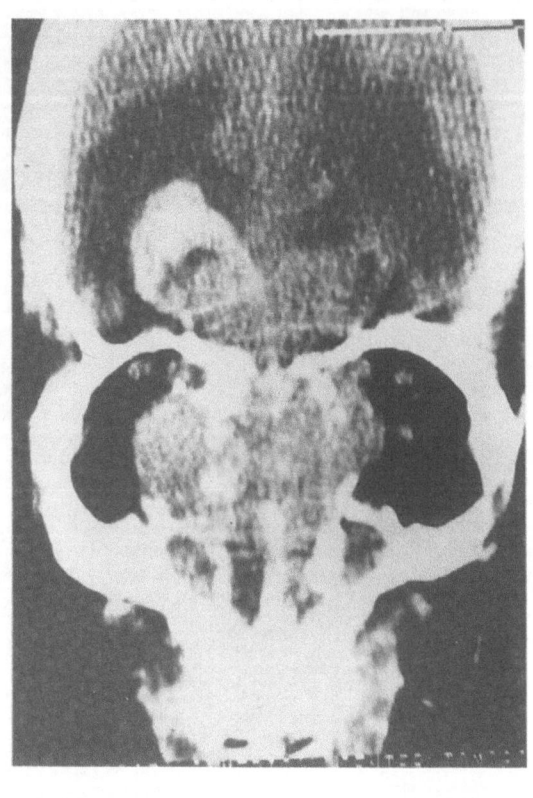

Fig. 3-35. (*A*) A 63-year-old male with 2-month history of pain and medial orbital swelling with nasal congestion and loss of smell. (*B*) CT scan showed midline tumor causing massive bone destruction and extension into the brain. Biopsy of the nasal mass showed esthesioneuroblastoma. The patient received palliative radiation.

have cuboidal or columnar luminal cells that are interspersed within the sea of primitive neuroblastic cells that are typical of esthesioneuroblastomas.

Management. Surgical ablation combined with radiation is the treatment of choice. The initial management should include incisional biopsy. Many times under local anesthesia, an incisional biopsy through the lid may be obtained. In other cases, a more direct biopsy route might be through the nose or via a Caldwell-Luc. We do not believe a fine needle aspiration biopsy should be the basis for radical surgery. Patients with extensive intracranial involvement may not be candidates even for palliative debulking; neurosurgical consultation is necessary for such patients.

Like other neuroblastic tumors, esthesioneuroblastomas are generally quite radiosensitive. Recurrences are common in approximately 50 percent of patients and may occur as long as 24 years after onset. In the largest ophthalmic series of esthesioneuroblastomas, 18 of 38 patients died of their disease.[143] Death results from local recurrence with intracranial extension; metastases to the local lymph nodes and lung occur in 20–60 percent of patients.

Cholesteatomas

Definition. The term cholesteatoma was introduced by Muller in 1938 to describe a tumor containing choles-

terol clefts. Histologically, a granulomatous reaction to blood breakdown products, that is, cholesterol, or to keratin lipids produced by epithelial elements is present. A primary cholesteatoma originates from a granulomatous reaction to keratin lipids produced by embryonal aberrant or entrapped squamous epithelium while a secondary cholesteatoma results from a posttraumatic or postsurgical epithelial inclusion.[144–148] Alternatively, the lining of the sinus that undergoes squamous metaplasia is the origin.

In some cases, epithelium is not present. Histologically, there is a granulomatous reaction to blood breakdown products that result from sequestered blood in any location. When no epithelium is present, the origin of such postinflammatory pseudotumors is even more obscure than when epithelial elements are present. Trauma may play a role in some cases. An intradiploic focus has been proposed since in some cholesteatomas that extend from the frontal bone toward the orbit, the inner and outer tables of the frontal bone are both eroded and the intraorbital extension is subperiosteal.

Clinical Features. Proptosis with limitation of upgaze and diplopia is the usual symptom. Pain is a variable symptom. Other sinuses including the ethmoid and maxillary sinus may also be involved.

CT Scan Findings. A mass lesion is present in the superonasal orbit with bone erosion of the frontal sinus; the posterior aspect of the sinus may be eroded. The lesion may be mistaken for a mucocele. However, with a mucocele, there is an expansile filling and outpouching of the entire sinus and its wall before the orbit is invaded. With a cholesteatoma, there is focal bone erosion with invasion of the orbit.

Tumors may also present in the superotemporal peripheral surgical space without sinus involvement but with significant thinning of the frontal bone with variable sclerosis. The lesion may appear circumscribed.

Management. Combined ophthalmologic and otolaryngologic expertise is necessary. Intraoperatively, a white, refractive nodular mass that represents cholesterol is often present. At other times, blood breakdown products may be visible as brown cheesy or greenish-brown material. Cholesterol will be evident as refractile bodies within the mass. When the mass spares the frontal sinus, the diagnosis of hematic cyst of the orbit should be considered. The latter lesion may also have an epithelial component.

Excision with curettage and placement of a drain that exits through the skin wound is usually curative. Those hematic cysts associated with epithelial elements rarely undergo malignant degeneration into squamous cell carcinoma; yet, the need for complete surgical excision is underscored by this possibility. Lesions that have epithelium may appear encapsulated at the time of surgery. Frozen sections are helpful in determining if there is an epithelial component. In some cases, packing of the frontal sinus with abdominal fat is necessary to ablate the sinus after the bone is burred with a drain to remove any epithelial remnants. It is logical that those cholesteatomas with epithelial elements are more likely to recur and may undergo malignant degeneration. In addition, these patients require greater follow-up and more radical surgery.

INTRAOCULAR TUMORS WITH ORBITAL EXTENSION

Basically, there are four intraocular tumors that may present with an orbital component: (1) retinoblastoma, (2) malignant melanoma of the choroid, (3) medulloepithelioma, and (4) carcinomas of the nonpigmented ciliary epithelium (Tables 3-17 and 3-18). A lymphoid infiltrate of the uvea, whether frankly malignant or totally benign, may have a noninflammatory clinical presentation with an orbital component. Similarly, leukemia may present with a predominantly uveal infiltrate and an orbital mass lesion. Rarely, granulocytic sarcoma, which almost always presents as an orbital mass with or without retinal straie, may also have iridic, choroidal, or vitreal involvement.

In addition, there are orbital tumors that invade the eye secondarily. These tumors include optic nerve gli-

Table 3-17
Secondary Tumors of the Orbit

Sinus Tumors
Intraocular tumors
   malignant melanoma of the choroid
   retinoblastoma
   medulloepithelioma
   carcinoma of the nonpigmented ciliary epithelium
   granulocytic sarcoma
   leukemia
   lymphoid
Lid Tumors with Orbital Extension (Skin)
   basal cell carcinoma
   squamous cell carcinoma
   sebaceous gland carcinoma
   adnexal carcinomas other than sebaceous
   melanoma
Conjunctival
   squamous cell carcinoma
   mucoepidermoid carcinoma
   melanoma
Lacrimal sac tumors with orbital extension (see Chapter 7).
   papilloma
   SCC
   lymphoma
   melanoma
Intracranial Tumors
   sphenoidal ridge meningioma
   chordoma
Metastatic from Distant Sites

oma, meningioma, and adenoid cystic carcinoma of the lacrimal gland. Each of these is discussed in the following sections.

Malignant Melanoma of the Choroid

Clinical Signs. Extraocular extension of choroidal melanoma occurs in 10–29 percent of cases.[149] Uveal melanomas that predispose to extraocular extension, in addition to being large epithelioid cell-containing tumors that often rupture through Bruch's membrane, are often diffuse.[150] In addition, orbital recurrence is likely when

Table 3-18
Orbital Tumors with Ocular Invasion

Optic nerve glioma
Optic nerve meningioma
Adenoid cystic carcinoma of the lacrimal gland

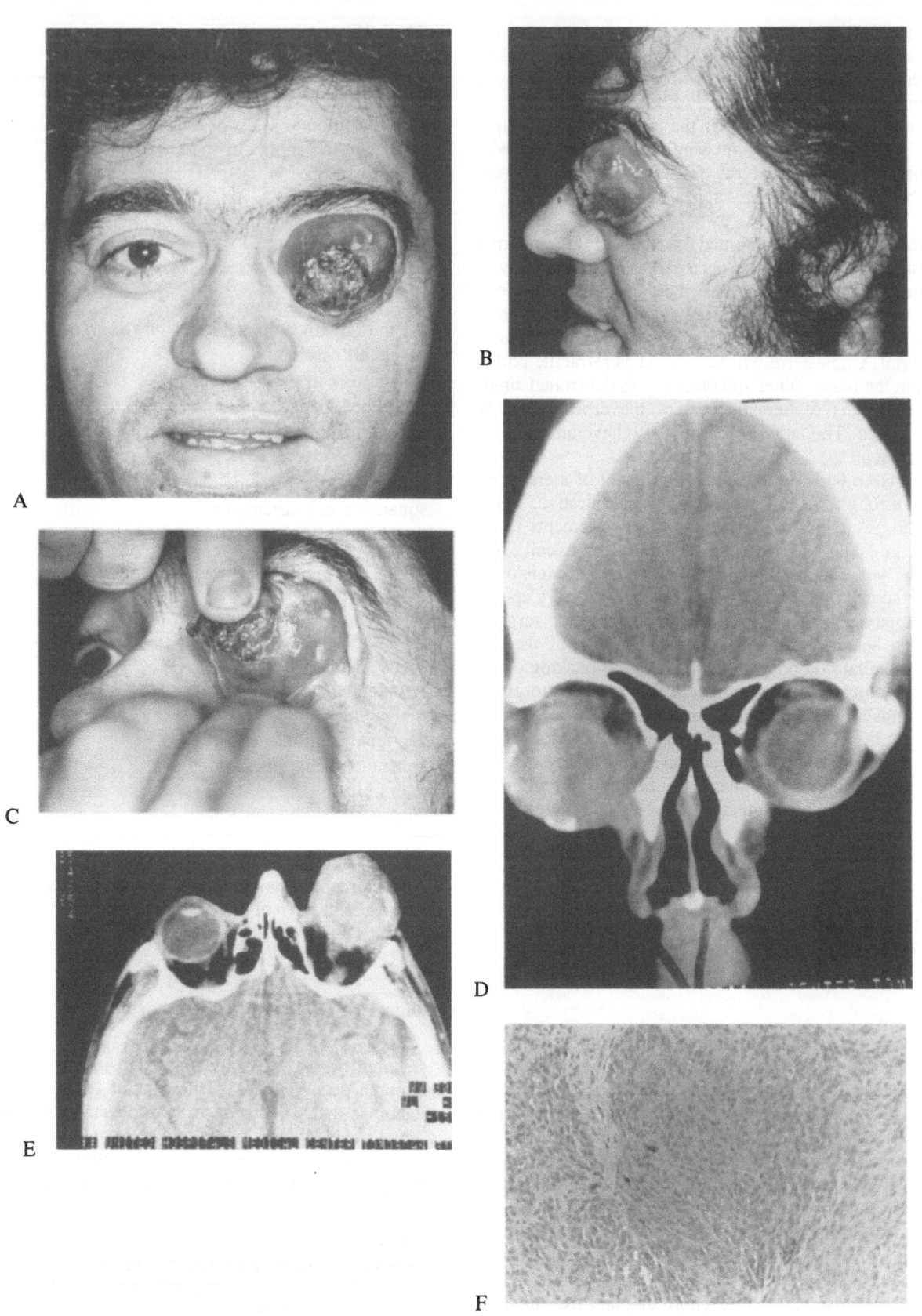

Fig. 3-36. (*A–C*) A 36-year-old male who presented with hemorrhage from the left eye for several days. On examination there was a fungating mass that emanated from the left eye. (*D,E*) Orbital CT scan showed calcified lens material and an intraocular tumor without extension to the bony orbital walls. (*F*) Biopsy showed spindle cells containing melanin consistent with malignant melanoma of the choroid with extrascleral extension. Work-up showed no evidence of metastases. Exenteration was performed.

an extraocular extension of a melanoma has not been completely removed with the globe. When tumor is suspected to be present on the episcleral surface, frozen sections should be obtained.

The most common initial signs of orbital extension of an intraocular malignant melanoma are those that relate directly to the eye. These signs include an intraocular or epibulbar mass (61%), glaucoma (61%), decreased vision (41%), retinal detachment (37%), or cataract (24%). Rarely is proptosis an initial sign.[151] At times, large untreated tumors present with hemorrhage (Fig. 3-36). Even more rarely, focal relatively small choroidal melanomas may be associated with an orbital component (Fig. 3-37).[152] The orbital component may have an area of central necrosis.[153] When there is massive necrosis, the clinical symptoms may resemble a bacterial orbital cellulitis and the CT scan may falsely suggest a localized walled-off abscess (Fig. 3-38).

An orbital mass may also be present years after enucleation of an eye containing a choroidal melanoma.[154–158]

CT Scan and Ultrasonic Findings. CT scan shows a choroidal mass with adjacent retrobulbar extension and may resemble an orbital cavernous hemangioma if the intraocular component is ignored. The orbital component may have a central area of necrosis.

B-scan ultrasonographic findings associated with choroidal melanoma include (1) mass lesion, (2) choroidal excavation, (3) acoustic "quiet zone," (4) shadowing of orbital fat, and (5) collar button configuration. Relative sonolucency immediately behind the sclera often occurs with extraocular extension.[149]

Management. The management of a choroidal melanoma with orbital extension is controversial.[159] Shammas

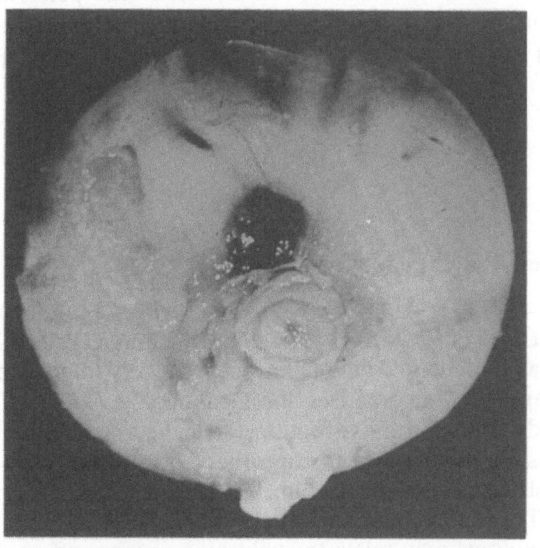

Fig. 3-37. Malignant melanoma with nodule of extrascleral extension.

and Blodi have advocated exenteration.[154] Starr and Zimmerman suggest that exenteration may not be curative but palliative, and they therefore advocate exenteration.[160] Still others question whether exenteration like enucleation may disseminate the tumor.[153,161] The presence of an encapsulated orbital mass may favorably influence prognosis. Melanomas with orbital spread usually are treated with exenteration because of factors that do not directly relate to improved prognosis such as lack of useful vision and severe proptosis and corneal exposure. Preoperative radiation may be of benefit.[162]

In any case, an oncologic work-up should be performed. When metastases from the choroid occur, the liver or lung is involved in 97 percent of cases. Therefore, liver function studies and chest x-rays should be obtained by the oncologist. Chemotherapy, immunotherapy, or radiation therapy may be of benefit with or without exenteration.

Retinoblastoma

Clinical Presentation. Of patients with retinoblastomas, 75 percent have the nonheriditary type, while 25 percent have the hereditary tumor.[163] Patients with bilateral hereditary retinoblastomas are more prone to local orbital spread than patients with unilateral disease. In addition, a retrobulbar tumor nodule may follow iatrogenic rupture of a globe containing a retinoblastoma during its enucleation (Fig. 3-38). Orbital recurrence tends to occur within the first 4 months after enucleation. Similarly, most patients with fatal outcomes die within 9 months of detection of their disease. The other important fact is that only 10 percent of patients survive with clinically apparent or biopsy-proven orbital spread.[164]

On examination, proptosis and lid swelling with or without ecchymosis may be present. Subconjunctival tumor nodules are soft and purple in color.

CT Scan Findings. Intraocular calcifications are often present (see Chapter 4).[165–167] In one study, every eye that presented with leukocoria due to retinoblastoma had calcifications. Coats' disease, persistent hyperplastic primary vireous (PHPV), and *Toxocara canis* may also have intraocular calcifications. Calcifications are easily seen on CT but not MRI scan. Other lesions including optic nerve head drusen, retinal astrocytoma, choroidal hemangioma, choroidal osteoma, retinopathy of prematurity, retinal dyaplasia, and trauma do not usually contain calcifications at the early age when retinoblastoma is diagnosed. Also, none of these simulating lesions show extraocular extension. CT scan of the head may also show central nervous system involvement, secondary orbital tumors, and pineal tumors such as that found in trilateral retinoblastoma.

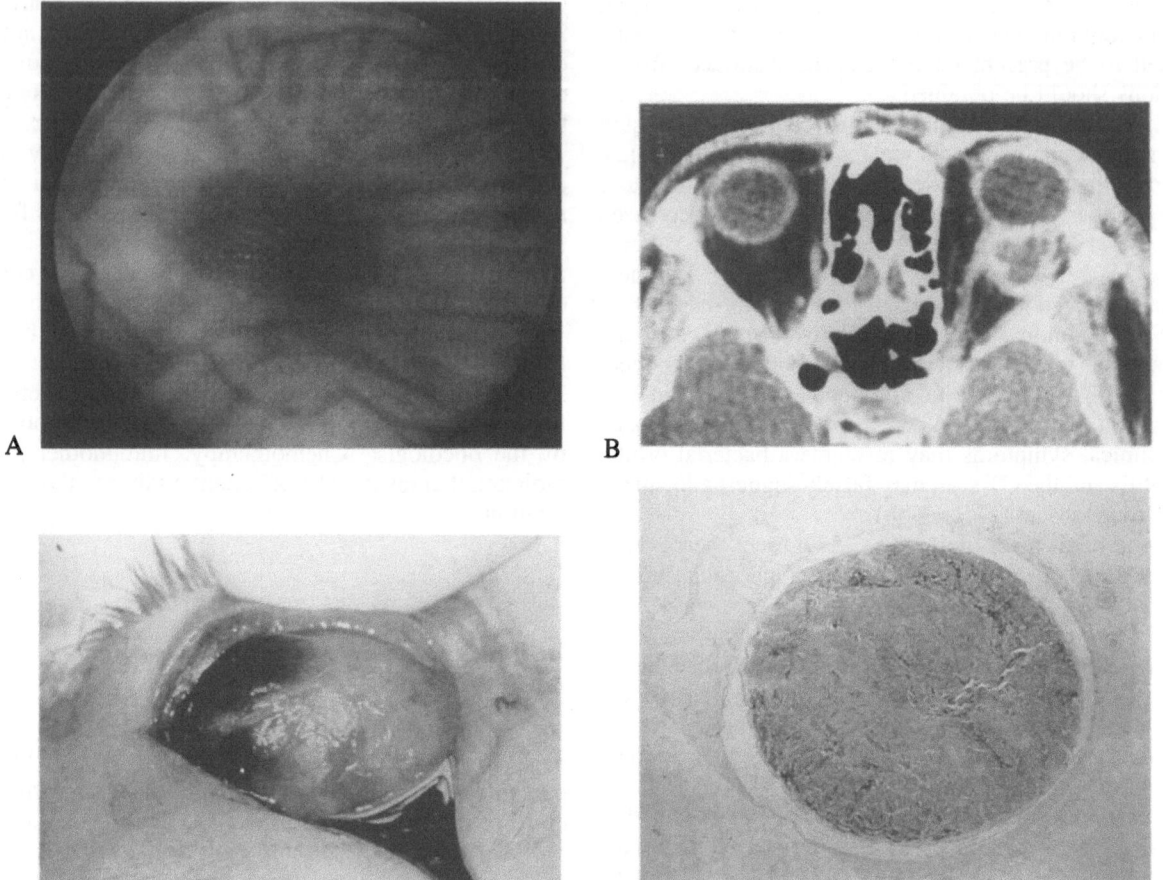

Fig. 3-38. (*A*) View of posterior pole of 63-year-old white male with a 3-month history of decreased vision to 20/100 in the left eye. He had an episode of decreased vision to 20/40 three months prior associated with conjunctival chemosis. Two semi-flat pigmented lesions were noted: (1) two disc diameters in width and submacular in location and (2) less than a disc diameter in width located superior to the disc. (*B*) Orbital CT scan showed an enhanced orbital mass adjacent to the temporal sclera with a central radiolucent necrotic lucency. Biopsy of the orbital mass showed malignant melanoma of the mixed cell type. Two weeks later an exenteration was performed. (Courtesy of Drs. Joel Kopelman and Norman Shorr, presented at the 11th Biennial Ophthalmic Alumni of the AFIP Meeting.) (*C*) Retinoblastoma with recurrence to orbit (AFIP ACC #1493394). (*D*) Retinoblastoma with extension into optic nerve (AFIP ACC #1182928).

Management. Patients with retinoblastoma and particularly those with extraocular extension should have a metastatic work-up including skull x-rays, long bone x-rays, cerebrospinal fluid examination, and bone marrow evaluation. Ophthalmologists, radiotherapists, and pediatric oncologists must aggressively treat patients with extraocular spread of retinoblastoma. Debulking of the tumor mass followed by appropriate chemotherapy and radiotherapy is the basic approach. We believe the management of these tumors is best performed at major centers where such patients are seen frequently. The exact treatment of such extraocular extension is beyond the scope of this book.

Medulloepithelioma

Clinical Features. Medulloepithelioma is an embryonal noninherited tumor almost exclusively found in children. The tumor arises most commonly at the ciliary body from primitive optic vesicle neuroepithelium or less commonly near the optic nervehead from persistent embryonal medullary epithelium.[168–169]

The median age of the patients is 5 years. Presenting symptoms may relate to strabismus or mass effect. The tumor itself appears as a white or partially pigmented mass. In general, orbital disease occurs several years after enucleation and is more common in those tumors that are located in the posterior pole because of the proximity of the posterior orbit.

CT Scan Findings. CT scan may be helpful in showing the intraocular tumor either at the ciliary body or optic nerve region. In the latter site, the absence of calcifications helps rule out the diagnosis of retinoblastoma.

Biopsy. Biopsy shows a tumor composed of two basic components. The first is a differentiated component of multilaminar cords and nests of columnar cells that create a netlike pattern, hence the old term, *diktyoma,* which is Greek for net. The cells may elaborate hyaluronic acid-like material detectable on special stains. The second component is a mass of poorly differentiated neuroblastic cells with scanty cytoplasm and hyperchromatic nuclei. Tumor buds may escape from the main mass of cells and form free-floating cysts in the aqueous. Teratoid elements including cartilage, striated muscle, and neuroglial tissue may be present. Depending on the degree of mitotic activity and cellular atypia, the tumor may be classified as benign or malignant. Metastases occur to orbital bones, brain, local lymph nodes, and lungs.

Management. Once extraocular extension is present, exenteration is probably the treatment of choice. Four of 33 patients with follow-up in the study by Broughton and Zimmerman died of their disease. The fact that three of the four patients with metastatic disease were adults suggests that such congenital tumors can be quiescent for years and become aggressive. Metastases may occur to orbital bones, brain, local lymph nodes, and lungs.

These tumors are generally not radiosensitive, and, therefore, surgical extirpation including exenteration is the treatment of choice as mentioned above. Those tumors that originate in the optic nerve are more likely to spread locally in the orbit than ciliary body medulloepitheliomas.

Carcinoma of the Nonpigmented Ciliary Epithelium

These rare tumors generally present as an epibulbar mass. Biopsy might suggest a metastatic carcinoma, but the presence of hyaluronic acid belies their origin. In addition, the presence of a PAS-positive basement membrane of the ciliary epithelium is diagnostic. The tumor may also present in phthisical eye.

Management. Exenteration is the treatment of choice. These tumors do not metastasise but are locally aggressive.[170–171]

LID AND CONJUNCTIVAL TUMORS WITH ORBITAL INVOLVEMENT

Lid tumors are discussed in a separate section. This brief discussion will focus on the management of the aggressive tumors. The reader is urged to review Chapter 8 in conjunction with this chapter.

Basal Cell Carcinoma

Clinical Presentation. Basal cell carcinoma of the eyelid represents approximately 19.3 percent of all lid tumors and 90 percent of malignant lid tumors. It is 40 times more common than squamous cell carcinoma in the eyelid region. Patients with neglected tumors will develop orbital invasion.[172]

Clinical proptosis is not common, but fixation to the orbital rim suggests orbital invasion (Fig. 3-39).

For histopathology, see Chapter 8.

Management. Surgical excision should be the primary mode of therapy. Orbital invasion often necessitates exenteration. Frozen sections on orbital fat are fairly reliable, but the question of bone invasion can only be answered to the level of the periosteum. Bone cannot be decalcified quickly enough for frozen section study. While CT scan may show soft tissue invasion, it is most helpful in determining whether the ethmoid sinus is involved.

Mohs' microsurgery has value in treating basal cell carcinomas of the eyelid in certain situations: (1) recurrent basal cell carcinoma of the eyelid, (2) tumors of the medial canthus, and (3) extensive tumors in young patients with multicentric tumors and morpheaform basal cell carcinomas.[173]

Postoperative radiation may be helpful in some patients but should not be the main therapy. Local and systemic chemotherapy using cisplatin (Platinol) and doxorubicin (Adriamycin) has been used successfully in some patients who have refused surgery.[172]

Squamous Cell Carcinoma of the Lid

See Chapter 8.

Sebaceous Gland Carcinoma

See Chapter 8.

Sebaceous gland (holocrine gland) carcinoma of the eyelid, unlike other tumors of the eyelid, is often multi-

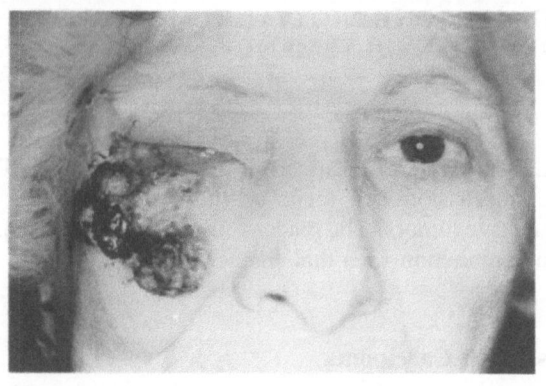

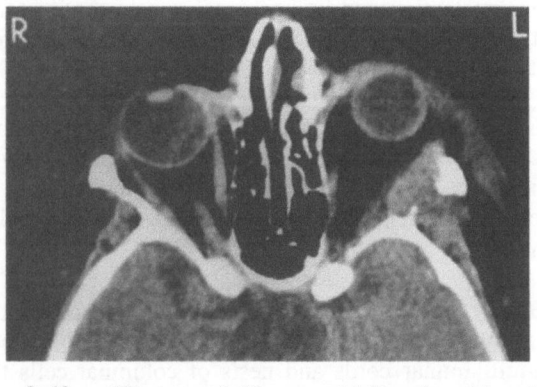

Fig. 3-39. A 69-year-old female with basal cell carcinoma causing cicatricial ectropion of the right lower lid that is most markedly laterally. Tumor was fixed to bone of lateral orbital rim. (Patient referred by Dr. A. Cinotti, Jersey City, NJ.)

Fig. 3-40. CT scan of 55-year-old female with orbital recurrence of adnexal sweat carcinoma removed from left lower lid 5 years before. Note extensive bony destruction of lateral orbital wall. (Patient referred by Dr. Louis Morrone, North Arlington, NJ.)

centric and shows diffuse pagetoid intraepithelial spread. For these reasons, more aggressive surgical treatment is necessary than is customary for treating basal cell carcinoma of the lid. Wider excision and earlier exenteration is indicated and may be life-saving. Because the tumor is often diffuse, multiple biopsies that sample the entire bulbar and palpebral conjunctiva are recommended. These biopsies should not be frozen sections but should be permanent sections and should precede radical surgery.[174]

Adnexal Carcinomas Other Than Sebaceous Gland Carcinoma

Sweat gland (eccrine) carcinomas tend to be more aggressive and more likely to metastasize than apocrine carcinoma of Moll's glands, which are almost always only locally aggressive and nonmetastasizing. Mucinous adenocarcinoma of the lids metastasizes with less frequency than eccrine carcinoma; yet a primary adenocarcinoma of the lid is rare and a work-up for metastatic disease is necessary (Fig. 3-40). A mucinous adenocarcinoma of the lid may arise from a breast or gastrointestinal primary. Similarly, a clear cell carcinoma of the lid is statistically more likely to represent metastatic renal cell carcinoma than clear cell cell carcinoma of the sweat gland.[175–176]

Malignant Melanoma of the Lids

Primary malignant melanoma of the eyelids is exceedingly rare. Nonetheless, primary malignant melanoma of the eyelids may spread locally to the orbit or metastasize via local lymph nodes or hematogenously. Rarely,

a cellular blue nevus associated with nevus of Ota may undergo malignant transformation and necessitate exenteration.

CONJUNCTIVAL TUMORS WITH ORBITAL EXTENSION

Squamous cell Carcinoma of the Limbus

Patients with advanced squamous cell carcinoma of the conjunctiva may have orbital extension. With the exception of patients with xeroderma pigmentosum or patients from tropical climates who may develop advanced squamous cell carcinoma at a young age, patients with advanced squamous cell carcinoma of the limbus are generally in their 50s and 60s. Death from orbital invasion is extremely rare.[177]

An unpublished study of squamous cell carcinoma precursor lesions by Drs. Ian McLean and Mauriello showed that such lesions could be divided into two basic types that have distinct clinical, histologic, and prognostic features: (1) "dysplasias," which are characterized by frequent recurrence and the tendency to become overt squamous cell carcinomas (Fig. 3-41), (2) "actinic keratoses," where recurrence and malignant transformation are exceedingly rare (Fig. 3-42), and (3) papillomas that are diffuse and frequently recur. Dysplasias clinically are diffuse, gelatinous-appearing lesions that histologically have a basaloid appearanace with little keratinization. Papillomas have a collagen vascular core and are composed of basaloid cells (Fig. 3-43). Actinic keratoses are focal, leukoplakic-appearing lesions that histologically have hyperkeratosis or parakeratosis and appear squamoid (Fig. 3-41).

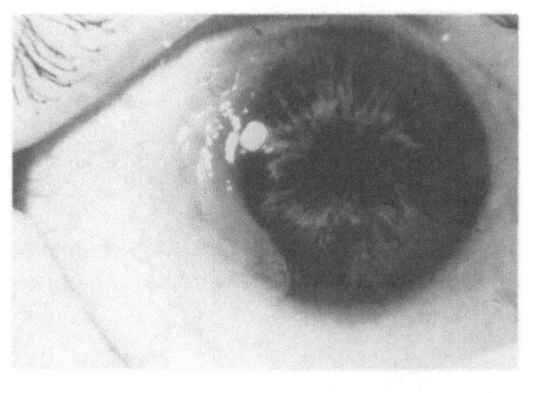

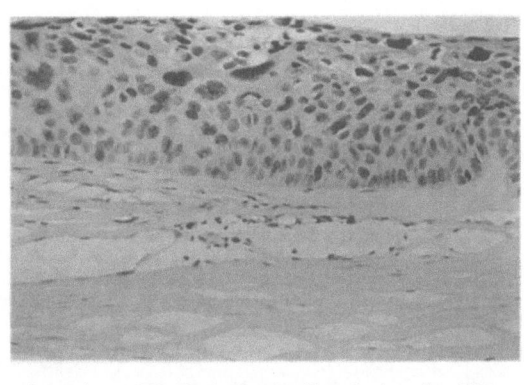

A

B

Fig. 3-41. (*A*) Note gelatinous appearance of dysplasia of conjunctiva. (*B*) Pathologically, lesion is diffuse and composed of basaloid cells with no parakeratosis or hyperkeratosis (AFIP ACC #1277391).

Mucoepidermoid carcinoma, a rare histologic variant of squamous cell carcinoma, tends to be more aggressive and deserves more aggressive surgical excision than the garden variety of squamous cell carcinoma of the limbus.[178-179]

Malignant Melanoma of the Conjunctiva

Malignant melanoma of the conjunctiva may arise de novo from a preexisting nevus or from acquired melano-

sis. A nevus, in turn, may be cystic and amelanotic and clinically resemble a lymphangioma of the conjunctiva. Nevi are composed of cells with ovoid nuclei arranged in nests at the junction of the epithelium and substantia propria (junctional nevus), in the substantia propria (subepithelial nevus), or in both locations (compound nevus).

Acquired melanosis of the conjunctiva is the skin equivalent of melanotic freckle of Hutchinson (Figs. 3-44 and 3-45). In the latter acquired condition in mostly adults over 50 years of age, there is a light brown or black macule of the skin of the face. As in the skin

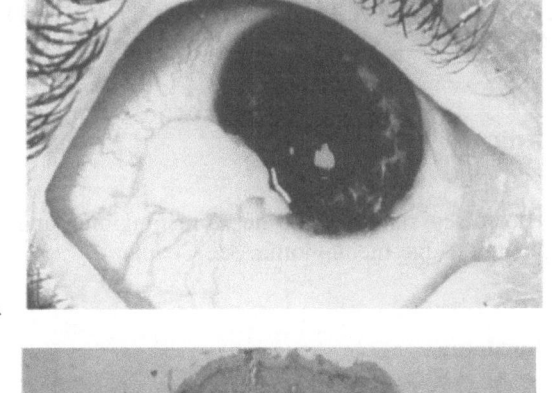

A

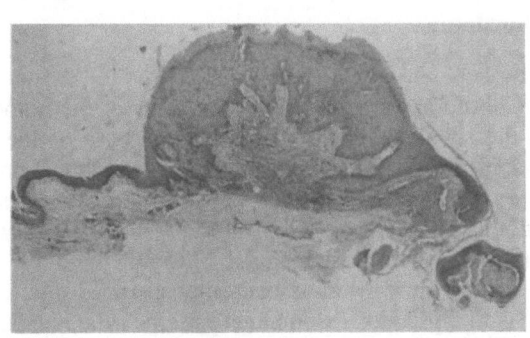

B

Fig. 3-42. (*A*) Actinic keratosis is a localized discrete tumor that appears leukoplakic due to hyperkeratosis or parakeratosis. (*B*) The lesion is squamoid rather than basaloid (AFIP ACC #114289).

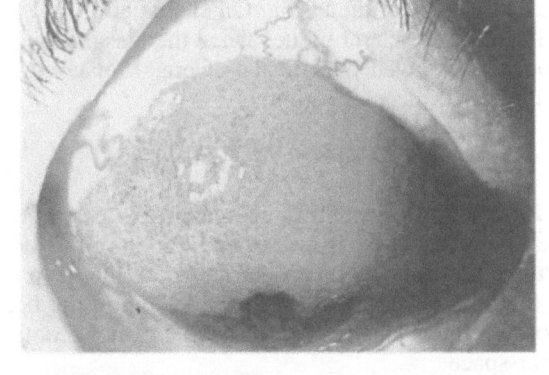

A

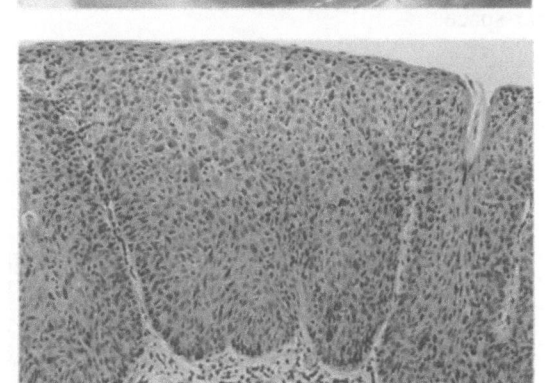

B

Fig. 3-43. Papillomatous lesion has many fibrovascular cores. Note marked acanthosis.

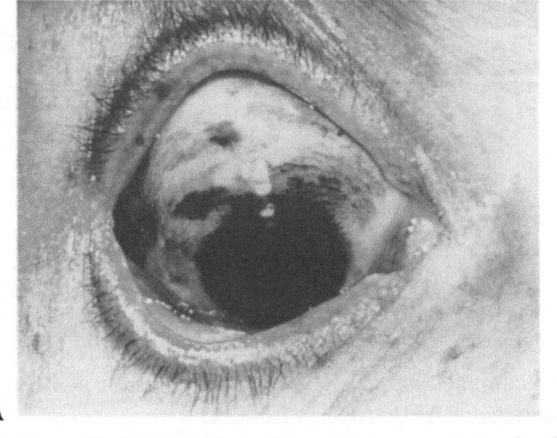
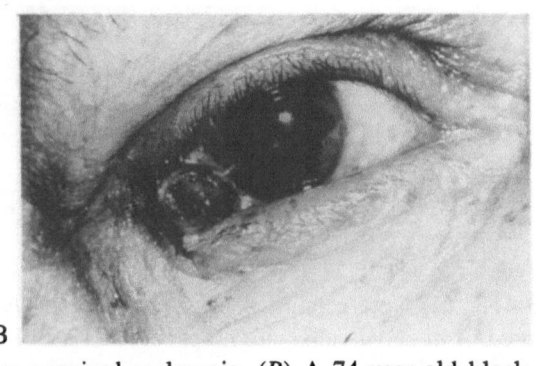

A   B

Fig. 3-44. (*A*) Light brown flat pigment typical of primary acquired melanosis. (*B*) A 74-year-old black male with a pedunculated mass arising from the temporal conjunctiva of the right eye. Biopsy of the main mass showed melanoma of the conjunctiva with spindle and epithelioid cells. Biopsy of the adjacent conjunctiva showed primary acquired melanosis confined to the epithelium. (Presented at the 11th Biennial Ophthalmic Alumni of the AFIP Meeting, Dr. Charles Barr, Louisville, KY.)

lesion, the conjunctival lesion is worrisome when a focal thickening papular or nodular formation is noted clinically. In this instance, the junctional component is accompanied by melanocytic cells that invade below the basement membrane.

Clinically, melanoma of the conjunctiva in the earlier stage may be distinguished from a nevus. Generally, patients with melanomas will have a history of documented growth of the lesion. On examination, the tumor is fixed to the scleral tissues when the anesthetized conjunctiva is moved over to the sclera. Melanomas tend to have a forniceal location.

Biopsy. Biopsy shows malignant spindle and or epithelioid cells. There is lack of maturation of the melanocytic cells from the superficial layers to the deep layers in that the cells at the base of the lesion do not become more spindle-shaped.[164] The nucleus often contains a clear space.

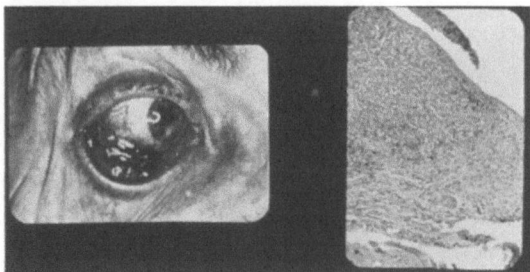

Fig. 3-45. A 55-year-old white male with melanoma arising in the conjunctival fornix.

LACRIMAL SAC TUMORS THAT INVADE THE ORBIT

See Chapter 7.

TUMORS FROM THE CRANIAL CAVITY THAT INVADE THE ORBIT

Meningioma

For discussion of optic nerve meningioma and adult sphenoid ridge meningioma, see Chapter 4.

Chordoma

Chordomas arise from the remnants of the notochord in the sphenooccipital regions of the base of the skull and in the clivus. Cranial nerve palsies are common. The tumors often extend into the bone of the sphenoid and maxillary sinus, nasopharynx, and nasal cavity. The tumors occur in patients aged 20 to 40.

Biopsy shows tumor cells that grow in chords and nests in a pseudoadenomatous pattern with abundant extracellular mucin. The individual cells often have a bubbly or vacuolated (physaliphorous) cytoplasm. Some cells have a granular, eosinophilic homogeneous cytoplasm. Chondrosarcomatous foci may make differentiation between chordoma and chondrosarcoma difficult.[164]

Treatment. These tumors are difficult to eradicate surgically because of their diffuse nature. Chordomas rarely metastasize.

Esthesioneuroblastoma

See "Nonosseous Sinusal, Oropharyngeal, and Nasal Tumors that Extend Secondarily into the Orbit" in this chapter.

METASTATIC TUMORS TO THE ORBIT (ADULTS)

Adult metastatic orbital tumors are discussed below, while pediatric metastatic orbital tumors are discussed in Chapter 4.

In adults, metastatic tumors are more common to the eyeball itself than to the orbit and are carcinomas from primaries of the breast in females and of the lungs in males. This pattern is quite the opposite in children, where the most common metastatic tumors involve the orbit and are neuroblastomas, Ewing's sarcomas, and Wilms' tumors (nephroblastomas).[180–184]

Symptoms most commonly include exophthalmos, periorbital swelling, and proptosis. Pain and ophthalmoplegia occur with many metastatic carcinomas more commonly than with primary orbital tumors except for adenoid cystic carcinoma of the lacrimal gland, where perineural tumor invasion and consequent pain are the rule. Enophthalmos, pain, ptosis, and ophthalmoplegia are quite characteristic of metastatic breast carcinoma. In addition, symptoms occur at an earlier stage than with primary orbital tumors. Left and right orbits are about equally affected.

Patients with a primary gastrointestinal carcinoid and liver metastases characteristically present with episodic flushing, asthma, diarrhea, and edema of the lower extremities.[185–186] Elevated urinary levels of 5-hydroxyindole acetic acid are present. Conjunctival vasodilation and lacrimation may occur with carcinoid tumors.

Of prime importance is a good general history and physical examination in any patient presenting with any orbital tumor. In metastatic breast carcinoma, the breast tumor precedes the recognition of the primary tumor in about 9 percent of cases. This finding contrasts to metastatic lung tumors, where in two-thirds of patients, ocular or orbital metastases occurred before the detection of the primary tumor. This finding is partially explained by the fact that breast tumors tend to metastasize late, while lung tumors metastasize early. Many orbital metastases will have concomitant pulmonary metastases in the case of metastatic breast carcinoma.[187]

While pulsating exophthalmos is most commonly cause by vascular malformations, arteriovenous fistulae, or cerebrospinal fluid pulsations transmitted through bony defects as in neurofibromatosis and meningoencephalocele, metastatic renal cell carcinoma may also cause pulsating exophthalmos duc to its rich vascularity.[188] Positional exophthalmos due to a varix is quite different from an arterial transmitted pulse. In the case of renal cell carcinoma, the palpable pulsations possibly result from the tumor's adoption of two arterial supplies, the ophthalmic artery and the terminal branches of the internal maxillary artery of the external carotid system. Pulsating cutaneous renal cell metastases have also been described. Renal cell carcinoma metastatic to the orbit often presents an average of 7 months before the primary has been discovered.

Bilateral exophthalmos due to possible hormonal influence has been documented in three patients with localized seminoma, although metastatic testicular carcinoma may rarely occur.[189]

CT Scan Appearance. Virtually any CT presentation of metastatic carcinoma is likely. For this reason, we have dedicated a small section to this topic.

The CT scan appearance is relatively nonspecific, consisting of an irregular infiltrating orbital mass. Bone erosion, enlargement of usually a single extraocular muscle with irregular borders, and focal as well as diffuse orbital involvement may occur.

ANCILLARY DIAGNOSTIC STUDIES

Decision and Method of Biopsy—The Role of Fine Needle Aspiration Biopsy

A discussion of the merits and disadvantages of fine needle aspiration biopsy (FNAB) is appropriate in this section since this technique may have its greatest application in patients with presumed metastatic disease.

FNAB is an alternative to the open biopsy of orbital tumors in certain clinical situations.[190–193] Kennerdell and colleagues have advocated the use of FNAB in diagnosing nonresectable deep orbital lesions that would otherwise require extensive surgery. Unfortunately, samples of orbital apex lesions are technically difficult to obtain and the procedure is not without danger because of the proximity of the superior orbital fissure and optic canal.

In general, FNAB may be diagnostic in patients with presumed metastatic disease. Certainly, in patients with a prior history of a tumor elsewhere in the body, FNAB may be diagnostic and save an open biopsy procedure. Certain scirrhous metastatic tumors that produce enophthalmos such as metastatic breast carcinoma are less likely to produce adequate pathologic material to render a diagnosis. Other primary tumors that have a significant fibrous component such as hemangioma, hemangiopericytoma, neurofibroma, fibrous histiocytoma, and dermoid cyst should probably not be needled. In addition, vascular lesions should not be needled because of possible retrobulbar hemorrhage. Lymphoid infiltrates should not be biopsied by FNAB simply because it is difficult for the ophthalmic pathologist to adequately study and diagnoses the benign or malignant nature of a lymphoid lesion with only a small specimen. In addition, solid epithelial tumors such as benign mixed tumor, malignant mixed tumor, and adenoid cystic carcinoma are difficult to diagnose. Also, a sampling error may lead to the misdiagnosis of a benign mixed tumor (L. E. Zimmerman, personal communication). Optic nerve tumors cannot be accurately diagnosed by FNAB. Arachnoidal hyperplasia that accompanies an optic glioma may easily be misdiagnosed as a meningioma.

The overall accuracy of the technique for histopathologic diagnosis is from 47 to 92 percent depending on how well the patients are selected. Patients should be told that if a needle biopsy is undertaken, a second procedure, an open biopsy, may be necessary. Since the procedure has limited morbidity, it should be part of the orbital surgeon's armamentarium.

Complications include orbital hemorrhage, which occurs in approximately 5 percent of patients and resolves without sequellae. Where the metastatic origin of the tumor is unclear, an open biopsy provides adequate tissue for examination of immunologic markers. We believe that an open biopsy should be performed in cases in which a primary orbital lesion is suspected.

In summary, the technique has greatest application in diagnosing (1) suspected metastatic tumors especially when the primary tumor is known, (2) recurrent orbital tumors, (3) a sterile abscess when it is not clear whether the primary process is an inflammation or a necrotic tumor abscess, and (4) secondary neoplasms such as sinus neoplasms that have already been biopsied.

Technique of FNAB. Kennerdell advocates use of a 20-ml disposable plastic syringe and a 22-gauge 3.75-cm needle. The length of the needle is determined by the tumor location and distance from the skin surface. The needle is introduced into the orbital lesion and the tissue is aspirated. Small to-and-fro movements within the lesion will harvest additional cells. The plunger is released to prevent further aspiration of material into the barrel of the syringe. The objective is to keep the aspirate in the needle. The aspirate may be immediately squirted onto slides, spread with another slide, and then fixed in alcohol for staining. Alternatively, the needle containing the specimen is removed from the syringe and connected to a second 5-cc syringe. The needle is then submerged into 3 cc of isotonic saline solution, and 1–2 cc of solution is aspirated. The particles of the specimen can be visualized in the suspension of the syringe. The contents are then brought to the laboratory for Millipore filtering or cell block technique. The need for an excellent cytopathologist cannot be overemphasized. The findings of the cytopathologist should be analyzed by an experienced ophthalmic pathologist and the orbital surgeon. The cytopathologic features of the various metastatic orbital tumors will not be discussed.

Other biopsy techniques, including orbital endoscopy, hold promise and but are not yet clearly established.

Possible Open Biopsy Results

Breast Carcinoma. Biopsy shows bland, uniform, histiocytic-like cells with a well-outlined ground-glass cytoplasm (Fig. 3-46). Indian-file columns of single cells that interdigitate between collagen fibers belie their epithelial origin. The presence of mucicarmine-positive intracytoplasmic vacuoles of mucin solidify the diagnosis. These tumors may be mistaken for benign conditions such as xanthoma, histiocytoma, and granular cell myoblastoma (granular cell tumors). When metastatic tumors infiltrate the extraocular muscle bundles, the tumor cells assume unusual configurations, and, in addition, the striated muscle cells themselves may be transformed by adjacent tumor and inflammation and may mislead the pathologist into making the erroneous diagnosis of a malignant striated muscle tumor.

Fresh tissue should be obtained for levels of estrogen and progesterone. Approximately 50–60 percent of women with breast tumors containing estrogen receptors, respond objectively to endocrine therapy, while only 15 percent of patients with tumors lacking estrogen receptors have a favorable objective response. The response rate increases to 78 percent if both estrogen and progesterone receptors are present. Fresh tissue is necessary for such studies on homogenized tissue, to which radioactive estradiol is added. More recently, fluorescent steroid histochemical techniques have been utilized to demonstrate progesterone and estrogen receptors in metastatic breast tumors.[187]

Oat Cell Carcinoma of the Lung. Biopsy shows undifferentiated small, round, or spindle cells with small nuclei and scanty cytoplasm. The tumor may be mistaken for lymphoma, but there are no other lymphoid cells present and lymphomas do not contain spindle cells. Oat cell carcinoma is a tumor found in adults, while neuroblastoma occurs in children.

Stomach Carcinoma. Biopsy shows signet-ring cells. Such cells are typical of a gastrointestinal origin. Alcian-blue stain may demonstrate the presence of intracytoplasmic mucin. Breast carcinoma may also be mucin-producing. The central cytoplasmic vacuole pushes the nucleus against the cell membrane.

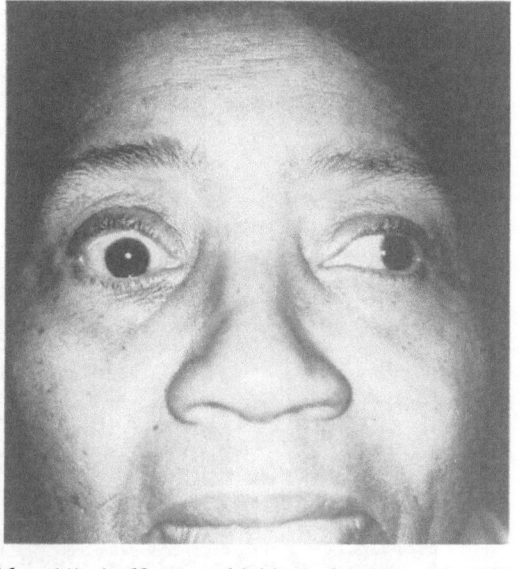 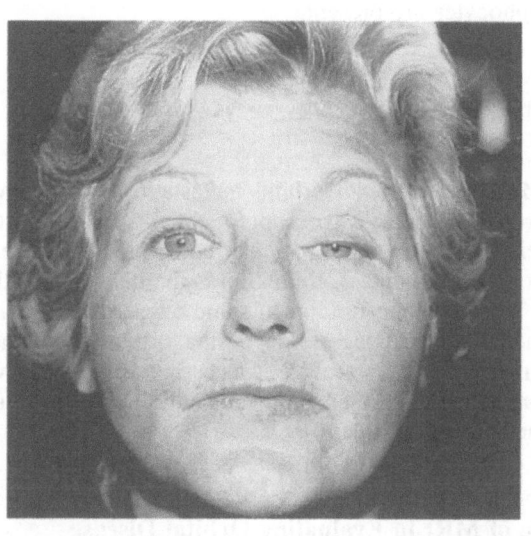

A   B

Fig. 3-46. (*A*) A 63-year-old black female with diffuse orbital metastatic breast carcinoma with enophthalmos and restricted motility. (*B*) Note similar presentation in 48-year-old female with metastatic breast carcinoma to the left orbit. Note ptosis without lid thickening and enlarged superior sulcus deformity.

Papillary Thyroid Carcinoma. Biopsy shows fronds with fibrovascular cores. The cores are lined by anaplastic epithelium that might pile up on the papillae or grow in solid masses. The same papillary histologic pattern may also occur in papillary carcinoma of the lung, kidney, or nonpigmented ciliary epithelium of the eye.

Renal Carcinoma. Biopsy shows nests of large, rich, clear cells compartmentalized by fibrovascular trabeculae in a circumscribed but not encapsulated mass. The cells have irregularly shaped, hyperchromatic nuclei with prominent nucleoli. The cytoplasm of the tumor cells contains large amounts of glycogen and occasional lipid droplets in some cells but no mucin.

Carcinoid of the Gastrointestinal Tract and Bronchial Tree. Biopsy shows a haphazard mixture of small cuboidal cells with two basic cell types, light and dark cells (Fig. 3-47). There is mild nuclear pleomorphism with inconspicuous nucleoli. Mitotic figures may be present. All bronchial tumors tend to give a negative argentaffin reaction; tumors that show a positive argentaffin reaction tend to demonstrate a positive argyrophilic reaction as well.[186]

Melanoma of the Skin. Biopsy shows multiple foci and sheets of cells composed almost entirely of epithelioid cells. Special stains for melanin show melanin in the cytoplasm of the epithelioid cells.

Testicular Seminoma. Biopsy shows sheets of malignant cells with large nuclei, prominent nucleoli, and mild nuclear anaplasia. The cells have clear cytoplasm

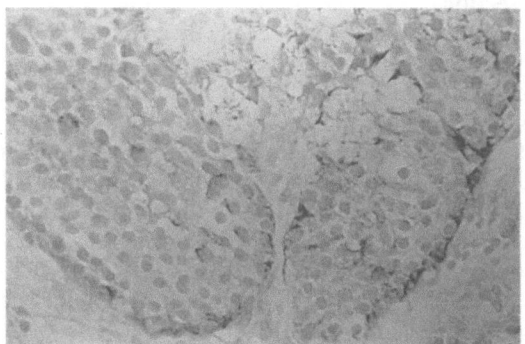

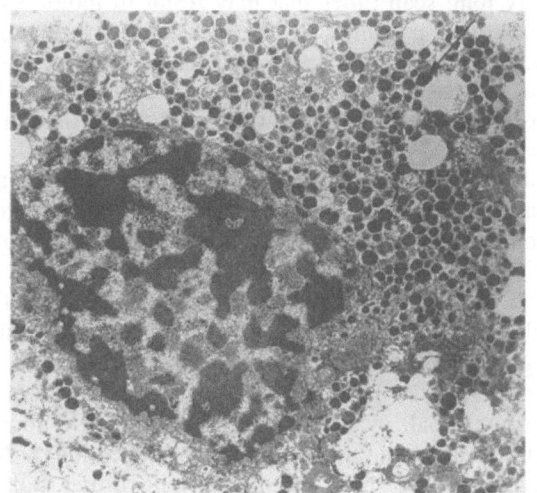

Fig. 3-47. (*A*) Organoid pattern typical of metastatic carcinoid tumor to orbit. (*B*) EM shows neurosecretory granules. (Courtesy AFIP, Washington, DC.)

with well-demarcated cytoplasmic borders. Scattered lymphocytes are present.

Management

Most patients with orbital metastatic disease have a short period of survival except for patients with metastatic carcinoid. In carcinoid patients, complete surgical excision is recommended. Radiation is the mainstay of therapy in most other tumors. In some cases, chemotherapy alone will cause regression of the orbital component. Exenteration may rarely be necessary in patients with intractable pain. An oncologist or radiotherapist is a necessary part of the team.

Role of MRI in Evaluating Orbital Disease

The exact role of MRI in the evaluation of orbital disease is still being delineated. The advantages and disadvantages of MRI versus CT scan are outlined in this section.

Advantages of MRI include (1) the avoidance of potentially harmful ionizing radiation in all patients as well as pregnant females, and (2) the high soft-tissue contrast resolution without the use of intravenous iodine in patients who are allergic to iodine or who are in renal failure. In addition, many sections in different planes including coronal and sagittal are obtained. Moreover, uncomfortable head positions necessary for CT coronal views are not required for coronal and sagittal MRI studies. Artifacts secondary to high-density dental materials are not a problem with MRI.

The general disadvantages of MRI include the relatively long scan times that may result in motor artifact because the patient is unable to keep from moving for a long period of time. MR is not as sensitive as CT scan in detecting calcifications and does not show bone erosion or bone tumors as well as CT scan. In addition, presently most surface coils allow study of only one orbit at a time. Study of both orbits doubles the examination time. Cosmetics that contain iron oxide pigment often produce metal artifacts in the images. In addition, patients with pacemakers should not have MRI scans since cardiac arrhythmias may be induced. In patients with possible metallic foreign bodies, especially ferromagnetic objects such as BBs, where MRI is contraindicated, CT scan should be utilized. Retinal tacks of titanium or cobalt nickel as well as metallic IOL loops of platinum and titanium are not a contraindication for MRI. Advancement of MRI technology will further widen its application to orbital disease.

Some theoretical considerations need to be outlined before the clinical applications of MRI are understood. In general, the advantage of MRI relates to its ability

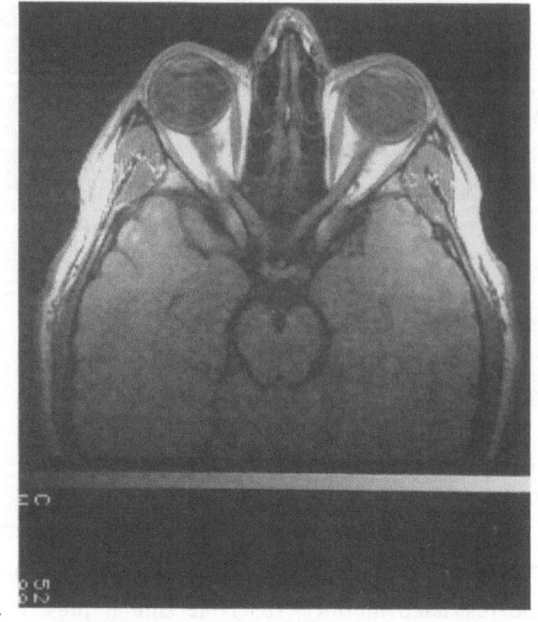

A

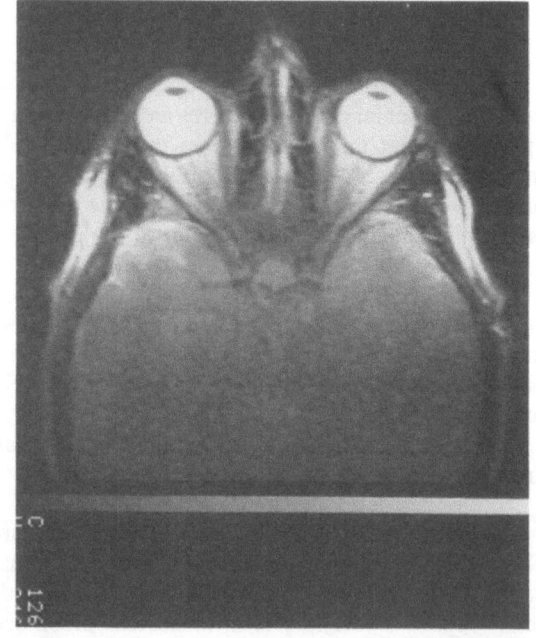

B

Fig. 3-48. (A) On T1-weighted image, the orbital fat has the highest signal and the vitreous the lowest signal. Optic nerve and muscle are intermediate. The lens shows a moderate signal and a low signal on T2-weighted images (B). A T2-weighted image demonstrates the highest signal from the vitreous. The orbital fat has moderate signal due to heavy T2-weighting. Normally some fluid can be seen within the dural sheath on the T2-weighted images. (Courtesy of Dr. Steven Harms, Dallas, TX.)

to characterize both normal and abnormal tissues by relaxation times.[194] Specifically, T1 and T2 relaxation times characterize hydrogen-proton alignment perturbations in

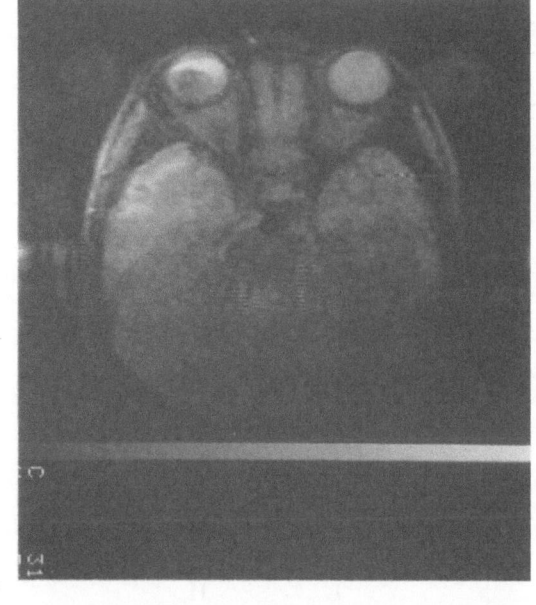

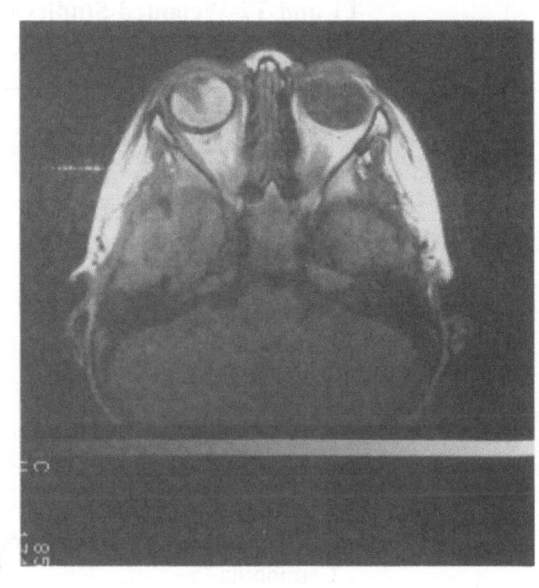

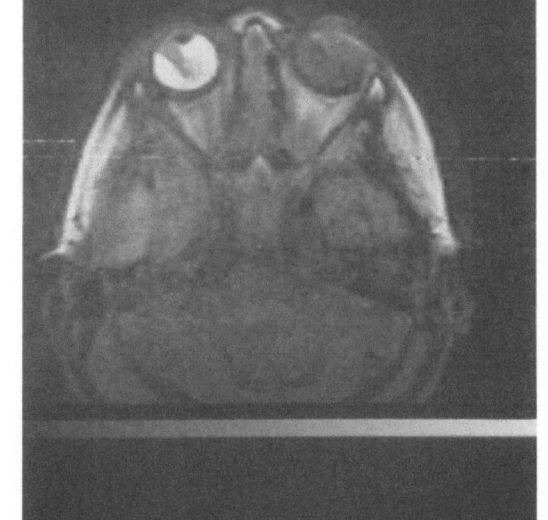

Fig. 3-49. (*A*) The T2-weighted image separates the high-signal subretinal effusion from the low-signal retinoblastoma. (*B–C*) T2-weighted image of a 4-year-old with Coats' disease. Note high-intensity signal due to lipoproteinaceous subretinal exudate characteristic of the disease. The T2 relaxation times of the subretinal exudate of Coat's are much longer than the T2 relaxation times of retinoblastoma. (Courtesy of Dr. Steven Harms, Dallas, TX.)

a magnetic field. Tissues with dissimilar molecular structures and proton densities can be differentiated by their own disparate relaxation times. Solids such as bone have a low proton content and thereby produce low-intensity signals and longer T1 and T2 relaxation times than do the soft tissue contents of the orbit. Shortened T1 and T2 relaxation times appear relatively hyperintense (Fig. 3-48). In general, subacute or chronic hemorrhage, subretinal exudate, and vascular tumors such as hemangioma appear hyperintense (Fig. 3-49). Fresh hemorrhage is hypointense in both T1- and T2-weighted images. Interestingly, melanin produces a stable free-radical signal that shortens both T1 and T2 relaxation values. Therefore,

in T1-weighted images, the lesion should be hyperintense and relatively hypointense compared with the vitreous on T2-weighted images. The contrast that occurs at the interfaces of tissues with different relaxation times enhances visualization of the various structures.

Increased signal:noise (S:N) ratios with the advent of surface coils have made thinner sections and increased spatial resolution possible.[195–196] Similarly, the lack of bony artifact because of bone's inherent low proton density is helpful. In other studies where tumor infiltrates bone, the CT scan is more helpful in showing bone erosion. CT visualization of the optic nerves, chiasm, and optic tract are somewhat hampered by the artifact

Table 3-19
T1 and T2-Weighted Studies in Patients with Orbital Neoplasms

	T1*	T2*
Normal Orbital Structures		
Orbital fat	H	M
Vitreous/Aqueous	L	H
EOMs	M	L
Brain—white matter	H	M
—gray matter	M	H
Air	L	L
Cortical bone	L	L
Orbital Inflammatory Disease		
Pseudotumor	L	L
Grave's ophthalmopathy	L	L
Lymphoma	L	H
Orbital abscess/cellulitis	L	H
Intraconal and Extraconal Tumors		
Carcinoma	L	H
Cavernous Hemangioma/Schwannoma	L	H
Hemorrhage (subacute)	H	H
Optic Nerve and Sheath Pathology		
Meningioma	L	L
Glioma of optic nerve	L	H
Optic neuritis	Isotense	High
Radiation change	Isotense	High
Tumors with Possible Adjacent Bone Involvement		
Mucocele	H	H
Dermoid cyst	H	H
Epidermoid cyst	L	H
Encephalocele	L	H
Bone Tumors		
Osteoma	L	L
Fibrous dysplasia	L	L†
Lacrimal Gland		
Adenoid cystic ca (lacrimal gland)	L	H
Intraocular Pathology—Children		
Retinoblastoma	H	L
Coats'	H	H
PHPV	H	H
Hemorrhage	H	H
Toxocara	H	H
Intraocular Pathology—Adults		
Melanoma	H	L
Metastatic carcinoma	L	H
Posterior scleritis	L	L
Hemorrhage	H	H
Phthisis bulbi	L	L

* L—low signal intensity; M—moderate; H—high

† The signal from fibrous dysplasia is not as low as that from a densely calcified osteoma.

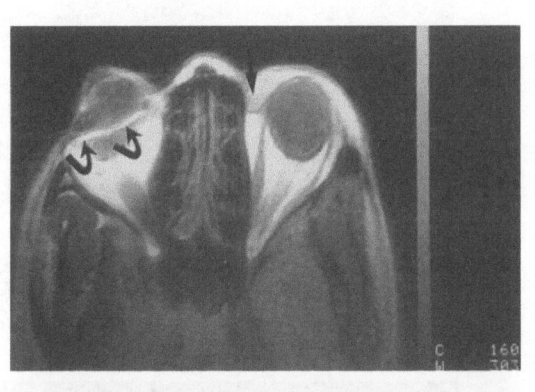

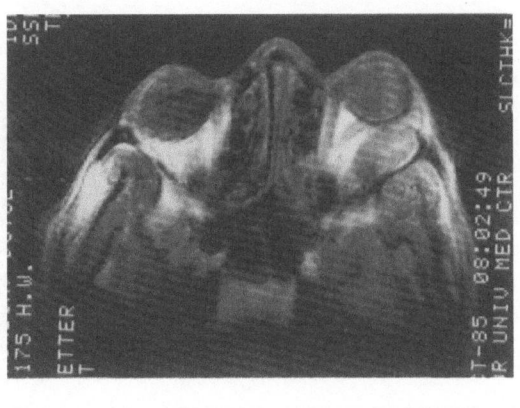

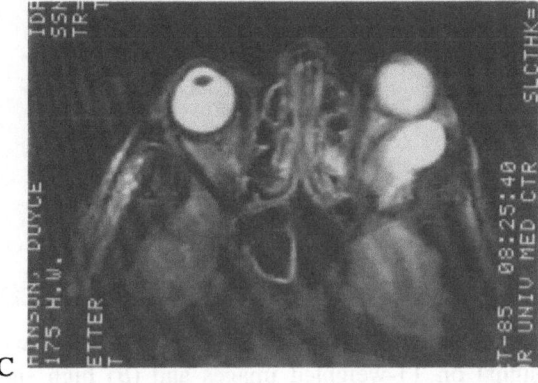

Fig. 3-50. (*A*) A fat-fluid level seen within well-defined dermoid cyst with dependent layer of water and cellular debris (arrow) and the free-floating fat layers. Note artefact (curved arrows) due to blue eyeshadow on right eye lids. (*B,C*) Epidermoid inclusion cyst on T1- and T2-weighted images. (Courtesy of Dr. Steven Harms, Dallas, TX.)

produced by the sella bone. No such artifactitious signal is seen on MRI because bones with their lower proton density produce no signal.

Subacute or chronic hemorrhage within a tumor that may appear homogeneous on CT scan is seen well as hyperintense on the T1- and T2-weighted images of MRI. Similarly, ischemic changes of the globe will be detected on MRI but not on CT scan, again because each tissue has its own relaxation time that varies with its physiologic state. Similarly, the CT scan better demonstrates calcification than MRI.

Intraocular tumors may be better visualized with MRI than CT scan because of the contrast between the vitreous and its high water content and the tumor (Fig. 3-49C).[197–198] However, CT scan will show calcifications that are specific for retinoblastoma and rarely found in Coats disease, PHPV, retinopathy of prematurity, and ocular toxocariasis.

In one study that evaluated patients with glioma of the optic nerve, intraconal optic nerve, chiasmal, and optic tract tumors were better visualized with MRI than CT scan.[199] Further experience with MRI will determine whether MRI will be helpful in differentiating parenchymal optic nerve diseases such as tuberculosis, multiple sclerosis, syphyllis, glioma, sarcoid, and optic neuritis, from extraneural processes such as meningioma and optic nerve sheath metastases. In one study,[195] neoplasms were graded as high-, moderate-, or low-signal intensity on T1- and T2-weighted examinations. The signal intensities

of retroorbital fat, vitreous, and extraocular muscles were used as internal standards (Table 3-19). In general, rhabdomyosarcomas and lymphomas have high signals and T2-weighted examinations and thyroid ophthalmopathy has a low signal on T2-weighted examinations (Fig. 3-50).

The signal characteristics were utilized to differentiate various neoplasms. Densely calcified lesions show a low signal intensity with T1- and T2-weighting due to the low mobile proton density. Again, CT is preferred for evaluation of orbital lesions that are heavily calcified or that involve bone.

Table 3-19 explains how MRI can be used to differentiate various lesions. The same principles outlined in this book for anatomically localizing the site of the disease process with the help of the CT scan may be utilized in the analysis of MRI (Figs. 3-51 and 3-52).[200–204]

ULTRASOUND

Application to Orbital Disease

With the refinement of high-resolution CT scan and the advent of MRI, ultrasonography has been somewhat underestimated. Its chief role is in tissue differentiation.

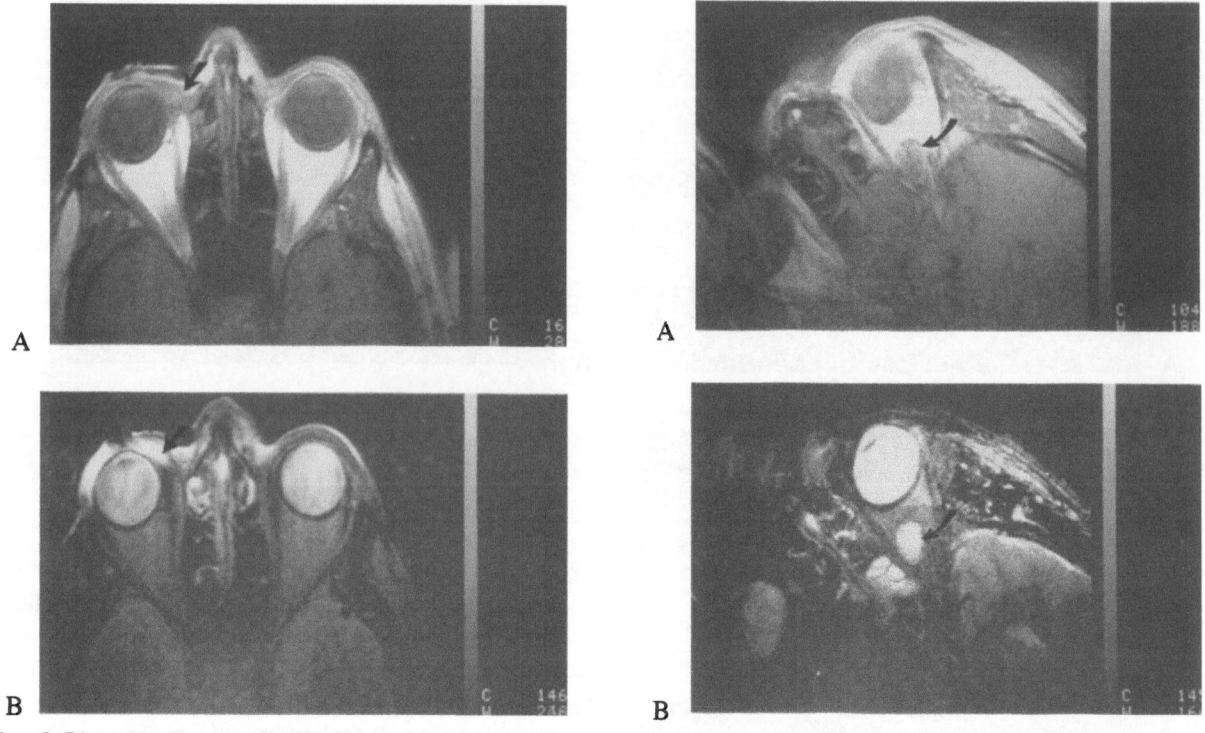

Fig. 3-51. (*A*) Preseptal cellulitis with low signal on T1-weighted image and (*B*) high signal on T2-weighted image. (Courtesy of Dr. Steven Harms, Dallas, TX.)

Fig. 3-52. (*A*) Well-defined intraconal mass with low signal on T1-weighted images and (*B*) high signal on T2-weighted image typical of cavernous hemangioma. (Courtesy of Dr. Steven Harms, Dallas, TX.)

In most clinical situations, we do not need more than a CT scan in order to make difficult decisions regarding biopsy and management. It is hoped that a general review of ultrasonographic principles followed by examples of clinical applications will guide the clinician in maximizing the selective use of ultrasonography.

Theory of Principles of A- and B-Scan Ultrasonography

Ultrasonography consists of the standardized A-scan and B-scan. Doppler ultrasound will not be considered in this section; it detects blood flow within orbital lesions.

The A-scan probe emits sound waves into orbital tissues that are then reflected from a wide cylindrical section of tissue. The reflected sound energy is registered on an oscilloscope. In the B scan, a larger probe obtains a two-dimensional cross-section of tissue. The A scan therefore employs a high sensitivity detector that allows tissue differentiation while B scan is primarily employed for delineating a lesion's size, shape, surface characteristics (i.e., well-defined or irregular borders), and its location (i.e., proximity to normal anatomic structures).[205–206] The latter function is better served by CT

scan. We believe that the main role of A scan is in its tissue differentiation.

In general, the normal orbital tissues are heterogeneous because the tissue gives high reflective echo spikes due to the presence of orbital fat and connective tissue septae. These high-amplitude echoes follow immediately after the posterior scleral echo and diminish in amplitude more posteriorly in the orbit due to the attenuation of the sound energy. This high-amplitude complex is then followed by another mid-amplitude spike representing the muscle and orbital wall. The orbital wall echo is usually not high in amplitude because the beam is not directly perpendicular to the orbital wall and the echoes are returned obliquely and not recorded by the probe. Once a concept of the normal A scan is obtained, the abnormal scan is more easily interpreted (Fig. 3-53).

Quantitative standardized A-scan echography is used to assess a lesion's (1) internal structure, (2) reflectivity, and (3) sound attenuation. The internal structure is the uniformity of the spike height and length and is termed *regular* or *irregular*. Reflectivity is the height of spikes from the baseline and is termed *high* or *low*. Lesions that contain a homogeneous distribution of cells and stroma without large interfaces such as large blood spaces or cystic spaces yield a pattern of regular internal structure and low reflectivity. The pattern is, therefore, regular

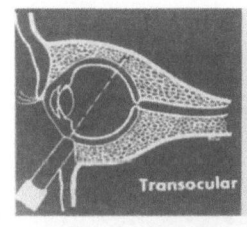
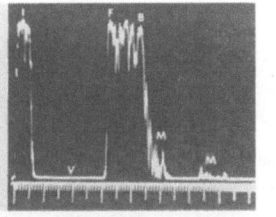

A

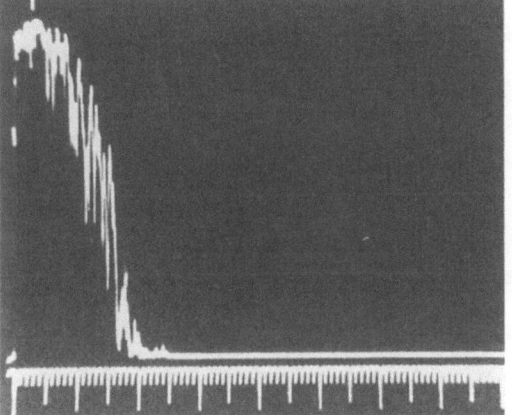

B

Fig. 3-53. (*A*) Transocular A scan shows initial spike (I), vitreous (V), fundus (F), bone spike (B), and multiple artefacts (M). (*B*) Paraocular A scan shows high reflectivity and heterogeneity of normal orbital tissues due to connective tissue septae and fat. (Reprinted with permission from Byrne SF, Glaser JS: Orbital tissue differentiation with standardized echography. *Ophthalmology* 90:1071–1090, 1983.)

and homogeneous. A regular arrangement of multiple interfaces produce regular internal structure and high reflectivity, making it regular and heterogeneous. An irregular arrangement of multiple interfaces produces irregular structure and high reflectivity. Sound attenuation is a measure of the scattering and absorption qualities of tissues. The angle kappa is formed by a line drawn through the peaks of the internal lesion's spikes and intersects the baseline.[205–206]

Topographic echography includes the location, shape, size, and surface characteristics or borders of the pathologic process. We believe that CT scanning is superior to ultrasound in these regards.

Kinetic echography is used to determine the consistency (compressibility), vascularity (blood flow), and mobility of the mass. Again, these parameters may be helpful in evaluating orbital disease. For example, a cystic lesion will be compressible and will show narrowed spikes as pressure is exerted perpendicular to the lesion. Experienced examiners appreciate the vascularity of a lesion by fast, spontaneous, mostly vertical flickering of internal lesion spikes during dynamic examination, that is, as the probe is moved. Stagnant blood such as that in a varix or cavernous hemangioma produces no

spike movement. Mobility or fixation to the periosteum or other structures may again be detected by the experienced ultrasonographer by observing the lesion echogram during eye-blinking. If the lesion is mobile, the echogram will blur during eye movement, and if fixed, it will not blur significantly.

Basic Examination Techniques

Screening is performed by directing the sound beam both through the globe—transocular—and adjacent to the globe—paraocular. The transocular examination starts at the limbus of the topically anesthetized globe and is continued radially toward the fornix of the same meridian. Six meridians are examined. With this limbus-to-fornix transocular examination, the extraocular muscles (EOMs) and posterior orbit are examined.

The paraocular examination is used to examine the anterior extraconal aspects of the orbit. Through closed lids, the probe is directed (1) anterior to posterior to the orbital apex, (2) toward the bony orbital wall, and (3) through the globe.

A-Scan Muscle Pattern of Thyroid Ophthalmopathy, Myositis, Metastatic Tumor Myopathy, and Congestive Myopathy

The normal A-scan pattern of the EOM is of lower reflectivity than adjacent soft tissues of the orbit due to its more homogeneous pattern than the surrounding tissues (Fig. 3-54).

In thyroid ophthalmopathy, the spindle-shaped fusiform thickening of the EOM that spares the muscle tendon is seen well on CT scan.[205–207] However, it is the pattern of A scan that depicts the inflammatory infiltrate that may be diagnostic in cases where the CT scan and clinical presentation are inconclusive. In most cases, however, clinical examination findings such as lid lag and lid retraction are diagnostic. The muscle infiltration is characteristically nonuniform and results in irregular, high internal muscle reflectivity (Figs. 3-55 and 3-56). In pseudotumor, the CT scan shows involvement of the tendon. However, the muscle belly thickening reflects the diffuse relatively uniform infiltration by inflammatory cells of low reflectivity and mimics the low internal reflectivity characteristic of a lymphoid infiltrate without other interfaces such as connective tissue septae or large blood vessels. This pattern is similar to the pattern of muscle infiltration seen in metastatic carcinoma. Congestive myopathy due to an arteriovenous fistula causes thickening of the belly of the muscle that spares the tendon; because there is no inflammatory cell infiltration, there is no significant change in internal muscle reflectivity.[208]

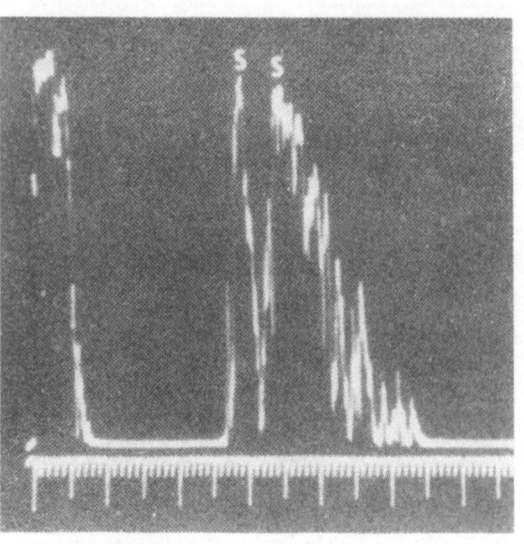

Fig. 3-54. Optic nerve substance has low reflectivity as well. Note spikes from optic nerve sheath. (Reprinted with permission from Byrne SF, Glaser JS: Orbital tissue differentiation with standardized echography. *Ophthalmology* 90:1071–1090, 1983.)

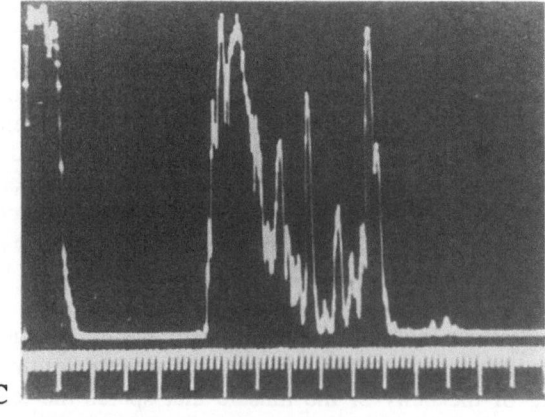

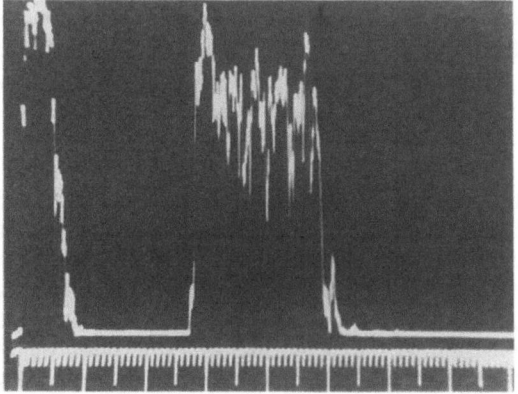

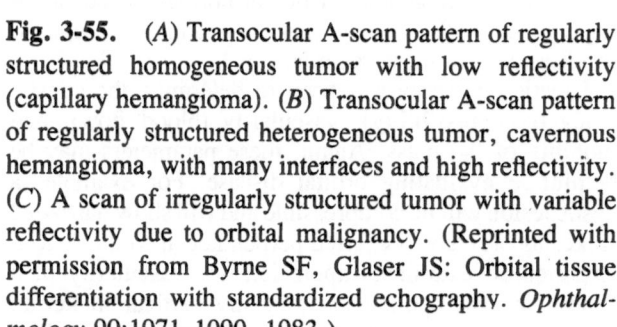

Fig. 3-55. (*A*) Transocular A-scan pattern of regularly structured homogeneous tumor with low reflectivity (capillary hemangioma). (*B*) Transocular A-scan pattern of regularly structured heterogeneous tumor, cavernous hemangioma, with many interfaces and high reflectivity. (*C*) A scan of irregularly structured tumor with variable reflectivity due to orbital malignancy. (Reprinted with permission from Byrne SF, Glaser JS: Orbital tissue differentiation with standardized echography. *Ophthalmology* 90:1071–1090, 1983.)

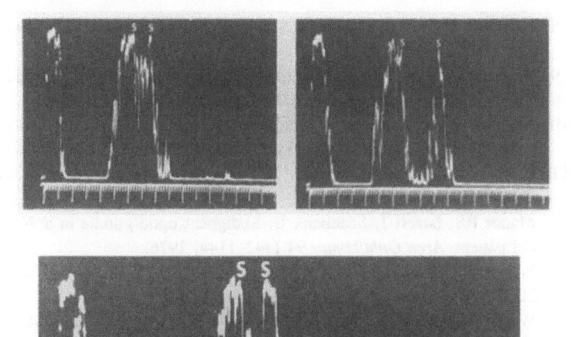

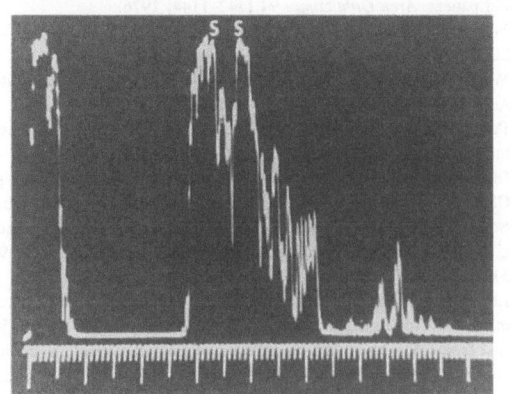

Fig. 3-56. (*A*) A scan shows muscle diameter between the sheaths. Normal muscle (left) shows higher reflective and narrow pattern compared with low reflectivity and marked thickening of an inflamed muscle (right) due to idiopathic myositis. (*B*) A scan of muscle enlarged from thyroid ophthalmopathy showing irregular and highly reflective echograms. Lymphoid lesions present as areas of low internal reflectivity due to homogeneity of tumor mass (Reprinted with permission from Byrne SF, Glaser JS: Orbital tissue differentiation with standardized echography. *Ophthalmology* 90:1071–1090, 1983.)

Pseudotumor

The ultrasonic pattern of pseudotumor as defined in this text is quite characteristic on both CT scan and ultrasound. Our definition of pseudotumor is limited to idiopathic inflammation that classically has an abrupt, painful onset; on CT scan, the EOMs show a myositis pattern that includes the tendon of the muscle. The margins of the muscles are ill-defined.[209] There is no mass lesion, and, therefore, biopsy is not indicated initially. Orbital B-scan ultrasonography shows a space between Tenon's capsule and the globe wall posteriorly. The edema usually extends along the optic nerve. A sonolucent crescent follows the contour of the globe posteriorly. Sclerosing pseudotumor will have bands of fibrous tissue and will present as an irregularly structured tumor mass.

Orbital Cellulitis and Abscess

The orbital fat will have an increased volume with echoes more widely spaced than normal. The EOMs may also be enlarged.

In its early stages, an abscess will produce focal changes consistent with inflammation. Later, as it becomes localized due to fibrosis, it may appear as a cystic cavity; at this stage, the cystic cavity on A scan will have moderate amplitude echoes from the internal debris.[206]

A-Scan Pattern of Lymphoid Infiltrate

A lymphoid infiltrate is a solid sheet of cells and therefore will appear as any solid tumor with well-demarcated contours, poor sound transmission, and internal echoes.

Optic Nerve Disease

Normally, like the muscle, the nerve pattern is recognized as a distinct defect that is less heterogeneous than the orbital fat. For optimal examination, the probe is placed close to the equator laterally and is aimed behind the globe perpendicular to the arachnoid sheaths.

Optic Nerve Tumors—Glioma vs. Meningioma. Glioma produces echograms of regular homogeneous low-to-medium reflectivity, while meningiomas are characteristically irregular in structure with higher reflectivity than gliomas.[206]

A-Scan Pattern of Orbital Tumors

In general, the A-scan pattern of tumors can be predicted based on knowledge of the histology of the given tumors. The location of the tumor, whether within the optic nerve substance, intraconal, extraconal, or subperiosteal, as well as the pattern of involvement, whether diffuse or well-localized, are key to establishing the differential diagnosis. This information is apparent on CT scan and B scan, and together with the history and physical examination usually provides the astute clinician with a fairly narrow differential diagnosis that leads to the appropriate management. However, in some cases, the A scan is the only modality that allows distinguishing histologic patterns.

Solid tumors such as neurofibroma and glioma have poor transmission, while cystic tumors such as dermoid cyst, cavernous hemangiomas, and mucocele have good transmission because they contain fluid; fluid transmits sound well.

A localized hemorrhage in the orbit might have the same pattern as a solid tumor. Tumors with good sound transmission will usually show a well-outlined posterior wall, while solid tumors often will not show a posterior wall because all the sound is attenuated in the tumor. Lymphangiomas have the same high-amplitude echoes and good sound transmission of dermoid cyst and cavernous hemangioma. However, because of their diffuse involvement of the orbit, finger-like projections of tumor are cut in cross-sections by the probe and the appearance of tiny cysts separate from the tumor mass may cause confusion of these tumors with a solid tumor.

Ultrasound—Ultimate Value

We do not feel that ultrasound replaces CT scan in any primary diagnostic problem. Its chief advantages are its immediate availability and low cost. The experience of the ultrasonographer influences the ultimate effectiveness of any study. On a practical level, it is most helpful in predicting the cellular pattern of a tumor. This information may be of some value in certain clinical situations. We do not employ ultrasound routinely.

REFERENCES

1. Rush JA, Younge BR, Campbell RJ, MacCarthy CS: Optic glioma. *Ophthalmology* 89:1213–1219, 1982.
2. Deen HG, Scheithauer BW, Ebersold M: Clinical and pathologic study of meningiomas of the first two decades. *J Neurosurg* 56:317–322, 1982.
3. Susac JO, Martins AN, Whaley RA: Intracanalicular meningioma with normal tomography. *J Neurosurg* 46:659–662, 1977.
4. Wilson MB, Gordon M, Lehman RA: Meningiomas confined to the optic canal and foramina. *Surg Neurol* 12:21–28, 1979.
5. Karp LA, Zimmerman LE, Borit A, Spencer WH: Primary intraorbital meningioma. *Arch Ophthalmol* 91:551–567, 1974.
6. Wright JE, Call MB, Liaricos S: Primary intraorbital meningioma. *Br J Ophthalmol* 64:553–558, 1980.
7. Miller NR, Iliff WJ, Green WR: Evaluation and management of gliomas of the anterior visual pathways. *Brain* 97:743–754, 1974.
8. Hoyt WF, Meshel LG, Lessell S, Schatz NJ: Malignant glioma of adulthood. *Brain* 96:121–132, 1973.
9. Spoor TC, Kennerdell JA, Martinez AJ, Zarub D: Malignant gliomas of the optic nerve pathways. *Am J Ophthalmol* 89:284–292, 1980.
10. Borit A, Richardson EP: The biologic and clinical behavior of pilocytic astrocytomas of the optic pathways. *Brain* 105:161–187, 1982.
11. Harper CG, Stewart-Wynne EG: Malignant optic gliomas in adults. *Arch Neurol* 35:731–735, 1978.
12. Manor RS, Israeli J, Sandbank U: Malignant optic glioma in a 70-year-old patient. *Arch Ophthalmol* 94:1142–1144, 1976.
13. Wilson B: Meningiomas of the anterior visual system. *Surv Ophthalmol* 26:109–125, 1981.
14. Wolter JR, Benz SC: Ectopic meningioma of the superior orbital rim. *Arch Ophthalmol* 94:1920–1922, 1976.
15. Pompili A, Caroli R, Cattani R, Iachetti M: Intradiploic meningioma of the orbital roof. *Neurosurgery* 12:565–568, 1983.
16. Stern J, DiGiacinto GV, Hosepian EM: Neurofibromatosis and optic glioma: Clinical and morphological correlations. *Neurosurgery* 4:524–528, 1979.
17. Stern J, Jakobiec FA, Houspian EM: The architecture of optic nerve gliomas with and without neurofibromatosis. *Arch Ophthalmol* 98:505–511, 1980.
18. Lewis RA, Gerson LP, Axelson KA, et al: von Recklinghausen neurofibromatosis. II. Incidence of optic gliomata. *Ophthalmology* 91:929–935, 1984.
19. Jakobiec FA, Depot MJ, Kennerdell JS, et al: Combined clinical and computed tomographic diagnosis of orbital glioma and meningioma. *Ophthalmology* 91:137–155, 1984.
20. Sibony PA, Krauss MR, Kennerdell JS, et al: Optic nerve sheath meningioma. *Ophthalmology* 91:1313–1326, 1984.
21. Charles NC, Nelson L, Brookner AR, et al: Pilocytic astrocytoma of the optic nerve with hemorrhagic and extreme cystic degeneration. *Am J Ophthalmol* 92:691–695, 1981.
22. Grimson BS, Perry DD: Enlargement of the optic disc in childhood optic nerve tumors. *Am J Ophthalmol* 97:627–631, 1984.
23. Foxman S, Cameron JD: Clinical implications of bilateral microphthalmos with cyst. *Am J Ophthalmol* 97:632–638, 1984.
24. Imes RK, Schatz H, Hoyt WF, et al: Evolution of optociliary veins in optic nerve sheath meningioma. *Arch Ophthalmol* 103:59–60, 1985.
25. Lloyd GAS: Primary orbital meningioma: A review of 41 patients investigated radiologically. *Clin Radiol* 33:181–187, 1980.
26. Mark LE, Kennerdell JS, Maroon JC, et al: Microsurgical removal of a primary intraorbital meningioma. *Am J Ophthalmol* 86:704–709, 1978.
27. Tenny RT, Laws ER, Younge BR, Rush JA: The neurosurgical management of optic glioma results in 104 patients. *J Neurosurgery* 57:452–458, 1982.
28. Cooling RJ, Wright JE: Arachnoid hyperplasia in optic nerve glioma: Confusion with orbital meningioma. *Br J Ophthalmol* 63:596–599, 1979.
29. Anderson DR, Spencer WH: Ultrastructural and histochemical observations of optic nerve gliomas. *Arch Ophthalmol* 83:325, 1970.
30. Mullaney J, Walsh J, Lee WR, Adams JH: Recurrence of astrocytoma of optic nerve after 48 years. *Br J Ophthalmol* 60:539–543, 1976.
31. Montgomery AB, Griffin T, Parker RG, Gerdes AJ: Optic nerve glioma: The role of radiation therapy. *Cancer* 40:2079–2080, 1977.
32. Dosoretz DE, Blitzer P, Wang C, Linggood R: Management of glioma of the optic nerve and/or chiasm: An analysis of 20 cases. *Cancer* 45:1467–1471, 1980.
33. Rosenberg LF, Miller NR: Visual results after microsurgical removal of meningiomas involving the anterior visual system. *Arch Ophthalmol* 102:1019–1023, 1984.
34. Wright JE, McDonald WI, Call NB: Management of optic nerve glioma. *Br J Ophthalmol* 64:545–552, 1980.
35. Marquardt MD, Zimmerman LE: Histopathology of meningiomas and gliomas of the optic nerve. *Human Pathol* 13:226–235, 1982.
36. Font RL, Cruxatto JO: Intracellular inclusions in meningothelial meningioma. *J Neuropathol Exp Neurol* 39:575, 1980.
37. Font RL, Wheeler T, Boniuk M: Intravascular papillary endothelial hyperplasia of the orbit and ocular adnexae. *Arch Ophthalmol* 101:1731–1736, 1983.
38. Ruchman MC, Flanagan JC: Cavernous hemangiomas of the orbit. *Ophthalmology* 90:1328–1336, 1983.
39. Cruxatto JO, Font RL: Hemangiopericytoma of the orbit: A clinicopathologic study of 30 cases. *Human Pathol* 13:210–218, 1982.
40. Jakobiec FA, Howard GM, Jones IS, Wolff M: Hemangiopericytoma of the orbit. *Am J Ophthalmol* 78:816–834, 1974.

41. Henderson JW, Farrow GM: Primary orbital hemangiopericytoma: An aggressive and potentially malignant neoplasm. *Arch Ophthalmol* 96:666–673, 1978.

42. Grant EG, Gronvail S, Sarosi TE, et al: Sonographic findings in four cases of hemangiopericytoma: Correlation with computed tomographic, angiographic and pathologic findings. *Ultrasound* 142:447–451, 1982.

43. Chilsholm IA, Polyzoidis K: Recurrence of benign orbital neurilemmoma (schwannoma) after 22 yeras. *Can J Ophthalmol* 17:271–273, 1982.

44. Konrad EA, Thiel HJ: Schwannoma of the orbit. *Ophthalmologica* 188:118–127, 1984.

45. Pereira LA, Choo YB: Schwannoma of the infraorbital nerve. *Ear Nose Throat J* 58:236–239, 1979.

46. Jones HS, Clwyd H: Benign schwannoma involving the infratemporal fossa and orbit. *Laryngoscope* 93:200–201, 1983.

47. Boniuk M, Messmer EP, Font RL: Hemangiopericytoma of the meninges of the optic nerve. A clinicopathologic report including electron microscopic observations. *Ophthalmology* 92:1780–1787, 1985.

48. Cappaert WE, Kiprov RV, Frank KE: Sector b-scan ultrasonographic 'hemangiomalike' pattern. *Arch Ophthalmol* 101:74–76, 1983.

49. Jakobiec FA, Jones IS: Neurogenic tumors, in Jones IS, Jakobiec FA (eds): *Diseases of the Orbit*. Hagerstown, MD: Harper and Row, 1979, pp 1–45.

50. Eggers H, Jakobiec FA, Jones IA: Optic nerve gliomas, in Jones IS, Jakobiec FA (eds): *Diseases of the Orbit*. Hagerstown, MD: Harper and Row, 1982, pp 1–17.

51. Krohel GB, Rosenberg PN, Wright JE, Smith RS: Localized orbital neurofibromas. *Am J Ophthalmol* 100:458–464, 1985.

52. Goldstein BG, Font RL, Alper MG: Granular cell tumor of the orbit: A case report including electron microscopic observations. *Ann Ophthalmol* 14:231–237, 1982.

53. Jakobiec FA, Font RL: Orbit, in Spencer WH (ed): *Ophthalmic Pathology* Vol 3. Philadelphia, PA: WB Saunders, 1986, pp 2476–2766.

54. Jakobiec FA, Jones IS: Mesenchymal and fibro-osseous tumors, in Jones IS, Jakobiec FA (eds): *Diseases of the Orbit*. Hagerstown, MD: Harper and Row, 1982, pp 1–42.

55. Enzinger FM, Harvey DA: Spindle cell lipoma. *Cancer* 36:1852, 1975.

56. Bartley GB, Yeatts RP, Garrity JA, et al: Spindle cell lipoma of the orbit. *Am J Ophthalmol* 100:605–609, 1985.

57. Font RL, Hidayat AA: Fibrous histiocytoma of the orbit. *Human Pathol* 13:199–209, 1982.

58. Font RL, Zimmerman LE: Nodular fasciitis of the eye and adnexae. A report of ten cases. *Arch Ophthalmol* 75:475–481, 1966.

59. Abramson DH, Ellsworth RM, Kitchin FD, Tung G: Second nonocular tumors in retinoblastoma survivors. Are they radiation-induced? *Ophthalmology* 91:1351–1355, 1984.

60. Font RL, Jurco S, Brechner RJ: Postradiation leiomyosarcoma of the orbit complicating bilateral retinoblastoma. *Arch Ophthalmol* 101:1557–1561, 1983.

61. Folberg R, Cleasby G, Flanagan JC, et al: Orbital leiomyosarcoma after radiation therapy for bilateral retinoblastoma. *Arch Ophthalmol* 101:1562–1565, 1983.

62. Leff SR, Henkind P: Rhabdomyosarcoma and late malignant melanoma of the orbit. *Ophthalmology* 90:1258–1260, 1983.

63. Hufnagel T, Ma L, Kuo T: Orbital angiosarcoma with subconjunctival presentation. Report of a case and literature review. *Ophthalmology* 94:72–77, 1987.

64. Guccion J, Font RI, Enzinger FM, et al: Extraskeletal mesenchymal chondrosarcoma. *Arch Pathol* 95:336–340, 1973.

65. Knowles DM, Jakobiec FA, Rosen M, Howard G: Amyloidosis of the orbit and adnexae. *Surv Ophthalmol* 19:367–384, 1975.

66. Marsh WM, Streeten BW, Hoepner JA, et al: Localized conjunctival amyloidosis associated with extranodal lymphoma. *Ophthalmology* 94:61–64, 1987.

67. Alper MG, Zimmerman LE, LaPiana FG: Orbital manifestations of Erdheim-Chester disease. *Trans Am Ophthalmol Soc* 81:64–85, 1983.

68. Ranchod M, Kempson RL: Smooth muscle tumors of the gastrointestinal tract and retroperitoneum. A pathologic analysis of 100 cases. *Cancer* 39:255–262, 1977.

69. Nasr AM, Blodi FC, Lindahl S, Hinkins J: Congenital generalized multicentric myofibromatosis with orbital involvement. *Am J Ophthalmol* 102:779–787, 1986.

70. Krohel GB, Wright JE: Orbital hemorrhage. *Am J Ophthalmol* 88:254–258, 1979.

71. Flanagan JC: Vascular problems of the orbit. *Ophthalmology* 86:896–913, 1979.

72. Winter J, Centeno RS, Bentson JR: Maneuver to aid diagnosis of orbital varix by computed tomography. *Am J Neuroradiol* 3:39, 1982.

73. Bullock JD, Bartley GB: Dynamic proptosis. *Am J Ophthalmol* 112:104–110, 1986.

74. Katz B, Carmody R: Subperiosteal orbital hematoma induced by the Valsalva maneuver. *Am J Ophthalmol* 100:617–618, 1985.

75. Rathbun JE, Hoyt WF, Beard C: Surgical management of orbitofrontal varix in Klippel-Trenaunay-Weber syndrome. *Am J Ophthalmol* 70:109, 1970.

76. Lamar L, Farber G, O'Quinn S: Klippel-Trenaunay-Weber syndrome. *Arch Dermatol* 91:58, 1965.

77. Mankad V, Gray G, Miller D: Bilateral nephroblastomatosis and Klippel-Trenaunay syndrome. *Cancer* 33:1462, 1974.

78. Sevel D, Rosales A: Orbital blood cyst. *Br J Ophthalmol* 62:571–574, 1978.

79. Skalka HW, Callahan MA: "Congenital" hematic cyst of the orbit. *Ann Ophthalmol* 11:1103–1107, 1979.

80. Cameron D: Hematic cyst of the orbit. Paper presented at the biannual AFIP Alumni Meeting, June, 1985.

81. Beyer R, Levine MR, Sternberg I: Orbital varices: A surgical approach. *Ophthalmic Plast Reconstr Surg* 1:205–210, 1985.

82. Blodi FC: Pathology of orbital bones. The XXXII Edward Jackson Memorial Lecture. *Am J Ophthalmol* 81:1–26, 1976.

83. Margo CE, Ragsdale BD, Perman KI, et al: Psammomatoid (juvenile) ossifying fibroma of the orbit. *Ophthalmology* 92:150–159, 1985.

84. Jakobiec FA, Potter GD, Mitchell J, Jones IS: Ossifying fibromas of the orbital roof. *Proc Third Int Symp on Orbital Disorders*, (Amsterdam) 325–333, 1977.

85. Shields JA, Nelson LB, Brown JF, Dolinskas C: Clinical, computed tomographic, and histopathologic characteristics of juvenile ossifying fibroma with orbital involvement. *Am J Ophthalmol* 96:650–653, 1983.

86. Jakobiec FA, Jones IS: Mesenchymal and fibro-osseous tumors of the orbit, in Duane T (ed): *Clinical Ophthalmology*. Hagerstown, MD: Harper and Row, 1976, pp 1–42.

87. Margo CE, Weiss A, Mutaz BH: Psammomatoid ossifying fibroma. *Arch Ophthalmol* 104:1347–1351, 1986.

88. Moore AT, Buncic JR, Munro IR: Fibrous dysplasia of the orbit in childhood. *Ophthalmology* 92:12–20, 1985.

89. Donoso LA, Magargal LE, Eiferman RA: Fibrous dysplasia of the orbit with optic nerve decompression. *Ann Ophthalmol* 14:80–83, 1982.

90. Jaffe HL: *Tumors and Tumorous Conditions of the Bones and Joints*. Philadelphia: Lea and Febiger, 1958.

91. Spjut HF, Dorfman HD, Fechner RF, Ackerman LV: Tumors of bone and cartilage. *Atlas of Tumor Pathology*, Fascicle 5. Washington, DC: Armed Forces Institute of Pathology, 1970, p 132.

92. Ronner HJ, Jones IS: Aneurysmal bone cyst of the orbit: A review. *Ann Ophthalmol* 15:626–629, 1983.

93. Jaffe HL, Lichtenstein L: Solitary unicameral bone cyst with emphasis on the roentgen picture. The pathologic appearance and the pathogenesis. *Arch Surg* 44:1004–1025, 1942.

94. Biesecker JL, Marcove RC, Huvos AG, Mike V: Aneurysmal bone cysts: A clinicopathologic study of 66 cases. *Cancer* 26:615–625, 1970.

95. Tillman BP, Dahlin DK, Lipscomb PR, Stewart JR: Aneurysmal bone cyst: An analysis of 95 cases. *Mayo Clin Proc* 43:478–495, 1968.

96. Powell JO, Glaser JS: Aneurysmal bone cyst of the orbit. *Arch Ophthalmol* 93:340–342, 1975.

97. Fu YS, Persin KH: Nonepithelial tumors of the nasal cavity, paranasal sinuses, and nasopharynx. A clinicopathologic study: III. Cartilaginous tumors (chondroma, chondrosarcoma). *Cancer* 34:453, 1974.

98. Shepherd WF, Maguire CJ, Bailey IC: Benign osteoblastoma of the orbit. *Irish J Med Sci* 146(abs):150, 1977.

99. Lowder CY, Berlin AJ, Cox WA, Hahn JF: Benign osteoblastoma of the orbit. *Ophthalmology* 93:1351–1354, 1986.

100. Babel J: Osteoclastome et granuloma a cellules geantes du rebord orbitaire. *Ann Ocul* 206:725, 1973.

101. Guccion J, Enzinger F: Malignant giant cell tumors of soft parts. *Cancer* 29:1518, 1972.

102. Mandel MR, Stewart WB: Periorbital osteosarcoma: An unusual case report

and review of the clinical and histopathologic features. *Ophthalmic Plast Reconstr Surg* 1:129–136, 1985.

103. Henderson JW: Osseous and cartilagenous tumors, in Henderson JW (ed): *Orbital Tumors*. Philadelphia: WB Saunders, 1980, pp 198–245.

104. Illif C, Ossofsky H: Infantile cortical hyperostosis: An unusual cause of proptosis. *Am J Ophthalmol* 53:976, 1962.

105. Naiman J, Green WR, d'Heurle D, et al: Brown tumor of the orbit associated with primary hyperparathyroidism. *Am J Ophthalmol* 90:565–571, 1980.

106. Hamlin WB, Lund PK: Giant-cell tumors of the mandible and facial bones. *Arch Otolaryngol* 86:658, 1967.

107. Ferry AP: Brown tumors (fibro-osseous bone replacement and overgrowth) of the orbit in hyperparathyroidism. *Metabolic Pediatric Ophthalmol* 3:67, 1979.

108. Kobayashi S, Kyoshima K, Nakagawa F, et al: Diploic meningioma of the orbital roof. *Surg Neurol* 13:277–281, 1980.

109. Wolter JR, Benz SC: Ectopic meningioma of the superior orbital rim. *Arch Ophthalmol* 94:1920–1922, 1976

110. Craig WM, Gogela LG: Intraorbital meningiomas, clinicopathological study. *Am J Ophthalmol* 32:1663–1680, 1949.

111. Gardner EJ: Follow-up study of a family group exhibiting dominant inheritance for a syndrome including intestinal polyps, osteomas, fibromas and epidermal cysts. *Am J Hum Genet* 14:376–390, 1962.

112. Blair NT, Trempe MD: Hyperplasia of the retinal pigment epithelium associated with Gardner's syndrome. *Am J Ophthalmol* 90:661–667, 1980.

113. Sherman RS, Wilner D: The roentgen diagnosis of hemangioma of bone. *Am J Roentgenol Radium Ther Nucl Med* 86:1146, 1961.

114. Brackup AH, Haller ML, Danber MM: Hemangioma of the bony orbit. *Am J Ophthalmol* 90:258–261, 1980.

115. Eretto P, Krohel GB, Shihab ZM, et al: Optic neuropathy in Paget's disease. *Am J Ophthalmol* 97:505–510, 1984.

116. Chen JR, Rhee RS, Wallach A, et al: Neurologic disturbances in Paget's disease of bone. Response to calcitonin. *Neurology* 29:448, 1979.

117. Ryan WG: Treatment of Paget's disease of bone with mithramycin. *Clin Orthop* 127:106, 1977.

118. Small ML, Green WR, Johnson LC: Lipoma of the frontal bone. *Arch Ophthalmol* 97:129–132, 1979.

119. Johnson LN, Krohel GB, Yeon EB, Parnes SM: Sinus tumors invading the orbit. *Ophthalmology* 91:209–217, 1984.

120. Jakobiec FA, Trokel S, Iwamoto T: Sino-orbital polyposis. *Arch Ophthalmol* 97:2353–2357, 1979.

121. Jakobiec FA, Rootman J, Jones IS: Secondary and metastatic tumors of the orbit in Jones IS, Jakobiec FA (eds): *Diseases of the Orbit*. Hagerstown, MD: Harper and Row, 1979, pp 503–569.

122. Spiro R, Huvos AG, Strong EW: Adenoid cystic carcinoma of salivary origin. A clinicopathologic study of 242 cases. *Am J Surg* 128:512–520, 1974.

123. Jakobiec FA, Mitchell J, Chauhan PM, Iwamoto T: Mesectodermal leiomyosarcoma of the antrum and orbit. *Am J Ophthalmol* 85:51–57, 1978.

124. Trautason OI, Felson SE: Cause of enophthalmos secondary to maxillary sinus mucocele. *Am J Ophthalmol* 95:838–840, 1983.

125. Frederick J, Braude AI: Anaerobic infection of the paranasal sinuses. *N Engl J Med* 290:135–137, 1974.

126. Kaufman SJ: Orbital mucopyoceles. Two cases and a review. *Surv Ophthalmol* 25:253–262, 1981.

127. Iliff CE: Mucoceles in the orbit. *Arch Ophthalmol* 89:392–395, 1973.

128. Tenzel RR, Groff J: Anterior ethmoidal mucocele. *Am J Ophthalmol* 62:160–161, 1966.

129. Fascenelli FW: Maxillary sinus abnormalities. *Arch Otolaryngol* 90:190–193, 1969.

130. Ritter FN: The surgical anatomy of the nasal sinuses. *Otolaryngol Clin N Am* 4:2–11, 1971.

131. Johnson LN, Hepler RS, Yee RD, et al: Sphenoid sinus mucocele (anterior clinoid variant) mimicking diabetic ophthalmoplegic and retrobulbar neuritis. *Am J Ophthalmol* 102:111–115, 1986.

132. Abrahamson IR, Baluyot ST, Tew JM, Scioville G: Frontal sinus mucocele. *Ann Ophthalmol* 11:173–178, 1979.

133. Ginsberg J, Polanco GB, Margolin HN, Pescovitz H: Malignant inverted papilloma characterized by proptosis. *Am J Ophthalmol* 82:129–135, 1976.

134. Hyams VJ: Papillomas of the nasal cavity and paranasal sinuses. *Ann Otolaryngol Rhinol Laryngol* 80(suppl 1–3):192, 1971.

135. Karcioglu ZA, Wesley RE, Greenidge KC, McCord CD: Proptosis and

pseudocyst formation from inverted papilloma. *Ann Ophthalmol* 14:443–448, 1982.

136. Lee KF, Hodes PJ, Greenberg L, Simotti A: Three rare causes of unilateral exophthalmos. *Radiology* 90:1009–1015, 1968.

137. Batsakis JG: *Tumors of the Head and Neck*. Baltimore: Williams and Wilkins, 1975, pp 76–85.

138. Snyder RN, Perkin KH: Papillomatosis of nasal cavity and paranasal sinuses (inverted papilloma, squamous papilloma). *Cancer* 30:668, 1972.

139. McGavran M, Sessions D, Dorfman R, et al: Nasopharyngeal angiofibroma. *Arch Otolaryngol* 90:68, 1969.

140. Christiansen T, Duvall A, Rosenberg Z, Carley R: Juvenile nasopharyngeal angiofibroma. *Trans Am Acad Ophthalmol Otolaryngol* 78:140, 1974.

141. Stern RM, Beauchamp GR, Berlin AJ: Ocular findings in juvenile nasopharyngeal angiofibroma. *Ophthalmic Surg* 17:560–564, 1986.

142. Skolnik EM, Massari FS, Tenta LT: Olfactory neuroepithelioma. Review of the world literature and presentation of two cases. *Arch Otolaryngol* 84:644–653, 1966.

143. Rakes SM, Yeatts P, Campbell RJ: Ophthalmic manifestations of esthesioneuroblastoma. *Ophthalmology* 92:1749–1753, 1985.

144. Parke DW, Font RL, Boniuk M, McCrary JA: 'Cholesteatoma' of the orbit. *Arch Ophthalmol* 100:612–616, 1982.

145. Hellquist H, Lundgren J, Olofsson J: Cholesterol granuloma of the maxillary and frontal sinuses. *J Otorhinolaryngol Relat Spec* 46:153–158, 1984.

146. Ramsey GS, Laws HW, Prichard JE, et al: Post-traumatic granuloma of the bony orbit simulating tumor. *Can Med Assoc J* 59:206–211, 1948.

147. Osborne DA, Wallace M: Carcinoma of the frontal sinus associated with epidermoid cholesteatoma. *J Laryngol Otolaryngol* 81:1921–1932, 1967.

148. Coates GM: Cholesteatoma of the frontal sinus. *Arch Otolaryngol* 26:29–37, 1937.

149. Martin JA, Robertson DM: Extrascleral extension of choroidal melanoma diagnosed by ultrasound. *Ophthalmology* 90:1554–1559, 1983.

150. Font RI, Spaulding AG, Zimmerman LE: Diffuse malignant melanoma of the uveal tract: A clinicopathologic report of 54 cases. *Trans Am Acad Ophthalmol Otolaryngol* 72:877–894, 1968.

151. Sassani JW, Weinstein JM, Graham WP: Massively invasive diffuse choroidal melanoma. *Arch Ophthalmol* 103:945–948, 1985.

152. Duffin RM, Straatsma BR, Foos RY, Kerman BM: Small malignant melanoma of the choroid with extraocular extension. *Arch Ophthalmol* 99:1827–1830, 1981.

153. Seiff SR, Shorr N, Kopelman J: Orbital extension of uveal melanoma. *Ann Ophthalmol* 18:171–173, 1986.

154. Shammas HF, Blodi FC: Orbital extension of choroidal and ciliary body melanomas. *Arch Ophthalmol* 95:2002–2005, 1977.

155. Shields JA, Augsburger JJ, Donoso LA, et al: Hepatic metastasis and orbital recurrence of uveal melanoma after 42 years. *Am J Ophthalmol* 100:666–668, 1985.

156. Saunders DH, Rodrigues MM, Shannon GM: Orbital recurrence of malignant melanoma of the choroid 24 years after enucleation. *Ophthalmic Surg* 8:31, 1977.

157. Donoso LA, Augsburger JJ, Sheilds JA, et al: Metastatic uveal melanoma: Correlation between survival times and cytomorphometry of primary tumors. *Arch Ophthalmol* 104:76–78, 1986.

158. Shields JA, Augsburger JJ, Dougherty MJ: Orbital recurrence of choroidal melanoma 20 years after enucleation. *Am J Ophthalmol* 97:767–770, 1984.

159. Shields JA: Current approaches to the diagnosis and management of choroidal melanomas. *Surv Ophthalmol* 21:443–463, 1977.

160. Starr HJ, Zimmerman LE: Extrascleral extension and orbital recurrence of malignant melanomas of the choroid and ciliary body. *Int Ophthalmol Clin* 2:369–384, 1962.

161. Zimmerman LE, McLean IW: An evaluation of enucleation in the management of uveal melanoma. *Am J Ophthalmol* 87:741–760, 1979.

162. Char DH, Phillips TL: The potential for adjuvant radiotherapy in choroidal melanoma. *Arch Ophthalmol* 100:247–248, 1982.

163. Shields JA, Augsburger J: Current approaches to the diagnosis and management of retinoblastoma. *Surv Ophthalmol* 25:347–372, 1981.

164. Jakobiec FA, Rootman J, Jones IS: Secondary and metastatic tumors of the orbit, in Duane TD, Jaeger EA (eds): *Clinical Ophthalmology*. Philadelphia, PA: Harper and Row, 1982, pp 1–67.

165. Char DH, Hedges TR, Norman D: Retinoblastoma CT diagnosis. *Ophthalmology* 91:1347–1350, 1984.

166. Haik BG, Louis LS, Smith ME, et al: Computed tomography of the nonrheg-

matogenous retinal detachment in the pediatric patient. *Ophthalmology* 92:1133–1142, 1985.

167. Haik BG, Louis LS, Smith ME, et al: Magnetic resonance imaging in the evaluation of leukocoria. *Ophthalmology* 92:1143–1152, 1985.

168. Broughton WL, Zimmerman LE: A clinicopathological study of 56 cases of intraocular medulloepitheliomas. *Am J Ophthalmol* 85:407–418, 1978.

169. Orellana J, Roberto AM, Font RL, et al: Medulloepithelioma diagnosed by ultrasound and vitreous aspirate. *Ophthalmology* 90:1531–1539, 1983.

170. Green WR, Iliff WJ, Trotter R: Malignant teratoid medulloepithelioma of the optic nerve. *Arch Ophthalmol* 91:451, 1974.

171. Zimmerman LE, Font R, Andersen SR: Rhabdomyosarcomatous differentiation in malignant intraocular medulloepitheliomas. *Cancer* 30:817, 1962.

172. Luxenberg MN, Guthrie TH: Chemotherapy of basal cell and squamous cell carcinoma of the eyelids and periorbital tissues. *Ophthalmology* 93:504–510, 1986.

173. Mohs FE: Micrographic surgery for the microscopically controlled excision of eyelid cancers. *Arch Ophthalmol* 104:901–908, 1986.

174. Putterman AM: Conjunctival map biopsy to determine pagetoid spread. *Am J Ophthalmol* 1022:87–90, 1986.

175. Aurora A, Luxenberg M: Case report of adenocarcinoma of glands of Moll. *Am J Ophthalmol* 70:984, 1970.

176. Miller WL: Sweat gland carcinoma. *Am J Clin Pathol* 47:767, 1967.

177. Zimmerman LE: The cancerous, precancerous, and pseudocancerous lesions of the cornea and conjunctiva, in Rycroft PV (ed): *The Poklington Memorial Lecture in Corneoplastic Surgery.* New York: Pergamon Press, 1969, pp 547–555.

178. Margo CE, Weitzenkorn DE: Mucoepidermoid carcioma of the conjunctiva: Report of a case in a 36-year-old with paranasal sinus invasion. *Ophthalmic Surg* 17:151–154, 1986.

179. Rao NA, Font RL: Mucoepidermoid carcinoma of the conjunctiva: A clinicopathologic study of five cases. *Cancer* 38:1696–1709, 1976.

180. Ferry AP, Font RL: Carcinoma metastatic to the eye and orbit. II. A clinicopathological study of 26 patients with carcinoma metastatic to the anterior segment of the eye. *Arch Ophthalmol* 93:472–484, 1975.

181. Ferry AP, Font RL: Carcinoma metastatic to the eye and orbit. I. A clinicopathologic study of 227 cases. *Arch Ophthalmol* 92:276–286, 1974.

182. Font RL, Ferry AP: Carcinoma metastatic to the eye and orbit. III. A clinicopathologic study of 28 cases metastatic to the orbit. *Cancer* 38:1326–1335, 1976.

183. Bloch RS, Gartner S: The incidence of ocular metastatic carcinoma. *Arch Ophthalmol* 85:673, 1971.

184. Albert DM, Rubenstein RA, Scheie HG: Tumor metastasis to the eye. Part II. Clinical study in infants and children. *Am J Ophthalmol* 63:727–732, 1967.

185. Rush JA, Waller RR, Campbell RJ: Orbital carcinoid tumor metastatic from the colon. *Am J Ophthalmol* 89:636–640, 1980.

186. Riddle PJ, Font RL, Zimmerman LE: Carcinoid tumors of the eye and orbit: A clinicopathologic study of 15 cases, with histochemical and electron microscopic observations. *Human Pathol* 13:459–469, 1982.

187. Reifler DM, Davison P: Histochemical analysis of breast carcinoma metastatic to the orbit. *Ophthalmology* 93:254–259, 1986.

188. Howard GM, Jakobiec FA, Trokel SL, et al: Pulsating metastatic tumor of the orbit. *Am J Ophthalmol* 85:767–771, 1978.

189. Rush JA, Older JJ, Richman AV: Testicular seminoma metastatic to the orbit. *Am J Ophthalmol* 91:258–260, 1981.

190. Kennerdell JS, Slamovits TL, Dekker A, Johnson BL: Orbital fine-needle aspiration biopsy. *Am J Ophthalmol* 99:547–551, 1985.

191. Spoor TC, Kennerdell JS, Dekker A, et al: Orbital fine needle aspiration biopsy with B-scan guidance. *Am J Ophthalmol* 89:274–277, 1980.

192. Krohel GB, Tobin DR, Chavis RM: Inaccuracy of fine needle aspiration biopsy. *Ophthalmology* 92:666–670, 1985.

193. Norris JL: Orbital endoscopy. *Oto-ophthalmol Soc* 59:145, 1978.

194. Hyman RA, Edwards JH: MR imaging versus CT in the evaluation of orbital lesions. *Geriatr Ophthalmol* 1:15–20, 1985.

195. Sullivan JA, Harms SE: Surface-coil MR imaging of orbital neoplasms. *Am J Neurorad* 7:29–34, 1986.

196. Holman RE, Grinson BS, Drayer BP, et al: Magnetic resonance imaging of optic glioma. *Am J Ophthalmol* 100:596–601, 1985.

197. Sobel DF, Kelly W, Kjos BO, et al: MR imaging of orbital and ocular disease. *AJNR* 6:259–264, 1985.

198. Char DH, Sobel D, Kelly WM, et al: Magnetic resonance scanning in orbital tumor diagnosis. *Ophthalmology* 92:1305–1310, 1985.

199. Haik BG, Louis LS, Smith ME: Nuclear magnetic resonance imaging in orbital disease. *Ophth Forum* 3:31–34, 1985.

200. Edwards JH, Hyman RA, Vacirca SJ: Magnetic resonance imaging of the orbit. *AJNR* 6:253–258, 1985.

201. Schenck JF, Hait HR, Foster IH, et al: Improved MR imaging of the orbit at 1.5 T with surface coils. *AJNR* 6:193–196, 1985.

202. Sobel DF, Moseley IF: Brant-Zawadzki M: Magnetic resonance imaging (MRI) of the eye and orbit, in Gonzalez CF, Becker MH, Flanagan JC (eds): *Diagnostic Imaging in Ophthalmology.* New York: Springer-Verlag, 1986, pp 99–114.

203. Sullivan JA, Harms SE: Characterization of orbital lesions by surface coil. *MR Imaging Radiographics* 7:9–28, 1987.

204. Mafee J, Peyman G, Peace J, et al: Magnetic resonance imaging in the evaluation and differentiation of uveal melanomas. *Ophthalmology* 94:341–348, 1987.

205. Byrne SF, Glaser JS: Orbital tissue differentiation with standardized echography. *Ophthalmology* 90:1071–1090, 1983.

206. Coleman DJ, Dallow RL: Orbital ultrasonography, in Duane TD, Jaeger EA (eds): *Clinical Ophthalmology, Vol. 2.* Philadelphia: Harper and Row, 1982, pp 1–16.

207. McNutt LC, Kaefring SL, Ossoinig KC: Echographic measurement of extraocular muscles, in White D, Brown RE (eds): *Ultrasound in Medicine, Vol 3A. Clinical Aspects.* New York: Plenum Press, 1977, pp 927–932.

208. Coleman DJ, Lizzi FL, Jack RL: Ultrasonography of the eye and orbit. Philadelphia: Lea and Febiger, 1977, p 331.

209. Ossoinig KC.: Orbital disorders, in deVlieger M (ed): *Handbook of Clinical Ultrasound.* New York: John Wiley & Sons, 1978, pp 884–904.

4

Pediatric Orbital Tumors

Joseph C. Flanagan
Joseph A. Mauriello, Jr.

This chapter considers both primary and metastatic orbital tumors unique to the pediatric age group. Pediatric fibroosseous tumors are discussed along with adult fibroosseous tumors in Chapter 3. Lacrimal gland tumors of adults and children are presented in a separate chapter.

Table 4-1 lists the differential diagnosis of tumors and inflammations that occur in the pediatric age group. The table attempts to classify these by CT-scan appearance and will serve as a guide for analyzing all pediatric patients with orbital tumors and inflammations. A further subdivision of pediatric tumors may be based on age of onset: congenital onset versus onset later in life. For example, causes of proptosis at birth are listed in Table 4-2, causes of massive unilateral proptosis are in Table 4-3, and causes of massive proptosis of a child at any age may be found in Table 4-4.[1] When the clinical features are combined with the CT-scan appearance, the practitioner may formulate a workable differential diagnosis.

As with adult tumors, pediatric tumors may have accompanying inflammation and mimic a primary inflammatory process. A trial of intravenous antibiotics may be necessary before biopsy is performed. While orbital pseudotumor is distinctly rare in the pediatric age group, the orbital myositis pattern is more common in children than other forms of pseudotumor. The necessity for CT scanning in such patients cannot be overemphasized. In addition, developmental anomalies such as microphthalmos with cyst and hamartomas such as lymphangioma may mimic tumors.

The clinical and CT-scan features of some more common congenital orbital tumors and anomalies are considered in Table 4-5.

CLINICAL FEATURES OF PEDIATRIC ORBITAL TUMORS AND DEVELOPMENTAL ANOMALIES

A summary of the salient diagnostic features of some of the above entities is considered below. Entities not considered below may be found in Chapter 3.

Microphthalmos with Cyst

Microphthalmos with cyst has three clinical presentations: (1) a cyst so small that it cannot be detected clinically with a microphthalmic eye, (2) a large cyst that is more clinically apparent than a microphthalmic eye, and (3) an excessively large cyst that deforms surrounding tissues and a microphthalmic eye so small that it is not clinically detectable. In patients with very large cysts, the cysts transilluminates. A bluish mass that distends the lower lid may be visible. The cyst may enlarge after birth. When microphthalmos with cyst is bilateral, often cardiac and central nervous system (CNS) abnormalities are present (Fig. 4-1).[1,2]

Children with microphthalmos with cyst may rarely present with proptosis as children or even as adults due to two basic mechanisms: (1) massive gliosis within the colobomatous cyst or (2) secondary glaucoma with buphthalmos in an infant with persistent hyperplastic primary vitreous (PHPV).[3]

Table 4-1
Pediatric Tumors and Inflammations—CT Scan Appearance

EOM Involvement
  Hyperthyroidism
  Pseudotumor

Intraconal
  Intrinsic Optic Nerve Tumors
  Glioma
  Meningioma
  Giant drusen (astrocytoma) of tuberous sclerosis
  Optic nerve sheath cyst—colobomatous arachnoid cyst
  Melanocytoma
  Blue nevus
  Juxtaneural Tumors
  Hemangioblastoma (von Hippel)
  JXG
  Leukemia

Inflammatory Optic Nerve Conditions That May Mimic Tumor
  Pseudotumor involving optic nerve
  Optic neuritis
  Thyroid ophthalmopathy
  Sarcoid

Miscellaneous Causes of Optic Nerve Enlargement
  Traumatic hematoma
  Optic nerve drusen

Localized Intraconal Tumors
  Cavernous hemangioma
  Hemangiopericytoma
  Schwannoma
  Neurofibromatosis (localized form)

Focal Cystic with Local Bone Involvement
  Dermoid cyst*
  Epidermoid cyst*
  Encephalocele†
  Meningocele†
  Mucocele‡

Focal Noncystic with Local Bone Involvement
  Alveolar soft part sarcoma (tends to involve EOM, well localized) #*

Diffuse Cystic without Bone Involvement
  Microphthalmos with cyst
  Congenital cystic eyeball
  Lymphangioma
  Teratoma‖ #

Diffuse (Intraconal and Extraconal) Noncystic—Usually without Bone Involvement
  Capillary hemangioma
  Pseudotumor
  Leukemia
  Lymphoid infiltrate (lymphoma rare)
  Granulocytic sarcoma‖ ††

  Rhabdomyosarcoma‖
  Sinus histiocytosis
  Endodermal sinus tumor‖
  Heterotopic brain tissue

Rare Spindle Cell Tumors (See Chapter 3)‖
  Fibrosarcoma
  Fibrous histiocytoma
  Leiomyosarcoma
  Malignant chondrosarcoma§
  Malignant schwannoma
  Malignant neurofibroma**
  Meningeal sarcoma
  Postradiation sarcoma
  Undifferentiated sarcoma

Diffuse (Noncystic) with Bone Involvement
  Metastatic neuroblastoma
  Metastatic Ewing's sarcoma

Sinus and/or Bone Involvement—Soft Tissue Tumors That Secondarily Involve Bone or Sinus
  Melanotic ectodermal tumor of infancy (retinal anlage tumor)
  Teratoma #
  Angiofibroma (also see Chapter 3)
  Alveolar soft part sarcoma (tends to involve EOM, localized)
  Esthesioneuroblastoma
  Unifocal or multifocal eosinophilic granuloma (histiocystosis X)
    Eosinophilic granuloma
    Letterer-Siwe disease
    Hand-Schüller-Christian disease
  Endodermal sinus tumor

Osseous and Other Tumors That Primarily Involve Bone (see Chapter 3)
  Ossifying fibroma
  Fibrous dysplasia
  Aneurysmal bone cyst
  Giant cell tumor
  Reparative granuloma
  Osteoblastoma

Intraocular Tumors with Orbital Spread (see Chapter 3)
  Retinoblastoma
  Medulloepithelioma
  Granulocytic sarcoma
  Leukemia

---

* are localized at suture lines with possible focal bone erosion

† at suture lines between maxillary, lacrimal, ethmoid, and frontal bones

‡ most often frontal and ethmoid sinus

§ very rare but adjacent to bone usually medial orbit

‖ may involve bone

may involve maxillary sinus and middle cranial fossa

** may extend from paranasal sinus into orbit

‡‡ 6 of 33 had orbital or adjacent sinus involvement, also may have choroidal involvement

Table 4-2
PROPTOSIS at Birth

Capillary hemangioma
Dermoid cyst
Ethmoiditis with orbital cellulitis
Hematoma
Pseudotumor
Thyroid ophthalmopathy
Craniostenosis
Rhabdomyosarcoma
Metastatic neuroblastoma
Ewing's sarcoma
Leukemia
Granulocytic sarcoma
Glioma of optic nerve
Optic nerve meningioma
Fibroosseus tumors
Lymphangioma
Unifocal or multifocal eosinophilic granuloma (*histiocytosis X*)
JXG
Meningocele
Encephalocele
Micropthalmos with cyst
Congenital cystic eyeball
Teratoma
Retinoblastoma or medulloepithelioma with extraocular
    extension

Table 4-3
Massive Unilateral Proptosis at Birth

Rhabdomyosarcoma
Undifferentiated sarcoma
Lymphangioma (chocolate cyst formation)
Metastatic neuroblastoma
Lymphangioma
Teratoma
Ruptured dermoid cyst
Hemorrhage (spontaneous or due to systemic disease)

Table 4-4
Massive Proptosis in Children

Orbital cellulitis
Leukemia
Granulocytic sarcoma
Histiocytosis X
Rhabdomyosarcoma
Burkitt's lymphoma
Metastatic neuroblastoma
Metastatic Ewing's sarcoma
Retinoblastoma
Endodermal sinus tumor

Capillary Hemangioma, Lymphangioma, and Varix

Both conditions, capillary hemangioma and lymphangioma, may be clinically confused.[4-9] Both may occur at birth or shortly after. Both are diffuse nonencapsulated tumors that may extend onto the face and palate. On clinical examination, capillary hemangiomas enlarge on Valsalva's maneuvers such as crying or placing the head in a dependent position, while lymphangiomas do not enlarge under such circumstances. Typically, lymphangiomas grow with the face until puberty while capillary hemangiomas grow the first 6 months of life and then regress until age 5 or 6 (Fig. 4-2). As they regress, white bands of fibrous tissue replace the bright red strawberry areas that are the pathologic counterpart of the endothelial-lined spaces of the capillary hemangioma (Figs. 4-3–4-5).

Table 4-5
Differentiating Features of Some Congenital Orbital Tumors and Developmental Anomalies

Clinical Findings	Micropthalmos with Cyst	Congenital Cystic Eye	Capillary Hemangioma
Laterality	30% bilateral	Usually unilateral	Usually unilateral
Typical location	Lower lid	Upper lid	Superonasal
Change in size with crying or Valsalva's maneuver	No	No	Yes
Ocular	Micropthalmos or deformed	None	Normal
CT scan finding	Calcifications, enlarged orbit	Normal	Occasional enlarged orbit

Table 4-5 (Continued)

Lymphangioma	Encephalocele/ meningocele	Rhabdo- myosarcoma	Teratoma	Neuroblastoma
Unilateral	Unilateral	Unilateral	Unilateral	May be bilateral
Diffuse	Nasal	Superonasal	Diffuse, may be maxillary sinus	Variable
No	Yes	No	No	No
Normal	Normal	Normal	Normal	Normal
Occasional enlarged, orbit	Defect in posterior or medial orbit	Occasional enlarged orbit, may involve bone	Occasional enlarged orbit	Soft tissue mass, may involve bone

A lymphangioma is a developmental malformation of vascular and lymphatic elements. A lymphangioma does not substantially communicate with the orbital circulation, although small arteries and veins are present in the connective tissue stroma that contain many endothelial-lined spaces with lymph fluid. These vessels may be the source of spontaneous hemorrhage. Because lymphangiomas do not have a significant connection to the systemic circulation, changes in head position have little effect on the tumor's size.

Chronic inflammatory cells and actual lymphoid follicles are a variable component; their presence explains why some lymphangiomas enlarge when the patient has an upper respiratory infection.

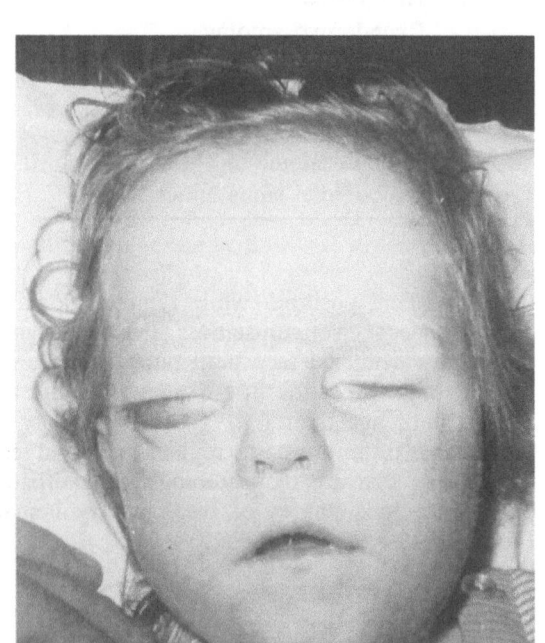

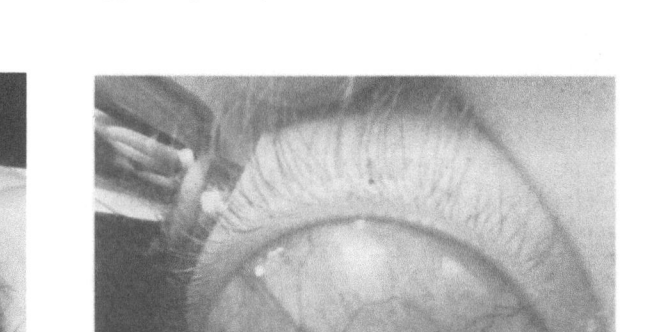

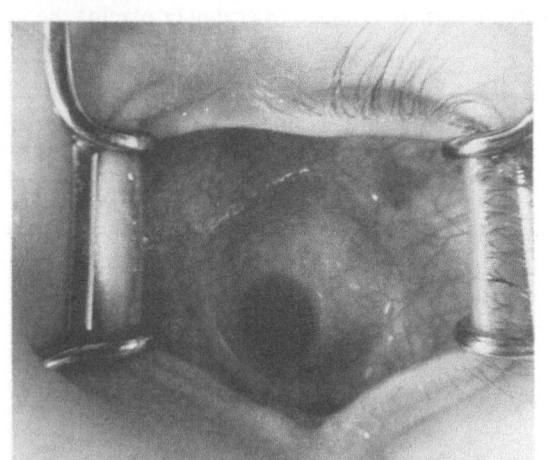

Fig. 4-1. (*A*) Child with microphthalmos with cyst on right side (*B*) and micropthalmic eye on the left side (*C*).

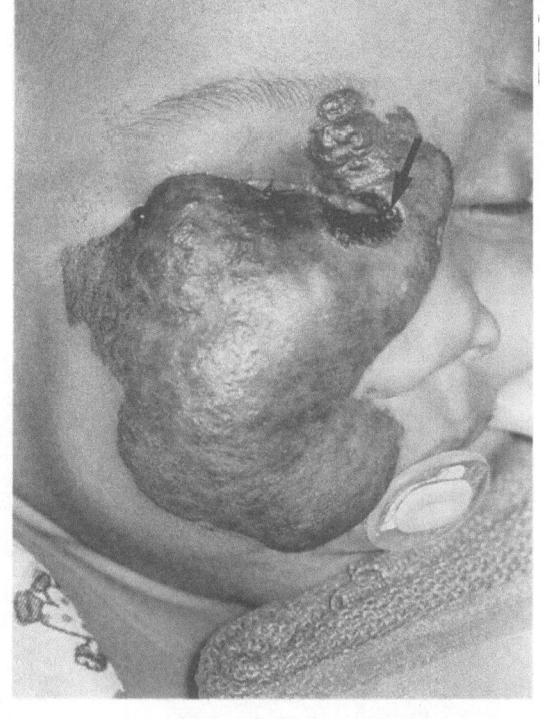

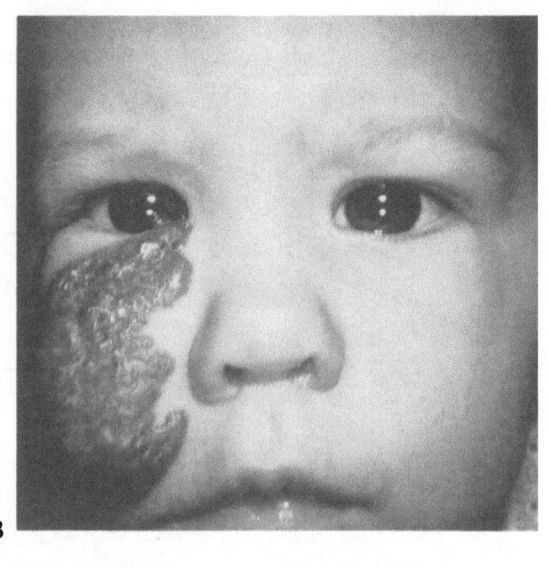

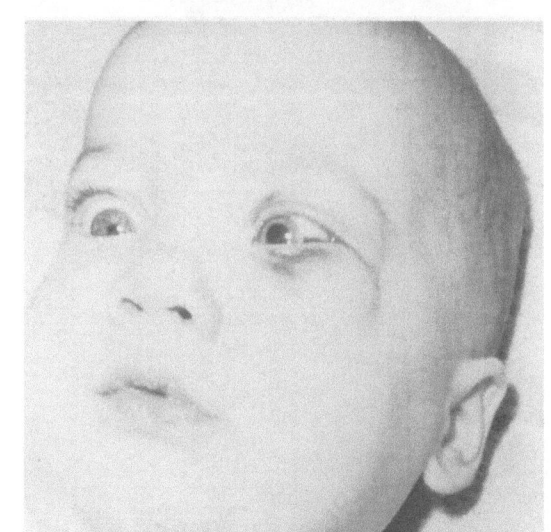

Fig. 4-2. (*A*) 6-month-old child with large capillary hemangioma with necrosis (arrow) of tumor. Patient underwent local steroidal injections because the tumor obstructed vision. (*B–C*) Patients with strawberry-colored capillary hemangiomas that did not necessitate treatment.

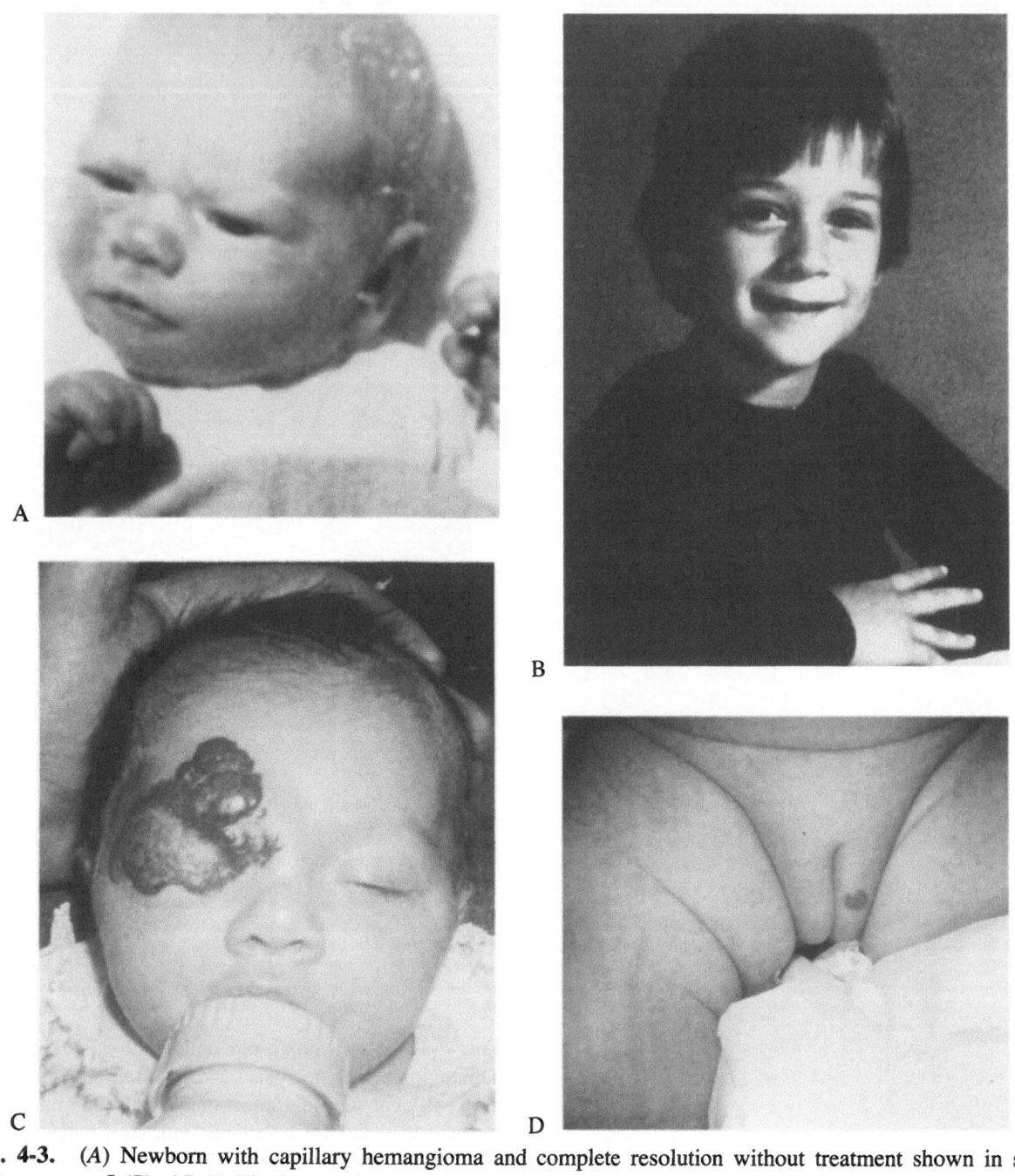

Fig. 4-3. (A) Newborn with capillary hemangioma and complete resolution without treatment shown in same patient at age 5 (B). (C–D) The hemangiomas may be multiple.

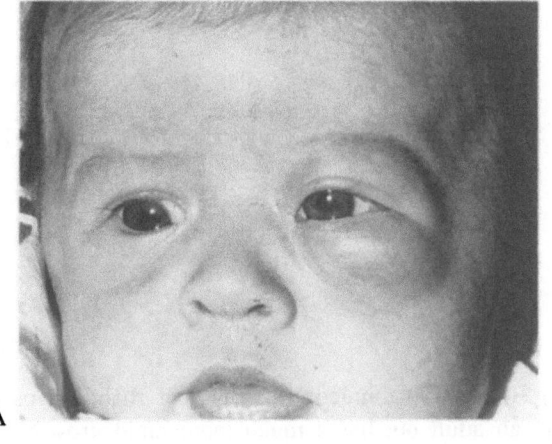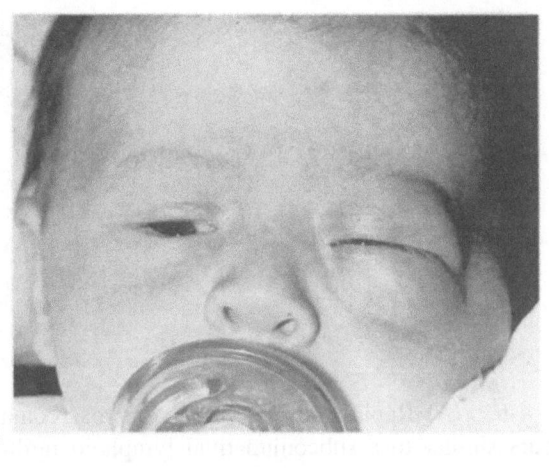

A   B

Fig. 4-4. (*A,B*) Unlike rhabdomyosarcoma and nevus flameus, when the child cries or otherwise performs a Valsalva's maneuver when sucking, the capillary hemangioma will enlarge. (*A*) is child before Valsalva's maneuver and (*B*) is during Valsalva's maneuver.

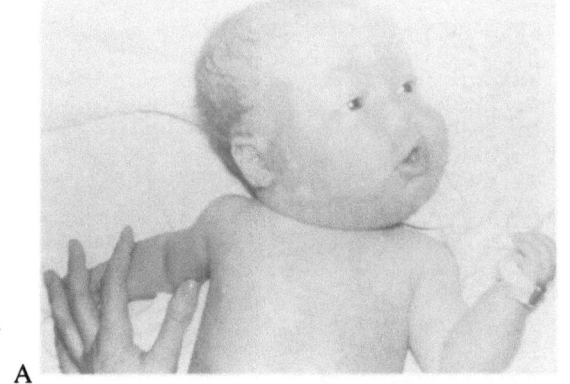

A

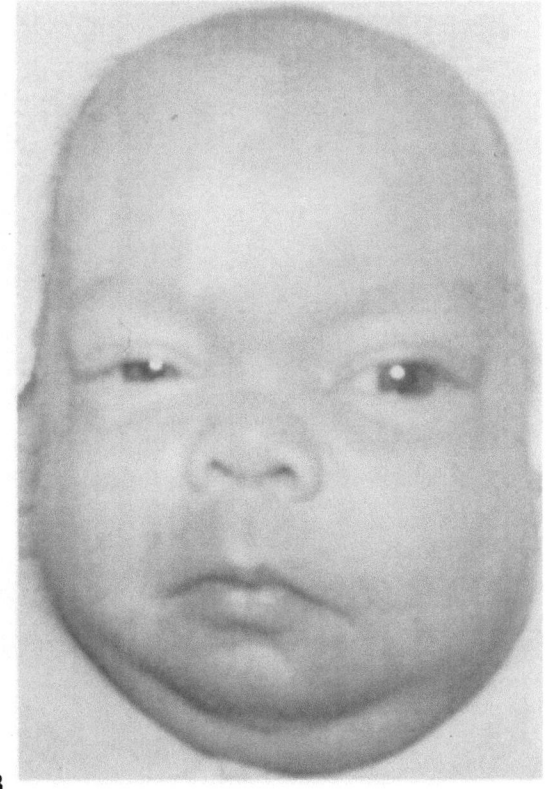

Fig. 4-5. (*A*) Nevus flameus grows proportionately to the size of the child. Newborn with Sturge-Weber syndrome. (*B*) At 4 months of age, the distribution of the macular lesion is the same as at birth.   B

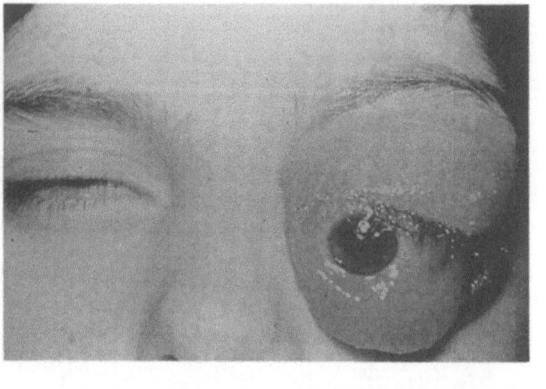

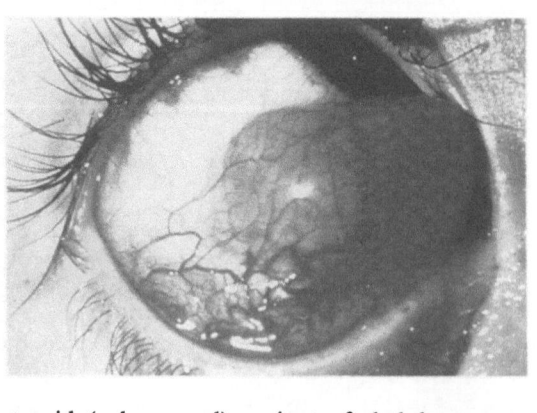

A   B

Fig. 4-6. (*A*) Rapidly growing rhabdomyosarcoma. (*B*) Botryoid (submucosal) variant of rhabdomyosarcoma appears similar to a subconjunctival lymphoid infiltrate in an adult but has a much more rapid growth. Unlike rhabdomyosarcoma, capillary hemangiomas grow slowly.

A capillary hemangioma or lymphangioma may be confused with a rhabdomyosarcoma, especially when hemorrhage occurs. The history of a mass enlarging over several days to weeks suggests a rhabdomyosarcoma (Figs. 4-6–4-8). In addition, rhabdomyosarcomas usually do not grow as rapidly as lymphangiomas that hemorrhage, unless there is severe tumor necrosis. Subconjunctival hemorrhage often accompanies orbital hemorrhage from a lymphangioma. Unfortunately, a subconjunctival hemorrhage is not a specific diagnostic sign, since subconjunctival hemorrhage may accompany any orbital tumor that grows rapidly and undergoes necrosis and hem-

orrhage. A botryoid or submucosal variant often presents as a salmon-colored mass that clinically resembles a subconjunctival lymphoid infiltrate in adults. The history of a rapid growth and the rarity of lymphoid infiltrates in children strongly favor the clinical diagnosis of rhabdomyosarcoma over lymphoid infiltrate.

Lymphangiomas are thought by some to represent a form of varix (Fig. 4-9).[9,10] A varix is a localized segmental ectasia of the orbital venous system. The dilated vein will enlarge on dependent position. The varix may be congenital or acquired due to a weakness of the vessel wall. A secondary varix may also develop distal to an

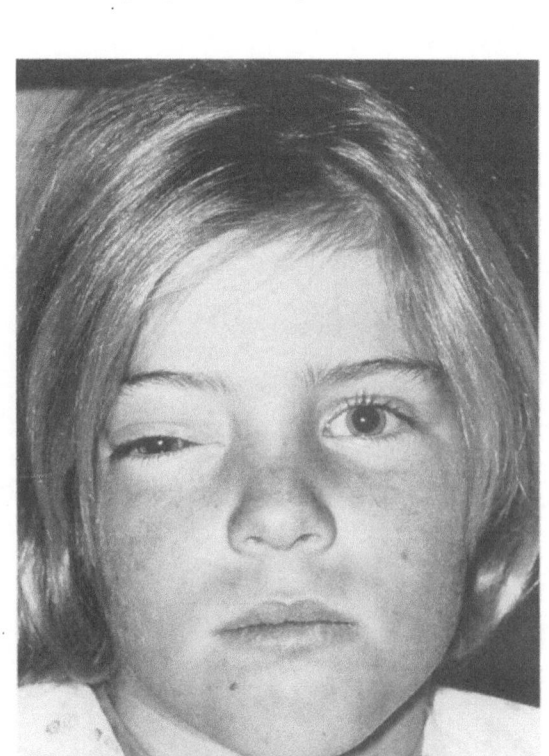

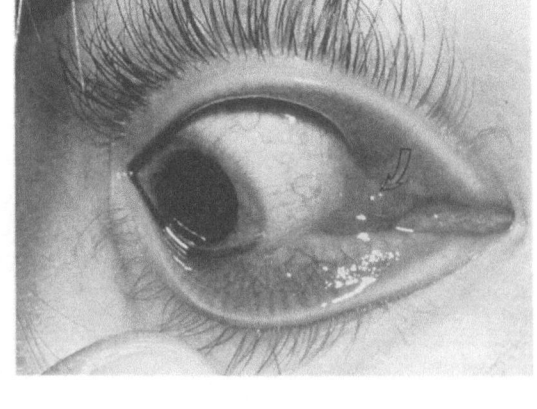

B

A

Fig. 4-7. (*A*) 9-year-old female who presented with 1-week history of ptosis of the right upper lid. (*B*) A subconjunctival mass was present (arrow). Biopsy showed a rhabdomyosarcoma.

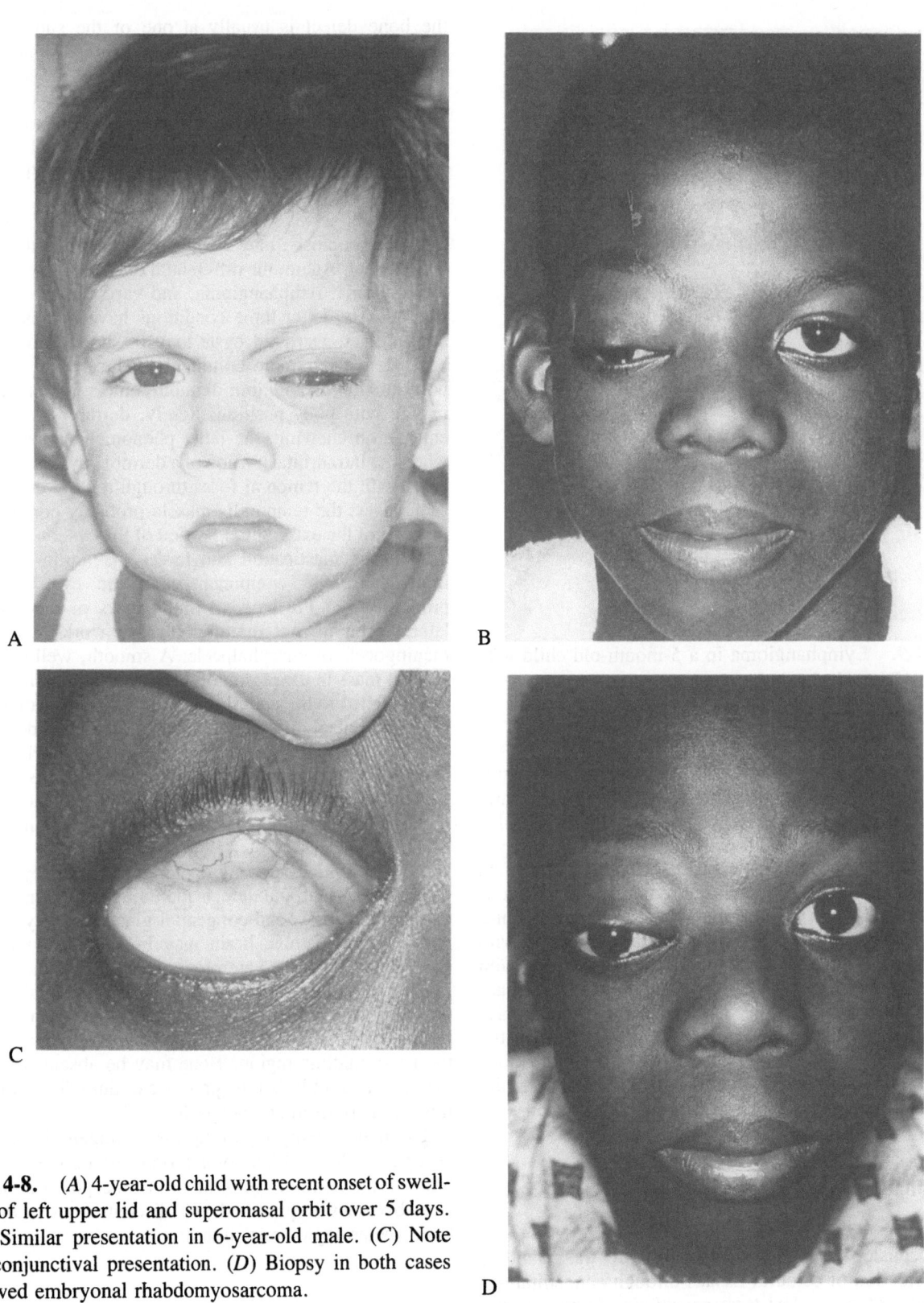

Fig. 4-8. (*A*) 4-year-old child with recent onset of swelling of left upper lid and superonasal orbit over 5 days. (*B*) Similar presentation in 6-year-old male. (*C*) Note subconjunctival presentation. (*D*) Biopsy in both cases showed embryonal rhabdomyosarcoma.

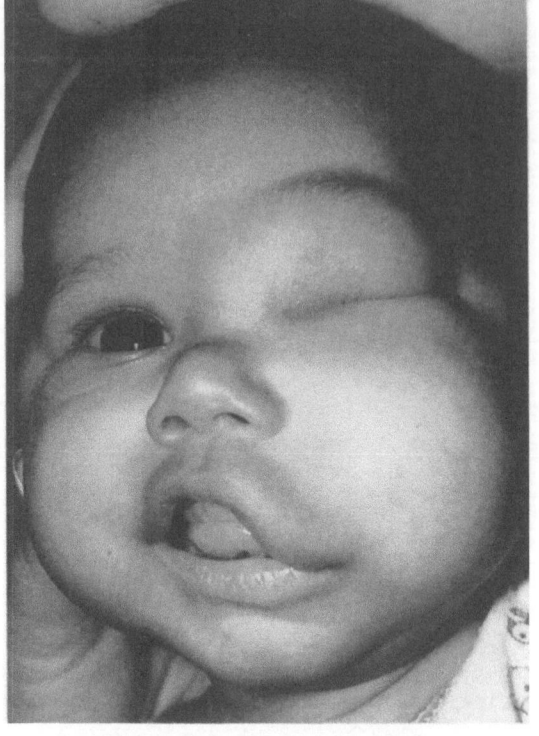

Fig. 4-9. Lymphangioma in a 5-month-old child with typical lid and cheek involvement. Patient underwent debulking of lid with frontalis suspension procedure.

abnormal communication and thereby occur in a structurally normal venous wall. Therefore, whenever a varix is present, an arteriovenous component should be ruled out. If there is an arterial bruit or pulsation, arteriography should be performed to exclude a secondary varix. In general, spontaneous bleeding from orbital varices is uncommon, while trauma may more commonly cause hemorrhage. Orbital CT scan should be performed with the patient assuming a dependent or prone position with contrast enhancement in order to demonstrate a primary varix. Ultrasound will also demonstrate the anomaly. In addition, orbital venography will also document the presence of a varix and is one of the few indications for venography since the advent of computed tomography (CT) and magnetic resonance imaging (MRI) scans.

Encephalocele and Meningocele vs. Dermoid Cyst

Encephaloceles and meningoceles are the result of the herniation of cerebral tissues through congenital dehiscences of bone. The term *encephalocele* refer to the herniation of brain tissue with its meningeal sac, while the term *meningocele* refers to the herniation that consists of only meninges and no brain tissue. Clinically, the mass is usually present superonasally in the orbit since

the bone defect is usually at one of the suture lines between the maxillary, ethmoid, and frontal bones.[11,12] Posterior protrusions may also occur through the sphenoid fissure or through a congenital dehiscence of the sphenoid wing. In this latter instance, symptoms do not occur until childhood or adolescence and consist of slowly progressing downward and forward proptosis (Figs. 4-10 and 4-11).

Pulsating as well as positional exophthalmos, that is, dynamic proptosis, may also be present due to the large bone defect. Again, the differential diagnosis of capillary hemangioma, lymphangioma, and varix should be considered. The latter three conditions have no associated bone defect. Dermoid cysts may be associated with a bone defect but more commonly induce focal smooth bone erosion; in addition, dermoid tumors do not change in size with body position. Rarely, dermoid cysts may enlarge on chewing; the latter phenomenon may occur when the intraorbital portion of a dermoid cyst communicates with the temporal fossa through a bony defect. In such cases, the temporalis muscle probably compresses the wall of the extraorbital portion of the cyst on contraction during mastication and forces the liquid contents into the orbital component, and the eye becomes proptotic.[12–16] Presumed dermoid cysts of the superolateral orbit do not require CT scan work-up to rule meningocele or encephalocele. A smooth, well-circumscribed mass in the region of the frontozygomatic suture and attached to the underlying bone is virtually diagnostic. The clinical differential diagnosis also includes eosinophilic granuloma or reparative granuloma, which are usually associated with focal punched-out destructive lesions of bone. Presumed dermoid cysts in the superomedial orbit require CT scan to rule out meningocele or encephalocele.

With encephaloceles and meningoceles, the eye itself usually is normal, but defects including coloboma, clinical anophthalmos, and congenital glaucoma may occur.

An orbital ectopic brain may be confused with an encephalocele. Brain heterotopia is defined as the occurrence of normal neural tissue outside the cranial cavity or spinal cord without continuity with the brain or meninges. This anomaly is most commonly reported in the nasal midline region. Bone may be absent between the brain and orbit, but the presence of dura distinguishes this anomaly from an encephalocele.[17]

The major theory regarding the pathogenesis of both encephaloceles and heterotopic brain tissue is that fetal brain tissue herniates into the orbit (encephalocele) and later becomes sequestered and discontinuous with the brain (heterotopic brain tissue).

Teratoma

A teratoma is by definition a congenital tumor that consists of tissues from more than one of the three germi-

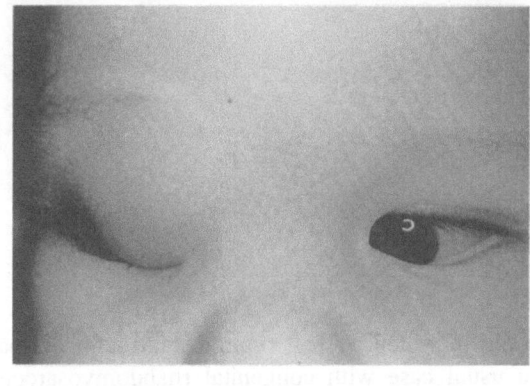

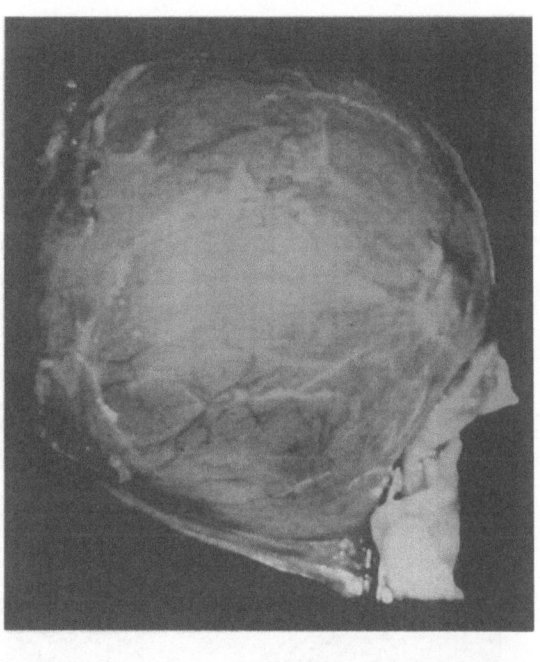

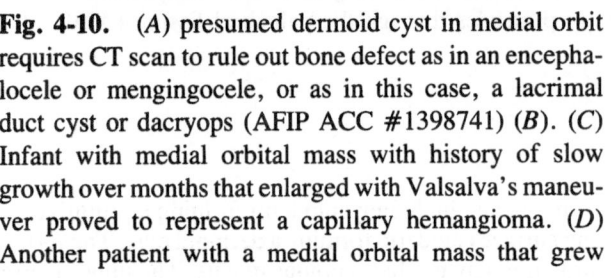

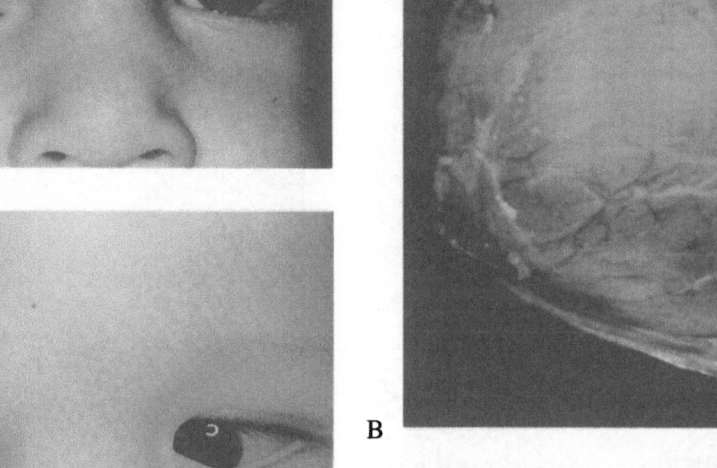

Fig. 4-10. (*A*) presumed dermoid cyst in medial orbit requires CT scan to rule out bone defect as in an encephalocele or mengingocele, or as in this case, a lacrimal duct cyst or dacryops (AFIP ACC #1398741) (*B*). (*C*) Infant with medial orbital mass with history of slow growth over months that enlarged with Valsalva's maneuver proved to represent a capillary hemangioma. (*D*) Another patient with a medial orbital mass that grew rapidly over a period of days. Biopsy showed an embryonal rhabdomyosarcoma.

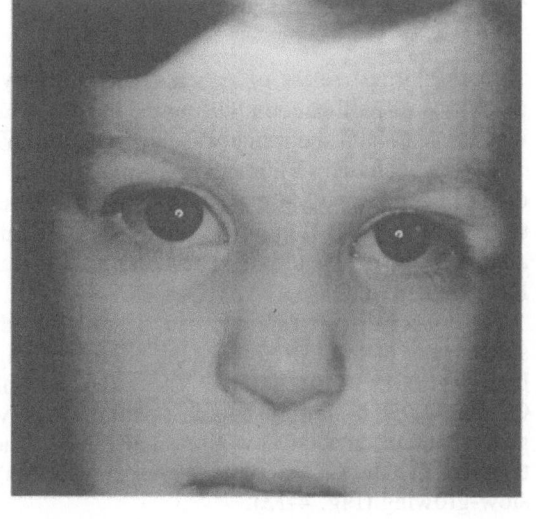

Fig. 4-11. Presumed dermoid cysts in area of frontozygomatic suture do not require CT scan work-up to rule out meningocele or encephalocele. However, eosinophilic granuloma must be considered, particularly if there is a focal osteolytic lesion of bone. Reparative granuloma often occurs in this area as well.

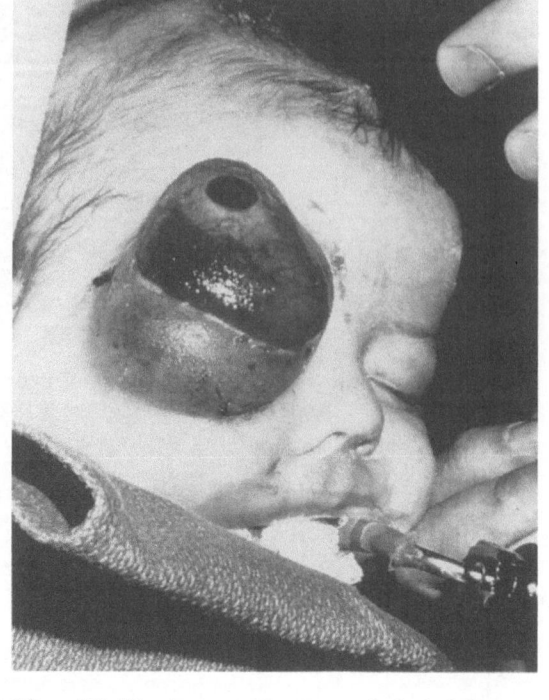

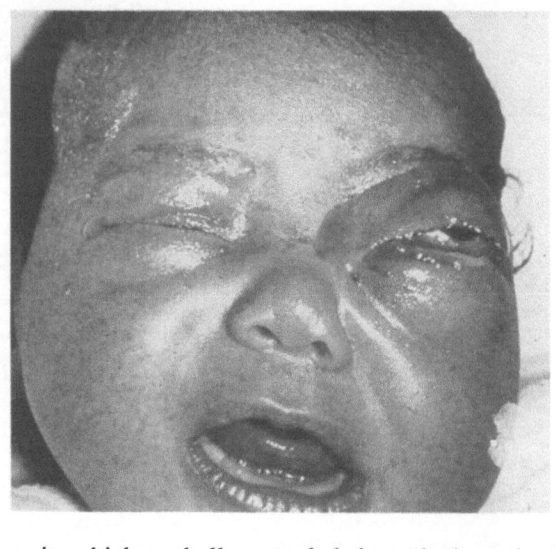

A   B

Fig. 4-12. (A) Newborn with congenital rhabdomyosarcoma in which eyeball protruded through the palpebral fissures rather than being covered by upper lid as is the usual case with congenital rhabdomyosarcoma. (B) Congenital orbital teratoma in which proptotic globe partially protrudes through the palpebral fissure (AFIP ACC #1367522).

nal layers: ectoderm, entoderm, or mesoderm.[13] The tumor is considered a choristoma. Ninety percent of teratoids consist of only ectodermal and mesodermal tissue, whereas 10 percent consist of only mesodermal and endodermal tissue. The tumor typically causes marked unilateral proptosis and upward displacement of the globe due to the rapid growth after birth in a full-term infant. In teratoma, at birth the proptotic globe tends to protrude through the palpebral fissure; in congenital rhabdomyosarcoma, the proptotic globe tends to be covered by the upper lid and does not protrude through the lids. There are, of course, exceptions to every rule (Fig. 4-12).[18]

Females with teratoma outnumber males by a ratio of 2:1.[19] A bilateral tumor has been reported.[19] Teratomas are generally confined to the orbit, but rarely extend into the middle cranial fossa or sinus. In one report, a rapidly growing orbital teratoma extended into the maxillary sinus, pterygopalatine fossa, nasal cavity, and middle cranial fossa.[20–21] The tumor may represent an abortive attempt at formation of the human body since a complete fetus has been found implanted in the orbit. Typically, the bony orbit has expanded without erosion so that its volume is doubled or tripled. Nasal and malar deformities result. The tumor may transilluminate due to its cystic

components, including entoderm forming a primitive gut and surface ectoderm forming a dermoid cyst. The former structure may produce copious mucus. The tumor is irreducible. Ependymal cells and even choroid plexus may also be present. Malignant teratomas may occur.

Alveolar Soft-Part Sarcoma

In the largest series of patients with primary orbital alveolar soft-part sarcoma (17 patients), the median age was 18 years and the range was 11 months to 69 years. The study included 13 females and 4 males. Two patients died of metastatic disease 14 years (lung and bone metastases) and 21 years (lung metastases) after orbital biopsy and excision of the tumor. The latter patients also had local radiation.[22–25]

Alveolar soft-part sarcoma usually involves the deep soft tissues of the extremities, including the thighs and buttocks. The histogenesis of the tumor is unknown. Clinically, the tumor presents as a painless pink vascular growth and often appears well-circumscribed. The tumor tends to invade the extraocular muscles (EOMs) and is slow-growing (Fig. 4-13).

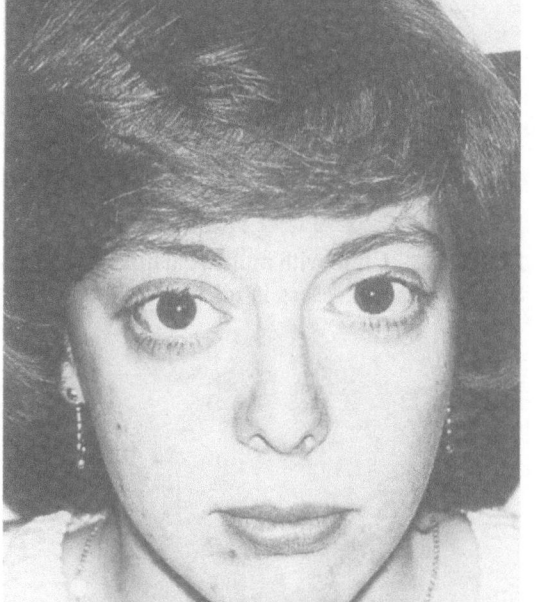

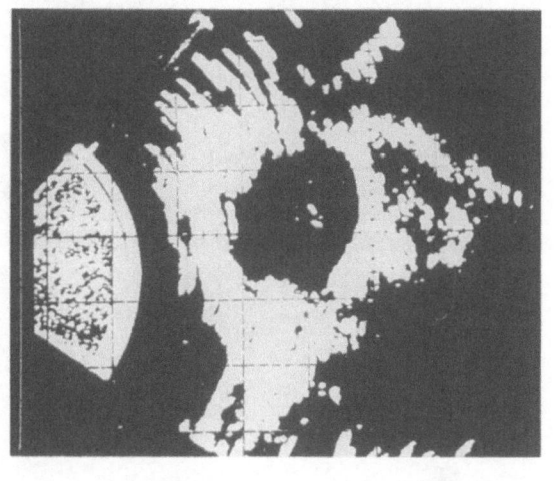

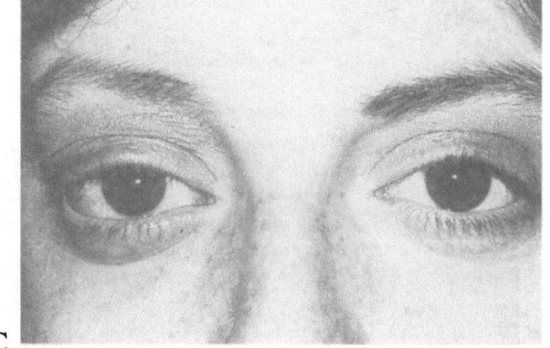

Fig. 4-13. (*A*) 22-year-old female with gradual onset of proptosis of right eye due to intraconal tumor that infiltrated the lateral rectus muscle. (*B*) B-scan ultrasonography shows well-demarcated intraconal mass. Alveolar soft-part sarcoma was treated with postoperative radiation. (*C*) Note slightly thickened right lower lid after surgery and radiation.

Unifocal or Multifocal Eosinophilic Granuloma

Eosinophilic granuloma, Letterer-Siwe disease, and Hands-Schüller-Christian disease are now under the umbrella term, *histiocytosis X.* The diseases are termed either *unifocal* (localized) or *multifocal* (systemic) in that there is skin, viscera, and lymph node involvement in addition to ocular or orbital disease. In general, the younger the patient, the more likely the disease will be multifocal (old Letterer-Siwe disease) (Figs. 4-14 and 4-15). Histologically, all three diseases are·indistinguishable and are characterized by the presence of histiocytic Langerhans' cells, normally present in the epidermis of skin, that contain Birbeck cytoplasmic granules or racquet bodies (Langerhans' granules) on electron microscopy.

The rare triad of lytic bone defects in the skull, proptosis, and diabetes insipidus are characteristic of Hand-Schüller-Christian disease.

Sinus Histiocytosis

This disease is most common in African children. The prognosis is good since the viscera and skin are spared unlike other histiocytic disorders. There is accompanying massive cervical adenopathy and retroperitoneal lymph node involvement.

Granulocytic Sarcoma

This tumor develops in the bones or periosteum of the skull in children. The tumor occurs at any time in the course of granulocytic leukemia as a localized orbital manifestation. Of the 33 cases reported by Zimmerman and Font, 7 of 33 showed evidence of orbital bone involvement (Fig. 4-16).[26] Two had bilateral orbital disease

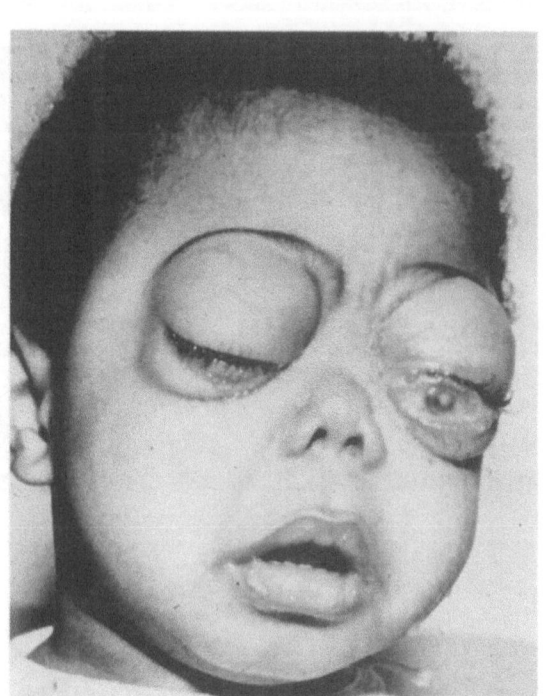

Fig. 4-14. Child with multifocal histiocytosis (Letterer-Siwe disease). Process is bilateral.

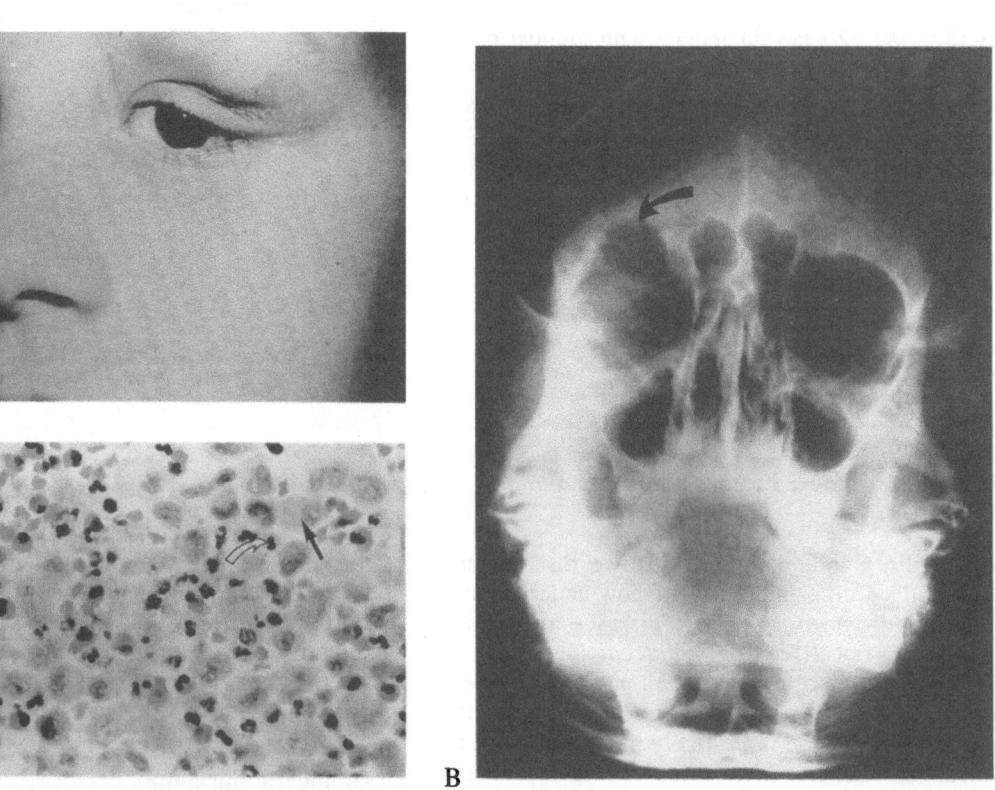

Fig. 4-15. (A) Child with localized superotemporal orbital mass. Differential diagnosis includes dermoid cyst, benign calcifying Malherbe tumor, or eosophilic granuloma. (B) Plain film shows osteolytic lesion (arrow) typical of eosinophilic granuloma. Systemic work-up for histiocytosis X was negative. Treatment included currettage. (C) Histologically, eosinophilic granuloma mimics reparative granuloma in that histiocytes (solid arrow) and eosinophils (open arrow) characteristic of eosiniophilic granuloma may be present in either entity. Eosinophilic granuloma is distinguished by the presence of Birbeck or Langerhans' granules (racket bodies) on EM found in the cytoplasm of the histiocytes. In reparative granuloma, there is often antecedent trauma, focal bone erosion, and histologically, a reaction to a subperiosteal hemorrhage.

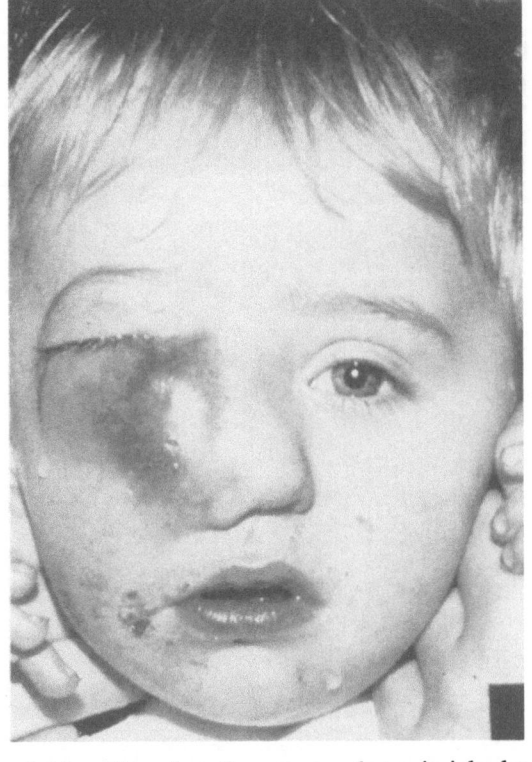

Fig. 4-16. Granulocytic sarcoma that mimicked a dacryocystitis. Note obvious distortion of nose and extension above the medial canthal tendon (AFIP ACC #1230223).

and a third had orbital and ocular involvement on one side and ocular involvement on the other side. Typically, as with neuroblastoma, patients with granulocytic sarcoma of the orbit already have well-recognized acute leukemia.[27,28]

Retinal Anlage Tumor (Melanotic Neuroectodermal Tumor of Infancy, Pigmented Retinal Choristoma)

Melanotic neuroectodermal tumor of infancy is probably of neural crest origin, although the exact cell of origin is unclear. Some believe the tumor arises from retinal cells, while others consider it of odontogenic origin. The tumor usually occurs in infants less than 1 year of age, although it may occur in older children and even adults. Ninety-two percent occur in the head and neck; however, the tumor may occur in any area of the body including the mediastinum, scapula, femur, epididymis, and shoulder. Orbital invasion is rare and usually results from secondary invasion from a tumor arising in the zygoma. The tumor may be multifocal and present as a subcutaneous facial or scalp mass. Less than 10 percent are malignant, but 10–15 percent recur.[29,30]

Metastatic Neuroblastoma

Neuroblastoma arises wherever embryonic neuroblastic tissue is found: (1) most commonly in the adrenal medulla (50%), (2) retroperitoneal parasympathetic and sympathetic tissue (25%), (3) and mediastinal (10%) and cervical sympathetic ganglion (2–5%).[31,32] The tumor generally presents in patients under 4 years of age and rarely in adults. Patients older than age 4 tend to have widespread disease, while patients who present at younger than age 1 tend to have a local disease.[32,33] In one series, 18 patients had unilateral orbital metastases while 23 had bilateral orbital disease.[32] Patients may develop a syndrome of rapid development of proptosis with hemorrhage and necrosis (Fig. 4-17). Bilateral blindness due to apparent optic nerve compression by metastatic tumor has been reported.[34] The patients most often present with periorbital ecchymosis. Some patients present with orbital cellulitis.[31–34]

Horner's syndrome results from involvement of the cervical or mediastinal sympathetic ganglion and may also occur as a complication of surgical trauma during removal of the tumor. Heterochromia may also occur. Ptosis and heterochromia that result from metastatic tumor to the sympathetic nerves in the neck is known as Hutchinson's sign. The latter sign has prognostic significance. Approximately 10 percent of patients with metastatic neuroblastoma have a 3-year survival rate. However, when Horner's syndrome is present alone, the survival rate is 79 percent at 3 years.

Opsoclonic wild, conjugate ocular movements result from a remote humoral effect, not metastatic disease, and are associated with a 100 percent three-year survival rates.[35] Patients with mediastinal and cervical disease in general do better than those with abdominal disease.[35] Liver metastases, Pepper form of metastasis, tend to occur in patients under age 1; osseous metastases, Hutchinson form of metastasis, occur in older patients.[36,37] Rarely, spontaneous regression of the primary tumor occurs. In one case report, a patient with bony orbital metastasis underwent spontaneous cure.[38]

Catecholamines byproducts may be present in the urine. Symptoms of flushing, diarrhea, and hypesthesias occur in these patients.

Ewing's Sarcoma

Ewing's sarcoma is a primary intramedullary tumor of bone, especially of the long bones and trunk in patients between ages 10 and 25. Metastatic orbital disease is heralded by rapid proptosis with hemorrhage and necrosis as in neuroblastoma. Both metastatic neuroblastoma and Ewing's sarcoma spare the globe. The bone is usually involved.[39,40] Unlike neuroblastoma, bilateral metastases are rare. Ewing's sarcoma that involves the roof of the orbit primarily has been reported.

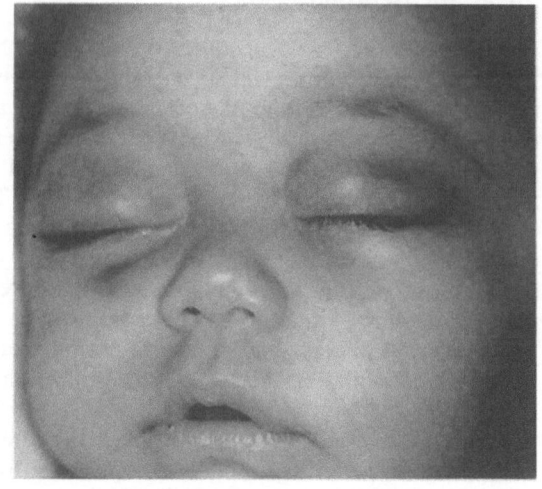

A

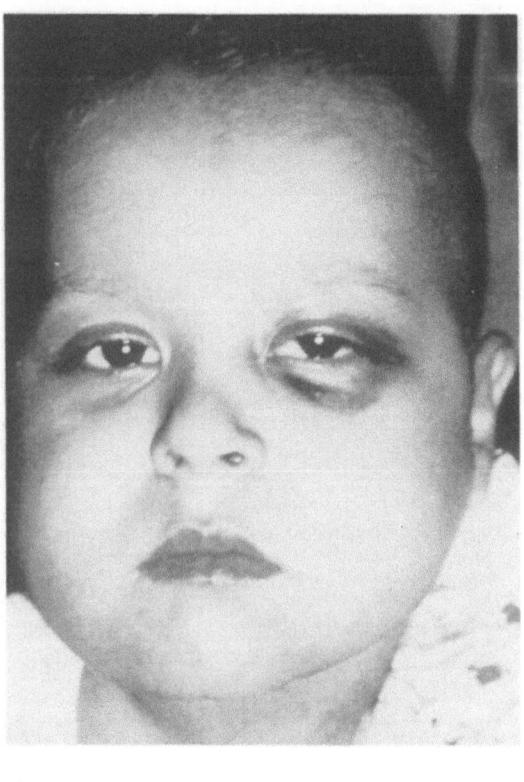

B

Fig. 4-17. (*A*) 10-month-old child with metastatic neuroblastoma with bilateral orbital involvement. Note infiltration of left temporal fossa. (*B*) Older child with similar presentations.

Rare Spindle Cell Tumors

There are a number of unusual spindle cell tumors that may occur in both children and adults. These tumors often occur after radiation for retinoblastoma and rhabdomyosarcoma. Leiomyosarcoma has not been reported in children. This occurred in two patients 23 and 28 years after radiation for retinoblastoma.[41–44] The clinicopathologic features of these tumors are discussed in Chapter 3. These include fibrosarcoma, fibrous histiocytoma, leiomyosarcoma, malignant chondrosarcoma, malignant schwannoma, malignant neurofibroma, hemangiopericytoma, meningeal sarcoma, and undifferentiated sarcoma.[45]

CT SCAN AND DIFFERENTIAL DIAGNOSIS

The differentiating clinical features above combined with the orbital CT scan often lead to a definitive diagnosis. Prior to any biopsy, orbital CT scan is imperative. Orbital exploration of a meningocele or encephalocele may result in meningitis, cerebral abscess, and death. We advocate orbital CT scan before surgical removal of a superonasal "dermoid cyst" because of the possibility of a meningocele. In cases of presumed rhabdomyo-

sarcoma, a preoperative CT scan will allow the oncologist and radiotherapist to properly evaluate the size and location of the lesion before surgery results in iatrogenic changes in the CT presentation. Immediate biopsy must be performed in patients in whom rhabdomyosarcoma is suspected.

Each of the subcategories listed in Table 4-1 will now be outlined.

EOM Involvement

Thyroid ophthalmopathy and pseudotumor have been discussed in Chapter 2. Pseudotumor typically causes an irregular thickening of the entire muscle and its tendon, while thyroid ophthalmopathy causes a fusiform thickening of the muscle that spares the tendon.

In children, pseudotumor often presents as a myositis with enlargement of a single EOM. At times, the process may present in the anterior orbit or as a diffuse swelling. The posterior sclera and the optic nerve may enhance.

Optic Nerve Tumors

These tumors have been discussed in Chapter 3 and include meningioma, glioma, hemangioblastoma, juvenile xanthogranuloma (JXG), metastatic disease, and melanocytoma.

Nonneoplastic enlargements of the optic nerve may be due to pseudotumor, sarcoid, traumatic hematoma of the nerve sheath, and optic nerve drusen. Calcifications may be evident in the latter condition.

Intraconal Tumors

See Chapter 3.

Focal (Cystic) Tumors with Bone Involvement

Several tumors are cystic and cause focal bone changes. Epidermal inclusions cysts do not usually extend to the bone and are continuous with the epidermis. Dermoid cysts tend to arise in the superotemporal or superonasal quadrant and cause adjacent erosion of bone or fossa formation, that is, a regular smooth excavation of the underlying bone. Mengingocele or encephalocele will show a bone defect in the superonasal roof of the orbit with herniation of meninges or brain tissue. Mucoceles are rare in children. As in adults, an eggshell-like expansion of the involved sinus wall will occur due to blockage of the sinus ostium (Fig. 4-18). An underlying tumor obstructing the sinus drainage should always be ruled out.

Focal Intraconal or Extraconal Noncystic Tumors

Alveolar soft-part sarcoma tends to be localized rather than diffuse and may involve the EOMs. Secondary bone involvement does not always occur (Fig. 4-19). In addition, the orbit may be secondarily invaded when the tumor originates in the nose or paranasal sinus. Primary involvement of bone alone is very rare.

Diffuse (Cystic) Tumors without Bone Involvement

Micropthalmos with cyst is a distinct entity on CT scan. A pseudopodic extension of a micropthalmic eye should be evident on serial axial and coronal views (Fig. 4-20). Calcifications may be present.

We have not observed a CT scan of congenital cystic eyeball. Single or multiloculations might be present. The EOM insertions are variably present on the wall of the cyst.

Lymphangiomas are diffuse tumors in that they are unencapsulated and usually extend both inside and outside the muscle cone. Cystic spaces are present and may

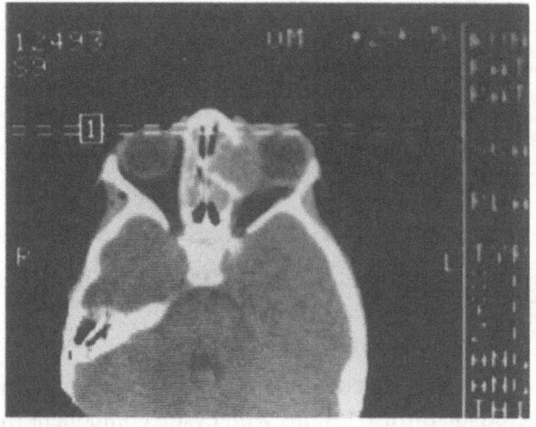

Fig. 4-18. 10-year-old female with 6-month history of lateral and upward displacement of left globe that worsens when child has an upper respiratory infection. CT scan shows mucocele of ethmoid sinus.

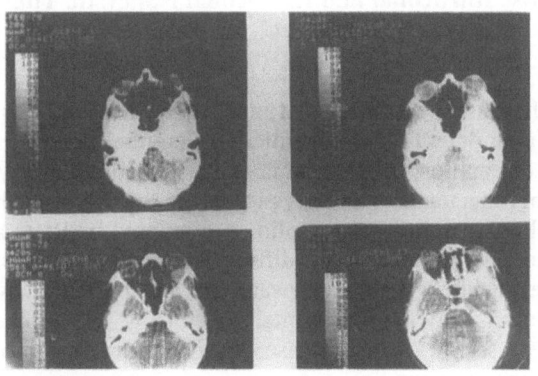

Fig. 4-19. CT scan of patient in Figure 4-13 showing tumor infiltrating lateral rectus muscle. There is no adjacent bone erosion.

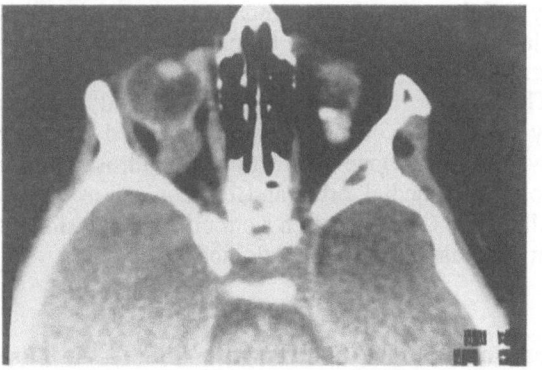

Fig. 4-20. CT scan of child with bilateral microphthalmos with cyst. Bilaterally, the cyst is smaller than the micropthalmic eye (Courtesy of Dr. Rudolph Wagner, Newark, NJ).

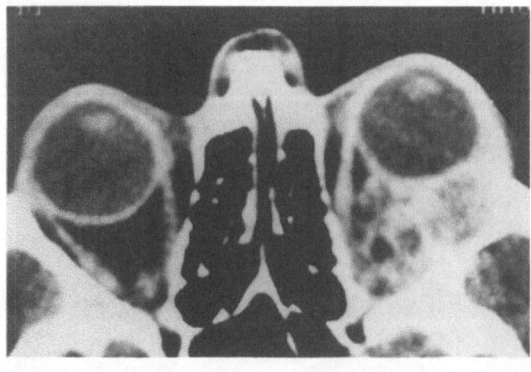

Fig. 4-21. CT scan of adult with lymphangioma shows characteristic diffuse lesions with cystic component from an adult with the tumor.

be enlarged due to hemorrhage. Bone erosion does not occur (Fig. 4-21).

Diffuse Intraconal and Extraconal Noncystic Tumors without Bone Involvement

The possible entities that tend to be diffuse are listed in Table 4-1. The main clinical differential diagnosis is that of capillary hemangioma and lymphangioma. Lymphangioma tends to have cystic spaces on CT scan, while capillary hemangioma is solid. A lymphoid infiltrate and leukemia all tend to be diffuse and spare the orbital bones, while granulocytic sarcoma and rhabdomyosarcoma may involve the orbital bones (Fig. 4-22). In the largest series, 6 of 33 cases of granulocytic sarcoma had bone erosion.

Diffuse Noncystic Tumors with Bone Involvement

Both metastatic neuroblastoma and Ewing's sarcoma may be bilateral and cause focal osteolytic lesions. Neuroblastoma has a tendency to metastasize to the zygoma (Fig. 4-23).

There are a number of rare spindle cell tumors that may cause either diffuse or rather localized disease with or without focal bone destruction. Chondrosarcoma may involve the medial orbit and ethmoid sinus in young adults.[45] On CT scan, often a circumscribed lesion rather than a diffuse lesion with calcification is noted.

Sinus and/or Bone Involvement—Soft Tissue Tumors

Melanotic ectodermal tumor in infancy commonly involves the maxillary sinus or zygoma and the orbit secondarily.

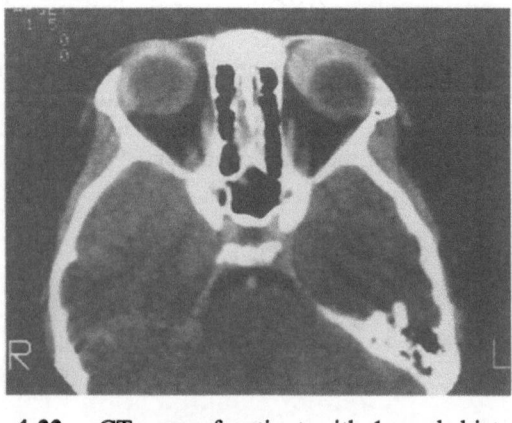

Fig. 4-22. CT scan of patient with 1-week history of enlarging superonasal mass of the left orbit. Biopsy showed undifferentiated rhabdomyosarcoma.

Esthesioneuroblastoma originates from the olfactory groove and extends from the nose or sinuses into the orbit.

Teratomas are congenital large multicystic masses that may fill the orbit and surround the eye; the tumor generally does not extend into the brain. Bone erosion and maxillary sinus involvement have been reported.

Histiocytosis X includes unifocal or multifocal eosinophilic granuloma. Eosinophilic granuloma may cause osteolytic lesions in the skull and orbital bones and tends to involve the superotemporal quadrant.

Angiofibroma, a rare vascular tumor of the oropharynx of adolescent males, locally erodes into the orbit, sinus, and base of the skull (see Chapter 3).

Intraocular Tumors with Orbital Spread

Retinoblastoma and medulloepithelioma are tumors of children, while malignant melanoma of the choroid

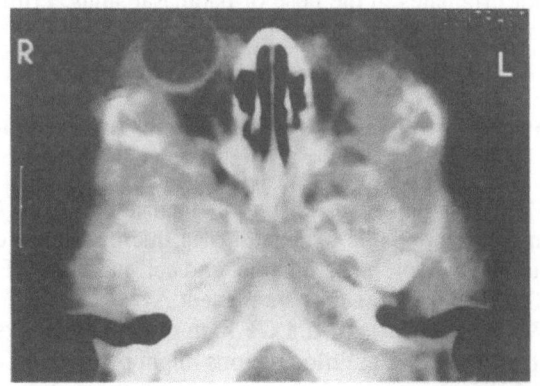

Fig. 4-23. CT scan from 10-month-old child with metastatic neuroblastoma. Note diffuse bilateral orbital involvement with bone destruction particularly involving lateral orbital wall.

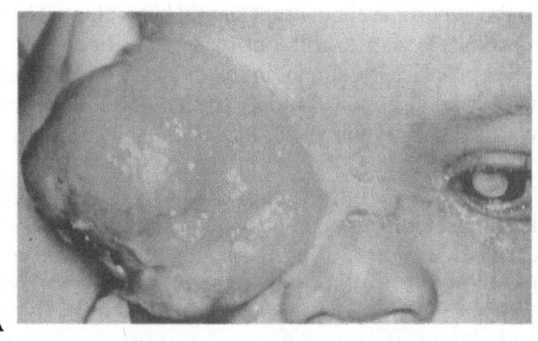

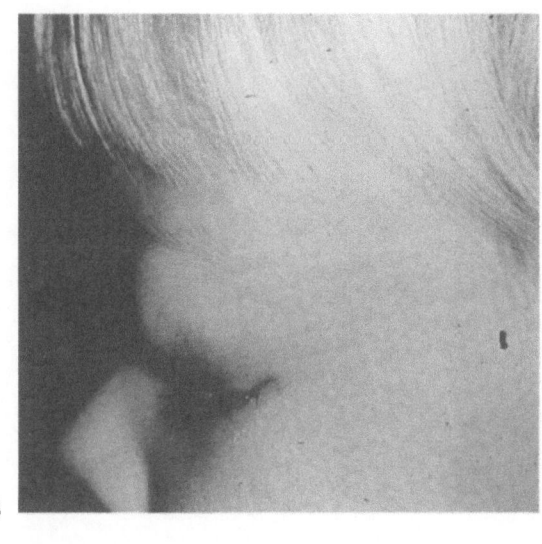

Fig. 4-24. (*A*) African child with advanced retinoblastoma with orbital extension (AFIP ACC #1036900). (*B*) Child with retinoblastoma extending into upper lid and orbit (AFIP ACC #1493394).

is basically a tumor of adults (Fig. 4-24). All three have been discussed in Chapter 3. Because intraocular tumors that spread into the orbit are of such a significant size, there is often accompanying tumor necrosis that may mimic an inflammatory process.

Calcifications typical of retinoblastoma may be seen on the CT scan in approximately 80 percent of the cases. Small tumors are often devoid of calcifications on CT scan.[46] Calcium complexes with denatured DNA from necrotic tumor cells. Such calcifications are present histologically in 95 percent of cases (Fig. 4-25).

We have seen a case of melanoma with intraocular calcifications due to a calcified dislocated lens (see Chapter 3). Tumors in the ciliary body might suggest medulloepithelioma or melanoma.

BIOPSY RESULTS AND MANAGEMENT

Many of the conditions have been discussed in other chapters. The discussion here will be limited to those not considered elsewhere.

EOM Involvement

See Chapter 2.

Optic Nerve Tumors

See Chapter 3.

Intraconal Tumors

See Chapter 3.

Focal Cystic Tumors with Local Bone Changes

Dermoid Cyst. Excisional biopsy shows a cystic mass containing keratin and lined by keratinizing stratified squamous epithelium and pilosebaceous units. Treatment requires complete surgical excision. The diagnosis is usually apparent on clinical examination. As with an epidermoid cyst, should rupture occur during excision, copious irrigation with balanced salt is sufficient to prevent a postoperative inflammatory course.

Other tumors that may be pathologically confused with dermoid cysts include orbital dermoid cyst of conjunctival origin, conjunctival cysts, dacryops (lacrimal gland duct cyst), and choristomatous cysts (Fig. 4-26). The dermoid

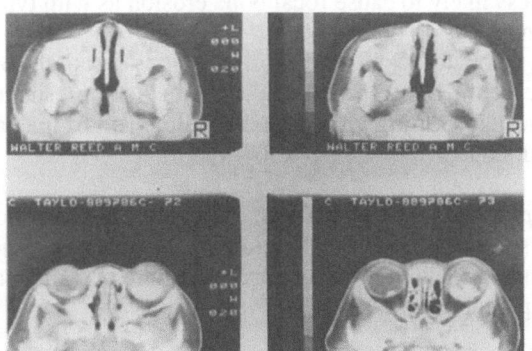

Fig. 4-25. Intraocular calcifications in child with bilateral retinoblastoma without orbital extension.

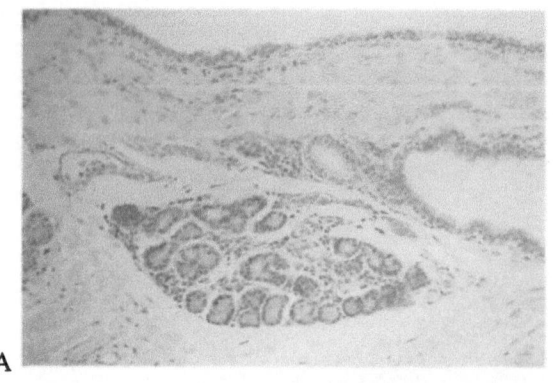

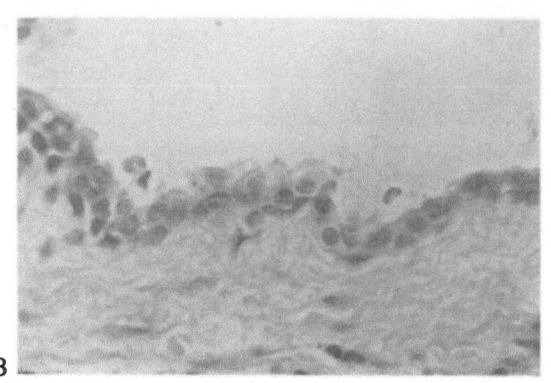

Fig. 4-26. (A) Lacrimal duct cyst with adjacent lacrimal tissue. (B) Cyst is lined by two layers of cuboidal epithelium (AFIP ACC #1972416).

cyst of conjunctival origin is a dermoid cyst lined by nonkeratinizing epithelium containing goblet cells like normal conjunctiva. Dermal adnexal structures are present in the walls and hair in the lumina.[47] Caruncular tissue, like all primitive conjunctiva, has the potential to differentiate toward sebaceous glands and hair follicles. This potential explains the origin of such cysts.

Conjunctival cysts are nonkeratinizing stratified squamous epithelium with goblet cells that presumably result from the sequestration of conjunctival tissue. In general, dermoid cysts of conjunctival origin and conjunctival cysts tend to be located away from bone and therefore are less likely to cause focal bone erosion as with typical dermoid cysts (Fig. 4-27).

A respiratory epithelial choristomatous cyst of the orbit is a cyst lined by respiratory epithelium that is presumably sequestered during intrauterine development of the paranasal sinuses.[47,48]

Epidermal Inclusion Cyst. Excisional biopsy shows a cystic mass lined by keratinizing stratified squamous epithelium without pilosebaceous units. Treatment is complete surgical excision.

Meningocele and Encephalocele. These anomalies should be clinically suspected and require the intervention of a neurosurgeon. Suspicious ''dermoid cysts'' located

in the superonasal quadrant should be evaluated by preoperative CT scan to rule out these conditions.

Appropriate treatment involves a combined orbitotomy with a craniotomy to repair any anatomic defects in the walls. Despite a bony defect, dura may remain intact.

Mucocele. Intraoperatively as soon as the epithelial lining is violated, copious mucus secretions should be evident. The entire lining should be removed and sent for biopsy to rule out an underlying tumor. Treatment consists of surgical extirpation of the involved sinus lining with establishment of drainage into the nose and/or obliteration of the sinus. ENT surgical collaboration is optimal.

Focal Noncystic Tumors with Local Bone Changes

Alveolar Soft-Part Sarcoma. Biopsy shows sheets of uniform cells arranged in a pseudoalveolar organoid pattern composed of nests of cells separated by thin fibrous septae containing delicate capillaries. The tumor cells are large and round to polyhedral with finely granular eosinophilic cytoplasm and distinct cell boundaries. The nests of cells are outlined by reticulin stain (Fig. 4-28). Occasional mitoses are present as well as scattered foci of hemorrhage or necrosis. PAS-positive diastase-resistant crystalline intracytoplasmic structures that may be rectangular, rhomboid, or needle-like in configuration are diagnostic. On electron microscopy (EM), the crystals have a periodicity of 8–10 nm. The tumor may be confused with renal cell carcinoma and vascular tumors such as angiosarcoma or hemangiopericytoma.[22]

Management includes complete surgical excision. Metastases to brain and lungs may occur years later. In the Zimmerman series, two patients died of metastatic disease. In one case, a patient died of lung metastases 21 years after orbital surgery, while one patient died of brain metastases 14 years after orbital exenteration and radiation. Local excision of pulmonary metastases

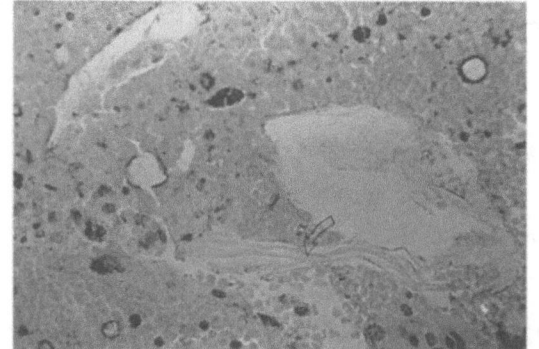

Fig. 4-27. Ruptured dermoid cyst with hemorrhage and giant cell reaction to keratin (AFIP ACC #1370892).

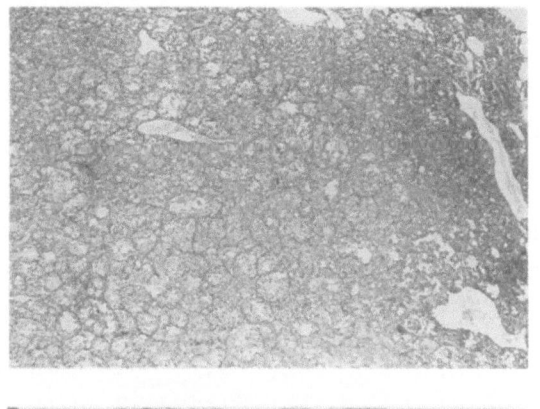

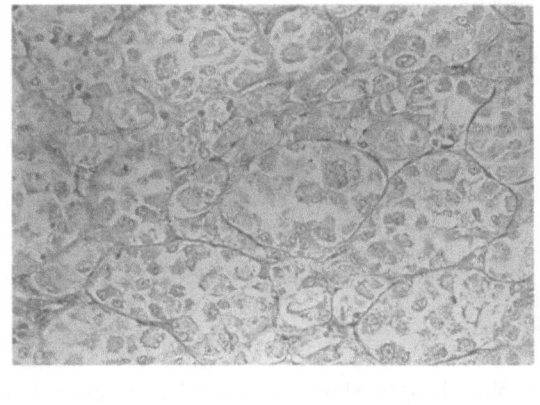

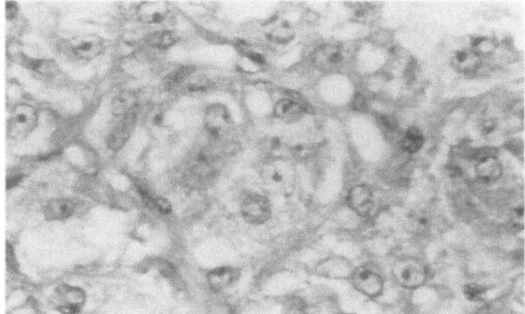

Fig. 4-28. (A) Tumor is composed of compartment of cells in a pseudoalveolar pattern. (B,C) The cells are large with finely granular eosinophilic cytoplasm and bland nuclei with nucleolus.

may prove effective. Radiation may be helpful after excision but there is no definite proof of its effectiveness.

Diffuse Cystic Tumors without Bone Involvement

Microphthalmos with Cyst. This is invariably a clinical diagnosis and does not require biopsy. Management depends on the clinical presentation.

Microphthalmos with cyst may be managed with a scleral lens; if clinical presentation warrants, combined excision of the cyst and enucleation may be followed by careful monitoring by an ocularist (Fig. 4-29). The fitting of progressively larger prostheses ensures orbital growth. The fitting of a prosthesis or scleral shell with or without surgery is mandatory to allow for growth of the involved orbit.[2]

Rarely, progressive proptosis may occur later in life due to massive gliosis within the micropthalmic eye; chronic inflammation possibly secondary to hemorrhage may also occur.

Congenital Cystic Eyeball. Again, as with micropthalmos with cyst, biopsy is not necessary. A congenital cystic eyeball usually requires enucleation and fitting with prostheses of consecutively larger sizes as the child develops. If the eye is small, conformers of increasing size may be placed to allow for orbital growth. In some cases, a cosmetic scleral lens may be fitted.[11,12]

Lymphangioma. Biopsy shows an unencapsulated tumor composed of endothelial-lined spaces separated by thin collagenous septae (Fig. 4-30). The spaces contain pink eosinophilic material that probably represents lymph fluid. Lymphoid follicles may be present. In general, unless there is occlusive or refractive amblyopia, lymphangiomas are best left untreated. Local steroidal injection has not been proven to benefit the condition. Theoretically, the lymphoid element would respond to steroids, but many of these tumors consist of endothelial-lined spaces that do not respond to injection.[8]

Surgical treatment when necessary appears to be the treatment of choice, although the alternative is less than

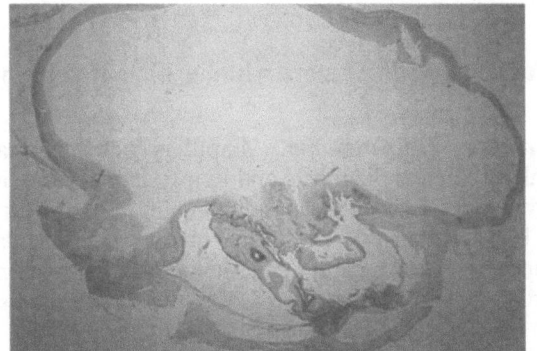

Fig. 4-29. Large cyst adjacent to microphthalmic eye is lined by glial elements (AFIP ACC #1554943).

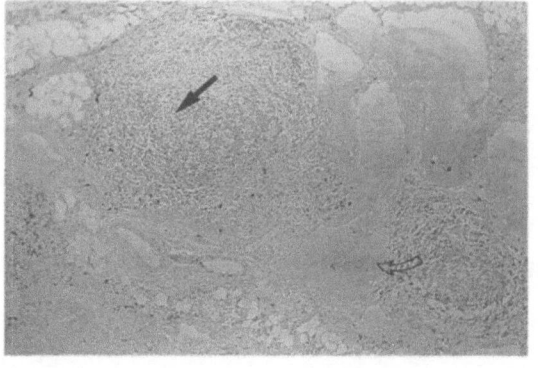

Fig. 4-30. Biopsy shows lymphoid aggregates (solid arrow) with endothelial-lined spaces (open arrow) that are filled with lymph fluid. These spaces are potential sites for hemorrhage that may occur spontaneously and form chocolate cysts or that may occur at the time of surgical excision (AFIP ACC #1493146).

satisfactory even if surgery is delayed until puberty when facial growth and concomitant tumor growth cease. since the tumor is not localized, it is difficult to resect. Surgical exploration does not generally result in profuse bleeding. The CO_2 laser is probably the treatment of choice to excise such tumors.

Teratoma. Biopsy shows a tumor that has a hyalinized fibrous connective tissue stroma and various epithelial elements that form multiple cysts. Some cysts are lined by keratinized stratified squamous epithelium. Others are lined by mucus-secreting cells resembling the epithelium of the gastrointestinal tract (Fig. 4-31). Other possible tissues include smooth muscle and cartilage. Surgical excision is the treatment of choice.[18] Rarely, structures resembling the choroid plexus of brain lined by ependymal cells, pancreas, parathyroid, liver, and mammary and lacrimal glands may also be present. Ovarian, testicular, or renal tissue has not been found in orbital teratomas, yet these tissues have been present in nonorbital teratomas. The eyeball should be retained if possible.

Diffuse Noncystic Tumors without Bone Involvement

Capillary Hemangioma. Capillary hemangioma is usually a clinical diagnosis and biopsy is not necessary. A strawberry-colored mass is evident on the skin surface or a bluish mass in the orbit. The tumor is histologically composed of many plump endothelial cells with varying degrees of fibrosis that increase as the tumor regresses with age (Fig. 4-32).

When the mass is too deep in the orbit to observe its color, the growth pattern will suggest the diagnosis. Capillary hemangiomas generally grow during the first

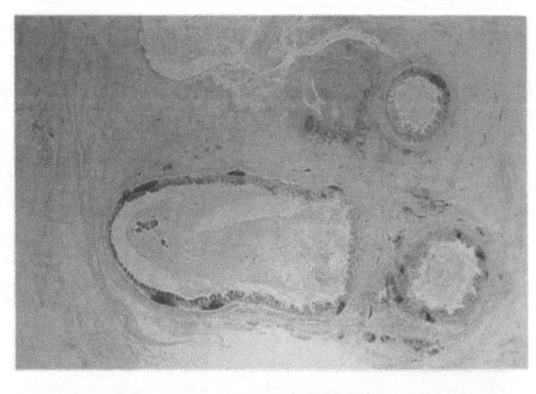

A

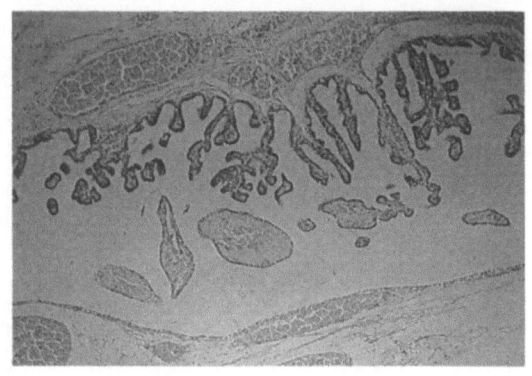

B

Fig. 4-31. (*A*) Teratoma in orbit with (*B*) choroid plexus (AFIP ACC #221088).

6 months of life and gradually regress over the next 5 years. In addition, Valsalva's maneuvers such as crying and dependent head position will cause enlargement that does not occur with lymphangiomas.[5]

Capillary hemangiomas are best not treated unless they cause occlusive amblyopia due to severe ptosis as evidenced by head position or refractive amblyopia. In one series, 46 percent of patients with capillary hemangiomas of the lid and orbit had asymmetric refractive error.[49]

When treatment is indicated, local injection of steroids

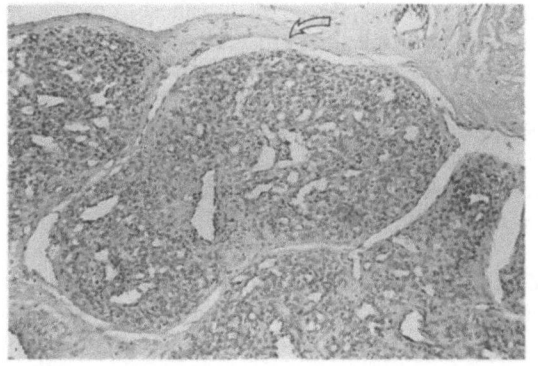

Fig. 4-32. Capillary hemangioma composed of endothelial cells that form an almost solid tumor mass. Note area of fibrosis (arrow).

is the treatment of choice. Injection into the lid component is well accepted, while intraorbital injection is somewhat controversial. The patients should be monitored by their pediatricians for systemic complications of steroids and for growth and development. A preparation of 3–4 cc Betamethasone sodium phosphate/betamethasone acetate (Celestone Soluspan, 6 mg/cc), which is rapid-acting, and 1–2 cc triamcinolone acetonide, (Kenalog 40 mg/cc), which has a prolonged action, is injected into the lesion under general anesthesia.[50] Systemic steroids are equally effective in treating infantile hemangiomas but growth delay and cushingoid features may result. Central retinal artery occlusion has been reported with periocular intralesional corticosteroid injections.[51] For this reason, 0.1 cc steroid alloquots injected slowly through a 30-gauge needle with avoidance of firm digital pressure on the lesion have been recommended. We dilate the pupils and evaluate the fundus at the time of injection for possible embolization of the retinal circulation.

Tumors that do not regress spontaneously or that do not respond to local steroidal injection may be treated with the CO_2, argon, or contact YAG laser. Surgical excision with a scalpel may result in significant hemorrhage and secondary postoperative scarring and a poor cosmetic result. Small localized lesions may be excised surgically.

Diffuse Noncystic Tumors without Bone Involvement

A diffuse infiltrate that molds about the orbital structures on CT scan in a child warrants biopsy. The differential diagnosis includes (1) lymphoma, which is rare in children except for Burkitt's lymphoma, which is very unusual in the United States, and Hodgkin's disease, which rarely affects the orbit; (2) leukemia; (3) granulocytic sarcoma; (4) rhabdomyosarcoma; (5) pseudotumor; (6) capillary hemangioma; (8) sinus histiocytosis; and (7) orbital hemorrhage due to any cause.

Biopsy shows a montonous population of immature lymphoid cells suggestive of malignant lymphoma. Systemic work-up for lymphoma by a pediatric oncologist is appropriate. A pathologist should be queried as to the possibility of granulocytic sarcoma.

Biopsy shows relatively uniform undifferentiated cells with scanty-to-moderately abundant eosiniophilic cytoplasm and round-to-reniform nuclei. Eosinophilic-type cells suggest the diagnosis of inflammatory pseudotumor, eosinophilic granuloma, and Hodgkin's disease.

Special stains for esterase show that the eosinophilic cells are of the granulocytic series and represent predominantly eosinophilic myelocytes or metamyelocytes (Fig. 4-33). Granules in the neutrophils and mast cells will also stain for esterase.[26,27] The diagnosis of granulocytic sarcoma is dependent on seeing the granules in the immature cells, not in the mature polyps. A negative stain for esterase is meaningless if the tissue has not been

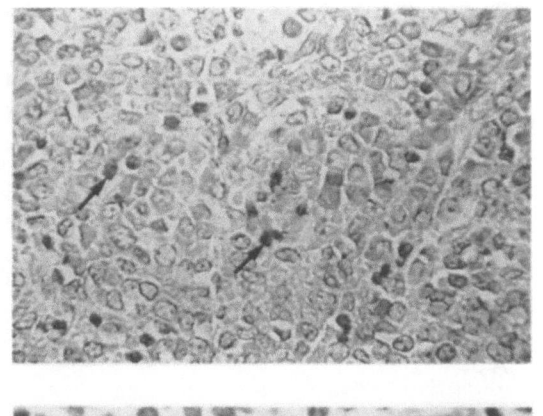

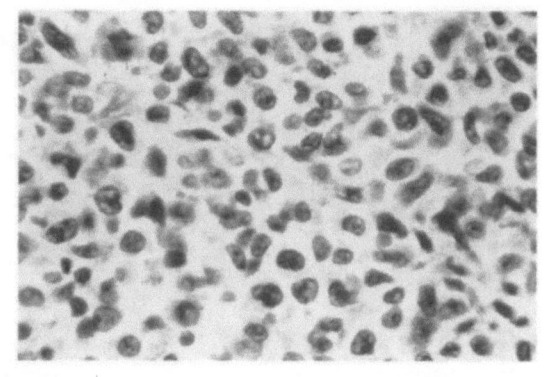

Fig. 4-33. (*A*) Biopsy shows uniform undifferentiated cells that (*B*) contain esterase granules consistent with granulocytic sarcoma.

adequately fixed in formalin and fresh tissue has not been properly stained.

Ancillary hematologic work-up including abdominal CT scan and bone marrow studies are indicated. Unfortunately, granulocytic sarcoma is almost uniformly fatal.

Rhabdomyosarcoma. Biopsy shows long, slender spindle cells with hyperchromatic nuclei and extensions of strongly acidophilic cytoplasm. Many small round cells with scanty cytoplasm and hyperchromatic nuclei also are present.

Histologic Variants. In the most common form, the embryonal form, the predominant cell is undifferentiated, small, and round, as described above (Fig. 4-34). There are some large cells with eosinophilic cytoplasm present. In the differentiated form, cells with acidophilic cytoplasm (rhabdomyoblasts) are present. The rhabdomyoblasts may have several different configurations. They may have a central nucleus with a thinly tapered, eosinophilic, cytoplasmic bipolar process. A racquet-shaped cell or tadpole cell has a nucleus located at one end. In a strap cell, two or more nuclei are arranged in tandem. Many longitudinal cross-striations may be present in the eosinophilic cytoplasm. The botryoid or submucosal form is a variation of the embryonal form in which there are

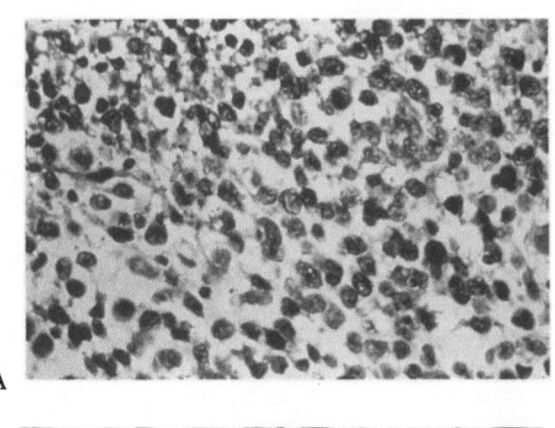

A

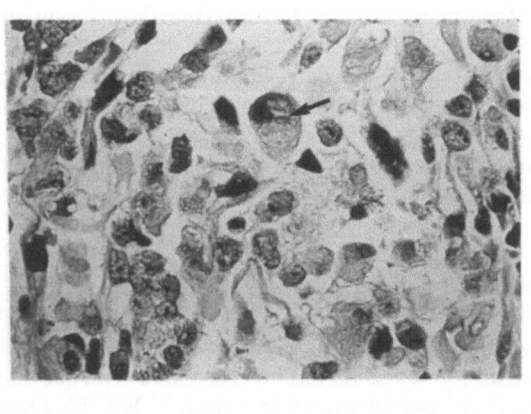

B

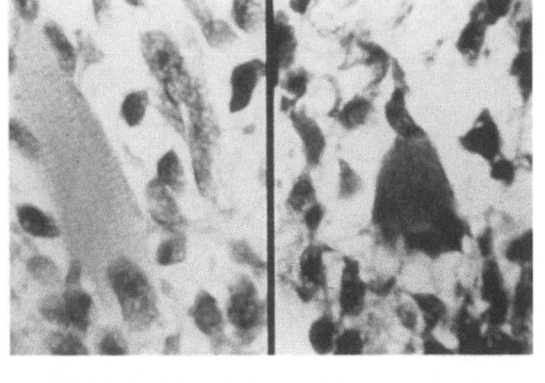

C

Fig. 4-34. (*A*) Low-power magnification shows diffuse sheets of cells. High-power magnification shows monotonous collection of small cells with bland hyperchromatic undifferentiated nuclei and scanty cytoplasm (AFIP ACC #808189). (*B*) Occasional cells with eosinophilic cytoplasm, rhabdomyoblasts, (arrow) are seen. (*C*) Among cells with eosinophilic cytoplasm, cross-striations may be found in rare differentiated tumors. PTAH stain shows cross-striations (AFIP ACC #71658).

polypoid grape-like clusters of tumors that have a subconjunctival or lid presentation (Fig. 4-35). In the alveolar form, connective tissue-vascularized trabeculae divide the tumor cells into "alveolar" clusters (Fig. 4-36). In each alveolus the cells are free-floating, while the peripheral cells line the alveolus. In general, the worst prognosis is associated with the alveolar form and the best prognosis with the differentiated form.

In the case of the poorly differentiated tumors, immunohistologic reactivity for desmin, myosin, and myoglobin may help confirm the diagnosis of rhabdomyosarcoma.[52]

Pathologically and clinically, rhabdomyoscarcoma and endodermal sinus tumor (yolk sac tumor) of the orbit may also be confused. Only five endodermal sinus tumors of the orbit have been reported. These occurred in patients ranging in age from 3 months to 4 years. Sudden proptosis develops and early metastasis may occur.

In all rhabdomyosarcomas, a work-up for lung and bone marrow metastases is appropriate before instituting therapy. Like most sarcomas, rhabdomyosarcomas spread hematogenously. Local lymph node spread is rare except with the most aggressive alveolar type. Prognosis is significantly worsened if sinus extension is present. Recurrences generally develop within 6 to 9 months. Radiotherapy often leads to long-term radiation complications to the eyeball including keratopathy, cataract, retinopathy, and optic neuropathy as well as a hypoplastic orbit. Secondary radiation-induced tumors have been reported in two cases: a lid melanoma and malignant fibrous

histiocytoma of the orbit. Exenteration is rarely necessary except for tumors unresponsive to radiation and chemotherapy.

Rare Spindle Cell Tumors. There are a number of unusual spindle cell tumors that may occur in children and adults whose pathology will not be discussed. These tumors occur in patients who have had hereditary retinoblastoma as children.

The spindle cell tumors in children include fibrosarcoma, fibrous histiocytoma, leiomyosarcoma, malignant chondrosarcoma, malignant schwannoma, malignant

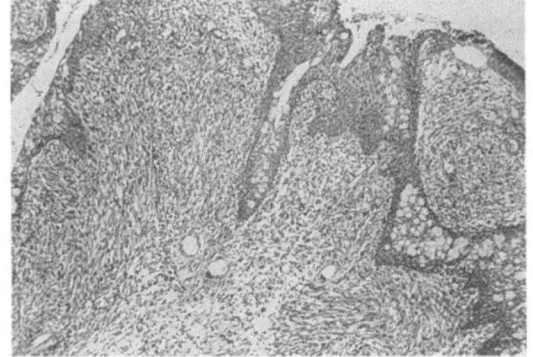

Fig. 4-35. Botryoid variant of rhabdomyosarcoma shows spindle cells in the subepithelial conjunctiva. Note numerous goblet cells.

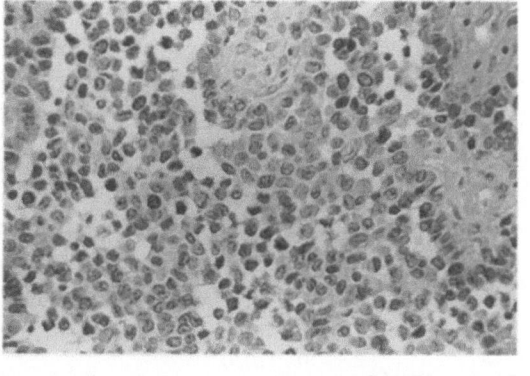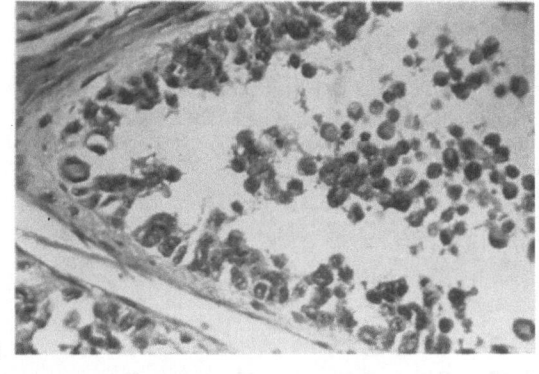

A   B

Fig. 4-36. (*A*) In alveolar form of rhabdomyosarcoma (AFIP ACC #1195919), connective tissue trabeculae create spaces that contain central free-floating tumor cells (*B*) with peripheral tumor cells adherent to the septae (AFIP ACC #983287).

neurofibroma, hemangiopericytoma, meningeal sarcoma, and undifferentiated sarcoma. Fibrosarcoma may occur as a congenital tumor, but is extremely rare at any age. All these tumors are quite rare, and scattered case reports appear in the literature. While leiomyosarcoma has not been reported in children, leiomyoma, hemangiopericytoma, malignant schwannoma, and neurofibroma have been reported. These may involve bone.

In general, all such tumors require incisional biopsy, followed by complete surgical extirpation that in some cases warrants exenteration. Radiation therapy consultation should be obtained.

Sinus Histiocytosis. Biopsy of sinus histiocytosis shows sheets of pale-staining histiocytes with vesicular nuclei and large cytoplasm that contain red blood cells or plasma cells, erythro- or lymphophagocytosis. Mature lymphocytes are also present. Follicles may be present. The disease is usually self-limited since there is no visceral involvement; radiation and chemotherapy are, therefore, generally not indicated.

Endodermal Sinus Tumor. The endodermal sinus tumor is a malignant germ-cell neoplasm of the ovary and testis that arises in extragonadal locations. Pathologically, endodermal sinus tumors are composed of a meshwork of spaces lined by flat-to-cuboidal epithelium that exhibits anaplasia and mitoses. Necrosis and hemorrhage are frequently present. In all five orbital cases, immunoperoxidase reaction for alpha fetoprotein was positive.[53]

Diffuse Noncystic Tumors with Sinus and Bone Involvement

Tumors of bone that involve the orbit secondarily are discussed in Chapter 3.

Granulocytic sarcoma and rhabdomyosarcoma are usually diffuse tumors that tend to involve the bone less

than metastatic neuroblastoma and Ewing's sarcoma. Alveolar soft-part sarcoma tends to be more localized than the above tumors but often involves the adjacent bone.[22]

Metastatic Neuroblastoma. Biopsy shows sheets of uniform small, round, undifferentiated cells with massive areas of necrosis. At the margin of the tumor, the cells grow in clusters. Neurofibrillary tangles (Homer-Wright rosettes) are rarely present (Fig. 4-37). EM may show neurotubules and dense core granules.[32]

Management consists of pediatric oncology consultation for orbital radiation and chemotherapy.

Metastatic Ewing's Sarcoma. Biopsy shows a uniform population of cells two to three times the size of lymphoma arranged in dense sheets or cords. The scanty cytoplasm may contain PAS-positive diastase-sensitive glycogen.

Treatment of Ewing's sarcoma is difficult because the primary tumor of the limb often produces early widespread disseminated emboli.[39] The primary intramedullary tumor often spreads to other bones and to the lungs. The eye itself is not involved. Treatment requires consultations from a pediatric oncologist.

Angiofibroma. See Chapter 3.

Esthesioneuroblastoma. See Chapter 3.

Melanotic Ectodermal Tumors of Infancy. Biopsy shows an unencapsulated tumor with a moderately cellular vascular stroma (Fig. 4-38). The tumor is composed of two types of cells: (1) cells with hyperchromatic round or oval nuclei and scanty cytoplasm that are arranged in nests or cords, and (2) cells with abundant cytoplasm that contain melanin pigment granules resembling those of the retinal pigment epithelium.[28] Tumors rarely have malignant cytologic features. Recurrences are possible. Surgical excision is the treatment of choice.

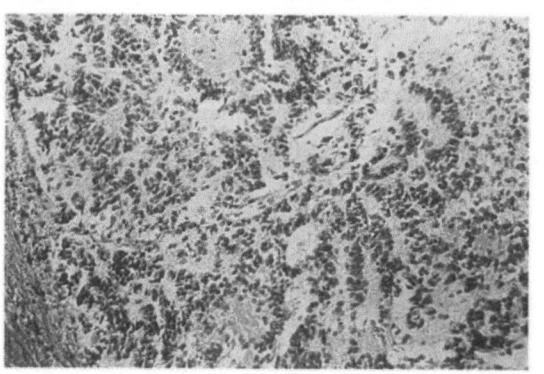

Fig. 4-37. Biopsy shows uniform small round cells with neurofibrillary tangles that are consistent with neuroblastoma.

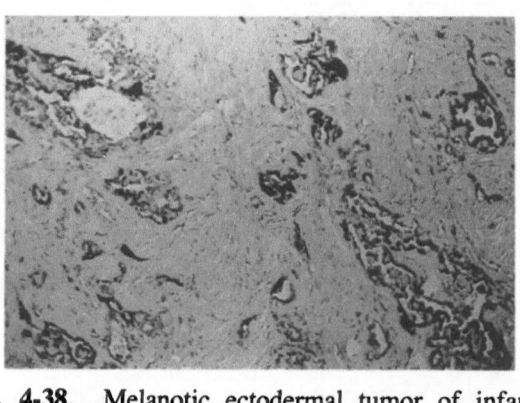

Fig. 4-38. Melanotic ectodermal tumor of infancy. Biopsy shows cells with melanin arranged in cords surrounded by a fibrous stroma.

Intraocular Tumors with Orbital Spread. See Chapter 3.

REFERENCES

1. Jakobiec FA, Nolan BT: Patient examination and introduction to orbital disease, in Duane TD, Jaeger EA (eds): *Clinical Ophthalmology*, Vol 2. Philadelphia: Harper and Row, 1982, pp 1–30.
2. Waring GL, Roth AM, Rodriguez MM: Clinicopathologic correlation of microphthalmos with cyst. *Am J Ophthalmol* 82:714, 1976.
3. Nowinski R, Shields JA, Augsburger JJ, Devenuto JJ: Exophthalmos secondary to massive intraocular gliosis in a patient with a colobomatous cyst. *Am J Ophthalmol* 97:641–643, 1984.
4. Jakobiec FA, Jones IS: Vascular tumors, malformations, and degenerations, in Duane TD, Jaeger EA (eds): *Clinical Ophthalmology*, Vol 2. Philadelphia: Harper and Row, 1982, pp 1–40.
5. Yee Rd, Hepler RS: Congenital hemangiomas of the skin with orbital and subglottic hemangiomas. *Am J Ophthalmol* 75:876, 1973.
6. Jones IS: Lymphangiomas of the ocular adnexa: An analysis of 62 cases. *Trans Am Ophthalmol Soc* 57:602, 1959.
7. Reese AB, Howard GM: Unusual manifestations of ocular lymphangioma and lymphangiectasis. *Surv Ophthalmol* 18:226, 1973.
8. Iliff WJ, Green WR: Orbital lymphangiomas. *Ophthalmology* 86:914–929, 1979.
9. Lloyd GA, Wright JE, Morgan G: Venous malformations in the orbit. *Br J Ophthalmol* 55:505–1971.
10. Wright JE: Orbital vascular anomalies. *Trans Am Acad Ophthalmol Otolaryngol* 78:606, 1974.
11. Pico G, Townsend W: Congenital and developmental anomalies of the orbit, in Duane TD, Jaeger EA (eds): *Clinical Ophthalmology*, Vol 2. Philadelphia: Harper and Row, 1982, pp 1–11.
12. Blodi FC: Developmental anomalies of the skull affecting the eye. *Arch Ophthalmol* 57:593, 1957.
13. Howard GM; Cystic tumors, in Duane TD, Jaeger EA (eds): *Clinical Ophthalmology*, Vol 2. Philadelphia: Harper and Row, 1982, pp 1–10.
14. Whitney CE, Leone CR, Kincaid MC: Proptosis with mastication: An unusual presentation of an orbital dermoid cyst. *Ophthalm Surg* 17:295–298, 1986.
15. MacDonald R, Byers JL: Dermoid tumor of the orbit simulating a neoplasm. *Am J Ophthalmol* 47:863–866, 1959.
16. Samuels B: Dermoid cysts of the orbit. *Arch Ophthalmol* 16:776–782, 1936.
17. Newman NJ, Miller NR, Green WR: Ectopic brain in the orbit. *Ophthalmology* 93:268–272, 1986.
18. Barber JC, Barber LF, Guerry D, Geeraets WJ: Congenital orbital teratoma. *Arch Ophthalmol* 91:45–48, 1974.
19. Levin ML, Leone CR, Kincaid MC: Congenital orbital teratomas. *Am J Ophthalmol* 102:476–481, 1986.
20. Georgiades P: Bilateral orbital teratoma. *Arch Ophthalmol* 5:106–108, 1956.
21. Ide CH, Davis WE, Black SP: Orbital teratoma. *Arch Ophthalmol* 96:2093–2096, 1978.
22. Font RL, Jurco SJ, Zimmerman LE: Alveolar soft-part sarcoma of the orbit: A clinicopathologic analysis of seventeen cases and review of the literature. *Human Pathol* 13:5669–5779, 1982.
23. Abrahams IW, Fenton RH, Vidone R: Alveolar soft-part sarcoma of the orbit. *Arch Ophthalmol* 79:185–188, 1968.
24. Altamirano-Dimas M, Albores-Saavedra J: Alveolar soft part sarcoma of the orbit. *Arch Ophthalmol* 74:496–499, 1966.
25. Varghese S, Nair B, Joseph TA: Orbital malignant non-chromaffin paraganglioma. Alveolar soft tissue sarcoma. *Br J Ophthalmol* 52:713–715, 1968.
26. Zimmerman LE, Font RL: Ophthalmologic manifestations of granulocytic sarcoma (myeloid sarcoma or chloroma). *Am J Ophthalmol* 80:979–990, 1975.
27. Davis JL, Parke DW, Font RL: Granulocytic sarcoma of the orbit: A clinicopathologic study. *Ophthalmology* 92:1758–1762, 1985.
28. Kincaid MC, Green WR: Ocular and orbital involvement in leukemia. *Surv Ophthalmol* 27:211–232, 1983.
29. Lamping KA, Albert DM, Lack E, et al: Melanotic neuroectodermal tumor of infancy (retinal anlage tumor). *Ophthalmology* 92:143–149, 1985.
30. Johnson RE, Scheithauer BW, Dahlin DC: Melanotic neuroectodermal tumor of infancy: A review of seven cases. *Cancer* 52:661–666, 1983.
31. Alfano JE: Ophthalmological aspects of neuroblastomatosis: A study of 53 verified cases. *Trans Am Acad Ophthalmol Otolaryngol* 72:830–848, 1968.
32. Albert DM, Rubenstein Ra, Scheie HG: Tumor metastasis to the eye. Part II. Clinical study in infants and children. *Am J Ophthalmol* 63:727–732, 1967.
33. Mortada A: Clinical characteristics of early orbital metastatic neuroblastoma. *Am J Ophthalmol* 63:1787–1793, 1967.
34. Shubert EE, Oliver GL, Jaco NT: Metastatic neuroblastoma causing bilateral blindness. *Can J Ophthalmol* 4:100–103, 1969.
35. Lopez-Ibor B, Schwartz AD: Neuroblastoma, in *Pediatric Clinics of North America*. Philadelphia: WB Saunders, 1985, 32:755–778.
36. Lingley JF, Sagerman RH, Santulli TB, Wolff JA: Neuroblastoma: Management and survival. *New Engl J Med* 227:1227–1230, 1967.
37. Diangio GJ, Evans AE, Koop CE: Special pattern of widespread neuroblastoma with favourable prognosis. *Lancet* 1:1046, 1971.
38. Carvalho L: Spontaneous regression of an untreated neuroblastoma. *Br J Ophthalmol* 57:832–835, 1973.
39. Johnson RE, Senyszyn JJ, Rabson AS, Peterson KA: Treatment of Ewing's sarcoma with local irradiation and systemic chemotherapy. Progress report. *Radiology* 95:195–197, 1970.

40. Jenkin RD, Rider WD, Sonley MJ: Ewing's sarcoma: Trial of adjuvant total-body irradiation. *Radiology* 96:151–155, 1970.

41. Leff SR, Henkind P: Rhabdomyosarcoma and late malignant melanoma of the orbit. *Ophthalmology* 90:1258–1260, 1983.

42. Font RL, Hidayat AA: Fibrous histiocytoma of the orbit: A clinicopathologic study of 150 cases. *Hum Pathol* 13:199–209, 1982.

43. Font RL, Jurco S, Brechner RJ: Postradiation leiomyosarcoma of the orbit complicating bilateral retinoblastoma. *Arch Ophthalmol* 101:1557–1561, 1983.

44. Folberg R, Cleasby G, Flanagan JC, et al: Orbital leiomyosarcoma after radiation therapy for bilateral retinoblastoma. *Arch Ophthalmol* 101:1562–1565, 1983.

45. Guccion J, Font RL, Enzinger FM, et al: Extraskeletal mesenchymal chondrosarcoma. *Arch Pathol* 95:336–340, 1976.

46. Char DH, Hedges TR, Norman D: Retinoblastoma CT diagnosis. *Ophthalmology* 91:1347–1350, 1984.

47. Shields JA, Augsburger JJ, Donoso LA: Orbital dermoid cyst of conjunctival origin. *Am J Ophthalmol* 101:726–729, 1986.

48. Newton C, Dutton JJ, Klintworth GK: A respiratory epithelial choristomatous cyst of the orbit. *Ophthalmology* 92:1754–1757, 1985.

49. Robb RM; Refractive errors associated with hemangiomas of the eyelids and orbit in infancy. *Am J Ophthalmol* 83:52–58, 1977.

50. Kushner BJ: Intralesional corticosteroid injection for infantile adnexal hemangioma. *Am J Ophthalmol* 93:496–506, 1982.

51. Shorr N, Seiff SR: Central retinal artery occlusion associated with periocular corticosteroid injection for juvenile hemangioma. *Ophthalm Surg* 17:229–231, 1986.

52. Cameron JD, Wick MR; Embryonal rhabdomyosarcoma of the conjunctiva: A clinicopathologic and immunohistochemical study. *Arch Ophthalmol* 104:1203–1204, 1986.

53. Jakobiec FA, Font FL: Orbit, in Spencer WH (ed): *Opthalmic Pathology*, Vol 3. Philadelphia: WB Saunders, 1986, p 2725.

54. Margo CE, Folberg R, Zimmerman LE, Sesterhenn IA: Endodermal sinus tumor (yolk sac tumor) of the orbit. *Ophthalmology* 90:1426–1432, 1983.

5

Surgical Approaches to the Orbit

Joseph A. Mauriello, Jr.
Joseph C. Flanagan

This chapter considers surgical approaches to orbital inflammations and tumors exclusive of lacrimal gland and lacrimal sac. Eyelid reconstruction after tumor resection is discussed in Chapter 8, "Management of Tumors and Inflammations of the Lids."

The optimal surgical approach to the orbit is dictated by the location of the tumor. The basic approaches include an (1) anterior orbitotomy that may be transconjunctival, transseptal, or transperiosteal, and in which one of the following quadrants is chosen: superonasal, superotemporal, inferonasal, and inferior; (2) lateral orbitotomy via a canthotomy of Krönlein approach; (3) medial orbitotomy via the Lynch incision and Weber-Ferguson for lesions in the apex of the orbit; and (4) neurosurgical transfrontal approach. Aside from the orbitotomy procedure, other procedures discussed in this chapter include (1) exenteration, (2) orbital surgery for surgical decompression due to thyroid opthalmopathy, including eyelid retraction and extraocular muscle (EDM) surgery, and (3) lacrimal gland surgery.[1-4]

GENERAL APPROACH TO ORBITAL SURGERY

Most orbital tumors require the skills of an orbital surgeon alone. However, tumors located in the apical orbit are best approached with the combined efforts of the neurosurgeon and opthalmologist. The neurosurgeon unroofs the orbit to allow access to the orbital apex. Paranasal sinus or oropharyngeal tumors that extend into the orbit require an incisional biopsy before definitive surgery is performed; an otolaryngologist's assistance is necessary if the tumor involves the sinus. Often an incisional biopsy through the lid or conjunctiva can be performed by the ophthalmologist. At other times, the otolaryngologist can obtain adequate tissue through the nose.

The skin incision and, therefore, the orbitotomy site is guided by the location of the tumor or inflammatory process. In addition, anatomic structures influence the exact surgical approach. Another consideration is the avoidance of a surgical tract for spread of a possible malignant tumor. For this reason, the ideal site of biopsy should be included in the resection at a later date.

WORKING SURGICAL ANATOMY

When a transperiosteal approach is utilized, an incision is made at the orbital rim; the periosteum is extremely adherent to the underlying bone adjacent to the orbital rim. The periosteum that covers the facial bones fuses with the periorbita at the arcus marginalis at the orbital rim. Once the adherent periosteum at the arcus marginalis is freed from the underlying bone, the periorbita is relatively easily lifted from the orbital bones. The anatomic features via the various approaches are outlined below.

Superonasal Quadrant

The superonasal quadrant is the most vascular quadrant because it contains the supratrochlear artery (with accompanying supratrochlear nerve) and dorsal nasal arterior (with accompanying infratrochlear nerve). The supratrochlear and dorsal arteries are above and below the trochlea, respectively (Plate 5-1). Surgery for lid retrac-

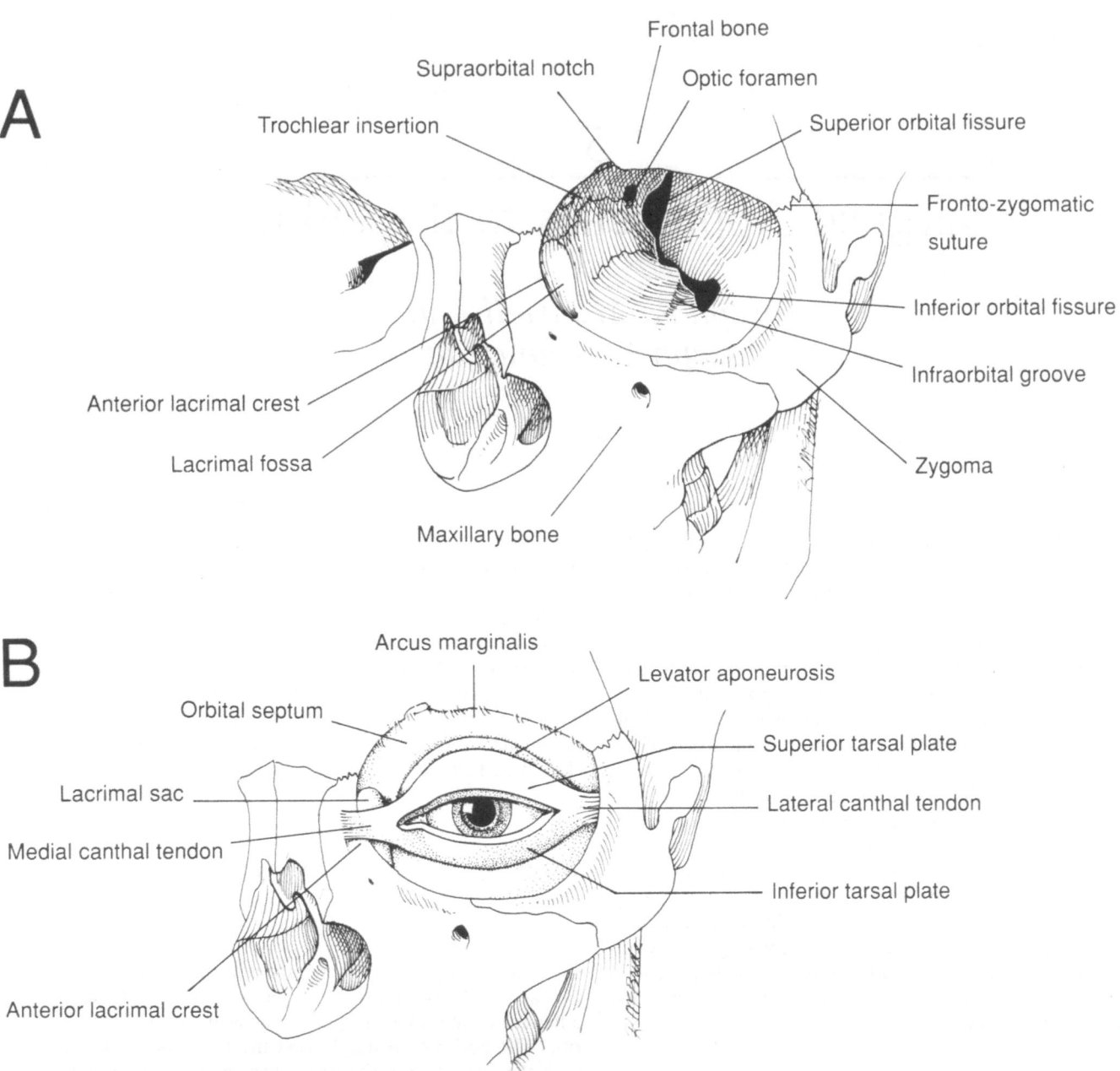

Plate 5-1. (*A*) Anatomy of orbital bones. (*B*) Soft tissue anatomy. Orbital septum inserts at the bony orbital rim as the arcus marginalis and fuses with the levator aponeurosis 6–8 mm above the superior border of the tarsal plate in the upper lid. Lateral canthal tendon inserts approximately 10 mm below the frontozygomatic suture inside the lateral orbital rim. Anterior crus of medial canthal tendon extends over lacrimal sac to insert at anterior lacrimal crest.

tion due to thyroid ophthalmopathy is also included in this chapter. The trochlea is located at the nasal aspect of the orbital roof 4 mm behind the rim. In addition, the supraorbital artery is located laterally and may perforate the orbital septum through a notch or a foramen. Inferonasally, the incision must be made medial to the lacrimal sac and canalicular system, which corresponds to the bone landmark of the anterior lacrimal crest to which the anterior crus of the medial canthal tendon inserts (Plate 5-1). The angular vein and artery course parallel to the lacrimal sac, 8 mm medial to the medial canthus, and superficially above the medial canthal tendon. If the angular vein is encountered, it should be clamped both superiorly and inferiorly since the facial and orbital vessels are valveless and blood may course in both directions. The entire lacrimal sac may be lifted out of the surgical field laterally. This maneuver requires severing the medial canthal tendon and all three of its attachments (1) just anterior to the anterior lacrimal crest and lacrimal sac at the suture of Notha, (2) superiorly on the frontal bone, and (3) posteriorly. The orbital septum and periosteum invest the lacrimal sac posteriorly where they fuse at the posterior lacrimal crest. The lacrimal sac is, therefore, located outside the orbit. A dacryocystitis is by definition a preseptal cellulitis.

The superior transverse ligament is the check or support ligament of the levator (Plate 5-2). Dissection in this area should be adjacent to bone and reattachment of the periorbita to the periosteum restores the normal relationship as long as these structures are not damaged during dissection. Superiorly, there is a thin layer of fat between the periorbita and the underlying levator and frontal nerve that branches into supraorbital and supratrochlear nerve of the ophthalmic division of the trigimenal nerve. The infratrochlear nerve is a branch of the nasociliary branch of the ophthalmic division of the trigeminal nerve.

The trochlea may need to be detached and tagged with a 4–0 silk suture. The periorbita and periosteum are resutured in order to restore the anatomy. An acquired

Brown's syndrome may occur and the patient should be made aware of this possible complication; in addition, a segmental ptosis may also occur.

The anterior ethmoidal artery is another structure that may be encountered. If this vessel is severed, massive bleeding will occur and because it is approximately 2 cm posterior to the posterior lacrimal crest, visualization and, therefore, control of its hemorrhage are difficult. Enlarging the incision superiorly and inferiorly may provide better exposure. A metal suction acting as an electrical conduit for the Bovie cautery may be helpful if the artery is partially severed. The vessel should be identified and surgical clips placed before it is cut between the previously placed clips. At times, the bipolar cautery with the long tips may be helpful. Identification of the anterior ethmoidal artery is necessary when performing ethmoidectomy for surgical decompression of the orbit. Just superior to the anterior ethmoidal foramen is the cribriform plate and brain. Inferior to the foramen is the ethmoid sinus anteriorly and sphenoid sinus posteriorly. The posterior ethmoidal foramen is a similar landmark and contains the posterior ethmoidal artery. The

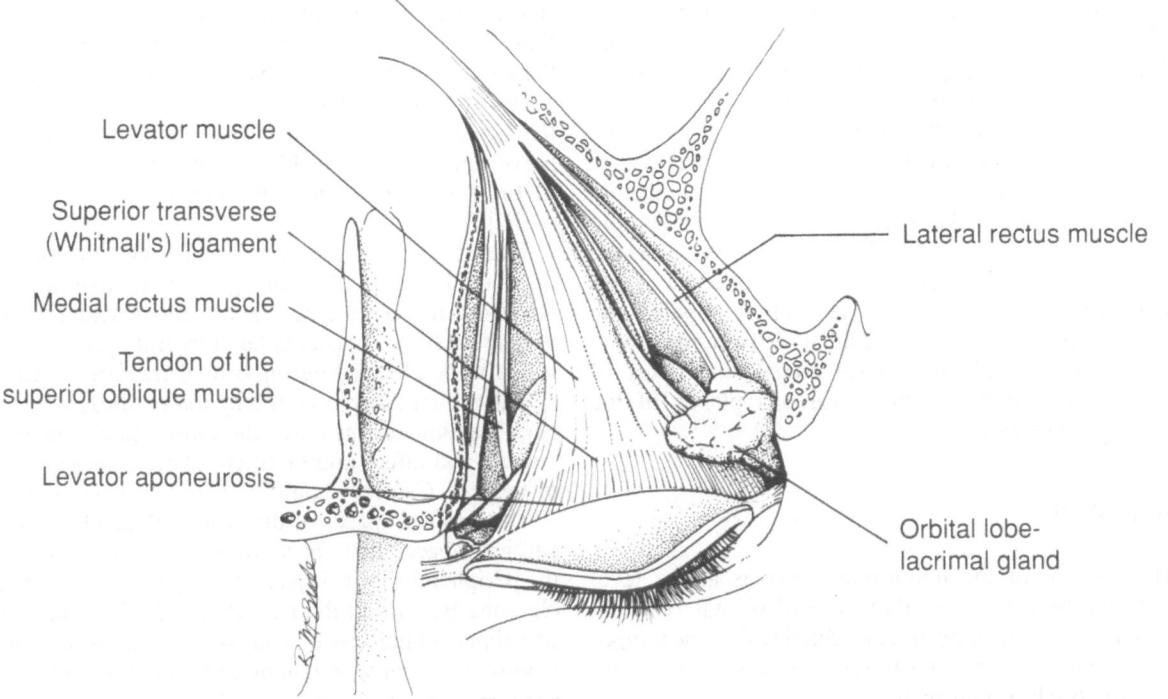

Levator muscle

Superior transverse (Whitnall's) ligament

Medial rectus muscle

Tendon of the superior oblique muscle

Levator aponeurosis

Lateral rectus muscle

Orbital lobe-lacrimal gland

Plate 5-2. Levator muscle changes from a horizontal to a vertical direction at the superior transverse (Whitnall's) ligament and forms the levator aponeurosis, which is 10–15 mm in vertical height. The lateral and medial horns of the levator are extensions of the superior transverse ligament. The lateral horn partially divides the lacrimal gland anteriorly into a superior orbital lobe and an inferior palpebral lobe, and the medial horn of the levator covers the reflected tendon of the superior oblique muscle. The lateral and medial recti are shown. The central (inner) surgical space is within the muscle cone, while the peripheral (outer) surgical space is between the external surface of the EOMs and the periorbita. The subperiosteal space is a potential space between the periorbita and the orbital bone, while episcleral or tenons space is a potential space between the sclera and tenons capsule.

bones between the foramen include, from anterior to posterior, (1) the frontal process of the maxillary bone, which contains the anterior lacrimal crest; (2) the lacrimal bone and the posterior lacrimal crest; (3) the ethmoid bone, and (4) the lesser wing of the sphenoid. Above these bones is the frontal bone with the frontal sinus medially and anteriorly and the cribriform plate and brain medially and posteriorly.

Superotemporal Quadrant

After the superonasal quadrant, this quadrant contains the second most number of structures of which the orbital surgeon needs to be aware. The lacrimal gland has fascial attachments to the frontal bone. Ignorance of these attachments may lead to prolapse of the inferior palpebral lobe of the lacrimal gland toward the limbus or prolapse of the superior orbital lobe of the lacrimal gland anteriorly toward the skin surface of the upper lid.[5] The gland extends laterally to the frontozygomatic suture and receives its blood supply from the lacrimal artery on its medial, posterior, and somewhat superior surface. In addition, a segmental ptosis may occur because the lateral fibers of the superior transverse ligament divide the lacrimal gland into its superior orbital lobe and inferior palpebral lobe. The same care utilized in the superonasal quadrant dissection with reinsertion of the periorbita to the periosteum is equally important here. If possible, the dissection should avoid the lacrimal gland and levator.

The optic foramen in the lesser wing of the sphenoid transmits the optic nerve, ophthalmic artery and sympathetic fibers from the carotid plexus. The superior orbital fissure between the greater and lesser sphenoid wings contains cranial nerves III, IV, and VI, the ophthalmic division of the fifth nerve, the ophthalmic vein, the orbital branch of the middle meningeal artery, and fibers of the ciliary ganglion and the cavernous plexus of the sympathetic system.

Lateral Wall

The equator of the nonproptotic eye is at the level of anterior aspect of the thick lateral orbital rim. On the external surface of the lateral orbital wall is the temporal fossa, which contains the temporalis muscle just posterior to the thick orbital wall.

The lateral canthal tendon inserts at the lateral orbital tubercle 10 mm inferior to the frontozygomatic suture, which is approximately 3 mm posterior to the lateral orbital rim. This structure is the attachment site for the lateral horn of the levator.

Approximately 8 mm inferiorly within the lateral rim are the zygomaticotemporal foramen, and a few millimeters below is the zygomaticofacial foramen; each of these foramen contain the respective artery and nerve. The structures enter the face through similar foramen into the temporal fossa and malar eminence, respectively.

Branches of both nerves and arteries are often disrupted while elevating the periorbita from the lateral canthal areas. Inside the orbit along the mid-aspect of the lateral wall is a branch of the zygomaticotemporal nerve, which supplies parasympathetic innervation to the lacrimal gland. The meningeal branch of the lacrimal artery may be large and pierces the greater wing of the sphenoid of the lateral orbital wall posteriorly. Excessive posterior dissection of the periorbita from the lateral wall in the areas of Hyrtl's canal in the greater wing of the sphenoid should be avoided.

The zygomatic bone extends 20 mm posterior, where it unites with the greater wing of the sphenoid. At this juncture, the lateral wall is 1 mm thick. The posterior wall of the greater wing of the sphenoid is the anterior aspect of the middle cranial fossa.

Inferior

The orbital floor is composed mainly of the maxillary bone and the tiny palatine bone posteriorly. The inferior orbital rim becomes continuous medially with the posterior lacrimal crest and the orbital septum attaches at these sites. The infraorbital nerve and artery exit onto the anterior surface of the maxillary sinus approximately 5 mm from the infraorbital rim, a thumb's width from the ala of the nose. The canal of the inferior orbital nerve and artery is visible as an elevation on the floor of the orbit. Posteriorly, the canal is a sulcus on the orbital floor.[6]

The inferior oblique muscle originates on the orbital floor just lateral to the opening of the nasolacrimal duct. An effort should be made to avoid this structure, although to date we have not encountered motility problems when it had to be elevated during orbital fracture repair.

The orbital fat is traversed by many fibrovascular septae. Traction on fat may, therefore, cause traction on vessels and affect important circulation through rupture of vessels. Cautery should be avoided if possible.

The surgical spaces of the orbit include (1) the central surgical space, that space within the muscle cone, (2) the peripheral surgical space, that space outside the muscle cone but within the periorbita, (3) the subperiosteal or subperiorbital space, and (4) the episcleral space or tenons space between tenons and underlying sclera. The subperiosteal space and episcleral space are potential spaces.

SURGICAL APPROACHES

A detailed knowledge of the anatomy is essential to any orbital exploration. The appropriate approach (Table 5-1) is dictated by the location of the tumor.

Table 5-1
Surgical Approaches to the Orbit

Anterior Orbitotomy (transconjunctival, transseptal,
transperiosteal)
    Superonasal
    Superotemporal
    Inferonasal
    Inferior
    Medial orbitotomy
Lateral Orbitotomy
    Canthoplasty
    Krönlein
    Transfrontal

Transconjunctival

A tumor that is subconjunctival or adherent to the globe and anterior to the equator is best approached transconjunctivally through the adjacent oblique quadrant (Plate 5-3).

The transconjunctival approach gives excellent access to the peripheral surgical space (outside the muscle cone but within the periorbita). It is particularly useful when an incisional biopsy is indicated for diffuse tumors such as lymphoid infiltrates. Biopsy can often be done under local or even topical anesthesia. As with extraocular

muscle (EOM) surgery, an incision is made parallel to the limbus with a Westcott scissor just behind the insertion of the EOMs. After tenons is incised with Westcott scissors, the recti are isolated in the appropriate quadrants and tagged with 4–0 silk sutures. If necessary, the tendon of the rectus muscle may be severed and later reinserted into the sclera using a double armed 5–0 chromicor vicryl suture. Retraction is aided by small malleable retractors or a Schepens retractor. This approach may be combined with a lateral orbitotomy to provide greater visualization medially for access to the optic nerve or lesions medial to the optic nerve. The approach is not advantageous when the lesion extends posteriorly toward the apex of the orbit.

Transseptal

Lid tumors that bulge through the septum anteriorly may be removed via a direct transseptal approach. The main disadvantage is that the levator aponeurosis must be identified; any large rent in the aponeurosis should be resutured. In either the upper or lower lid, such resuturing may result in lid pull down or cicatricial ectropion due to scarring of the orbital septum (Plate 5-4). For these reasons, it is best to go through the septum 8 mm above the tarsus in the upper lid where the levator and septum are separated by the preaponeurotic fat pad.

At least on a theoretic basis, the transseptal approach

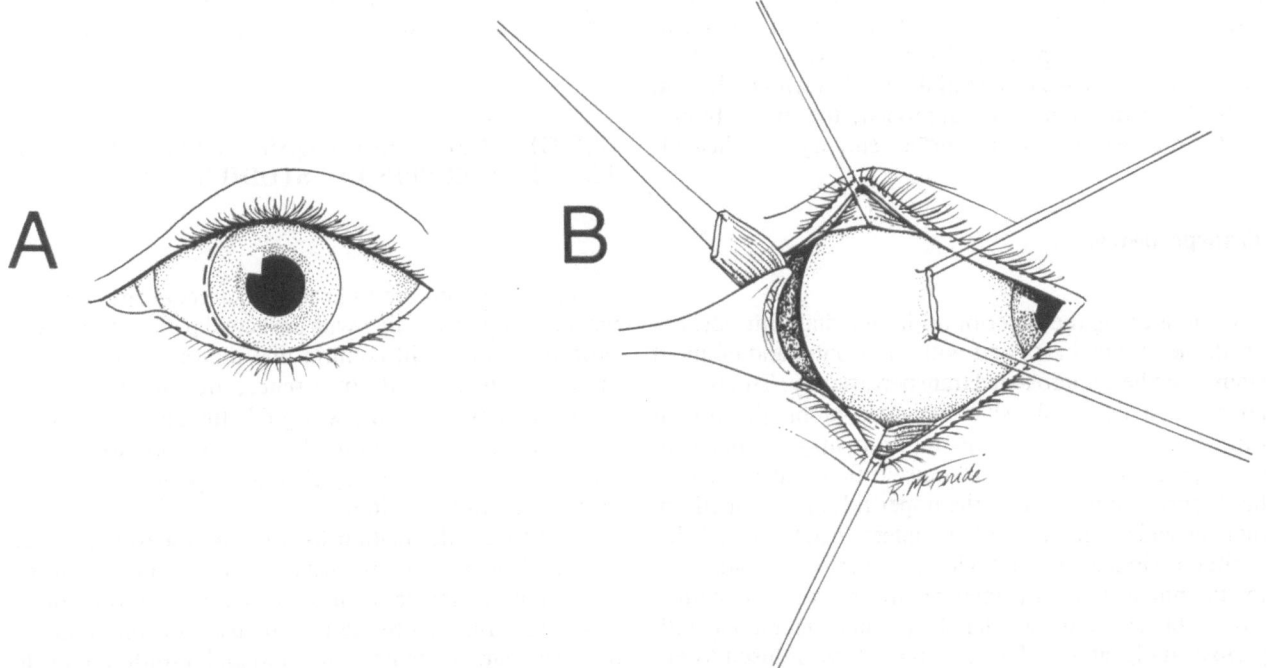

Plate 5-3. (A–B) Transconjunctival approach may be limbal or forniceal. The medial conjunctival approach provides exposure to the anterior half of the inner surgical space by disinsertion of the medial rectus muscle. A Schepens retractor assists exposure.

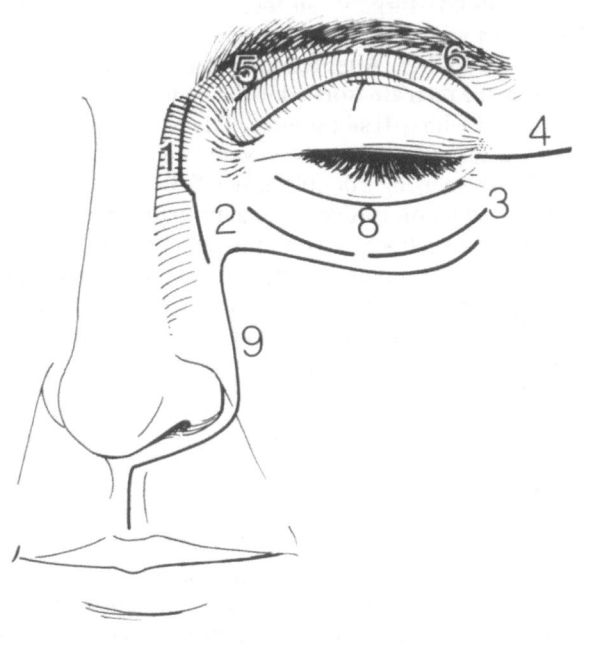

Plate 5-4. Anterior orbitotomy incisions: (1) medial orbitotomy, (2) inferior orbitotomy (medial), (3) inferior orbitotomy (lateral), (4) lateral orbitotomy (lateral canthal approach), (5) superior orbitotomy (medial), and (6) superior orbitotomy (lateral). (1) through (6) represent transperiosteal approaches. (7) and (8) represent transeptal incisions in upper and lower lids. (9) represents Weber-Fergusson approach.

is favored in cases where a malignant lacrimal gland tumor is suspected. With an extraperiosteal approach, the integrity of the periosteal barrier is violated and the extraperiosteal space is potentially seeded with malignant cells. With the transseptal approach, the entire biopsy tract can be excised if any further surgery is indicated.

Transperiosteal

Lesions along the superior orbit—medial, inferior, beneath the lacrimal sac, and with the frontal and ethmoid sinus—are best approached transperiosteally. Tumors are approached by ample skin incisions along the orbital rim. Alternatively, the skin incision may be made in the superior lid fold, a skin muscle flap undermined to the superior orbital rim in the upper lid, and a subciliary incision and a skin muscle flap undermined to the inferior orbital rim in the lower lid. Next, the periosteum adherent to the rim is freed by incising the periosteum with a No. 15 blade and using a hand-over-hand technique with periosteal elevators. Malleable retractors are used to expose the periorbita, while four-prong rakes of appropriate size are used to retract the skin in the desired quadrant. A 4–0 silk baseball stitch is used as a traction suture at

the detached arcus marginalis. Depending on the orientation of the tumor and the adjacent anatomic structures, an anterior-posterior (A-P) incision or transverse incision into the periorbita at the appropriate distance from the orbital rim is made. An A-P incision is less likely to affect the underlying orbital structures. A buttonhole incision is made into the periorbita with a No. 11 blade and the incision is extended with Stevens or Westcott scissors with one blade on the orbital side of the periorbita and the other blade on the bone side of the periorbita. Pressure is always made away from the orbit. An extra assistant is helpful for retraction. The microscope can be helpful. Muscle hooks serve to retract the periorbita and orbital fat. Cotton tip applicators are used to bluntly dissect the tumor from the orbital fat.

The central retinal artery enters the optic nerve 10–15 mm behind the globe inferiorly. At the orbital apex, the chance of nerve damage becomes more likely since there is less space and more vital structures. An encapsulated tumor is secured with a hammerhead cryoprobe. Diffuse tumors are debulked, and an incisional biopsy is performed using a No. 15 blade and Westcott scissors. A 0.5-mm Castroviejo forceps may be helpful for fixation. The pupil should be monitored. The ciliary ganglion lies just temporal to the optic nerve near the orbital apex and pupillary dilation may occur if this structure is manipulated.

Hemostasis may be achieved with bipolar cautery and cottonoids soaked in topical thrombin. Lidocaine with epinephrine, 1:200,000, may also be injected anterior to the orbital septum to enhance hemostasis when performing skin and muscle incisions but should be avoided in the deep orbit. Inadvertent retrobulbar injection may result in pupillary dilation from retrobulbar block.

USE OF FROZEN SECTIONS AND FIXATION OF TISSUES FOR SPECIAL STUDIES

Frozen sections are indicated if surgeons are not sure whether they are dealing with the actual pathologic tissue. Frozen sections will confirm that the proper tissue has in fact been biopsied. In essence, frozen sections are used if they will in some way guide the operative procedure. In general, we do not believe exenteration or any radical extirpative surgery should be performed on the basis of a frozen section.

Glutaraldehyde fixation for electron microscopy may be useful in special circumstances, especially when the pathologist is unable to make a light microscopic diagnosis. Fresh-frozen tissue may be used for immunoperoxidase marker studies on lymphoid proliferations to determine the monoclonal and polyclonal pattern of immunoglobulin production. Monoclonal tumors tend to be malignant, while polyclonal tumors are often benign. In addition, immunohistologic identification of un-differentiated tumors may disclose the cell origin and solidify the diagnosis. For example, the 100S antigen is found in neural tumors; both desmin found in skeletal and smooth muscle tumors and myoglobin found in skeletal muscle tumors may be found in rhabdomyosarcomas. Similarly, hormonal receptor assays are helpful in determining which patients with metastatic breast and prostatic carcinoma will respond to hormonal therapy.[7]

LATERAL APPROACH

The lateral approach should be an extension of a lateral canthotomy. In this manner, the lymphatic drainage of the lids is least affected. A horizontal incision is made toward the upper aspect of the ear at the lateral canthus. Next, an incision is made into the periosteum at the lateral orbital rim. An extensive tumor requires the wider exposure afforded by the Krönlein approach. Apical tumors are most accessible by this route.

Lateral (Modified) Krönlein Approach

Using Wright's approach, the skin incision is similar to that of the lateral orbitotomy and extends approximately 35 mm toward the upper helix of the ear and, therefore, continues over the lateral orbital rim of bone and over the temporalis fascia (Plate 5-5). A 4–0 silk suture is placed in the belly of the lateral rectus muscle for its identification. The periosteum is incised parallel to the lateral orbital rim 2–3 mm from the anterior aspect of the lateral orbital rim. Attachments of the lateral canthal tendon are bluntly severed with a periosteal elevator, and the periorbita is freed from the lateral orbital wall. The periosteum is also freed over the entire anterior surface of the bone of the lateral orbital wall. In this manner all of the exposed bone is freed of periosteum.

Next, the lateral wall is removed by making osteotomies (1) superiorly parallel to and 5 mm above the fronto-zygomatic suture and (2) inferiorly at the superior margin of the zygomatic arch. The osteotomy may be made with the small blade of the Stryker saw with the assistant protecting the globe with a malleable retractor. An osteotome and mallet may also be used. Then, using an end-cutting rongeur, the bony aspect of the lateral orbital wall is grasped. Attachments of the temporalis muscle are severed with a No. 15 blade and the bone is removed. Deep bone fragments of the lateral wall are removed, and the edges of the osteotomy are made smooth with an end-cutting rongeur. According to Reese, the lateral wall breaks about 12 mm posteriorly and another 12 mm can be removed with a rongeur.[7] Alternatively, if

exposure is adequate, the lateral wall may be left-hinged at its posterior aspect. Depending on the location of the tumor as determined by computed tomography (CT) scan, the orbit is entered above or below the lateral rectus. The inferior approach below the lateral rectus is preferred because there is less chance of affecting levator and causing a postoperative ptosis than with a superior approach.

A fiberoptic headlight is almost essential for all orbitotomies. Magnification provided by loupes or the operating room microscope are also extremely valuable.

The periorbita is incised with a No. 15 blade parallel to the lateral rectus muscle. Once the orbit is entered, blunt dissection is necessary. In general, an encapsulated tumor or well-circumscribed tumor is removed in toto and delivered with a cryoprobe. Diffuse tumors are biopsied and, depending on the clinical setting, are debulked or simply biopsied. Frozen sections are helpful in the latter regard. It is our belief that all tumors should be debulked as long as there is no risk to the surrounding structures (Table 5-2).

After removal of the tumor, the bone flap is reposited or removed. A small Penrose drain or suction drain is inserted into the wound to allow for egress of hemorrhage. The periorbita is not closed. Deep tissues in the lateral canthus and temporalis fossa are reapproximated with 4–0 chromic sutures. A 4–0 silk suture closes the lateral canthus. A horizontal mattress suture from upper lid margin at the gray line to lower lid margin at the gray line is used.

APPROACH TO APICAL TUMORS

Combined Lateral and Medial Approach for Apical Medial Tumors

Tumors located in the apical orbit, particularly the superior medial orbit, may be approached by a combined lateral orbitotomy with removal of bone and medial approach through either the skin if the lesion is extraconal or through the conjunctiva if the lesion is intraconal and relatively small. However, the Krönlein or neurosurgical approach affords better apical exposure. In the latter case, a generous peritomy is performed, and the superior and inferior recti are isolated with 4–0 silk sutures. The medial rectus tendon is disinserted after the tendon is sutured with a double armed 5–0 vicryl suture; the medial rectus is reflected medially. Various ribbon retractors and Schepens retractors allow gentle retraction of the soft tissues and orbital fat. The inferior oblique muscle is encountered and limits exposure if the tumor is inferonasal.

The lateral orbitotomy allows for adequate displacement of this tissue. After removal of the tumor, the

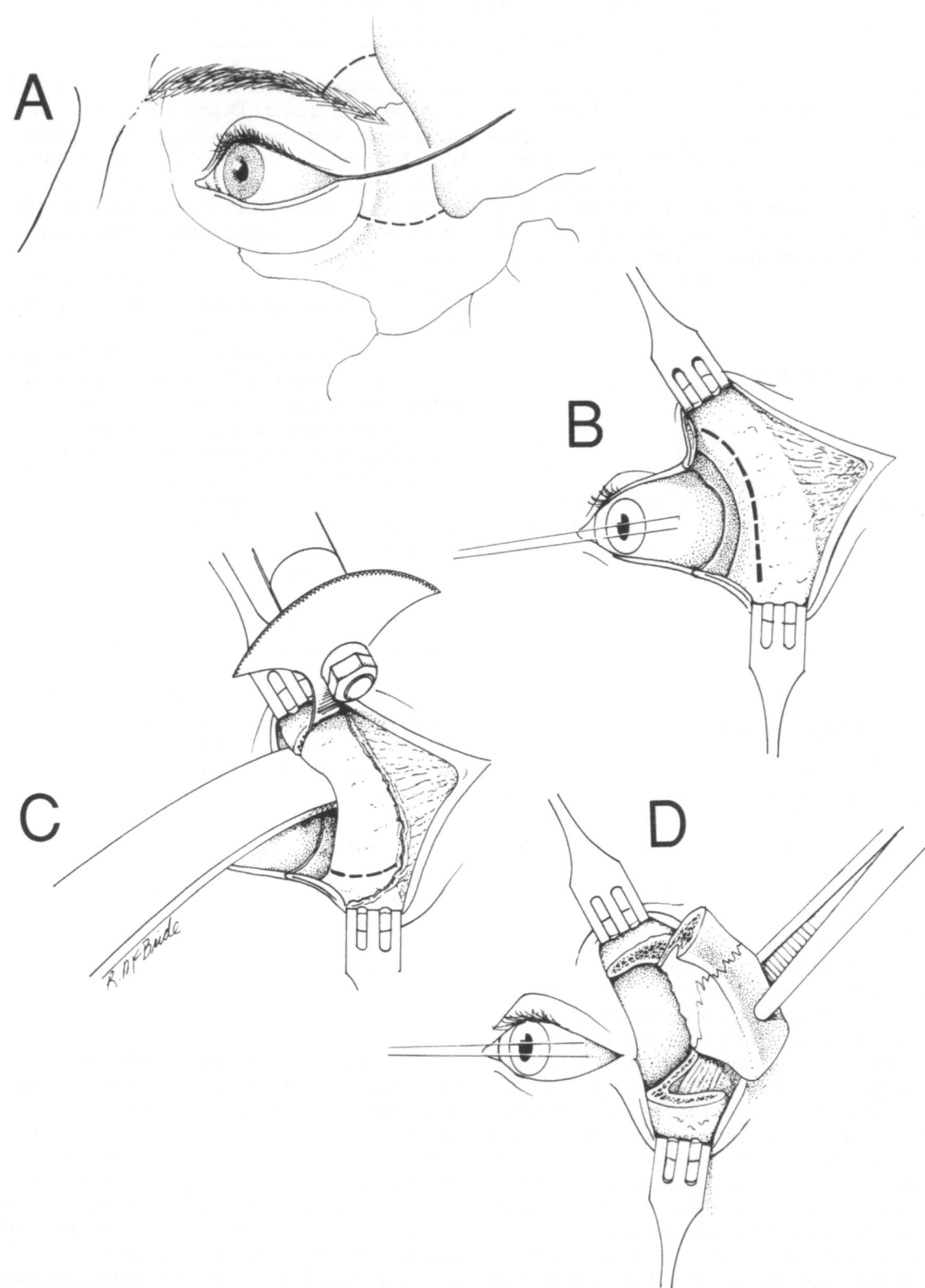

Plate 5-5. (*A*) Lateral orbitotomy after lateral canthal incision. Bone flap to be mobilized or removed is outlined. (*B*) Suture passed through lateral rectus and extent of bone flap is outlined. Incision (dotted line) is shown through periosteum at anterior aspect of orbital rim. Underlying bone is exposed. (*C*) Stryker saw or osteotome is used to osteotomize orbital rim. (*D*) Bone flap mobilized with large hemostat includes thinner posterior aspect of lateral orbital rim with attached temporalis muscle on its external surface. Ribbon retractor is used to expose orbital contents.

Table 5-2
Guide to Intraoperative Management of Orbital Tumors

Total Excision
   cavernous hemangioma
   hemangiopericytoma
   schwannoma
   dermoid cyst
Incisional Biopsy
   lymphoid lesions
   rhabdomyosarcoma
   metastatic tumor
Debulk
   neurofibroma
   lymphangioma

medial rectus is reinserted with a 5–0 vicryl suture and the peritomy is closed with 6–0 plain suture.[8]

Medial Orbitotomy

In the medial orbitotomy, the incision is made 5 mm medial to the medial canthus. A horizontal step is made in the Lynch incision to decrease webbing of the skin. The periosteum is incised with a No. 15 blade and is elevated from the underlying bone. The lacrimal sac is elevated and displaced laterally. The anterior ethmoidal vessels are identified and surgically clipped 2.5 mm behind to the posterior lacrimal crest. Dissection above the vessels is avoided so as not to penetrate the cribriform plate. For apical orbital tumors or when combined with maxillectomy, the incision is extended inferiorly allow the side of the nose, under the nostril, and to the lip.

The Lynch or Weber-Ferguson incisions for medial orbitotomy may, therefore, obviate the need for lateral orbitotomy.

Large Superior Orbitotomy for Medial Apical and Superior Apical Tumors

A large superior orbitotomy from canthus to canthus may also be attempted for apical medial tumors and especially for superiorly located apical tumors.[9] This approach avoids the necessity to perform the lateral Krönlein incision and may provide better exposure than through the peritomy site. Ptosis and EOM imbalance may arise because of the detachment of the levator and trochlea, respectively.

Transfrontal Approach to Apical Tumors

The transfrontal or neurosurgical approach is appropriate for tumors at the orbital apex and optic canal that are too posterior or medial to be accessible by a lateral or medial orbital approach. The approach is mandatory for lesions that involve both the intraorbital and intracranial compartments or for lesions, such as glioma or meningioma, in which intracanalicular extension is suspected.[10] The periorbita of the orbital apex and the dura, after the optic canal is unroofed, are incised. The levator and superior rectus may be detached to enhance exposure. The levator and superior recturs are later reattached with 5–0 chromic sutures. A bicoronal flap is raised (Plate 5-6). The frontal bone is removed and the dura is reflected superiorly. The orbital roof and periorbita are then opened. Just beneath the incised periorbita, the frontal nerve and artery, the trochlear nerve medially, and the levator-superior rectus complex are gently retracted medially or temporally with a muscle hook. For optic nerve tumors, the periorbita is incised medial to the frontal nerve from anterior to posterior, and the levator-superior rectus complex are reflected laterally. For tumors in the lateral orbit, the periorbita is incised lateral to the frontal nerve, and the levator is reflected medially. The periorbita is closed at the end of the procedure. Various materials, autogenous or alloplastic, may be placed over the orbit to prevent pulsating exophthalmos. Such materials include fascia lata, wire mesh, aluminum, and polymethylmethacrylate. Other neurosurgical considerations are beyond the scope of this book.

COMPLICATIONS OF ORBITAL SURGERY

Respect for the blood supply to the globe is crucial in all surgical manipulations. The intraocular blood supply is derived from (1) the central retinal artery that pierces the inferior aspect of the optic nerve 12–15 mm posterior to the posterior aspect of the globe, and (2) the posterior ciliary arteries that are located at the posterior aspect of the globe, especially temporally. Excessive traction on orbital structures as well as external pressure on the globe that might compromise intraocular circulation should be avoided.[10] The pupil should be monitored throughout the procedure. The fundus may be examined in the operating room using the coaxial fiberoptic headlight and an indirect lens. The risk of pharmacologic pupillary dilation as it influences postoperative evaluation must be considered in each individual situation. In the postcataract extraction eye, excessive pressure on the globe may result in limbal rupture with a wound leak, flat chamber, and intraocular lens (IOL) dislocation.

All patients who have had an orbitotomy should be

examined by the surgeon the night of surgery for possible retrobulbar hemorrhage and external compression of the optic nerve circulation. A short, 3-day course of prednisone at 60 mg/day with rapid taper the first, second, and third days, respectively, is helpful in reducing postoperative swelling if not medically contraindicated. In addition, pupil checks by the nurses every hour the first 24 hours are indicated. Any dressing should be loose to avoid external pressure on the globe. Any sudden pain or proptosis may be a sign of orbital hemorrhage, and the nurses should be instructed to call the surgeon if any such signs develop.

Ophthalmologic findings consistent with retrobulbar hemorrhage include "tight" lids and poor ocular motility. Fundoscopy may show poor perfusion of the nervehead. Corneal clouding may be due to external pressure on the eye and secondary rapid elevation of the intraocular pressure. Treatment of retrobulbar hemorrhage includes intravenous mannitol and acetazolamide to decrease intraocular pressure. Oral prednisone is helpful in reducing orbital edema. In patients with retrobulbar hemorrhage in which medical treatment fails, a generous lateral canthotomy may be necessary with lysis of the inferior crus and, if necessary, superior crus of the lateral canthal tendon. Such patients should be advised that a lateral canthoplasty may be necessary. The original wound may need to be opened with evacuation of blood and cauterization of any any bleeding vessels. A Penrose or Jackson-Pratt drain should be inserted to decompress the orbit should any further bleeding occur.

Internal ophthalmoplegia may be due to damage to the ciliary ganglion or third nerve. In the former situation, an Adie's or tonic pupil results. The latter is supersensitive to dilute solutions of pilocarpine and is slow to react to light and accommodation. Improvement and resolution may occur gradually. Such patients may require a plus lens for reading and possibly distance vision. The nerves to the various recti muscles and superior oblique muscle generally pierce the given muscle approximately 26 mm posterior to the muscle's insertion. The inferior oblique nerve enters the muscle as it crosses the inferior rectus at its lateral border approximately 12 mm posterior to the inferior rectus insertion in the area of the Lockwood's ligament (inferior transverse ligament). External ophthalmoplegia may also be caused by muscle injury. Motility disturbances after surgery should be observed for 6 months without significant improvement before repair is undertaken. Prisms may be helpful.

The most common cause of diplopia is a fibrous adhesion of the lateral rectus to the canthotomy scar. An acquired pseudo-Duane's syndrome with retraction on adduction may occur.

Surgical trauma to the sensory nerves may result in hypesthesia in the nerve distribution. Supraorbital nerve damage may result in hypesthesia in the forehead, while infraorbital anesthesia may occur after inferior orbitotomy. Anesthesia of the nasal region may follow injury to the ethmoidal nerves. Similarly, an incision near the lateral orbital rim may injure the zygomaticotemporal or zygomaticofacial nerves. Nasociliary nerve damage at the apex of the orbit may result in neuroparalytic keratopathy.

Ptosis may be segmental or may involve the entire upper lid and is generally due to mechanical injury to the levator or its supporting ligament, the superior transverse ligament of Whitnall. Therefore, in performing all superior orbitotomies, surgeons should not damage the periorbita in their dissection at the orbital rim. Repair should not be considered for 6 months after the orbital surgery, especially if there is evidence of recovery of levator function.

Other complications include cerebrospinal fluid leaks from violation of the dura, most commonly in the medial orbit in the area of the cribriform plate. Small leaks may be sealed with Gelfilm or butyl-2-cyanoacrylate. Large tears may be sutured with 5–0 silk. Tears too large to be sutured are reconstructed with lyophilized cadaver dura or autogenous fascia. Slow virus infection has been reported for lyophilized cadaver dura. Neurosurgical consultation should be sought. Infectious disease consult is also helpful in guiding antibiotic therapy.[10]

EXENTERATION

The ophthalmologist is able to manage tumors confined to the orbit; however, the assistance of an ENT, head and neck, or neurosurgeon may be required for tumors that extend beyond the orbit.

Techniques of Exenteration

The basic technique of exenteration involves removing the entire orbital contents including lids and conjunctiva.

The procedure is performed under general anesthesia. A skin incision is marked at the orbital rim. Hemostasis is augmented by local infiltration of 1 percent lidocaine with 1:200,000 epinephrine at the orbital rim. An incision is made with a No. 15 blade about the entire orbital rim. Freshly diluted epinephrine may also be used. The dissection to the periosteum of the orbital rim may be completed with the Bovie in the cutting mode or contact YAG laser. The plastic sleeve of the Bovie protects the superficial skin. The lids may be sutured together with a 4–0 silk suture for traction. Care is taken in the superonasal orbit and medial orbit to cauterize the supraorbital artery and angular vessels respectively.[11]

The periosteum is incised with a No. 15 blade or contact YAG laser, while exposure is obtained with

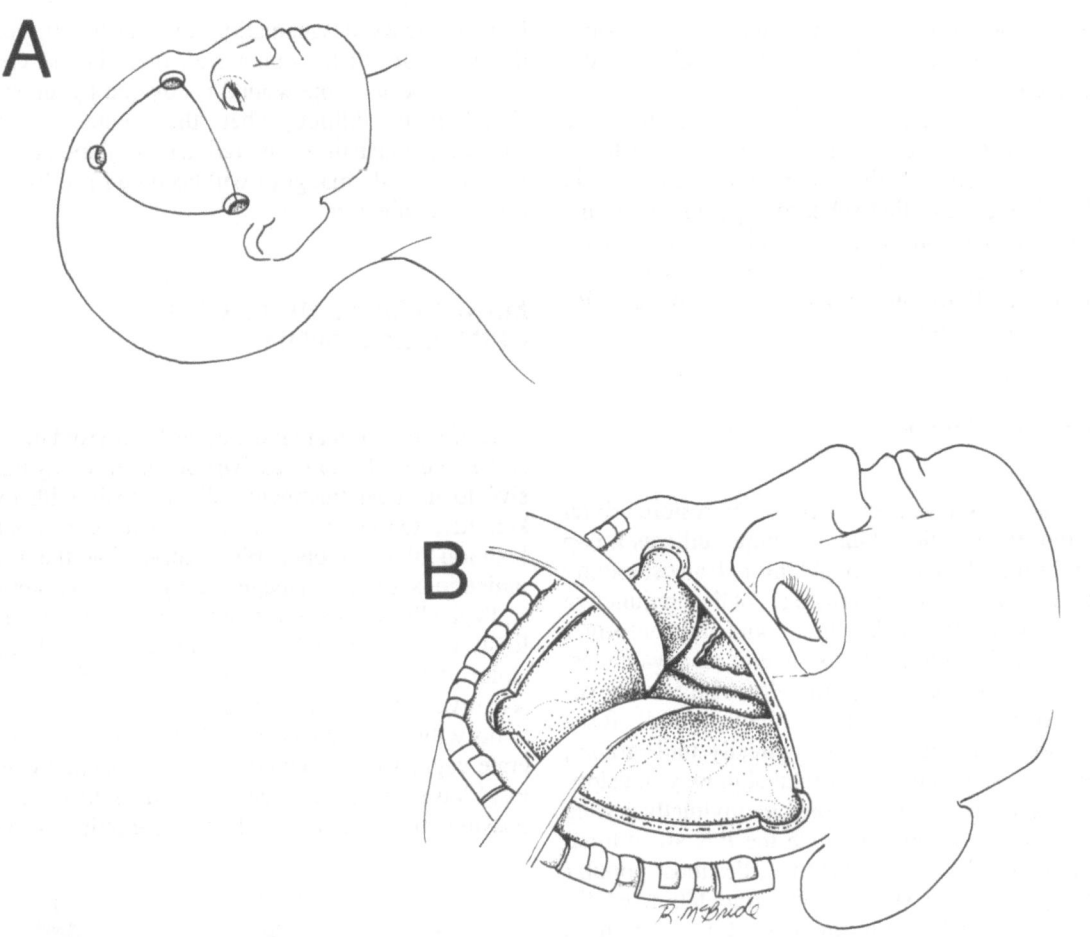

Plate 5-6. Cranial approach to orbital tumors. (*A*) Frontal is removed. (*B*) Dura is reflected exposing orbital roof (partially removed).

malleable retractors and rake retractors. A periosteal elevator is used to free the periosteum from the underlying bone at the orbital rim. Next, using a hand-over-hand technique with two elevators and/or malleable retractors, the surgeon lifts the periorbita from the underlying orbital bones. The dissection is carried out in the medial orbit last because it is the most vascular quadrant. The anterior ethmoidal atery may be identified and surgically clipped before it is cut. The vessel may also be severed with the Bovie cautery or contact YAG laser. The thin bone of the medial and inferior orbital walls are retracted gently to avoid bone perforations. Fistula formation into the sinuses and nasal cavity is thereby minimized. The periorbita tends to be more adherent at the following areas: (1) trochlea, (2) origin of the inferior oblique muscle, (3) superior and inferior orbital sulcus, and (4) medial and lateral canthal tendons. The latter structures are generally incised with a No. 15 blade. The lacrimal sac is included in the specimen. The nasolacrimal duct may be ligated or included in the specimen after dissection along its bony course.

A large curved hemostat is used to grasp the structures at the orbital apex for hemostasis. Large curved enculea-

tion scissors are used to amputate the specimen at the orbital apex. The spatula tip of the Bovie cautery may be bent at 30 to 40 degrees to accomplish this task. There is also an angle tip for the YAG contact laser. Areas of involved bone are removed and sent for permanent pathologic sections. Frozen sections cannot be performed on calcified bone.

The orbit is lined with rectangular strips of telfa and then packed with xeroform gauze. The patch is removed in 3 days to 1 week. The socket is lavaged every week with diluted 50:50 hydrogen peroxide and dressed with topical antibiotic ointment and telfa for a period of 2–3 months until granulation is complete.

Several techniques may be utilized when performing the exenteration, depending on the type of tumor. Since the procedure is radical, total excision of the mass should take precedence over reconstruction. For apical masses such as optic nerve meningiomas, the anterior lid structures and lids and conjunctiva may be spared and the dissection started with a limbal peritomy. Alternatively, the lids, except the lid margin, may be spared by dissecting from the lid margin to the orbital septum. The skin flaps may be mobilized to line the orbital walls.[12]

Another method is to make an incision in the tarsoconjunctiva about 3 mm parallel to the lid margin in order to preserve cilia.

For basal cell carcinomas requiring exenteration, the lids and conjunctiva must be sacrificed. The posterior orbit may be retained since the tumor originates anteriorly in the skin. We believe that sebaceous gland carcinoma and malignant melanomas of the conjunctiva, because of their inherent aggressiveness and multifocal character, should have "total" exenteration as opposed to the "subtotal" procedures outlined above.

Reconstruction of the Exenterated Orbit

Various methods have been employed to restore orbital volume after exenteration. One technique utilizes a flap of temporalis muscle that is brought through an osteotomy in the lateral orbital wall. The cut edges of the conjunctiva are then sutured to each other, and a conformer inserted.[13,14] This technique has several disadvantages: (1) recurrence is masked, (2) difficulty with jaw movements may occur, (3) depression of the temporalis fossa on the involved side may be cosmetically undesirable, and (4) paresthesias in the periorbital skin may develop. Similarly, we do not employ Gass' methylmethacrylate implant to restore volume in which the lids are sutured over the implant.[15] In our experience, the most popular techniques include (1) spontaneous granulation or (2) lining of the orbit with split-thickness skin (epidermal) or dermal grafts.[16]

The technique using a split-thickness graft allows for less postoperative care compared with spontaneous granulation. The technique employs harvesting a split-thickness epidermal skin graft 15/1000 of an inch in thickness. We prefer to harvest the graft from the outer aspect of the thigh (Fig. 5-1). The dermatome is slowly advanced from the lower aspect of the upper thigh while the assistant holds a tongue depressor to apply traction and a smooth surface as the dermatome is advanced. Downward countertraction is supplied toward the feet from the knee area. Toothless forceps are used to grasp the harvested split-thickness epidermal graft. The harvested graft is cut into rectangular sections to cover the four quadrants of the orbit. The raw donor surface is treated with topical antibiotic ointment, petrolatum gauze, or xeroform gauze, and a 4-inch cling is used to wrap the thigh.

Alternatively, a second dermal graft may be harvested from the bed of the epidermal graft, which is left-hinged at one end. The edges of the split-thickness epidermal graft are sutured to the skin edges.

The epidermal or dermal graft techniques are advantageous in that once the donor dressing is changed every week for a month, the postoperative care is usually complete. With spontaneous granulation, healing does not occur for 2–3 months.

The dermal graft has advantages over the epidermal graft. The main advantage at the recipient site is the lack of greasy desquamation and the heartiness of the dermal graft. At the donor site, there is less chance of infection because the wound is covered by an epidermal skin flap. In addition, where the exenteration involves sinuses, as when the exenteration is combined with maxillectomy, the dermal graft will become lined by nonkeratinizing epithelium.

MANAGEMENT OF THYROID OPHTHALMOPATHY

There are four main indications for thyroid decompression surgery: (1) compressive optic neuropathy unresponsive to medical treatment, (2) proptosis with exposure keratitis, (3) cosmetic, and (4) recurrent spontaneous luxation of the globe. We assume that the last three indications are not manageable by eyelid surgery alone.

Typically, compressive optic neuropathy occurs painlessly with insidious loss of vision and central scotomas. Color plates and visual fields with color objects are most sensitive.[17] Occasional optic neuropathy develops in patients with severe congestion, but surprisingly only moderate degress of exophthalmos are associated with visual loss. Visual loss may occur over days to weeks.[18] It is possible that patients with less compliant orbits and,

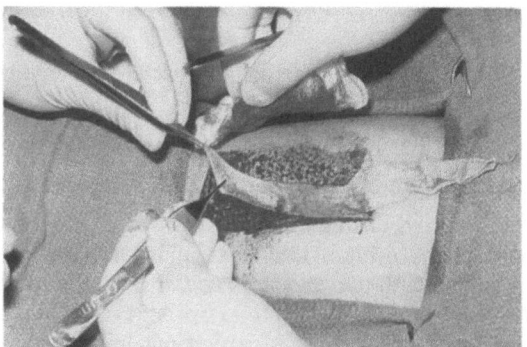

A

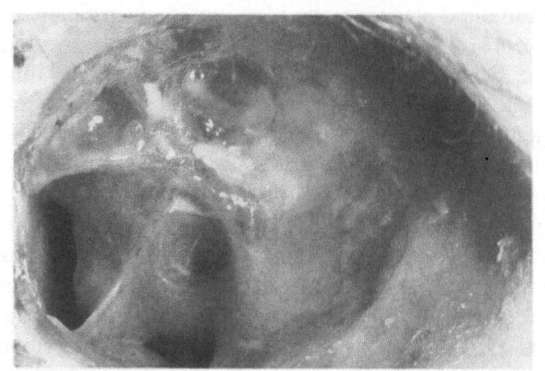

B

Fig. 5-1. (A) Harvesting of split-thickness dermal graft after epidermal flap has been hinged. (B) Three months after surgery, dermal graft has reepithelialized. There is no evidence of keratinization.

therefore, less proptosis suffer greater visual loss when their orbital tissues become acutely congested.[19]

The surgical approaches include (1) a translid, with or without an external ethmoidectomy, and (2) a transantral (Caldwell-Luc) approach. As with any orbitotomy, the patient should be cautioned about the possibility of loss of vision, worsening of double vision, or the onset of new diplopia. Patients with long-standing thyroid ophthalmopathy may have more inelastic orbits that respond less effectively to decompression.

In general, when exophthalmos is greater than 25 mm and there is no evidence of compressive neuropathy, orbital decompression rather than simple eyelid surgery is necessary for cosmetic considerations. Lid retraction surgery for cosmetic purposes may camouflage moderate degrees of exophthalmos with Hertel measurements less than 25 mm.

The history of thyroid decompressive surgery dates back to 1889 when Krönlrein advocated a lateral orbitotomy that he had first used for the removal of orbital tumors.[20] In 1936, Sewall applied an external approach in a frontoethmoidectomy to decompress the orbit.[21] In 1950, Hirsch advocated a transantral removal of the orbital floor.[22] In 1957, Walsh and Ogura combined a transantral removal of the floor and the medial wall.[23]

The goal of surgery—removal of the inferior and medial walls—may also be accomplished through a translid approach by either a subciliary incision or an incision through the conjunctiva and fornix after a lateral canthotomy.

For patients with severe exophthalmos of 35 mm or more, a four-wall decompression that involves the lateral and superior wall may also be performed.[24] This technique is best done in collaboration with a neurosurgeon; during the operation a lateral Krönlein orbitotomy is combined with removal of the orbital roof outside the frontal sinus. The greater wing of the sphenoid bone in the lateral wall of the orbit and the lateral half of the orbital roof are removed, exposing dura and relieving 14–16 mm of proptosis.

Translid Vs. Transantral Approach to Decompression of the Floor and Medial Wall

The translid procedure is probably the better choice when decompressions are performed for cosmetic reasons. Studies have shown that the incidence of postoperative motility disturbances are significantly greater with the transantral than the translid approach.[25] In fact, after the translid approach, motility imbalances may be improved. This improvement occurs because more of the posterior ethmoid sinus is removed with the transantral technique than is removed with the translid approach. The posterior ethmoids probably give support to the inferior and medial recti. For the same reason, the excision of greater amounts of posterior ethmoids than is possible with the transantral approach may be better suited for

compressive optic neuropathy. In one study, the need for postoperative radiation was significantly greater following translid surgery than was needed following transantral surgery. The translid procedure may be combined with an external ethmoidectomy.

The lateral orbitotomy alone does not improve proptosis as well as the inferior and medial wall decompression through either the translid or transantral approach (25). The lateral approach improves proptosis by 2 to 3 mm while the translid or transantral approach reduces proptosis by 4 to 6 mm. The lateral technique does not relieve the compressive optic neuropathy at the orbital apex. Of course, the lateral wall surgery may be combined with the medial and inferior wall decompression but the addition of the third wall does not significantly enhance the decompressive effect overall and especially not at the apex.

Translid—Surgical Technique. The translid approach is performed through a subciliary incision after local infiltration of 1 percent lidocaine with 1:200,000 epinephrine. A skin muscle flap is mobilized inferiorly to the orbital rim. A No. 15 blade is used to incise the periosteum 1–2 mm below the orbital rim. The orbital floor is exposed by using a hand-over-hand technique with periosteal elevators. The infraorbital neurovascular bundle is identified as a slight convexity on the medial aspect of the orbital floor running from anterior to posterior. The floor is fractured medial to the neurovascular bundle using blunt pressure with the tip of an elevator or using a small osteotome and mallet. A surgical needle holder or hemostat may be used to remove fragments of bone. The bone of the orbital floor can then be "peeled off" the underlying mucosa of the maxillary sinus and the infarorbital nerve and artery. Several techniques for "peeling off" the bone are helpful. The elevator can be placed between the bone of the floor and the maxillary sinus mucosa at the cut edge of the bone. The elevator is gently raised; a second elevator may be placed against the bone fragments from above. Alternatively, a small end-cutting rongeur found on "hand sets" in the general operating room may be used. A straight hemostat or surgical needle holder may be used as a well as a Kerrison punch to remove the medial wall (Plate 5-7). The orbital rim is not removed because of the possibility of developing cicatricial ectropion. The periorbita is incised from anterior to posterior to allow for prolapse of the orbital contents. The periorbita may also be stripped with toothed forceps. We prefer not to incise the mucosa of the maxillary sinus if the orbital contents prolapse sufficiently through the orbital osteotomy because of the increased chance of infection. A nasal antrostomy is not performed unless there was previous evidence of poor maxillary sinus drainage or if significant intraoperative bleeding occurs.

The same surgery may be performed through a conjunctival cul-de-sac approach after a lateral canthotomy with the advantage of not having an external scar on the lower eyelid.

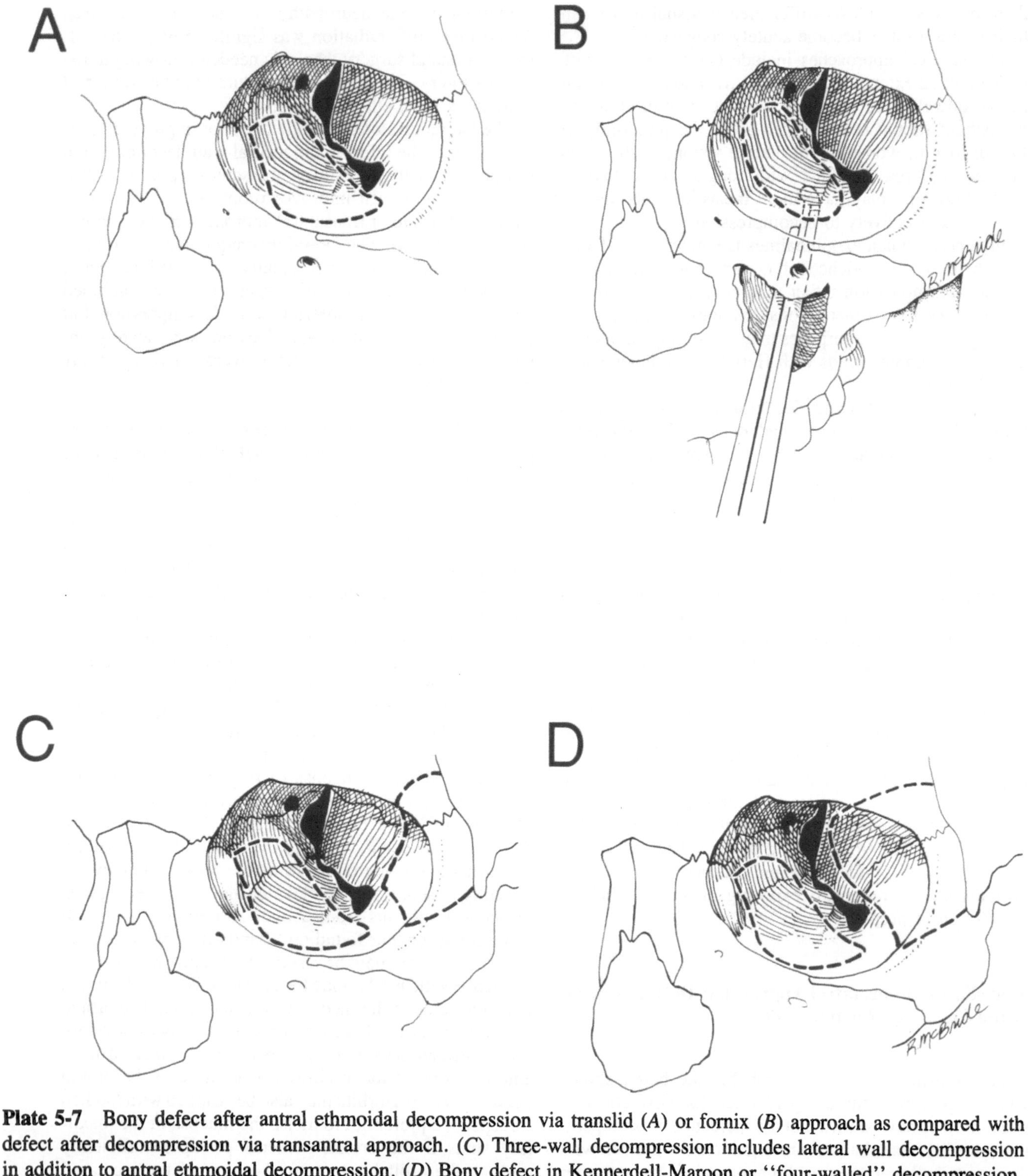

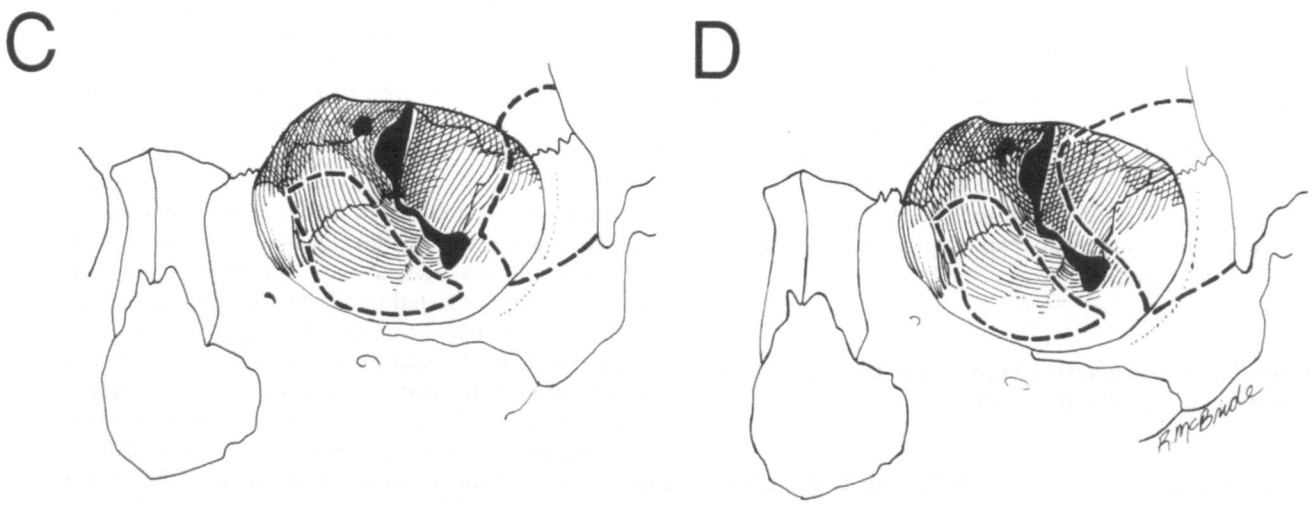

Plate 5-7 Bony defect after antral ethmoidal decompression via translid (*A*) or fornix (*B*) approach as compared with defect after decompression via transantral approach. (*C*) Three-wall decompression includes lateral wall decompression in addition to antral ethmoidal decompression. (*D*) Bony defect in Kennerdell-Maroon or "four-walled" decompression. The third or lateral wall decompression includes removal of a large portion of the greater wing of the sphenoid bone and the lateral portion of the roof. A five-wall decompression includes the roof of the orbit.

Transantral Approach—Surgical Technique. The canine fossa is infiltrated with lidocaine with epinephrine for hemostasis and is incised with a No. 15 blade for a standard Caldwell-Luc procedure. The mucosa of the mouth is elevated from the anterior wall of the maxillary sinus. The infraorbital nerve is identified and preserved. An osteotomy is made into the anterior wall of the maxillary sinus with a osteotome and mallet. Using a Kerrison punch, the anterior wall is removed. The infraorbital neurovascular bundle is avoided. In the medial superior portion, the bone is removed up to the orbital rim to provide visualization.

Attention is directed to the superior medial corner of the antrum. An inferior-based mucosal flap is mobilized. The ethmoid sinus is entered by breaking the thin bone, and the medial orbital floor is removed. The infraorbital nerve must be carefully preserved. The orbital contents are retracted laterally. The floor is removed before the medial wall because the medial wall prolapse may obscure the view of the floor. Using an operating room microscope, the medial and inferior aspect of the orbital apex is removed. Takahashi forceps are helpful in removing the thin bone of the medial wall.

After completing the osteotomy, the periorbita is opened and orbital fat is teased through the periorbita. Longitudinal incisions from anterior to posterior may be made. Cross-hatching may also be done if the anterior-to-posterior incisions do not allow for adequate prolapse of orbital fat. Stripping of the periorbita with toothed forceps may be helpful.

A nasal antral window is made with a small chisel that is used to elevate the mucosa from the lateral wall of the nose just below the inferior turbinate posterior to the osteum of the nasolacrimal duct. An osteotomy is then performed with a chisel, and the cut may be enlarged using a curved hemostat. Care must be taken not to damage the osteum of the nasolacrimal duct. This nasoantral window allows for sinus drainage since significant trauma may damage the normal maxillary sinus ostea. The window also allows for egress of any postoperative hemorrhage (Plate 5-7).

Translid and External Ethmoidectomy. The translid and external ethmoidectomy approach may be combined. We have found that this technique affords the greatest exposure and therefore ensures the decompressive effect at the orbital apex. A Lynch incision is made, through which the anterior and posterior ethmoidectomy is performed. The anterior ethmoidal artery is surgically clipped and severed.

Complications of Orbital Decompressive Surgery

The complications of surgical orbital decompression include those of any orbitotomy: loss of vision, diplopia, and ptosis. In addition, cerebrospinal fluid (CSF) leakage may occur after the ethmoidectomy, particularly if the cribriform plate is located more inferiorly than normal. The ethmoidal vessels are the landmark for the cribriform plate. Surgery should not be performed above the ethmoidal vessels. Its anterior counterpart is the superior aspect of the lacrimal fossa.

Infection is increased when the maxillary sinus is entered as well as when a nasoantral window is opened. Prophylactic antibiotics are recommended, particularly when either of these surgical maneuvers is performed. We give several intravenous dosages of a cephalosporin for 1–2 days followed by oral antibiotics for 1 week. Leakage of CSF is not an indication for prophylactic antibiotics, and an antibiotic that crosses the blood-brain barrier should be utilized. An infectious disease consult may be indicated if CSF is noted at the time of surgery.

In addition, nasolacrimal duct obstructions has been reported after transantral decompression.[26] In general, lid retraction, if present, is improved in the lower lid because of the postoperative downward displacement of the globe; upper lid retraction may be slightly aggravated for the same reason.

Diplopia is more often worsened with transantral surgery, while diplopia is often improved following translid surgery.

If necessary, EOM surgery is performed after orbital decompression but prior to any surgery for eyelid retraction, fat herniation, lacrimal gland resuspension, and canthopexy.[5]

Role of Radiation Therapy

External beam radiation therapy is generally the third choice after steroid therapy and surgical decompression have failed. However, other than steroid failure, indications for radiation therapy include (1) medical contraindication to steroids, (2) steroid side-effects, or (3) poor patient compliance or refusal to take medication.

Some studies have shown that only a minority of patients will respond to radiation therapy, with only moderative improvement in optic neuropathy, motility, and other soft tissue signs such as periorbital edema, hyperemia, and a subjective feeling of less orbital pressure and discomfort.[27] More recent studies indicate that when 2000 rad over 10-day treatment period is administered in the early stages of the disease (within 6 months of onset), radiation can be quite effective. Radiation is least effective when used in mild long-standing thyroid ophthalmopathy.[28] A positive response usually occurs within 6 weeks, and maximum benefit from radiation therapy occurs within 4–6 months but may take as long as 2 years. Therefore, close monitoring of patients is essential.

Leone reported no progression or reactivation of the inflammation in 24 of 25 patients who had undergone radiotherapy.[29] In his series, a linear accelerator is the preferred source since it delivers a finely columnated beam with little scatter. The dose is 2000 rad, 1000 rad from each lateral port, over a 10-day period of 200 rad per day. Steroids, if already started, are continued during the treatment, then gradually tapered.

Complications of radiation include transient skin erythema, keratitis due to dry eye, punctal occlusion, cataract, radiation retinopathy, and radiation-induced neoplasm (see Chapter 8).

Extraocular Muscle Surgery in Thyroid Ophthalmopathy

Extraocular muscle surgery should be performed after orbital decompression, usually approximately 2 months later. Because of the restrictive nature of the myopathy, the strabismus is noncomitant. The patient should be aware that after strabismus surgery there will be residual diplopia in some fields of gaze and that the goal of the surgery is to restore binocularity in the primary position. In general, recessions of the muscles are performed. Adjustable sutures are helpful in that the muscles are extremely tight and the results are somewhat unpredictable. Conjunctival recessions and bare scleral closure are employed.[30] Resections are not indicated because motility will be restricted. Generally, for vertical deviations of over 15–20 prism diopters, two vertical recti will need to be recessed. Similarly, for horizontal deviations of greater than 30 prism diopters, two horizontal recti need to be recessed. The oblique muscles generally do not need to be treated.

Eyelid Surgery for Thyroid Ophthalmopathy

Eyelid retraction with scleral show both superiorly and inferiorly is a common sequella of thyroid ophthalmopathy. Like compressive optic neuropathy, medical management is the initial mainstay of therapy. Ocular lubricants, drops during the day and ointments at bedtime, are essential. Sometimes copious ointment at bedtime sealed with plastic wrap and a light eye patch to keep the plastic wrap in place are necessary. Retraction is the result of several complex factors: (1) sympathetic stimulation of Muller's muscle from the systemic thyroid disease, (2) recurrent bouts of inflammation and edema resulting in scarring and secondary contraction, (3) fibrosis and retraction of the inferior rectus causing lower lid retraction because of the attachment of the inferior rectus to the lower lid via the capsulopalpebral fascia, (4) overaction of the levator and superior rectus complex to counteract the inferior rectus contractures, and (5) gravitational effects that exacerbate lower lid retraction.

Steroids, because of their systemic side-effects, probably play no role in the treatment of lid retraction. Topical sympatholytics may result in tachyphylaxis and have inherent corneal toxicity. Unless corneal exposure is a serious problem, eyelid retraction surgery should be delayed for at least 1 year to ascertain the stability of the degree of lid retraction.

Upper eyelid retraction surgery may be performed through a skin or conjunctival approach. We prefer a skin approach when there is excessive fat herniation. When no significant fat herniation is present, we utilize a conjunctival approach. In the past, spacer materials such as sclera, fascia, ear cartilage, and nasal septum have been used. We no longer use these substances because of their tendency to resorb and to cause persistent lid edema and their occasional unsightly and bulky appearance.

Skin Approach. An incision 10 mm (8–9 mm in males) from the lid border is marked in the superior palpebral furrow with a marking pen. Local infiltration with 1 cc of 2 percent lidocaine and ½ percent Marcaine is adequate. Although the lids are quite vascular, we prefer not to use epinephrine because of its effect on Muller's muscle. A 4–0 silk transmarginal traction suture facilitates dissection. A skin muscle flap is mobilized inferiorly over the tarsus (Plate 5-8). Superiorly, dissection is initiated at least 8 mm above the superior tarsal border through the preseptal orbicularis muscle. The orbital septum is incised, the preaponeurotic fat pad is identified, and the fat is teased from its septal and levator attachments using blunt dissection with cotton tip applicators. The fat is clamped, cut, and cauterized.

Westcott scissors are used to undermine and elevate the levator aponeurosis and Muller's muscle from the superior tarsal border and conjunctiva. Muller's muscle may be excised to enhance the recession effect. Dissection is facilitated by local injection of anesthetic under the levator to free the levator from Muller's muscle and conjunctiva. Inadvertent perforations of conjunctiva are sutured with interrupted 6–0 plain sutures with the knot away from the conjunctiva. Muller's muscle may be excised. The edge of the levator aponeurosis is sutured to the conjunctiva with interrupted 6–0 chromic sutures. For each millimeter of retraction, the levator needs to be recessed approximately 2 mm. Because the lid retraction is more marked laterally in thyroid disease, the lateral horn of the levator is cut. The lid position may be adjusted for contour and position on the operating room table. The skin is closed with interrupted 6–0 silk sutures. Three of these sutures should include a bite through the deep tissues in order to create a lid fold.

Grove has described a marginal myotomy technique for lid retraction repair.[31] The levator-Muller's muscle complex is isolated at least 20 mm above the upper tarsal margin; Muller's muscle extends only 10 mm from the upper tarsal border. Two incisions are made in the medial and lateral aspect of the levator and Muller's muscle. These cuts are parallel to the lid border. The lower cut is 2–3 mm above the superior tarsus and the second cut is 5–10 mm above the first. Both cuts extend just across the midline. In general, the levator should

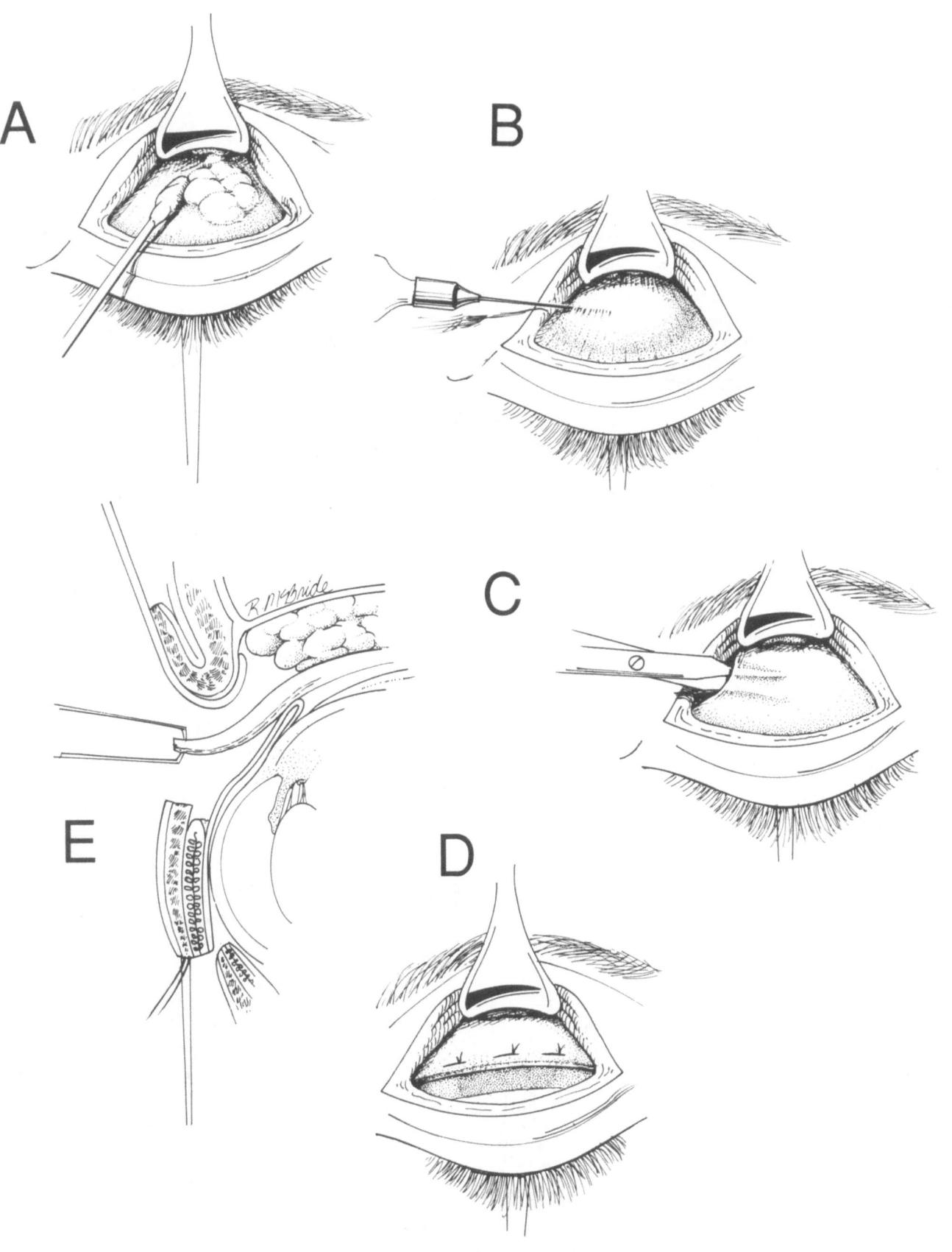

Plate 5-8. Levator and Muller's muscle recession—skin approach. (*A*) Lid fold incision exposes tarsus inferiorly. Preaponeurotic fat pad has been dissected from underlying levator aponeurosis. (*B*) Dissection of levator and Muller's muscle from underlying conjunctiva is enhanced by ballooning subconjunctival tissue with fluid. (*C*) Levator and Muller's muscle are dissected from conjunctiva and buttonholes in conjunctiva are repaired with interrupted or running 6–0 plain sutures. (*D*) Superiorly, the levator muscle is bluntly dissected from conjunctiva posteriorly and orbital fat anteriorly (not shown). The lateral horn of the levator is cut. (*E*) The levator is recessed 2 mm for each millimeter of retraction with three interrupted 7–0 chromic sutures.

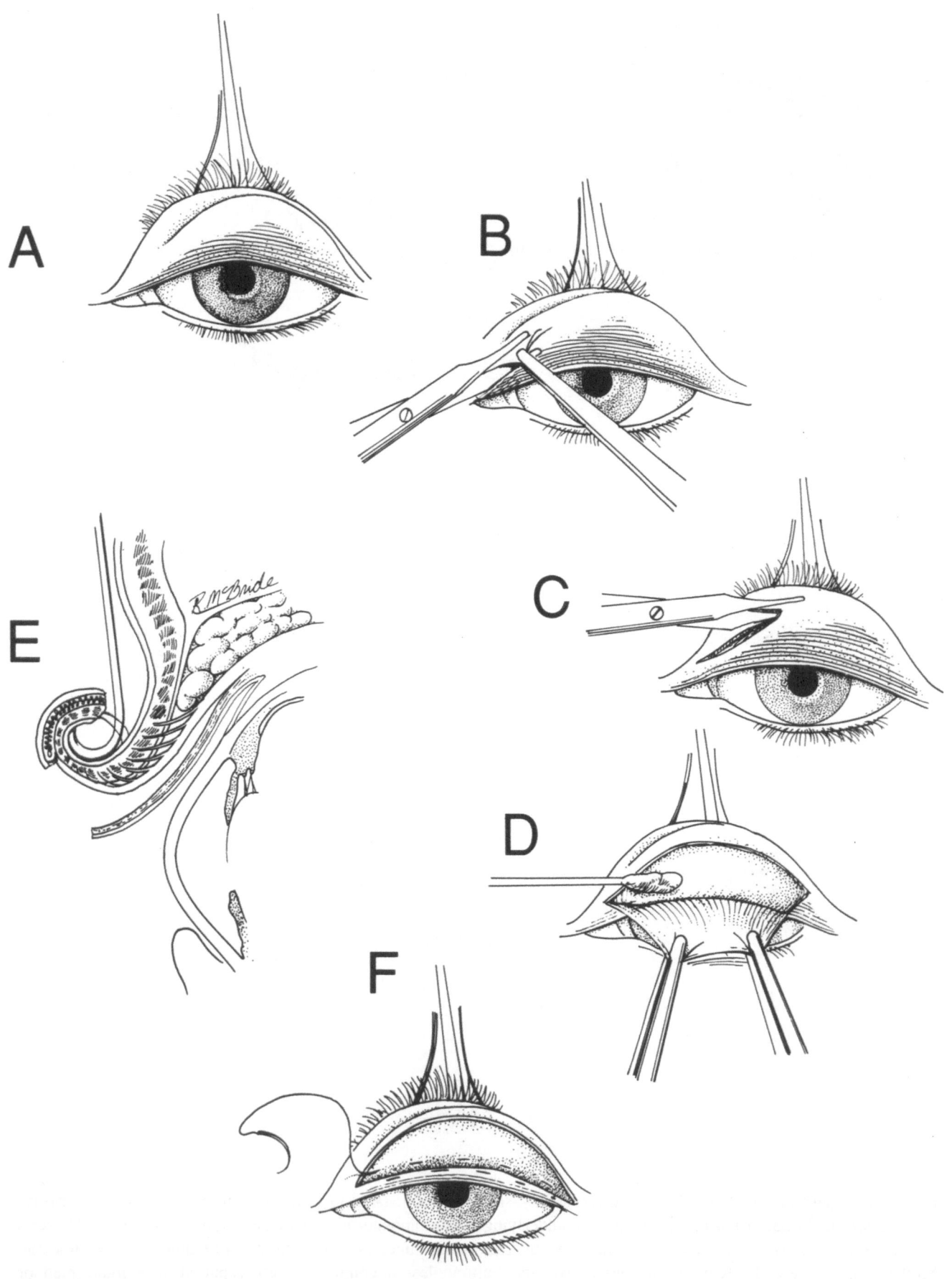

Plate 5-9. Muller's muscle recession—conjunctival approach upper lid. (*A*) Lid has been everted on Desmarres lid retractor after applying a transmarginal traction suture. (*B*) Conjunctival incision just above superior tarsal border. (*C*) Muller's muscle and conjunctiva are dissected (*D–E*) from levator aponeurosis and recessed 7–8 mm from the superior tarsal border (*F*) using a running horizontal mattress 7–0 vicryl suture.

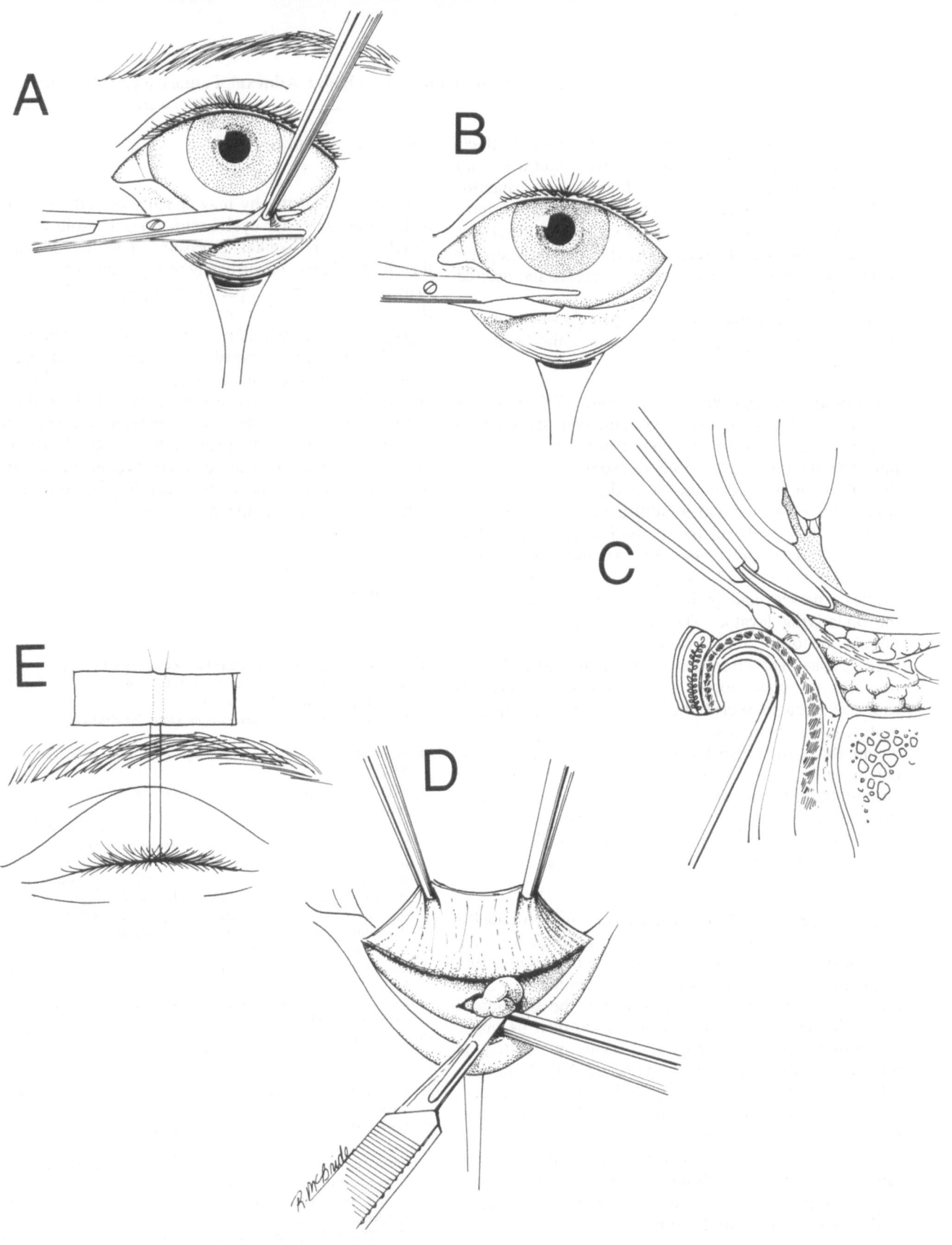

Plate 5-10. Recession of lower lid retractors—conjunctival approach. (*A*) Lid is everted on a Desmarres lid retractor. Conjunctival, Muller's muscles, and capsulopalpebral fascia are severed at the mid aspect of the inferior tarsal border. (*B*) With one blade within the conjunctiva and one blade outside, conjunctiva, Muller's muscle, and capsulopalpebral fasia are cut across the lower tarsal border. (*C*) Dissection is carried down to the orbital rim in the suborbicularis plane between the orbicularis muscle and the capsulopalpebral fascia. (*D*) Herniated orbital fat that is exposed between the capsulopalpebral fascia and orbital septum is excised. (*E*) With 4–0 black silk sutures, the lower lid is pulled upward to the eyebrow.

be lengthened by 1.25 to 1.50 times the desired effect. A temporary suture placed at the tarsus, and a second temporary suture placed 15 mm higher in the anterior levator guides the procedure. At the end of the procedure, the upper lid traction suture is taped to the cheek for 1–2 days. The lid is, therefore, often left at the midpoint of the pupil or lower and gradually rises to the desired height after surgery.

Another skin approach utilizes a pedicle of tarsus that is rotated superiorly in order to lengthen the levator.[32]

Conjunctival Approach—Upper Lid. When there is 1–3 mm of lid retraction, a conjunctival approach in which Muller's muscle and conjunctiva are recessed 7 mm from the upper tarsal border is somewhat more predictable than the procedures just described.[33] After a frontal nerve block and local infiltration, a transmarginal traction suture is placed and the lid is everted on a Desmarres lid retractor (Plate 5-9). An incision is made just above the tarsus by grasping the conjunctiva and Muller's muscle and pulling these tissues away from the underlying levator. The conjunctiva and Muller's muscle are disinserted across the entire extent of the upper tarsus. The dissection is then extended at least 7 mm into the upper fornix. A 7–0 polyglactin (vicryl) suture is used to secure the conjunctiva and Muller's muscle to the internal surface of the levator aponeurosis 7 mm above the upper tarsal border. The effect can be enhanced by dissecting the levator attachments from the anterior tarsal surface and thereby creating a small levator dehiscence. This dissection should be carried out laterally where the retraction is usually most marked. Too aggressive a dissection will lead to overcorrection and ptosis.[34]

Skin Approach to Lower Lid Retraction. A subciliary skin incision is made after local infiltration with 1 percent lidocaine with epinephrine. We use epinephrine in the lower lid for hemostasis but not in the upper lid; epinephrine will have little or no effect on the capsulopalpebral fascia, which is less of a muscle than its upper lid Muller's muscle analogue. A skin muscle flap is mobilized down to the orbital rim (Plate 5-10). Prolapsing orbit fat is removed. If decompressive surgery is necessary, it may be performed at this time. Next, the lower lid retractors, Muller's muscle, and capsulopalpebral fascia are disinserted from their attachment to the lower tarsal border by button-holing all the tissues posterior to the skin muscle flap. The traction suture may be taped to the brow or the lower lid supported with ¼-inch steristrips.

Conjunctival Approach to Lower Lid. In this approach, Muller's and conjunctiva may be recessed 7 mm as in the upper lid technique. A lateral canthotomy may be performed and the decompression performed without a skin incision. .

Lateral Canthoplasty

A lateral tarsorrhaphy may enhance the effect of any of the procedures for eyelid retraction. Thyroid disease lengthens the horizontal dimension of the eyelids and, therefore, a lateral tarsorrhaphy restores anatomy. A permanent tarsorrhaphy is performed by splitting the lid at the gray line and mobilizing apposing tarsal conjunctival flaps and skin muscle flaps. The mucosal epithelium at the lid margin of the tarsal strip is excised. The tarsal conjunctival flaps are then sutured end-to-end with 5–0 chromic sutures. The lid margin, including the follicles in the skin muscle layer, are excised and the apposing lids are sutured with vertical mattress 6–0 silk sutures in order to ensure that the cilia are everted away from the globe. The tarsorrhaphy may later be opened to effect a desired horizontal palpebral fissure.

REFERENCES

1. Jones IS, Jakobiec FA, Nolan BT: Patient examination and introduction to orbital disease, in Duane TD (ed): *Clinical Ophthalmology*, Vol. 2. Philadelphia: Harper and Row, 1982, pp 1–30.
2. Beard C, Quickert MH: *Anatomy of the Orbit.* Birmingham, AL: Aesculapius, 1977.
3. Zide BM, Jelk GW: *Surgical Anatomy of the Orbit.* New York: Raven Press, 1985.
4. Warwick R: *Eugene Wolff's Anatomy of the Eye and Orbit.* Philadelphia: WB Saunders, 1976.
5. Mauriello JA, Flanagan JC: Lacrimal gland prolapse, in Smith B, Bosniak SL (eds): *Lacrimal Disorders, Advances in Ophthalmia Plastic and Reconstructive Surg*, Vol 3. New York: Pergamon, 1984, pp 341–347.
6. Mauriello JA, Gonzalez CF, Grossman CB, Flanagan JC: Orbital trauma in diagnostic imaging, in Gonzalez CF, Becker MH, Flanagan JC (eds): *Ophthalmology.* New York: Springer-Verlag, 1985, pp 323–342.
7. Reese AB: *Tumors of the Eye.* Hagerstown, MD: Harper and Row, 1976, pp 407, 413, 456.
8. Leone CR: Surgical approaches to the orbit. *Ophthalmology* 86:930–940, 1979.
9. Leone CR: Surgical approach to the medial retrobulbar space. *Am J Ophthalmol* 96:1–5, 1983.
10. Cooper WC, Harris GJ: Orbital surgery, in Duane TD, Jaeger EA (eds): *Clinical Ophthalmology,* Vol 5. Philadelphia: Harper and Row, 1982, pp 1–24.
11. Kennedy RE: Indications and surgical techniques for orbital exenteration. *Ophthalmology* 86:967–973, 1979.
12. Fox SA: *Ophthalmic Plastic Surgery.* Philadelphia; Grune & Stratton, 1976, pp 557–564.
13. Reese AB, Jones IS: Exenteration of the orbit and repair by transplantion of the temporalis muscle. *Am J Ophthalmol* 51:217, 1961.
14. Naquin HA: Orbital reconstruction utilizing temporalis muscle. *Am J Ophthalmol* 41:519, 1956.
15. Gass JDM: Technique of orbital exenteration utilizing methyl methacrylates implant and temporalis muscle flaps. *Arch Ophthalmol* 82:789, 1969.
16. Mauriello JA, Han K, Wolf R: Use of split-thickness dermal graft to line the exenterated orbit. *Am J Ophthalmol* 100:465–467, 1985.
17. Linberg JV, Anderson RL: Transorbital decompression. *Arch Ophthalmol* 99:113–119, 1981.
18. Trobe JD, Glaser JS, La Flamme P: Dysthyroid optic neuropathy. *Arch Ophthalmol* 96:1199–1209, 1978.
19. Frueh B, Musch DL, Grill R, et al; Orbital compliance in Graves' eye disease. *Ophthalmology* 92:657–665, 1985.

20. Kronlein RU; Zur Pathologie und operativen Behandlung der Dermoidcysten der Orbita. *Beitr Klin Chir* 4:149–163, 1889.
21. Sewall EC: Operative control of progressive exophthalmos. *Arch Otolaryngol* 24:6214, 1936.
22. Hirsch O: Surgical decompression of malignant exophthalmos. *Arch Otolaryngol* 51:325–334, 1950–1951.
23. Walsh TE, Ogura JH: Transantral orbital decompression for malignant exophthalmos. *Laryngoscope* 65:544, 1957.
24. Kennerdell JS, Maroon J: An orbital decompression for severe dysthyroid exophthalmos. *Ophthalmology* 89:467–472, 1982.
25. McCord CD: Current trends in orbital decompression. *Ophthalmology* 82:21–33, 1985.
26. Colvard DM, Waller RR, Neault RW, DeSanto LW: Nasolacrimal duct obstruction following transantral-ethmoidal orbital decompression. *Ophthalm Surg* 10:28, 1979.
27. Teng CS, Crombie AL, Hall R, Ross WM; An evaluation of supervoltage orbital irradiation for Graves' ophthalmopathy. *Clin Endocrinol* 13:545, 1980.
28. Hurbli R, Char DH, Harris J, et al: Radiation therapy for thyroid eye disease. *Am J Ophthalmol* 99:633–636, 1985.
29. Leone CR: The management of ophthalmic Graves' disease. *Ophthalmology* 91:770–779, 1984.
30. Shorr N, Seiff SR: The four stages of surgical rehabilitation of the patient with dysthyroid ophthalmopathy. *Ophthalmology* 93:476–483, 1986.
31. Grove AS: Upper eyelid retraction and Graves' disease. *Ophthalmology* 88:507–512, 1981.
32. Kohn R: Treatment of eyelid retraction with two pedicle tarsal rotation flaps. *Am J Ophthalmol* 95:539–544, 1983.
33. Henderson JW: Relief of eyelid retraction: A surgical approach. *Arch Ophthalmol* 74:205–216, 1965.
34. Putterman AM: Surgical treatment of thyroid-related upper eyelid retraction. *Ophthalmology* 188:507–512, 1981.

6

Lacrimal Gland Tumors and Inflammations

Joseph C. Flanagan
Joseph A. Mauriello
Thaddeus Nowinski
Mark Ruchman

INTRODUCTION

As in other areas of the orbit, the clinician must attempt to distinguish tumors from inflammations when dealing with lacrimal gland enlargements. This chapter is placed after Chapters 3 and 4 on orbital tumors because many of the processes that affect the orbit similarly affect the lacrimal gland. This chapter will concentrate on inflammations and tumors that are unique to the lacrimal gland area and do not occur elsewhere in the orbit or tumors and inflammations that have a unique expression in the lacrimal gland area.

A discussion of lacrimal gland anatomy will provide insight into the clinical manifestations of lacrimal gland tumors and inflammations.

ANATOMY OF THE LACRIMAL GLAND

The unencapsulated lacrimal gland is composed of two lobes that are flat and shaped like pancakes: the larger superior, orbital lobe and the smaller, inferior palpebral lobe. The two lobes are continuous posteriorly and divided anteriorly by Whitnall's ligament. The superior surface of the gland's orbital lobe is convex and covered by periosteum; the inferior surface is slightly concave and rests on the lateral expansion of the levator aponeurosis. The anterior border of the orbital lobe is in contact with the orbital septum. The palpebral lobe is approximately one-third the size of the orbital lobe and lies just below the orbital lobe in the superior fornix on the conjunctiva (Fig. 6-1). The ductules pass from the orbital lobe to the palpebral lobe into the upper fornix. Muller's muscle is present in the lateral aspect of the lacrimal gland.

Tumors tend to develop in an individual lobule, mostly in the orbital lobe, while inflammation affects all lobes and lobules. Inflammatory cells are normally present to some extent in the lacrimal gland.

During inflammation, the secretory cells succumb first and the duct cells survive and proliferate. In benign lymphoepithelial syndrome, the end result is the solid proliferation of terminal duct cells, epimyoepithelial islands in a sea of lymphocytes. The duct cells make secretory IgA, which binds to epithelial cells and thereby prevents bacteria from attaching to and injuring epithelial cells. Acinar cells make tears via eccrine secretion and contain PAS-positive zymogen granules.

DIFFERENTIAL DIAGNOSIS AND NOMENCLATURE

The differential of lacrimal gland tumors and inflammations is summarized in Table 6-1.

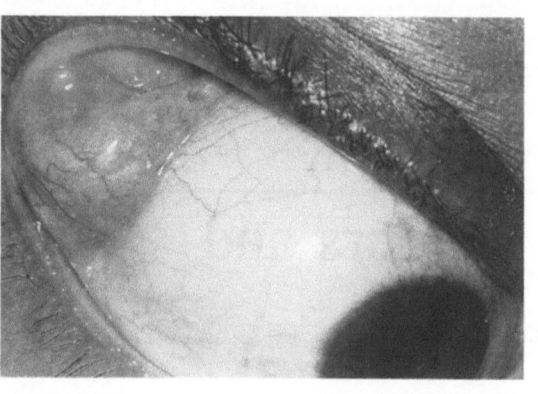

Fig. 6-1. Palpebral lobe of lacrimal gland is normally visible in upper fornix. Note lack of accompanying orbital fat prolapse.

Classic studies from referral centers and pathologic institutes report that 50 percent of lacrimal gland tumors are epithelial and 50 percent are inflammatory or lymphoid.[1-3] In clinical practice, probably greater than 95 percent of lacrimal gland enlargements are due to

Table 6-1
Lacrimal Gland Inflammations and Tumors

Pseudotumor (acute, subacute, or chronic dacryoadenitis)
Lymphoid infiltrate
Leukemia
Sarcoid
Sjögren's syndrome
Benign lymphoepithelial lesion
Wegener's granulomatosis
Cholesterol granuloma
Eosinophilic granuloma
Thyroid ophthalmopathy
Tumors
  epithelial (Benign)
    pleomorphic adenoma (benign mixed tumor, BMT)
  epithelial (Malignant)
    malignant mixed tumor
    adenoid cystic carcinoma
    mucoepidermoid carcinoma
    squamous cell carcinoma
    undifferentiated carcinoma
  cystic tumors
    dermoid cyst
    lacrimal gland duct cyst (dacryops)
  other tumors
    cavernous hemangioma
    neurofibroma
    schwannoma
    oncocytoma (also see Chapter 3)

inflammation and less than 5 percent are due to lacrimal gland tumors.

For the purposes of our discussion, dacryoadenitis and idiopathic pseudotumor are synonomous. Some of these patients will have bacterial dacryoadenitis; however, viral infections including infectious mononucleosis and mumps are more common.

HISTORY AND CLINICAL FEATURES

Lacrimal gland inflammations and tumors present as superotemporal quadrant masses. The chief historical questions concern duration of enlargement and presence of pain.

In general, processes that have been symptomatic for less than 6 months are either an inflammation or an epithelial malignancy. Inflammatory pseudotumors often have duration of only weeks, while lymphoid infiltrates have a more gradual onset over months. Pleomorphic adenomas will occur as a slowly enlarging lacrimal gland mass over years. Patients with a malignant mixed tumor became symptomatic within a 6-month period or had a preexisting benign mixed tumor that became malignant with a fulminant growth manifested by a history of less than 6 months.

Painful masses are pseudotumors and adenoid cystic carcinoma. Pain accompanies adenoid cystic carcinomas because of the propensity for the tumor to invade nerves. In one series, 9 of 10 patients had pain. Painless masses are lymphoid infiltrates, pleomorphic adenomas, chronic sclerosing pseudotumor or sarcoid.[4]

Pseudotumors with greater degrees of chronicity will have proportionately a greater duration of symptoms, less associated pain, and greater sclerosis or fibrosis on pathologic examination.

Lymphoid infiltrates do not present with pain as a rule and have a gradual onset (see Chapter 2). For the purposes of this discussion, lymphoid infiltrates are best conceptualized as tumors and not inflammation even though pathologically, they may be composed of chronic inflammatory cells.

In general, age can be a helpful part of the differential diagnosis. Pleomorphic adenoma is a disease of the 30- and 40-year age group, while adenoid cystic carcinoma appears in younger patients. In the largest series of patients with adenoid cystic carcinoma of the lacrimal gland, the mean age was 39.4 years with a range of from 12 to 74 years. Females predominate 59 percent to 41 percent males.[5] Lymphoid infiltrates occur in patients in the 50s and 60s.

Dermoid cysts occur in infants, children, and middle-aged adults. A history of trauma or inflammation may suggest why the dermoid has become recently symptomatic in an older patient.

OPHTHALMOLOGIC EXAMINATION

In general, vision is not affected in lacrimal gland inflammations or tumors. In one series, in a patient with acute dacryoadenitis, an accompanying scleritis and chorioidal effusion was responsible for decreased vision. In one patient with a lymphoid infiltrate, an afferent pupillary defect was present in the affected eye with a vision of 20/50. Another patient with advanced adenoid cystic carcinoma with frozen globe and decreased pupillary reaction had 20/200 vision.[6] The exact cause of the loss of vision in this patient is unclear from the report. Both situations are clearly the exception.

In general, patients with true tumors of the lacrimal gland, including patients with lymphoid infiltrates, are more likely to demonstrate displacement of globe, downward and inward, than patients with inflammatory disease of the lacrimal gland and are, therefore, likely to have diplopia. In contrast, patients with inflammatory processes will show a visible palpebral lobe of the lacrimal gland. The "s-shaped" curve of the swollen lid with a significant mechanical temporal ptosis is typical.

Patients with systemic disease such as sarcoid and thyroid ophthalmopathy often have bilateral palpebral lobe swellings. The palpebral lobe of the gland may be also visible by elevating the lids and observing the prolapsing palpebral lobe of the lacrimal globe on the conjunctival side.

Patients with inflammatory processes of the lacrimal gland such as pseudotumor, sarcoid, or thyroid ophthalmopathy with lacrimal gland enlargement, the lobular architecture of the gland is often preserved when palpated. This lobule architecture is less likely to be preserved with chronic sclerosing inflammations.

In tumors of the lacrimal gland such as pleomorphic adenoma or lymphoid infiltrates, the enlarged gland has a smooth palpable surface; individual lobules cannot be palpated.

Patients with bilateral lacrimal gland enlargement should have a medical work-up for systemic disease (Table 6-2). Bilateral disease is never due to an epithelial tumor. A complete ocular examination should include Schirmer's test for Sjögren's syndrome. A history of dry eye, dry mouth, and arthritis should also be obtained. Systemic lupus erythematosus should always be considered in the differential diagnosis. Infectious mononucleosis may present with lacrimal gland enlargement, and medical work-up is necessary in suspicious cases.

Patients with adenoid cystic carcinoma may develop symptoms of an orbital apex syndrome. Because of its tendency to grow along nerves, the tumor may invade the lacrimal nerve and ultimately involve the superior orbital fissure. The clinical spectrum of the orbital apex syndrome includes third, fourth, and sixth nerve deficit, ocular sympathetic paralysis, proptosis, and sometimes conjunctival chemosis. In addition, pain may result from

Table 6-2
Systemic Causes of Bilateral Lacrimal Gland Enlargement

Sarcoid*
Pseudotumor
Lymphoid*
Leukemia*
Thyroid
Sjögren's syndrome*
Benign lymphoepithelial lesion*
Wegener's granulomatosis
Systemic lupus erythematosus*
Tuberculosis*
Syphyllis*

* May have parotid or submandibular gland enlargements

tumor infiltration of the first and second divisions of the fifth nerve.

Patients with cystic masses in the lacrimal gland area will have a dermoid cyst or a lacrimal gland duct cysts (dacryops). A discussion of dermoid cysts is found in Chapter 4. Lacrimal gland duct cysts occur after trauma, infection, or inflammation or may arise spontaneously. When they arise in the palpebral lobe of the lacrimal gland, they may be seen clinically in the temporal cul de sac and are known as simple dacryops. They may also arise in the orbital lobe of the lacrimal gland, in the accessory lacrimal glands of Krause (fornix) and Wolfring (superior border of the tarsus), and in ectopic lacrimal gland tissue.

A simple dacryops or cyst of the palpebral lobe is often preceded by a history of inflammation or trauma. Pain may be present. The cyst will increase in size dramatically in response to weeping or exposure to cold. There may be a history of episodic decompression of the cyst associated with a rapid gush of tears. Symptoms of dry eye do not occur unless there is persistent or recurrent cyst since the integrity of the remainder of the lacrimal gland is preserved. The cyst is mobile, bluish-gray in color, and transilluminates. Cysts of the accessory lacrimal glands have a similar presentation to cysts of the palpebral lobe except that their location is not limited to the superotemporal quadrant; these cysts are quite rare.

Orbital lobe cysts are very rare and are often congenital, but clinical appearance may not occur for several years. The cyst often presents as a tense mass in an infant or young child with proptosis and downward nasal displacement of the globe.

All of the entities listed in Table 6-2 have been discussed in Chapter 2 except for Sjögren's syndrome and benign lymphoepithelial lesion. The latter is more common in the parotid than the lacrimal gland.

The gallium scan is extremely sensitive in detecting

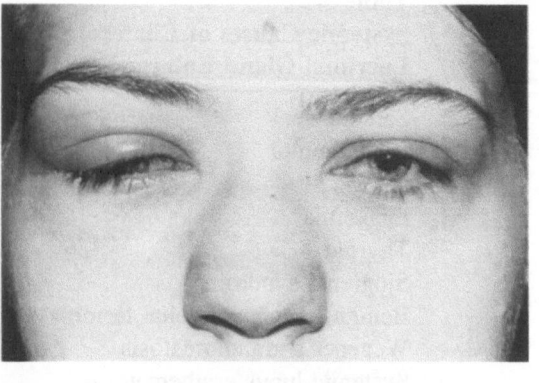

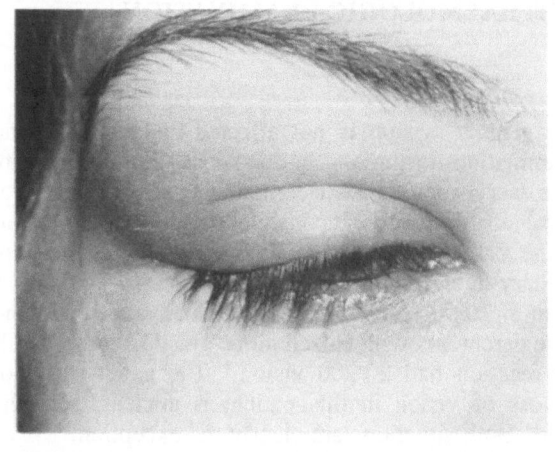

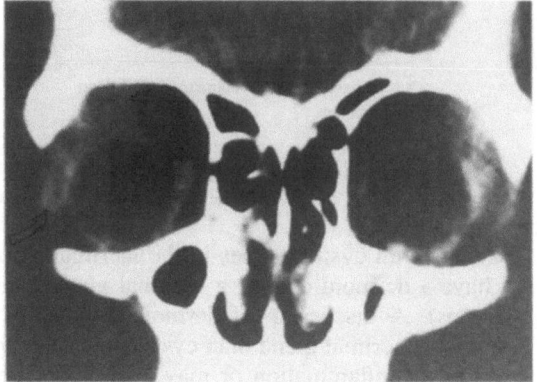

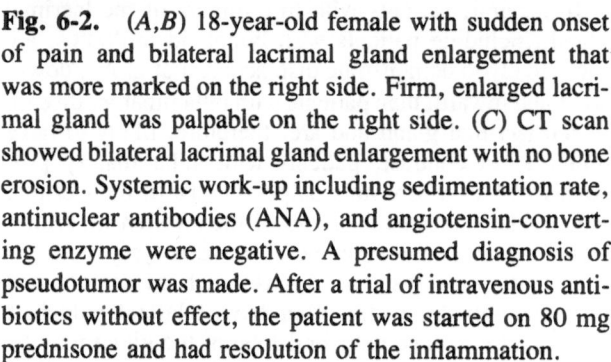

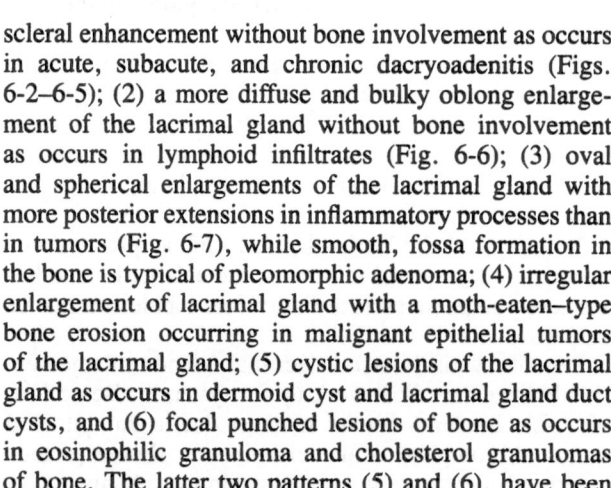

Fig. 6-2. (*A,B*) 18-year-old female with sudden onset of pain and bilateral lacrimal gland enlargement that was more marked on the right side. Firm, enlarged lacrimal gland was palpable on the right side. (*C*) CT scan showed bilateral lacrimal gland enlargement with no bone erosion. Systemic work-up including sedimentation rate, antinuclear antibodies (ANA), and angiotensin-converting enzyme were negative. A presumed diagnosis of pseudotumor was made. After a trial of intravenous antibiotics without effect, the patient was started on 80 mg prednisone and had resolution of the inflammation.

lacrimal gland enlargement in sarcoid. Serum angiotensin-converting enzyme and chest x-ray demonstrating hilar adenopathy should be obtained. Patients with bilateral lymphoid disease affecting the lacrimal glands should have a systemic work-up for lymphoma including bone marrow, serum protein electrophoresis, and abdominal computed tomography (CT) scan, along with a general medical evaluation as in all patients with bilateral lacrimal gland enlargement.

Patients with lacrimal gland enlargement may have thyroid ophthalmopathy. The presence of lid lag will separate this group of patients from patients with pseudotumor and myositis.

Patients with Wegener's granulomatosis may also have bilateral lacrimal gland swelling. This diagnosis should always be ruled out whenever there is concomitant sinus disease. Other systemic signs include pulmonary, kidney, or skin involvement.

CT SCAN FINDINGS

There are several possible CT scan patterns of inflammations and tumors involving the lacrimal gland area. These include: (1) oblong, contoured, diffuse enlargement of the lacrimal gland with or without a ring of scleral enhancement without bone involvement as occurs in acute, subacute, and chronic dacryoadenitis (Figs. 6-2–6-5); (2) a more diffuse and bulky oblong enlargement of the lacrimal gland without bone involvement as occurs in lymphoid infiltrates (Fig. 6-6); (3) oval and spherical enlargements of the lacrimal gland with more posterior extensions in inflammatory processes than in tumors (Fig. 6-7), while smooth, fossa formation in the bone is typical of pleomorphic adenoma; (4) irregular enlargement of lacrimal gland with a moth-eaten–type bone erosion occurring in malignant epithelial tumors of the lacrimal gland; (5) cystic lesions of the lacrimal gland as occurs in dermoid cyst and lacrimal gland duct cysts, and (6) focal punched lesions of bone as occurs in eosinophilic granuloma and cholesterol granulomas of bone. The latter two patterns (5) and (6), have been described in Chapters 3 and 4.

Calcifications occur in dermoid cysts, malignant lacrimal gland tumors, and vascular lesions (Table 6-3, Chapter 3).

Differential Diagnosis Based on CT Pattern, Biopsy Technique and Results

CT Pattern of Oblong and Contoured Enlargement of the Lacrimal Gland without Bone Involvement. This pattern is observed in dacryoadenitis. In

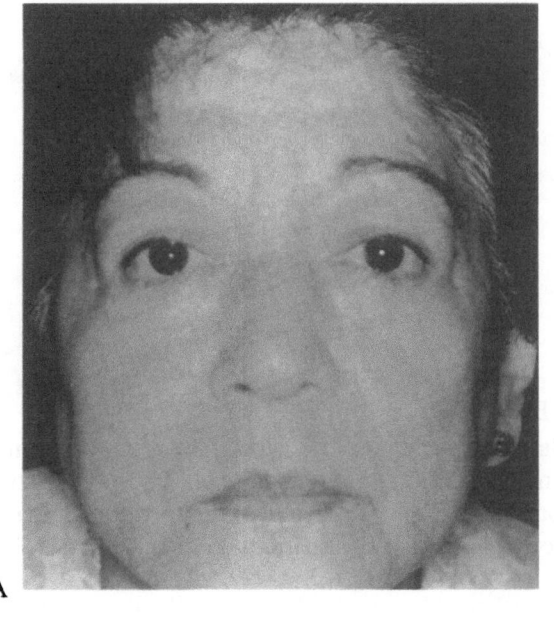

A

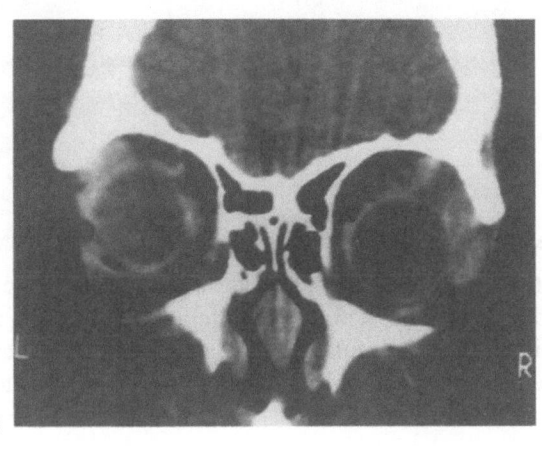

B

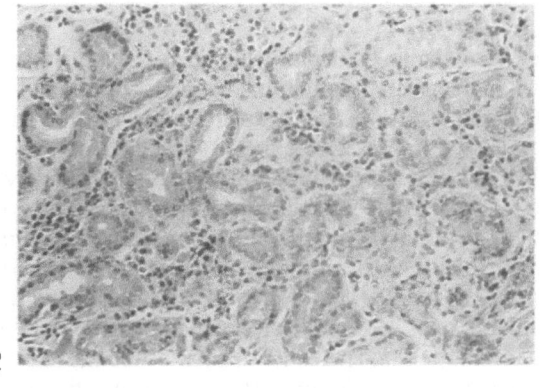

C

Fig. 6-3. (A) 55-year-old female with moderate bilateral lacrimal gland and submandibular gland enlargement. (B) CT scan showed bilateral lacrimal gland enlargement. (C) Biopsy showed nonspecific dacryoadenitis consistent with pseudotumor. Work-up showed evidence of systemic lupus erythematosus. Lacrimal gland enlargement responded to trial of prednisone. (Patient referred by Dr. D. Cinotti, Jersey City, NJ.)

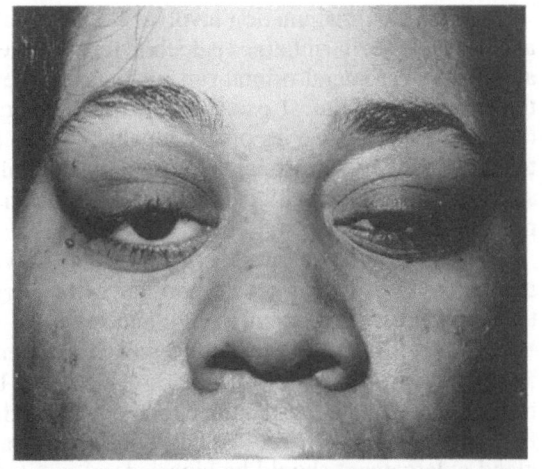

A

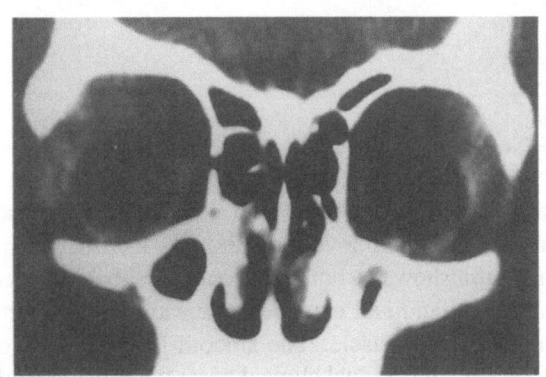

B

Fig. 6-4. (A) 36-year-old female with bilateral lacrimal gland enlargement seen on coronal CT scan. (B) Elevated serum angiotensin-converting enzyme suggested clinical diagnosis of sarcoid that was also supported by a conjunctival biopsy of the lacrimal gland showing noncaseating granuloma consistent with sarcoidosis.

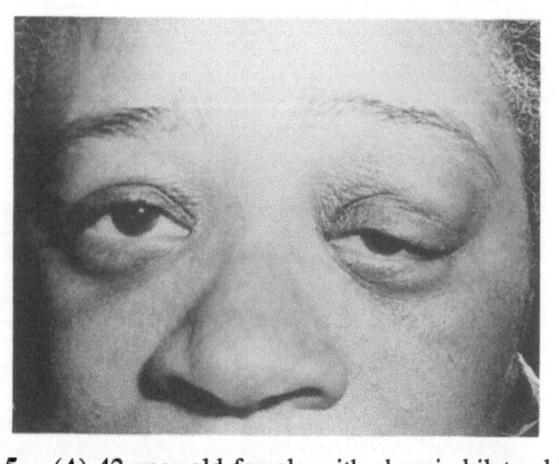

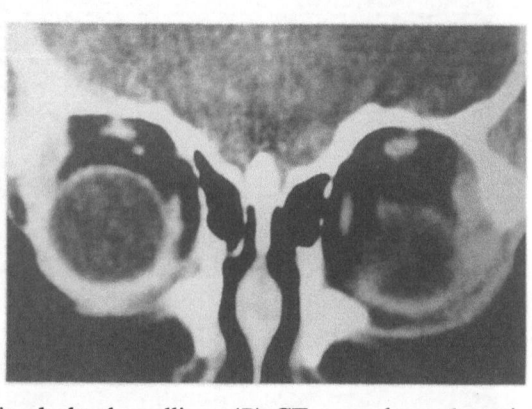

Fig. 6-5. (A) 42-year-old female with chronic bilateral lacrimal gland swelling. (B) CT scan showed a minimal infiltrate that suggested a pseudotumor rather than a lymphoid infiltrate. Systemic work-up was negative for sarcoid, collagen vascular disease, and Wegener's granulomatosis. Biopsy (not shown) shows lacrimal gland with marked sclerosis and only minimal chronic inflammatory cells present. Patient partially responded to steroid trial.

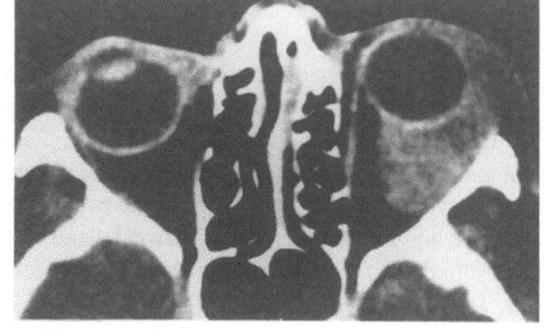

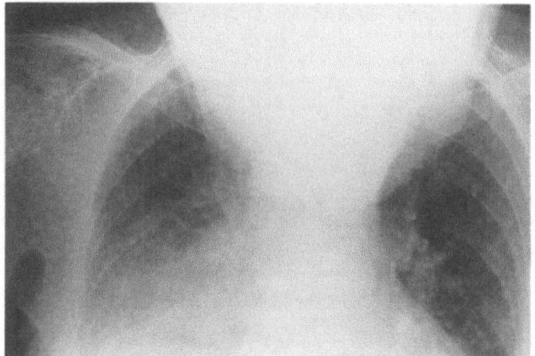

Fig. 6-6. (A) CT scan of 82-year-old female with onset of painless proptosis involving the left lacrimal gland area and orbit showed a homogeneous mass that involved the lacrimal gland and extended posteriorly, infiltrating the lateral rectus muscle. The smooth borders, lack of bone erosion, and gradual clinical onset favor the diagnosis of lymphoid infiltrate. Biopsy showed a well-differentiated lymphoma. (B) Chest x-ray showed evidence of hilar adenopathy consistent with lymphoma.

dacryoadenitis the architecture of the gland is preserved, and edema anal inflammatory cells fill both lobes of the gland. The gland is enlarged but at the same time appears compressed between the globe and the bone. In the acute stage, inflammation often spills over and affects the adjacent lateral rectus in a myositis-type pattern. With myositis, there is an irregular fluffy involvement of the entire muscle and its tendon with irregular margins, unlike thyroid myositis which causes a fusiform enlargement of the muscle with smooth borders and inflammation that spares the tendon of the muscle. Scleral enhancement with contrast is a nonspecific finding in inflammatory lesions that occurs along the epibulbar plane. Scleral enhancement is more likely to occur with acute dacryoadenitis than with chronic forms as in sarcoid.

Because the inflammation involves both the palpebral and orbital lobe, the inflamed palpebral lobe often extends anterior to the lateral orbital rim in the axial view. For this reason, on clinical examination the palpebral lobe of the lacrimal gland is often palpable. Since tumors tend to involve the orbital lobe of the lacrimal gland and spare the palpebral lobe, most of the expansion occurs posteriorly.

The key to this diagnosis is the fact that on viewing the lesion on CT scan, there appears to be very little to biopsy other than an enlarged gland.

In bilateral disease or recurrent unilateral disease, an appropriate work-up for systemic disease should be performed. Biopsy of recurrent unilateral cases is indicated. In addition, patients with parotid gland or submaxillary gland enlargement should be biopsied.

The biopsy results will be similar to those of pseudotumors elsewhere in the orbit. Noncaseating granuloma may strongly suggest a diagnosis of sarcoid; clinical

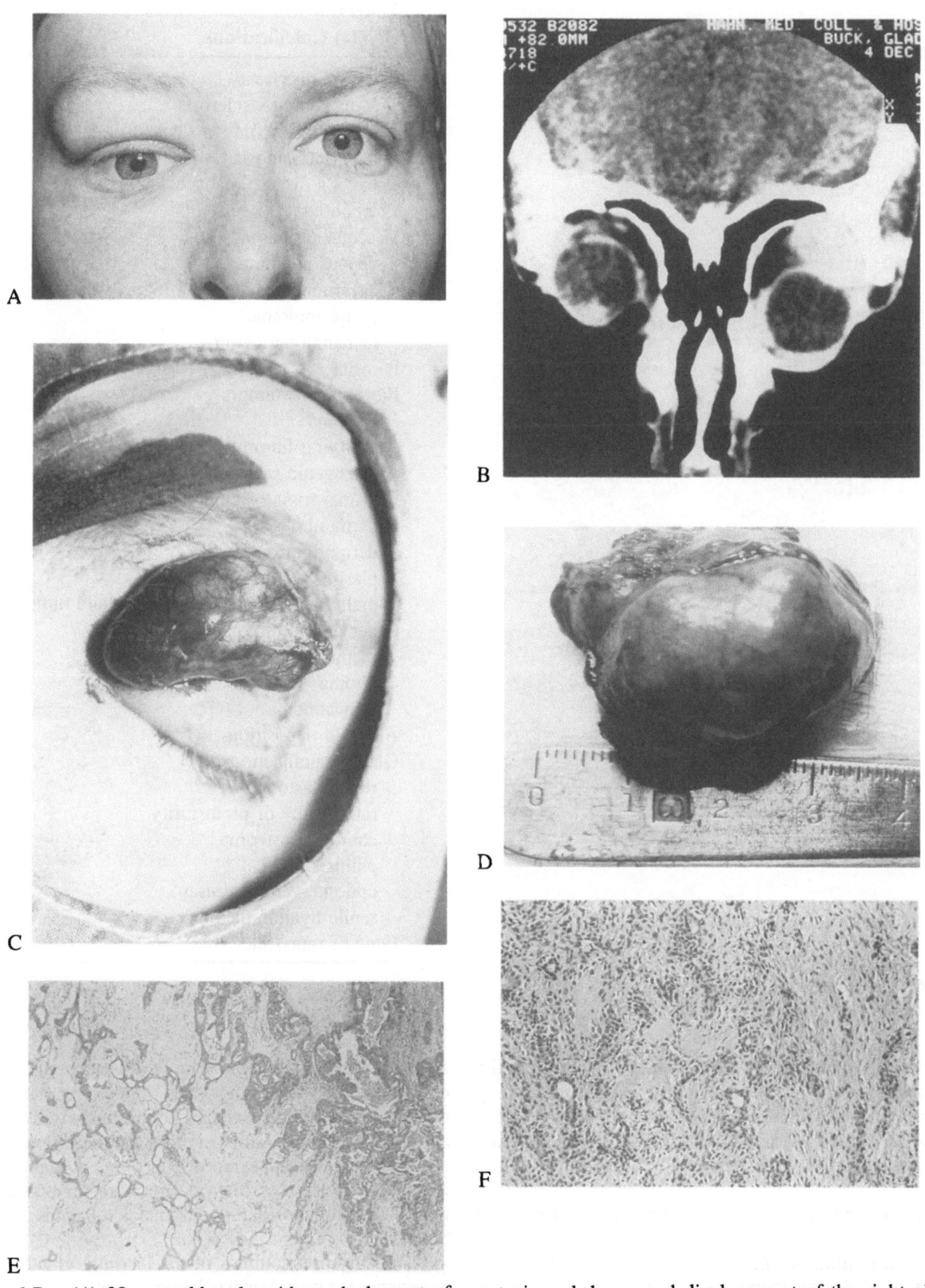

Fig. 6-7. (*A*) 38-year-old male with gradual onset of proptosis and downward displacement of the right globe. (*B*) CT scan showed a well-localized lacrimal gland mass without bone erosion. (*C,D*) Intraoperatively, an encapsulated mass was removed. Excisional biopsy showed a benign mixed tumor of the lacrimal gland. (*E,F*) The tumor is composed of epithelial cells that form ductule elements. There is a myxoid stroma. (*G*) Note thin pseudocapsule with abutting epithelial elements. (*H*) Compare CT scan in above patient (*B*) with that of patient with adenoid cystic carcinoma. Note bone erosion of lateral orbital wall. (*I*) Multinodular recurrent benign mixed tumor. Each nodule represents a focus of recurrent tumor.

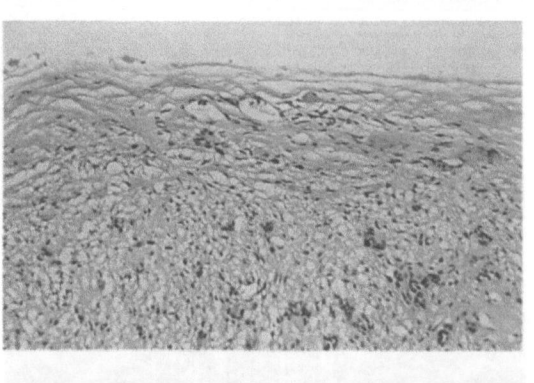

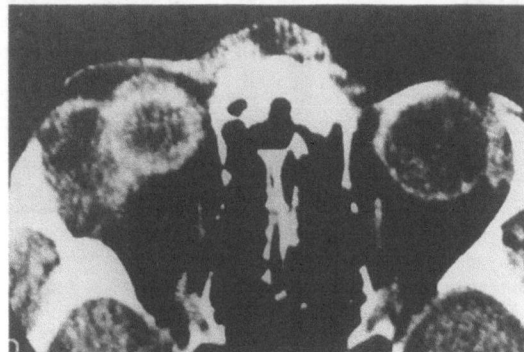

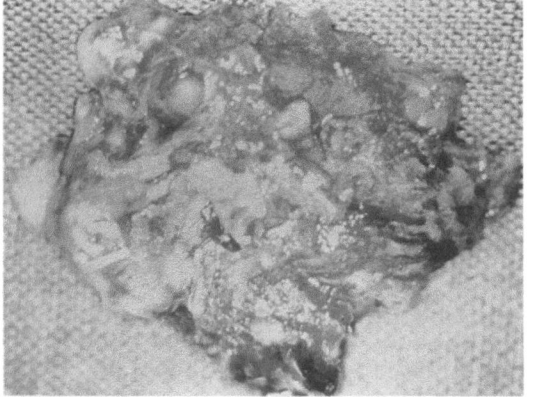

Fig. 6-7 (continued)

Table 6-3
Orbital Calcifications

Systemic disease
   Monckeberg's sclerosis
   hyperparathyroidism
   hypervitaminosis
   Paget's disease of bone
Phleboliths
Vascular lesions
   venous angioma
   cavernous hemangioma
   lymphangioma
   hemangiopericytoma
Parasite
Fibroosseous tumors
   osteoma
   ossifying fibroma
   osteogenic sarcoma
Lacrimal fossa calcifications
   dermoid cysts
   dermolipoma
   plasmacytoma
   malignant epithelial lacrimal gland tumor
Other orbital tumors
   meningioma
   glioma
   schwannoma
Amyloid deposition
Ocular calcifications
   retinoblastoma
   retinopathy of prematurity
   choroidal osteoma
   phthisis bulbi
   optic nervehead drusen
   senile hyaline plaque
Edge of mucocele

correlation and work-up are necessary to confirm the diagnosis.

Oral prednisone, 60–80 mg/day rapidly tapered after 10–14 days, may be instituted after a trial of systemic antibiotics as outlined in Chapter 2.

Diffuse and Bulky Enlargement of the Lacrimal Gland. The difference between a dacryoadenitis and lymphoid infiltrate of the lacrimal gland on CT scan is a matter of degree (compare Fig. 6-2C, 6-4, or 6-5B with Fig. 6-6B. In the case of a lymphoid infiltrate, there is a mass to biopsy. The lymphoid infiltrate mass enlargement appears larger on axial and coronal views than does dacryoadenitis, but the lacrimal gland enlarge-

ment tends to be more oblong and diffuse than the spherical enlargement of a tumor. The oblong enlargement is evident on viewing the edges of the mass on coronal and axial CT scans. This pattern is quite different from the round-to-oval appearance of a tumor. Again, there is no bone erosion as often occurs with tumors. There may be inflammation of the adjacent lateral rectus muscle. Scleral enhancement may occur.

Sclerosing pseudotumor of the lacrimal gland in our experience is a more localized process than its counterpart elsewhere in the orbit. Sclerosing pseudotumor of the lacrimal gland tends to enlarge the lacrimal gland but does not fill the orbit as much as a lymphoma of the orbit. The presence of streak densities on CT scan that are due to fibrosis are helpful in differentiating patients with sclerosing pseudotumor from those with lymphoid infiltrate. In the lacrimal gland, sclerosing pseudotumor is more likely to be confused with a benign mixed tumor that has not caused bone erosion than with a lymphoid infiltrate of the lacrimal gland since the latter is more diffuse.

Bilaterality is also an extremely helpful diagnostic feature. Bilateral involvement does not occur with epithelial tumors, is rare with lymphoid infiltrates, and is more common with pseudotumor of the lacrimal gland or systemic diseases such as sarcoid and thyroid ophthalmopathy.

Incisional Biopsy Technique. Incisional biopsy of a presumed lymphoid infiltrate of the orbital lobe of the lacrimal gland is indicated through a lid transseptal incision. The palpebral lobe may be utilized to perform a snip biopsy of the palpebral lobe of the lacrimal gland. Care must be taken not to injure the lacrimal gland ductules in the superotemporal conjunctival fornix. The orbital septum and levator may be opened in a vertical fashion to avoid lagophthalmos from septal scarring and ptosis.[7] Alternatively, a brow incision may be performed and a superior orbitotomy via a transperiosteal approach may be utilized.

Biopsy results will parallel those elsewhere in the orbit and so may show reactive lymphoid hyperplasia, atypical reactive lymphoid hyperplasia, or malignant lymphoma. Appropriate oncologic work-up for systemic disease and treatment as outlined in Chapter 3 is necessary. Hodgkin's disease may affect the lacrimal gland.

In addition, benign lymphoepithelial lesion will show proliferating terminal duct cells to form epimyoepithelial islands within a sea of lymphocytes (Fig. 6-8). This rare histologic pattern is consistent with Sjögren's syndrome. Lymphomas rarely have been documented to develop from inflammatory infiltrates associated with Sjögren's syndrome. The term *Mickulicz's disease* or *syndrome* is confusing and should be abandoned.

CT Pattern of Oval and Spherical Enlargement of the Lacrimal Gland with Fossa Formation. In pleomorphic adenoma, the enlargement occurs more posteriorly and the edges of the tumor are rounded and regular. The compressed bone in the lacrimal fossa may be smoothly excavated.

A lateral orbitotomy should be performed for total excision of the tumor. An anterior orbitotomy is not recommended because it often leads to a subtotal or piecemeal removal of the lesion with possible seeding of the incision site. Recurrence has been definitely linked to incisional biopsy where multiple tumor nodules result. The recurrence rate for incisional biopsy of incomplete excision is ten times higher than excision within an intact pseudocapsule.[8] The chance of malignant transformation of incompletely excised and recurrent benign mixed tumors increases with length of time. Removal of the unin-

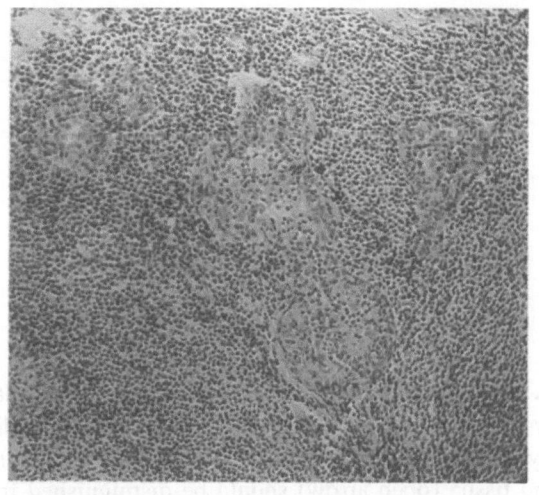

Fig. 6-8. Biopsy of benign lymphoepithelial lesion shows proliferating ductule composed of epithelial cells in sea of lymphocytes.

volved palpebral lobe, adjacent tarsus, conjunctiva, and aponeurosis has been advocated by some authors. The importance of careful preoperative evaluation to avoid a mistaken diagnosis and inappropriate incisional biopsy of a pleomorphic adenoma cannot be overemphasized.

Biopsy shows a bosselated multilobulated mass that has a pseudocapsule. A mixture of epithelial and connective tissue elements are present. Tubular structures are arranged in an irregular anastomosing pattern in a myxoid stroma. The ducts are lined by a double layer of epithelium. The inner layer of epithelial cells may secrete mucus or undergo squamous metaplasia. The outer layer of epithelial cells may undergo metaplasia to form myxoid, fibroid, and cartilaginous stromal tissue.[9] Tumors that are histologically identical to benign mixed tumors of the lacrimal gland may arise from the sweat glands of the lid skin. Other tumors such as capillary hemangioma may mimic a benign mixed tumor (Fig. 6-9).

Recurrence is best treated by complete surgical excision through a lateral orbitotomy, since malignant degeneration may occur (Fig. 6-10).

Biopsy may also show cavernous hemangioma,[10] and may show localized neurofibroma or schwannoma.[11]

Biopsy shows cells arranged in a glandular pattern or as sheets of cells. The cells are large, uniform cells that are polyhedral in shape and have abundant granular eosinophilic cytoplasm. The nuclei are small, round, and paracentral with a single nucleolus. Mitoses are infrequent. The diagnosis is oncocytoma or oxyphilic adenoma. The oncocyte cells are thought to be derived from myoepithelial cells and are often found normally in the salivary, parathyroid, thyroid, pituitary, adrenal glands, gastrointestinal tract, and other locations.[12] Isolated nontumorous aggregates of these cells have been reported in 7 of 20 normal lacrimal glands at autopsy.[13]

Oncocytomas are more common in the caruncle than

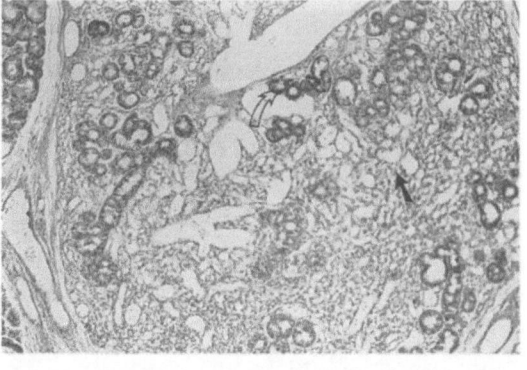

Fig. 6-9. Capillary hemangioma of the lacrimal gland may present similar to a benign mixed tumor both clinically and on CT scan (AFIP ACC #1428113). Lacrimal gland tissue (open arrow) should be distinguished from capillary hemangioma (solid arrow).

in the lacrimal gland or orbit and are generally benign. Five reported malignant onocytomas have involved the ocular adnexa: three involved the lacrimal gland, two of which had intracranial extension, and two involved the lacrimal sac, one of which had maxillary sinus involvement.[13,14]

CT Pattern of Irregular Enlargement of Lacrimal Gland with Motheaten Bone. With malignant mixed tumor or adenoid cystic carcinoma as with benign mixed tumor, the mass generally does not extend anteriorly beyond the orbital rim since all tumors begin from one focus within the lacrimal gland. While a pleomorphic adenoma has rounded and sharply demarcated edges in all directions with smooth excavation of bone in the lacrimal gland fossa, adenoid cystic carcinoma and malignant mixed tumors have irregular serpiginous contours with a motheaten destructive infiltrating tumor pattern much like advanced metastatic carcinoma elsewhere in the orbit (Figs. 6-10 and 6-11). In 75 percent of cases of adenoid cystic carcinoma of the lacrimal gland, bone involvement was present; in 7 percent of cases, the sinuses were involved.[5]

In general, the presence of calcifications in the fossa of the lacrimal gland indicates a malignant process.[4,6,15–18] A recent report stresses that clinical correlation is warranted. Progressive symptoms must be correlated with the CT scan findings. Other cases of orbital and ocular calcifications are listed in Table 6-3.

Unlike cases of presumed pleomorphic adenoma where excisional biopsy is indicated, in suspected cases of adenoid cystic carcinoma or malignant mixed tumor, incisional biopsy is indicated. The following biopsy results are possible. In 9 of 79 tumors reported by Font and Gamel, a preexisting pleomorphic adenoma was found.[5] This fact underlines the need for follow-up in all patients with benign mixed tumors.

Biopsy shows several possible forms of adenoid cystic carcinoma:

1. "Swiss cheese" cribriform appearance in which biopsy shows multiple lobules with a prominent cribriform pattern (Fig. 6-12). The tumor is composed of aggregates of small, tightly packed cells. The cells are undifferentiated and contain hyperchromatic nuclei and scanty cytoplasm. Mucin is contained in the cystic foci.
2. Sclerosing pattern that shows alternating hyalinized cylinders of connective tissue and elongated epithelial cords. It is this type that arose from the mucous glands of the accessory nasal sinuses that Billroth termed "cylindroma" in 1859.[19] When compressed in the pathology lab, such tumors express the hyalinized cylinders of connective tissue much like when toothpaste is expressed from its tube.
3. Basaloid or solid nests of cells without cribriform pattern (see Fig. 6-11*D*).
4. Comedocarcinoma, which is characterized by large epithelial lobules with foci of central necrosis.
5. Tubular pattern, which is composed of elongated and comma-shaped epithelial tubules lined by two or three layers of cells. Some tubules may show lumens that contain acidophilic material.

Other biopsy results include:

1. Malignant mixed tumors, which have the basic pattern of a benign mixed tumor but have sufficient malignant cytologic features to be labelled malignant and adenocarcinomas. In approximately 25 percent of the cases, the tumor may appear as an adenoid cystic carcinoma. These tumors may also undergo squamous differentiation and form squamous cell carcinoma or sebaceous differentiation to form sebaceous gland carcinomas. Sarcomatous malignant deterioration is the least common form. Malignant mixed tumors may arise from a preexisting benign mixed tumor that had been present for years, after a surgical debulking or incomplete excision of a benign mixed tumor, or de novo. In all cases, there is a rapid onset of symptoms within 6–12 months.
2. Mucoepidermoid carcinoma, undifferentiated carcinoma, and squamous cell carcinoma. All of these tumors share a poor prognosis and require radical treatment.

Management of all suspected malignant epithelial tumor of the lacrimal gland includes incisional biopsy followed by radical surgery.[20] Such surgery includes exenteration with removal of orbital bone adjacent to the tumor and requires a team approach with a neurosurgeon and orbital surgeon. Overall, in the case of adenoid cystic carcinoma, the 10-year actuarial survival is approximately 20 percent. Radical surgery appears to signifi-

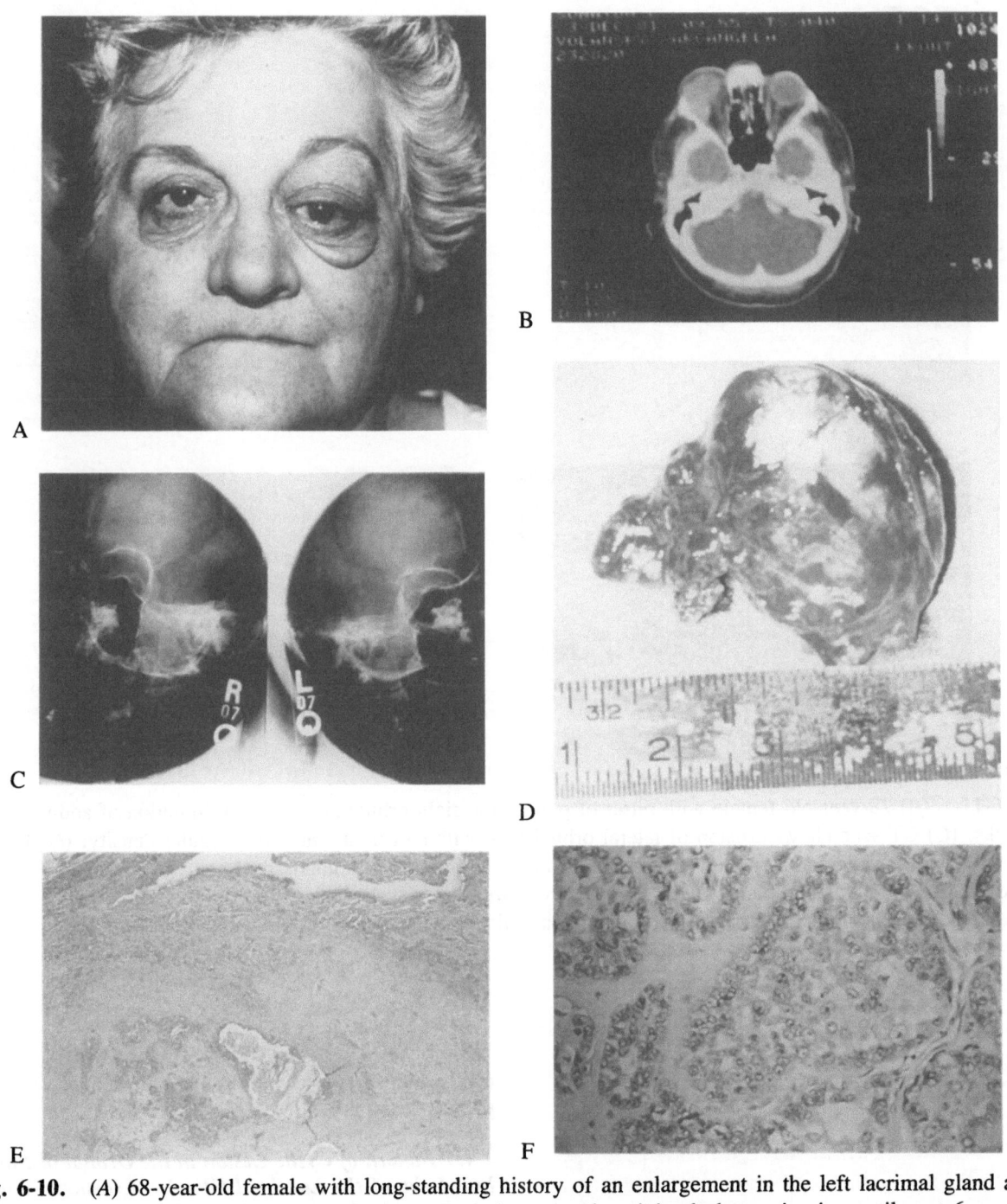

Fig. 6-10. (*A*) 68-year-old female with long-standing history of an enlargement in the left lacrimal gland area. The mass had been present for at least 10 years and showed only minimal change in size until past 6 months, during which the mass almost doubled in size. (*B*) CT scan shows a lacrimal mass extending along the lateral orbital wall posteriorly with possible bone erosion. (*C*) Plain x-ray shows bone erosion in lacrimal gland fossa on left side. (*D*) Intraoperatively, an irregular mass was found. (*E,F*) Biopsy showed aggregates of cells that resembled a mixed cell tumor. However, cytologic atypia suggested the diagnosis of malignant mixed tumor.

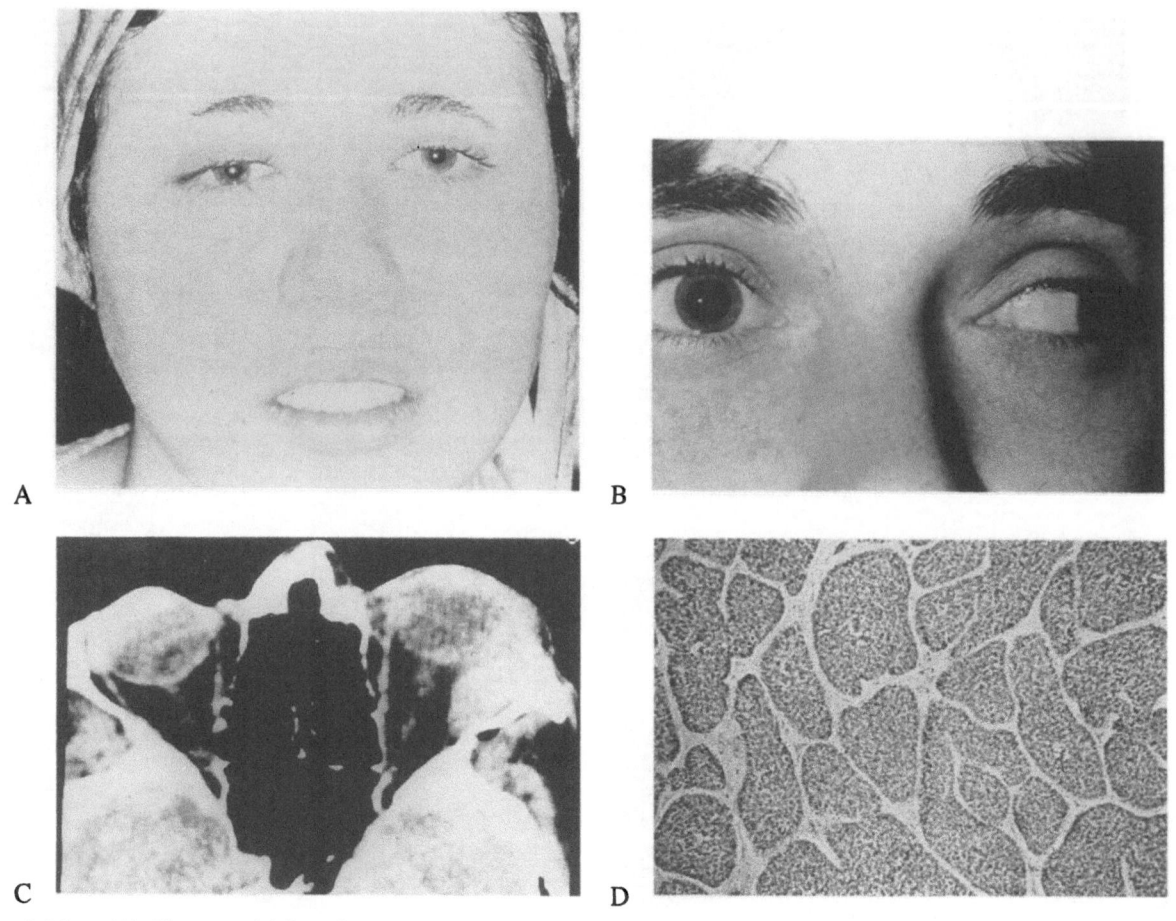

Fig. 6-11. (*A*) 28-year-old female with onset of pain in the right orbital area and (*B*) limitation of adduction for 3 weeks. (*C*) CT scan shows erosion of lateral orbital wall with soft tissue mass of irregular density. (*D*) Biopsy showed adenoid cystic carcinoma of the lacrimal gland. The tumor was composed of aggregates of small, tightly packed cells with hyperchromatic nuclei and scanty cytoplasm. Hyalinized stroma is present between the cell aggregates. The histologic pattern is typical of the basaloid form of adenoid cystic carcinoma.

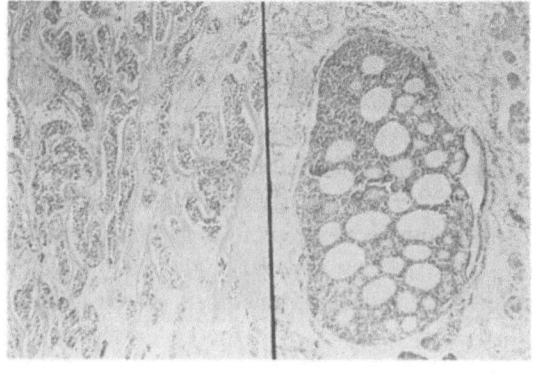

Fig. 6-12. Note "swiss cheese" pattern within nests of tumor cells on the right. Note baseloid pattern of adenoid cystic carcinoma on the left (AFIP ACC #482842).

cantly influence survival. Radiotherapy appears to be palliative and not curative.

CT Pattern of Cystic Lesion in the Orbital or Palpebral Lobe of the Lacrimal Gland. Excisional biopsy of palpebral lobe cyst is best performed via a transconjunctival cul-de-sac approach.[21–23] Lateral cantholysis may enhance exposure. Vigorous surgical manipulation may damage the lacrimal ducts. A lateral orbitotomy may be required in some cases where the cyst extends posteriorly. Tumors of the orbital lobe are best approached via a lateral orbitotomy. A dry eye may result from excision. A preoperative Schirmer's test is necessary. In patients with dry eye, marsupialization of the cyst has been recommended.[22]

Biopsy shows usually two layers of epithelium, an inner low cuboidal layer and an outer myoepithelial layer.

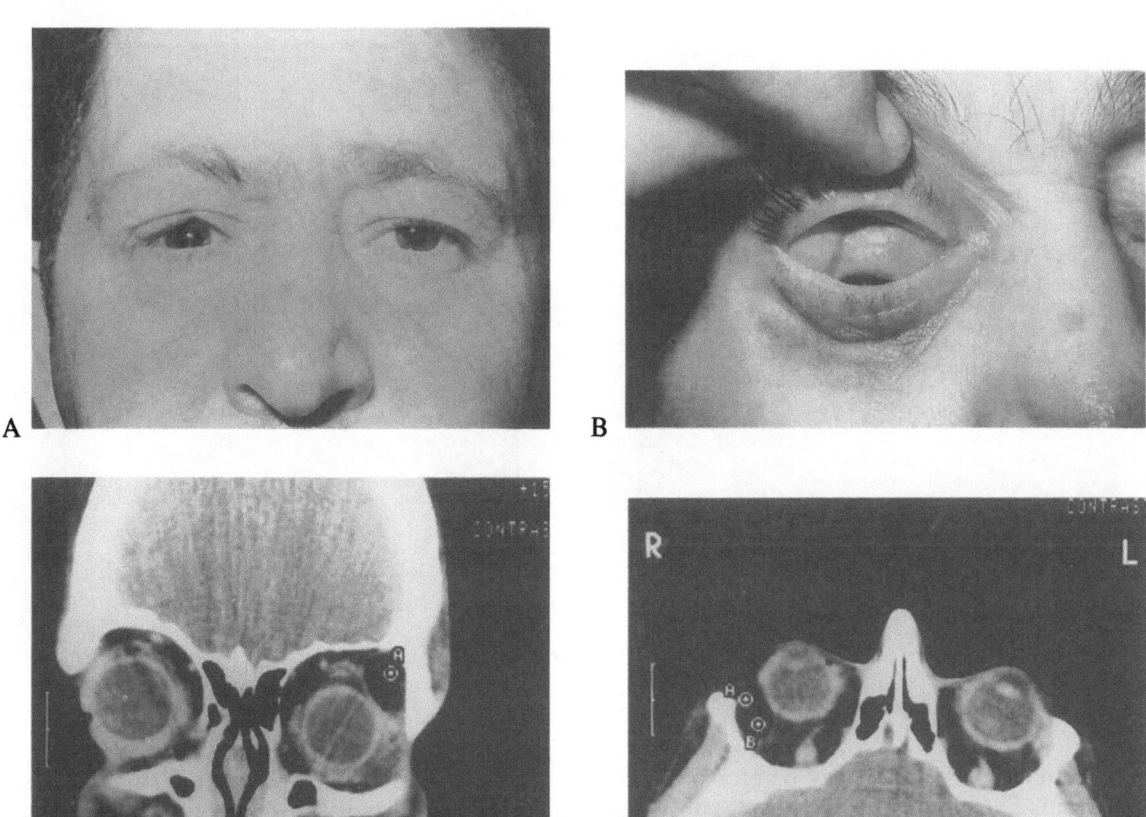

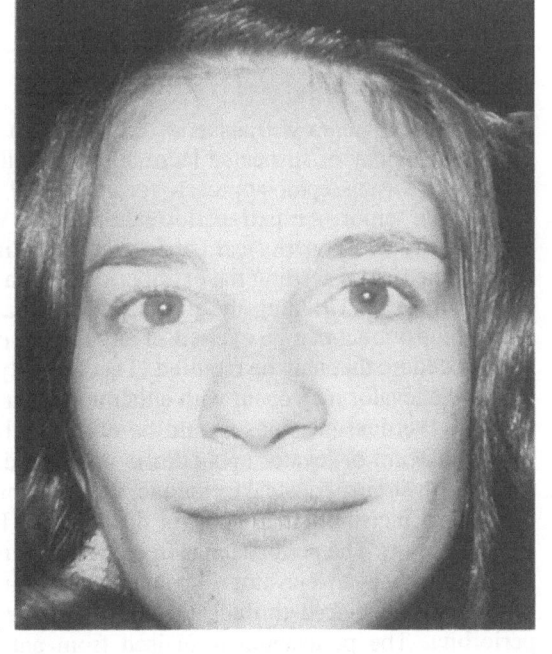

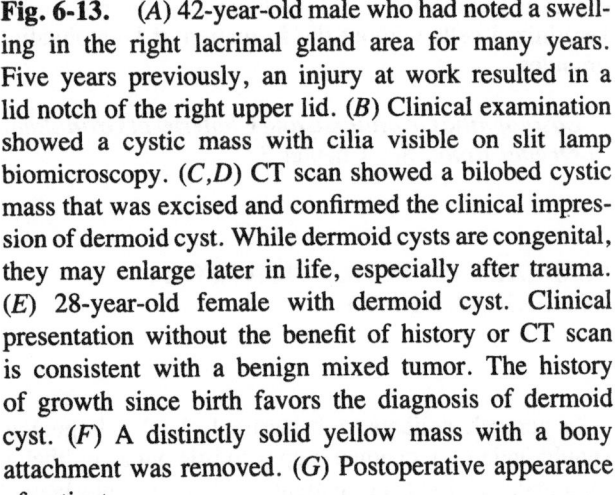

Fig. 6-13. (*A*) 42-year-old male who had noted a swelling in the right lacrimal gland area for many years. Five years previously, an injury at work resulted in a lid notch of the right upper lid. (*B*) Clinical examination showed a cystic mass with cilia visible on slit lamp biomicroscopy. (*C,D*) CT scan showed a bilobed cystic mass that was excised and confirmed the clinical impression of dermoid cyst. While dermoid cysts are congenital, they may enlarge later in life, especially after trauma. (*E*) 28-year-old female with dermoid cyst. Clinical presentation without the benefit of history or CT scan is consistent with a benign mixed tumor. The history of growth since birth favors the diagnosis of dermoid cyst. (*F*) A distinctly solid yellow mass with a bony attachment was removed. (*G*) Postoperative appearance of patient.

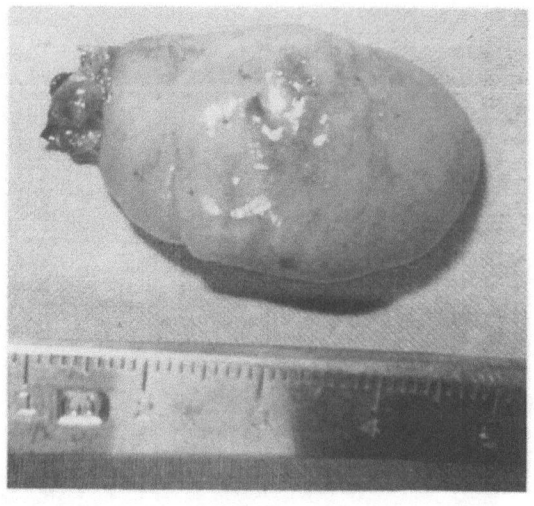

F

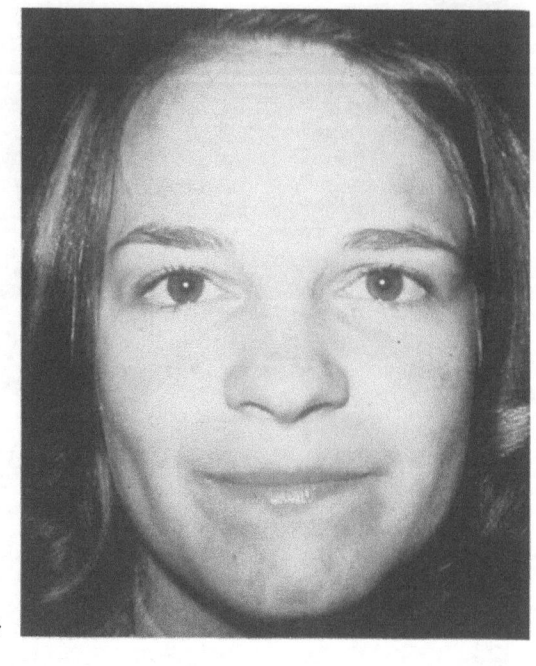

G

Fig. 6-13 (continued)

Adjacent lacrimal gland tissue may be present. A conjunctival cyst is lined by nonkeratinizing stratified squamous epithelium with variable numbers of goblet cells. A mucocele is lined by respiratory-type epithelium with pseudostratified columnar cells with cilia. An epidermoid inclusion cyst is lined by epidermis, that is, keratinizing squamous epithelial cells with a superficial granular layer containing keratohyaline granules, and a dermoid cyst is lined by epidermis with pilosebaceous units, eccrine (sweat glands) glands, and sometimes apocrine glands (Figs. 6-13 and 6-14). Tricholemmomal keratinization associated with pilar cysts produces large homogeneous keratinized cells without the formation of keratohyaline granules.

Eosinophilic Granuloma and Cholesterol Granuloma of Orbital Bone. See Chapter 3.

SUMMARY OF INDICATIONS FOR INCISIONAL BIOPSY

In general, patients with lacrimal gland enlargement should undergo incisional biopsy to rule out an epithelial malignancy. However, patients with a possible benign mixed tumor should have an en-block excision to avoid multinodular recurrence. In addition, patients with a short history (less than one month) with infectious signs should have a trial of oral antibiotics prior to incisional biopsy. Patients with a presumed inflammatory pseudotumor may receive a trial of oral prednisone. In both instances, lesions that do not show resolution require incisional biopsy.[16]

SPECIAL CONSIDERATIONS IN GLAND LACRIMAL SURGERY

We favor a subbrow transperiosteal approach for the incisional biopsy of suspected lacrimal gland inflammations and a transseptal approach for incisional biopsy of possible tumor. An extraperiosteal approach violates the integrity of the periosteal barrier and potentially increases the risk of seeding the extraperiosteal space with malignant cells. Utilizing the transseptal approach, the entire biopsy tract can be excised in any further extirpation procedure that may be required. Theoretically, damage to the levator may occur with either approach. When possible, vertical incisions should be utilized whenever the periosteum or levator aponeurosis is violated.[7]

Using the transperiosteal technique, the surgeon makes a subbrow incision that is brought down to the bone at the orbital rim. The periosteum is freed from the underlying bone using an elevator. A running traction suture of 4–0 silk is placed through the anterior edge of the periorbita. The periosteum is incised from anterior to posterior. We suture periorbita to periosteum at the orbital rim at the end of the procedure. This approach clearly does not allow for complete excision of posterior tumors (see Chapter 5).

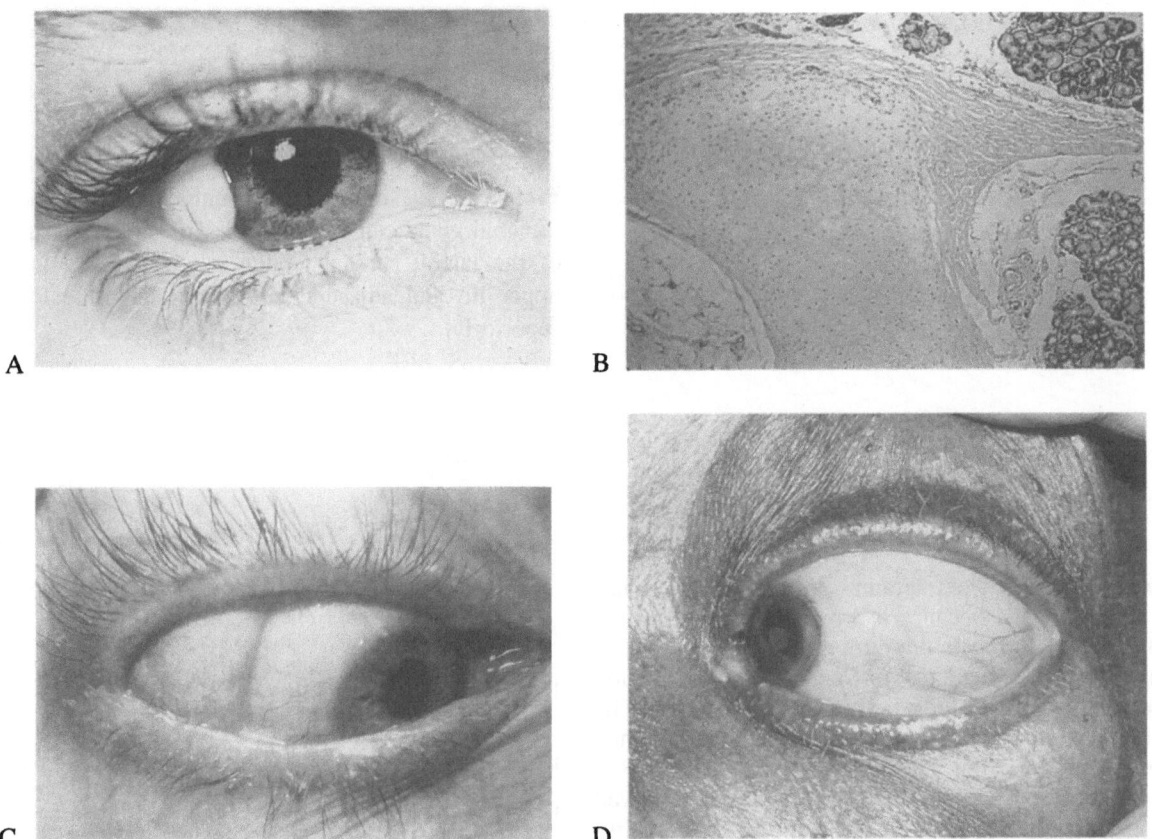

Fig. 6-14. (*A*) A dermoid of the limbus is a solid tumor and is to be distinguished from a dermoid cyst. (*B*) Most often this tumor is composed of fat and collagen. The limbal tumor is termed a *complex choristoma* when cartilage and lacrimal gland tissue are present. (*C*) Dermoids may also be located away from the limbus. The mass is firm, well-defined, and whitish-pink in color as compared with (*D*) prolapsed orbital fat, which is soft with less-defined margins and is distinctly yellow in color due to its fat content. Unlike a solid dermoid, there are no cilia present on its surface. Compare the clinical appearance of these entities, dermoid cyst, solid dermoid, and prolapsed orbital fat, with the prolapsed palpebral lobe of lacrimal gland in Figure 6-1.

The techniques of lateral orbitotomy outlined in Chapter 5 apply to the en-bloc removal of benign mixed tumors. Krönlein's original lateral orbitotomy procedure is no longer used. We prefer a superior lateral approach as described by Stallard and popularized by Wright because it provides greater exposure and avoids a lateral canthotomy (see Chapter 5).[24] A lateral canthal approach may also be used (Plate 6-1). When encountering a benign mixed tumor, the gland is removed with its overlying periorbita. The periosteum is incised at the superolateral orbital rim and elevated posteriorly. Forward traction on the periorbital edge with a 4–0 silk suture facilitates exposure of the gland. The lateral horn of the levator, if incised, should be resutured to the periosteum with a 4–0 chromic suture.

The surgeon must use care when making the osteotomy above the frontozygomatic suture because of its close proximity to the anterior cranial fossa superiorly. Exposure of the orbital space is significantly enhanced by further removal of the lateral portion of the greater wing of the sphenoid with rongeurs. Brisk bleeding can be controlled with bone wax. Care should be exercised in the area of the branches of the zygomatic nerve and vessels and middle meningeal artery. The gland should be removed with its overlying periorbita. The periosteum is incised at the superotemporal rim and elevated from the lacrimal fossa. A traction suture is helpful. The periorbita is incised at the posterior extent of the gland. The lacrimal artery enters the gland posteromedially.

Malignant tumors will require exenteration with en-bloc removal of involved bone (see Chapter 5). The amount of bone resected is determined on the basis of preoperative tomograms but mainly on its appearance at the time of surgery. Since malignant tumors require radical, aggressive surgery, the dura may become exposed when resecting the posterior portion of the tumor. For these reasons, neurosurgical collaboration in the operating room is almost mandatory. Specifically, a radical

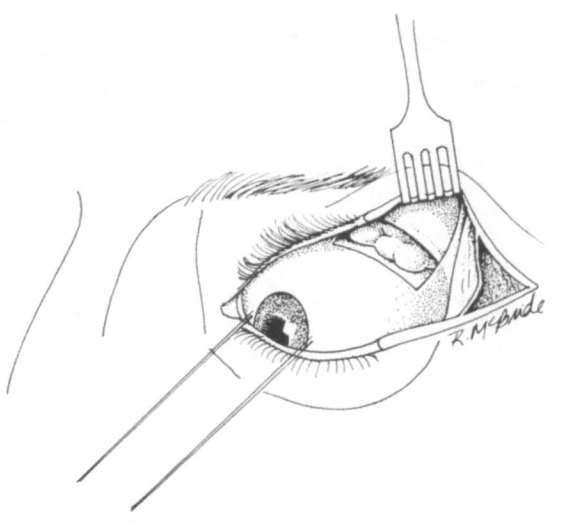

Plate 6-1. Using a lateral canthal incision, the lacrimal gland can be explored. The superior crus of the lateral canthal tendon is severed and the upper lid and adjacent soft tissues are reflected superiorly.

combined intra- and extracranial en-bloc resection has been recommended because it proves better assessment of resectability, protects the dura and underlying cortex during resection, and allows for frozen section evaluation of the tumor spread along cranial nerve routes.[25] The initial biopsy site should be included in the final specimen to avoid tumor seeding.

Radiotherapy and chemotherapy alone have not proved to be effective in the treatment of lacrimal gland malignancies, but are indicated for microscopic residual tumor after attempted resection.

REFERENCES

1. Henderson JW: *Orbital Tumors.* ed 2. New York: Thieme-Stratton, 1980, pp 261–324, 394–424.

2. Jakobiec FA, Jones IS: Neurogenic tumors, in Jones IS, Jakobiec FA (eds): *Diseases of the Orbit.* Hagerstown, MD: Harper and Row, 1979, pp 371–415.

3. Font RL, Gamel JW: Epithelial tumors of the lacrimal gland: An analysis of 265 cases, in Jakobiec FA (ed): *Ocular and Adnexal Tumors.* Birmingham: Aesculapius, 1978, pp 787–505.

4. Wright JE: Factors affecting the survival of patients with lacrimal gland tumors. *Can J Ophthalmol* 17:3–9, 1982.

5. Font RL, Gamel JW: Adenoid cystic carcinoma of the lacrimal gland. A clinicopathologic study of 79 cases, in Nicholson D (ed): *Ocular Pathology Update.* New York: Masson, 1980, p 272.

6. Jakobiec FA, Yeo JH, Trokel SL, et al: Combined clinical and computed tomographic diagnosis of primary lacrimal fossa lesions. *Am J Ophthalmol* 94:785–807, 1982.

7. Nowinski T, Anderson RL: Advances in orbital surgery. *Ophth Plast Reconstr Surg* 1:211–217, 1985.

8. Jakobiec FA: Lacrimal gland tumors, in Fraunfelder FT, Roy FH (eds): *Current Ocular Therapy.* Philadelphia: WB Saunders, 1980, p 492.

9. Hogan MJ, Zimmerman LE: *Ophthalmic Pathology. An Atlas and Textbook.* Philadelphia: WB Saunders, 1962.

10. Seiff SR, McFarland JE, Shorr N, Simons KB: Cavernous hemangioma of the lacrimal fossa. *Ophthalm Plast Recon Surg* 2:21–24, 1986.

11. McDonald P, Jakobiec FA, Hornblass A, Iwamoto T: Benign peripheral nerve sheath tumors (neurofibromas) of the lacrimal gland. *Ophthalmology* 90:1403–1413, 1983.

12. Forest AW: Lacrimal gland tumors, in Duane TD, Jaeger EA (eds): *Clinical Ophthalmology,* Vol 2. Philadelphia: Harper and Row, 1982, pp 1–40.

13. Shields CL, Shields JA, Arbizo V, Augsburger JJ: Oncocytoma of the caruncle. *Am J Ophthalmol* 102:315–319, 1986.

14. Biggs SL, Font RL: Oncocytic lesions of the caruncle and other ocular adnexa. *Arch Ophthalmol* 95:474, 1977.

15. Stewart WB, Krohel GB, Wright JE: Lacrimal gland and fossa lesions: An approach to diagnosis and management. *Ophthalmology* 86:886–895, 1979.

16. Wright JE, Stewart WB, Krohel GB: Clinical presentation and management of lacrimal gland tumors. *Br J Ophthalmol* 63:600–606, 1979.

17. Hurwitz JJ: A practical approach to the management of lacrimal gland lesions. *Ophthalm Surg* 13:829–836, 1982.

18. Krohel GB, Stewart WB, Chavis RM: Orbital disease: A practical approach. Philadelphia: Grune & Stratton, 1981, p 72.

19. Billroth T: Beobachtungen uber Geschwulste der Speicheldrusen, in Virchow R (ed): *Archiv fur Pathologische Anatomie and Physiologie und fur Klinische Medicin.* Berlin: Georg Reimer, 1859, pp 357–376.

20. Henderson JW: *Orbital Tumors.* Philadelphia: WB Saunders, 1980, pp 394–425.

21. Hornblass A, Herschorn BJ: Lacrimal gland duct cysts. *Ophthalm Surg* 16:301–306, 1985.

22. Harris GJ: Marsupialization of a lacrimal gland cyst. *Ophthalm Surg* 14:75–78, 1983.

23. Bullock JD, Fleishman JA, Rosset JL: Lacrimal ductal cysts. *Ophthalmology* 93:1355–1360, 1986.

24. Wright JE: Orbital surgery in ophthalmic plastic surgery, in *American Academy of Ophthalmology Manual,* ed 3. Rochester: American Academy of Ophthalmology, 1977, p 213.

25. Marsh JL, Wise DM, Smith M, Schwartz H: Lacrimal gland adenoid cystic carcinoma: Intracranial and extracranial en bloc resection. *Plast Reconstr Surg* 68:577, 1981.

7

Lacrimal Sac Tumors and Inflammations

Joseph C. Flanagan
Joseph A. Mauriello, Jr.
Mary Stefanyszyn

INTRODUCTION AND OVERVIEW

As with other tumors and inflammations of the ocular adnexae, diagnosing lacrimal sac tumors first requires determining whether the patient has an underlying inflammation or a tumor.

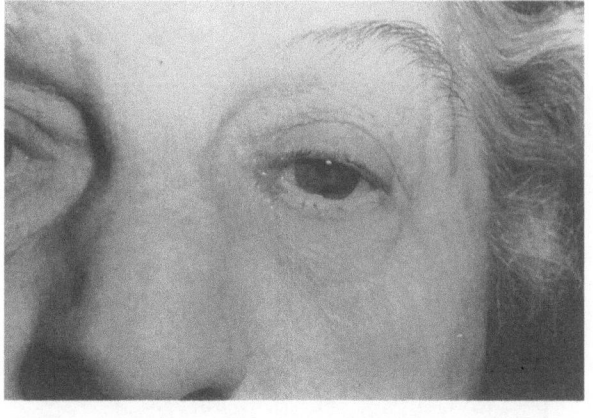

Fig. 7-1. 67-year-old female with 3-month history of bloody tears in the left eye. On irrigation of the left lacrimal system, there is a block where the lacrimal sac meets the nasolacrimal duct. Orbital CT scan showed no tumor mass. Note the lack of clinical evidence of a tumor mass. Dacryocystorhinostomy was performed and no mass was identified intraoperatively; biopsy of the lacrimal sac showed no evidence of tumor. The patient is asymptomatic 4 years after dacryocystorhinostomy. (Patient referred by Dr. A. Cinotti, Jersey City, NJ.)

In the lacrimal sac area, a tumor should be considered in all patients who present with bloody tears and a painless mass in the lacrimal sac area (Fig. 7-1). Preoperative dacryocystography and computed tomography (CT) scan may be helpful in evaluating patients suspected of harboring a lacrimal sac tumor. Although many different types of tumors originate in the lacrimal sac, epithelial tumors are most common. Determination of the benign or malignant nature of epithelial tumors is difficult even for the most experienced pathologist (Fig. 7-2). In general, malignant epithelial tumors are locally invasive and rarely metastasize. Treatment of lacrimal sac tumors usually involves complete surgical excision followed by local radiotherapy.[1-8]

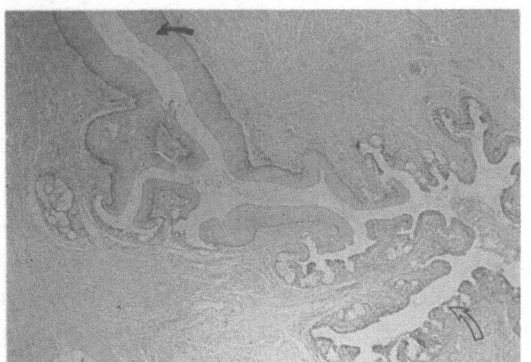

Fig. 7-2. Canaliculus is lined by relatively (solid arrow) thick stratified nonkeratinizing epithelium. The sac appears collapsed on itself and is lined by columnar epithelium (open arrow). (Courtesy AFIP, Washington, DC.)

HISTORY AND OPHTHALMOLOGIC EXAMINATION

Lacrimal sac tumors are rare, yet the diagnosis must be suspected in any patient with a history of chronic dacryocystitis.[1,2] Two ancillary diagnostic signs are (1) the history or presence of bloody tears that occur sponta-

neously after irrigation of the lacrimal system or after pressure over the lacrimal sac, and (2) a painless mass that extends above the medial canthal tendon (Fig. 7-3). The inability to reduce the mass by digital pressure over the lacrimal sac mass favors a tumor, although recurrent bouts of dacryocystitis may result in an inflamed, palpable, and tender lacrimal sac. Sometimes, there are no signs or symptoms of inflammation. In addition, congenital amnioceles of the sac may be irreducible. In any case, inflammations do not cause enlargement of the sac above the level of the medial canthal tendon.

Spratt has divided the evolution of lacrimal sac tumors into the following clinical stages.[8] In the first stage, epiphora is the only symptom. In the second stage, a round hard mass, not reducible by digitial pressure, is present (Fig. 7-4). Usually the lacrimal system is patent when irrigated. A dacryocystogram that shows a lacrimal sac with a narrowed lumen favors the diagnosis of a tumor, while a large dilated sac with a thin stretched wall suggests an inflammatory process. In the third stage, the lids and orbit are involved and the diagnosis should be apparent. At this point, the mass generally adheres firmly to surrounding structures. Epistaxis and nasal ob-

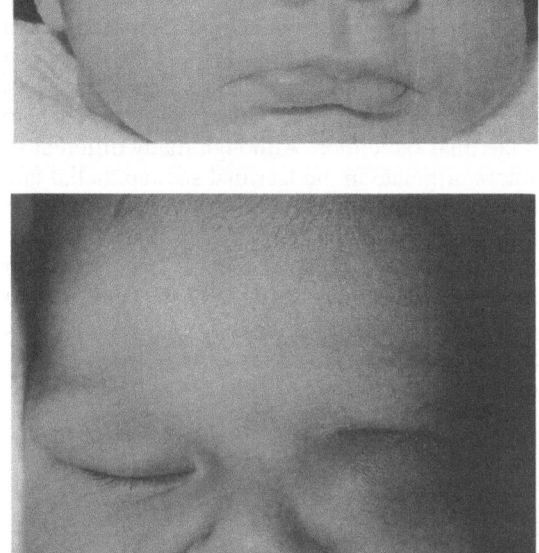

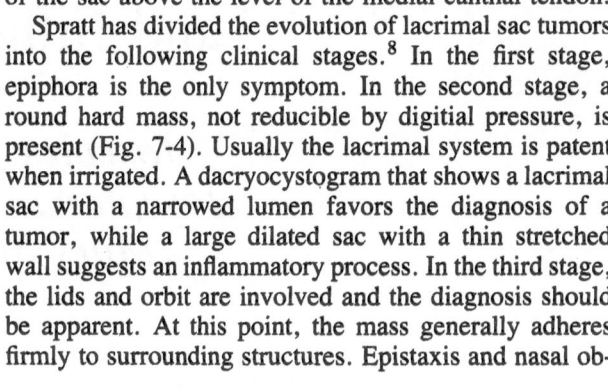

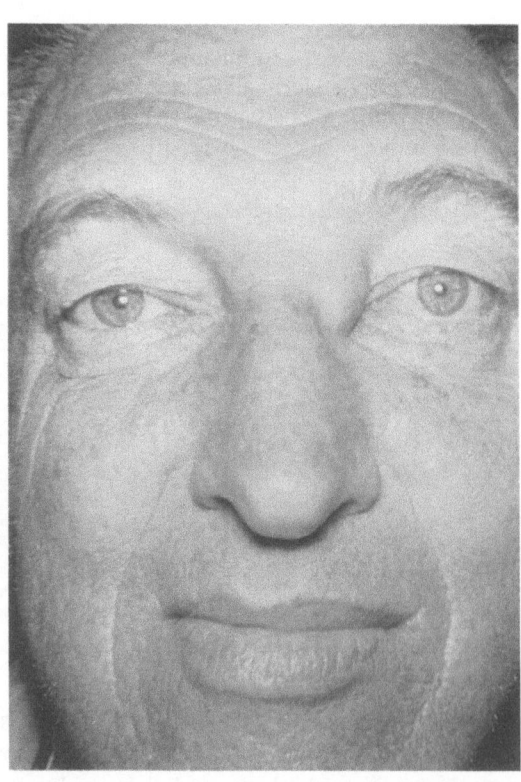

Fig. 7-3. (A) Newborn with congenital amniocele of sac due to obstruction at level of common internal punctum and Hasner's valve at end of nasolacrimal duct. Note that the mass is localized beneath the medial canthal tendon. Patient was treated with simple probing. (B) Newborn with infected amniocele of sac. Patient responded to course of intravenous and topical antibiotics and did not require probing. Lacrimal sac tumors are extremely rare in newborns and children.

Fig. 7-4. 62-year-old male with lacrimal sac tumor that extends above the medial canthal tendon. Frozen section biopsy showed a lymphoid infiltrate that on permanent section diagnosis was evaluated as a well-differentiated lymphoma. Systemic work-up for lymphoma was negative. Treatment included local radiation.

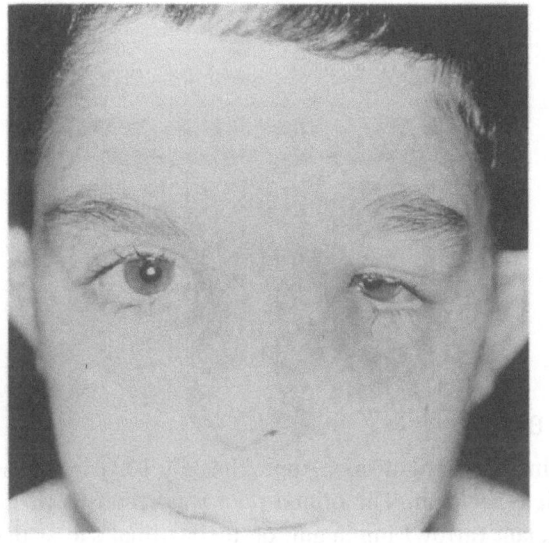

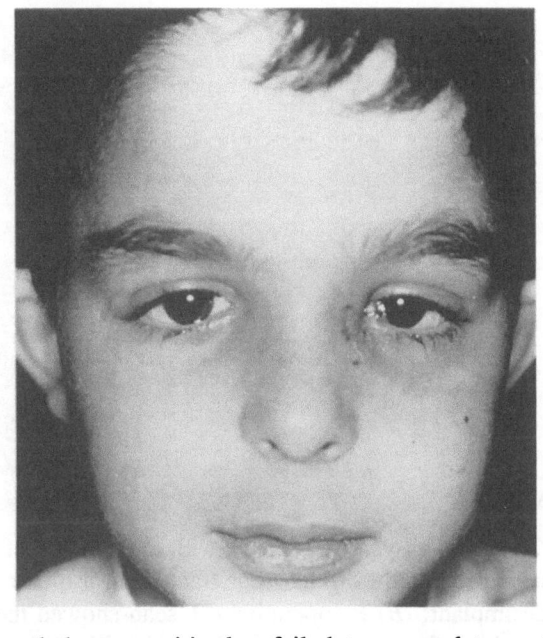

A   B

Fig. 7-5. (*A*) 7-year-old male with 1-year history of bilateral dacryocystitis that failed to respond to medical management. Disease was most severe on the left side. Patient had no history of congenital nasolacrimal duct obstruction but had had a bout of systemic Kawasaki's disease that preceded the onset of the tearing and lacrimal sac infections. History of a systemic inflammatory vasculitis, lack of bloody discharge, and bilateral total block of the lacrimal systems strongly favor diagnosis of inflammation over tumor. In addition, the inflammation was mostly inferior to the medial canthal tendon. Patient underwent dacryocystorhinostomy on the left side and a probing on the right side. The patient has been asymptomatic for 3 years. (*B*) Postoperative appearance of patient after 1 month with Johnson wire in place in inferior canaliculus. (Reprinted with permission from Mauriello JA, Stabile CS, Wagner RS: Acute dacryocystitis associated with Kawaskaki's disease. *Ophthalm Plast Reconstrct Surg* 2:209–211, 1987.)

struction suggest involvement of the nose and warrant a complete ear, nose, and throat (ENT) evaluation.

As in the work-up of orbital inflammatory disease, failure to respond to a trial of antibiotics will favor the diagnosis of tumor over inflammation (Figs. 7-5 and 7-6). In addition, unusual conditions such as Kawasaki's disease and obstruction of the lacrimal sac by an orbital floor implant may cause dacryocystitis.[9,10]

DIFFERENTIAL DIAGNOSIS

The different types of lacrimal sac tumors are summarized in Table 7-1.

The origin of lacrimal sac tumors is most commonly the epithelial lining of the lacrimal drainage apparatus (Fig. 7-2). The lining of the normal canaliculus consists of nonkeratinizing stratified squamous epithelium; the lacrimal sac is lined by stratified columnar epithelium that contains scattered goblet cells with foci or ciliated respiratory epithelium. The nasolacrimal duct and nose contain ciliated respiratory epithelium. These various epithelial elements are the source of several types of epithelial tumors.

Benign papillomatous lesions as well as carcinomas can be divided by cell type into squamous or transitional types. Squamous papillomas contain acanthotic stratified squamous epithelium, whereas transitional lesions contain stratified columnar apithelium. Papillomas may also be divided into two subtypes on the basis of their growth pattern: (1) exophytic and (2) endophytic or inverted. Exophytic tumors grow into the sac lumen, while inverted or endophytic papillomas grow into the sac wall and appear invasive.

In the largest single pathologic review of lacrimal tumors (184 cases), 86 tumors were of epithelial origin, 46 were pseudotumors, 31 were mesenchymal tumors, 6 were melanocytic tumors, and 15 were lymphomas.[3] Ryan and Font studied 27 primary epithelial tumors of the lacrimal sac.[4] In their series, the papillomas were divided into three types: (1) Squamous papillomas containing squamous cells, (2) transitional cell papillomas containing stratified columnar epithelium, and (3) mixed papillomas with both transitional and stratified columnar cell elements. Carcinomas included squamous cell carci-

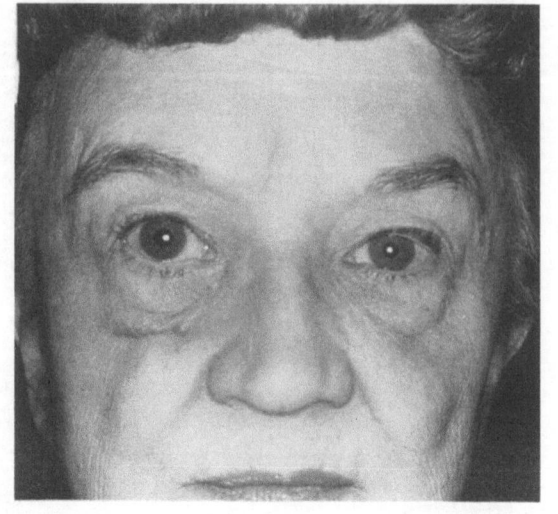
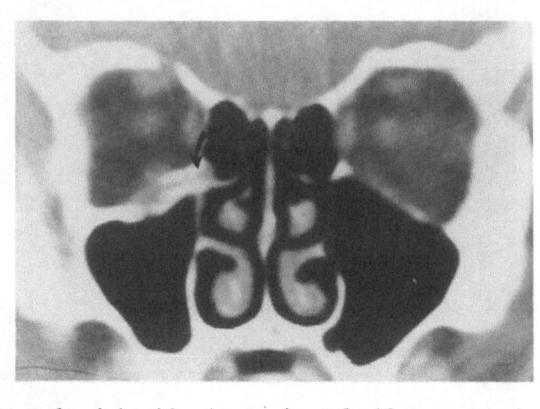

Fig. 7-6. (*A*) 68-year-old female with long history of tearing on the right side. Approximately 10 years previously, she sustained a right orbital floor fracture in a motor vehicle accident. The orbital floor was reconstructed with a silastic implant. (*B*) Preoperative CT scan showed the implant (arrow) impinging on the lacrimal sac at the level of the orbital floor. Intraoperatively, on probing, the orbital floor implant was found to obstruct the lacrimal sac. Removal of the implant combined with dacryocystorhinostomy has resulted in a resolution of the patient's symptoms. Orbital floor implants should (1) not be so large as to obstruct the lacrimal sac, (2) not be placed too medially or anteriorly near the lacrimal sac, and (3) be fixed so they do not migrate. (Reprinted with permission from Mauriello JA, Fiore P, Kotch M: Dacryocystitis: Late complication of orbital floor fracture repair with silicone implant. *Ophthalmology* 94:248–250, 1987.)

Table 7-1
Lacrimal Sac Tumors

I. Epithelial Tumors
   A. Benign papillomas—exophytic (grow into lumen of sac) and endophytic (inverted)
      1. squamous
      2. transitional
      3. mixed
   B. Carcinomas—de novo or within papillomas
      1. squamous
      2. transitional
      3. mixed
      4. mucoepidermoid
II. Grandular Tumors
   A. Adenoma/oncocytoma
   B. Adenocarcinoma
III. Mesenchymal Tumors
   A. Fibrous histiocytoma
   B. Hemangiopericytoma
   C. Fibroma/fibromyxoma
   D. Hemangioma
IV. Malignant Melanoma
V. Lymphoid Infiltrates (benign, atypical, malignant)
VI. Inflammatory pseudotumor

noma, transitional cell carcinoma, papillomas with carcinoma, adenocarcinoma of the oncocytic cells, and mucoepidermoid carcinoma. Mucoepidermoid carcinomas arise from a mixture of squamous cells and goblet cells and are extremely rare in the lacrimal sac.

Various mesenchymal tumors of the lacrimal sac may occur such as fibrous histiocytoma, hemangiopericytoma, fibroma, fibromyxoma, and hemangioma.

Lymphoid proliferations are not uncommon in the lacrimal sac area. In addition, malignant melanomas rarely occur (Fig. 7-4).

Overall, 25 percent of lacrimal sac tumors are pseudotumors. Of the true neoplasms of the sac, 73 percent are malignant.

Secondary tumors may arise from the nose, paranasal sinuses, skin, and conjunctiva. Isolated metastases to the lacrimal sac area are very rare.[3] If present, adjacent structures such as the eyelid, nose, sinuses, and orbit are also involved. Evaluation of biologic behavior is diffcult.[4]

Malignant tumors in the lacrimal area tend to be more common than benign tumors. In one large series of 28 cases, 90 percent were malignant.[7] The lack of clear-cut criteria and the rarity of these tumors make histologic determination of the benign or malignant nature of these lesions difficult even for the most experienced pathologist.[4]

RADIOLOGIC WORK-UP OF SUSPECTED LACRIMAL SAC TUMORS

If there is any suspicion of a lacrimal sac tumor, radiologic preoperative examination is important and may include plain films of the sinus, dacryocystogram, and CT scan. Sinus x-ray examinations may be of value in all patients who undergo routine dacryocystorhinostomy in order to rule out tumor or other sinus pathology. We favor CT scans over plain films if a tumor is suspected.

If a series of 63 malignant tumors of the lacrimal sac, bony destruction was found in 31 cases on plain films.[7] Only 10 of the 63 patients had normal x-ray findings. A dacryocystogram is a helpful ancillary test when a lacrimal sac mass is suspected.[8,11] A filling defect is often noted on dacryocystogram of a patient with a lacrimal sac mass. Similarly, if the clinical suspicion is high, a CT scan is critical in evaluating intranasal or paranasal involvement, and in certain instances it replaces the dacryocystogram (Fig. 7-7). The CT scan may be used with the injection of contrast material into the lacrimal sac. Coronal views are extremely helpful. The raidologist should be asked to concentrate on the lacrimal fossa area. Ear, nose, and throat consultation should be obtained when nasal or paranasal involvement is present.

INITIAL BIOPSY OF LACRIMAL SAC MASS

The surgical approach and technique of biopsy is based on the CT scan appearance. For example, if there is a localized mass that does not appear to invade the bone of the lacrimal fossa, an excisional biopsy should be performed However, if there is an extensive mass with local bone destruction, an incisional biopsy through the standard dacryocystorhinostomy (DCR) type incision should be performed before definitive radical extirpation is performed. The former procedure may sometimes be done under local anesthesia.

If there is a large mass with intranasal extension, the simplest mode of biopsy might be by an otolaryngologist through a nasal approach. Fine needle aspiration biopsy should also be considered in all instances.

Management Based on Biopsy Results

Case Study. Biopsy shows montonous population of lymphoid series consistent with lymphoma. Any patient with an orbital or lacrimal sac lymphoid infiltrate should be evaulated with a complete general physical examination and studies including a serum protein electrophoresis, bone marrow examination, and abdominal CT scan to rule out other foci of possible lymphoma. An oncologist/hematologist and radiologist should be consulted. The diagnosis of leukemia should always be considered and will become apparent based on the blood tests and bone marrow examination.

Case Study. Biopsy shows an epithelial tumor with benign features. Management includes complete surgical excision.

Case Study. Biopsy shows a malignant spithelial tumor. Management includes complete surgical extirpation with radiation therapy if residual tumor is thought to be present (Fig. 7-8).

Other Biopsy Results. The major types of tumors and their management are listed above. The other possible more rare tumors will not be considered in this chapter. Their management can be found in Chapter 3.

INTRAOPERATIVE TECHNIQUE AND TREATMENT

In general, treatment requires complete surgical excision of the tumor.[12-16] Reconstruction of a drainage system should not be considered for at least 5 years after the patient is found to be free of tumor. Any reconstructive technique is a potential path of spread for tumor cells. Therefore, an osteotomy, although performed in routine dacryocystorhinostomy, should not be done when a lacrimal sac tumor is suspected because the osteotomy provides the tumor with an iatrogenic entrance into the nose. If the bones of the lacrimal sac are involved on clinical or radiologic examination, they should be removed by wide surgical excision and submitted for pathologic examination. If there is any nasal or paranasal sinus involvement, the assistance of an ENT surgeon is helpful.

Theoretically, the entire canalicular system, the lacrimal sac, and nasolacrimal duct should be excised. The rationale for total excision of the lacrimal drainage system is twofold: (1) if the tumor is epithelial, all of the structures including the canaliculi, lacrimal sac, and nasolacrimal duct are continuous and may be involved and (2) prevention of recurrence requires complete excision of the tumor.

The operative technique involves the standard dacryocystorhinostomy incision.[16] We prefer a vertical incision about 2 cm in length and 11 mm medial to the medial canthal angle in order to avoid the angular vessels. The incision is carried down through muscle to the periosteum. The lacrimal fossa is exposed by freeing the perios-

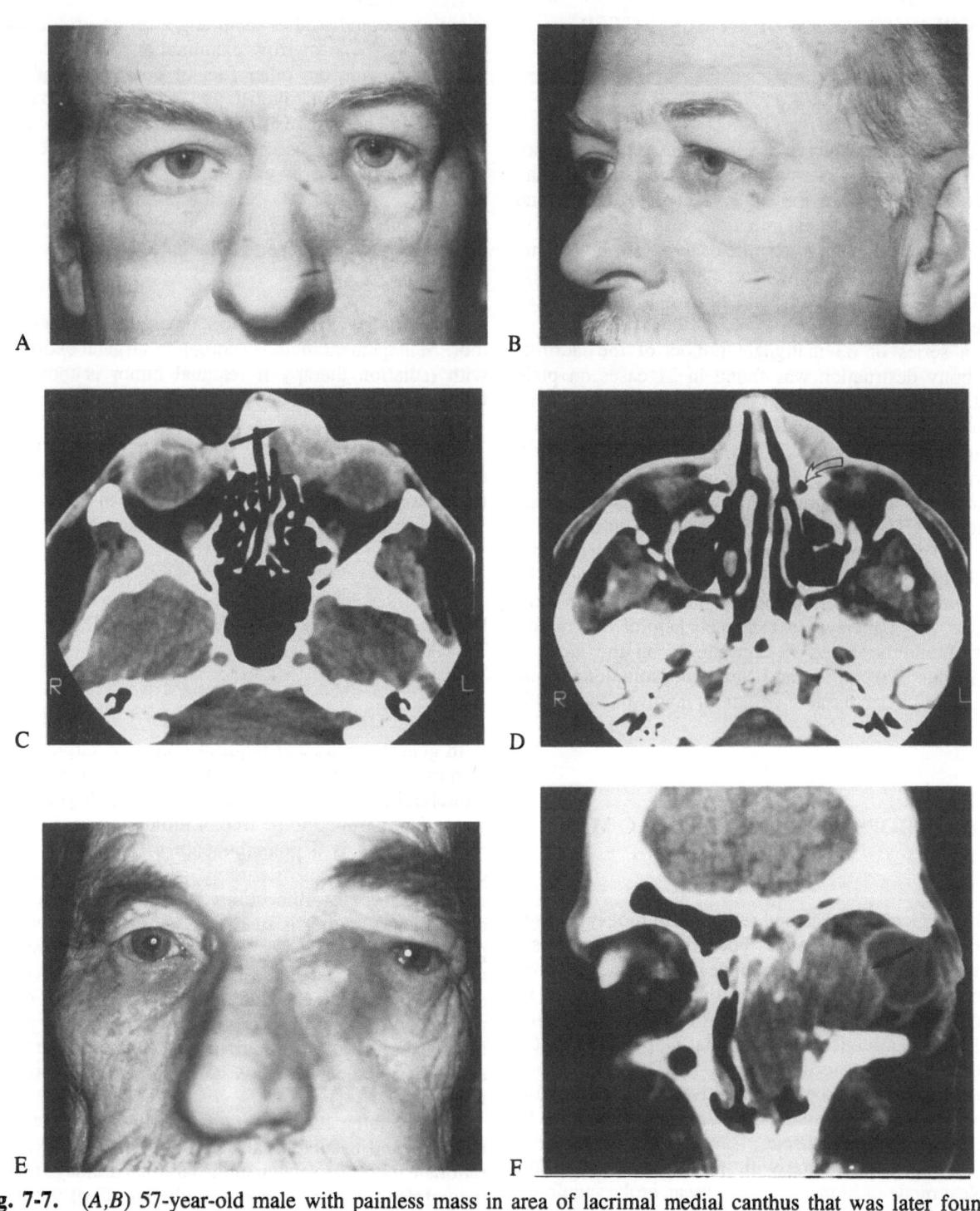

Fig. 7-7. (*A,B*) 57-year-old male with painless mass in area of lacrimal medial canthus that was later found to be due to squamous cell carcinoma. (*C*) CT scan shows focal bone erosion (arrows) at the level of the lacrimal sac. (*D*) the nasolacrimal duct does not contain tumors (open arrow). (*E*) 68-year-old male with rapid growth over 3–4 weeks of painless mass. Irrigation of lacrimal system showed a total blockage. (*F*) CT scan showed a mass that impinged on the globe (arrow) and involved the nose—frontal, ethmoid, maxillary sinuses. The lacrimal sac was found to be filled with undifferentiated adenocarcinoma.

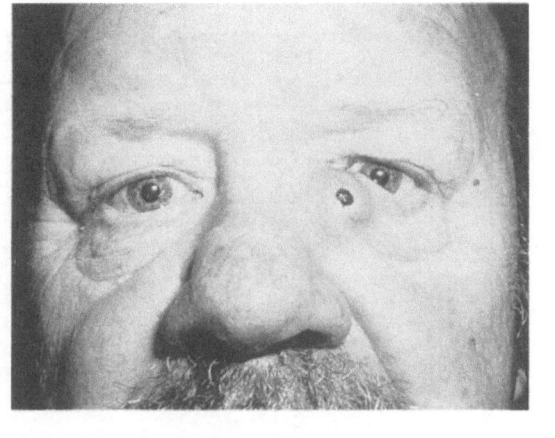

A

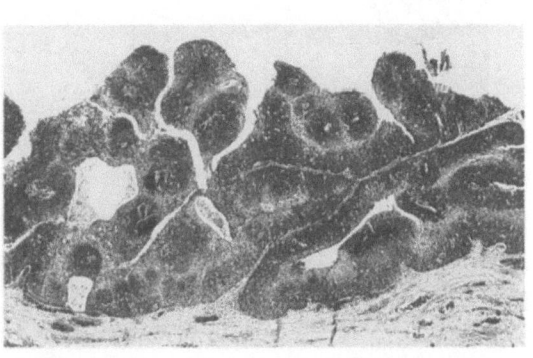

B

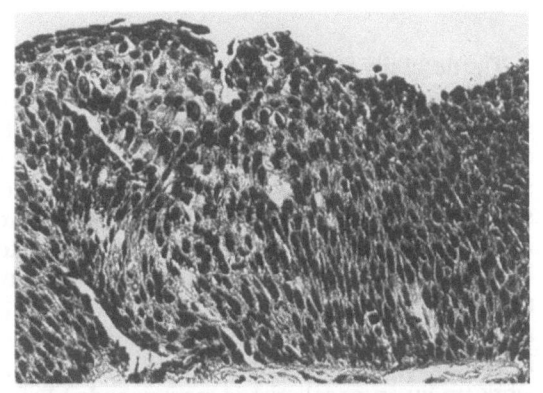

C

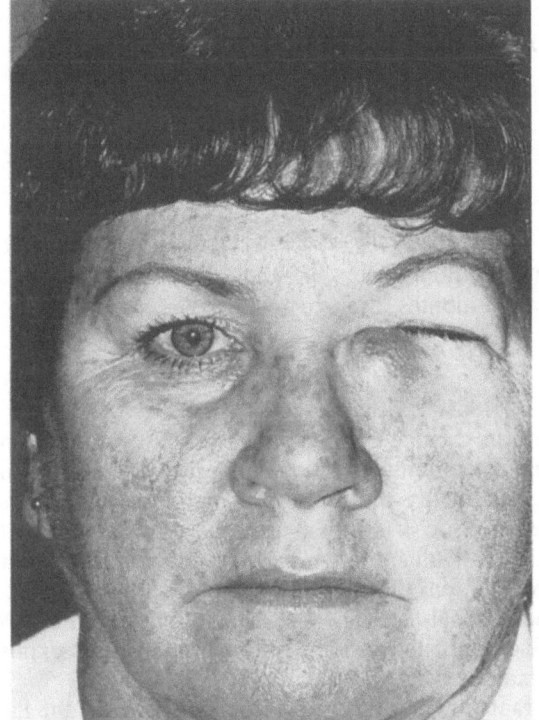

D

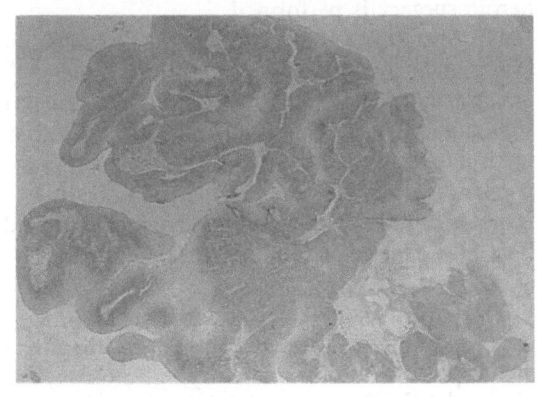

E

Fig. 7-8. (*A*) 68-year-old male with painless swelling in lacrimal sac area with a draining fistulous tract. Probing showed a narrowed inferior canaliculus, but on irrigation of the lower canalicular system, fluid was recovered in the nose as well as through the fistulous tract. At the time of surgery, a tumor was identified within the lacrimal sac; the bone was not violated by tumor. The lining of the nasolacrimal duct was removed. (*B,C*) Biopsy showed a squamous cell carcinoma of the lacrimal sac. Postoperative radiation was performed. The patient has had no recurrence of tumor after 5 years. (*D*) 57-year-old female with lacrimal sac tumor. (*E*) Biopsy showed squamous cell carcinoma that was treated by local surgical extirpation and radiation.

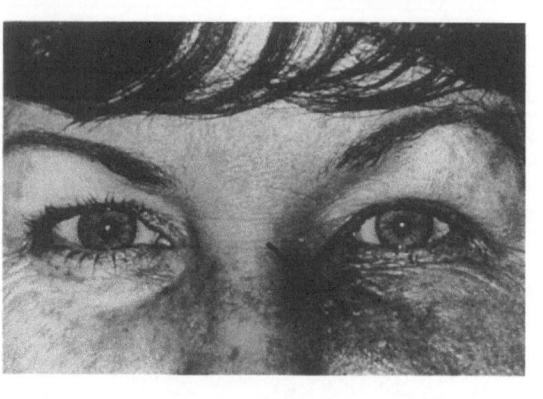

F

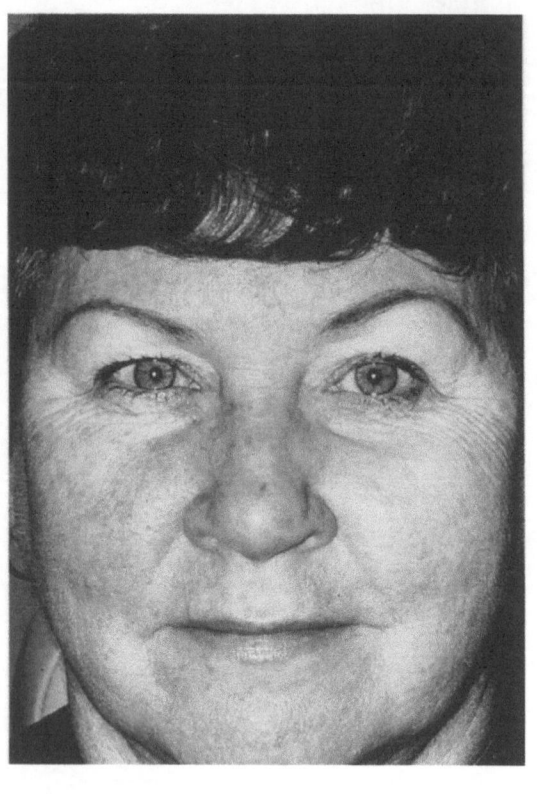

G

Figure 7-8 (continued)

(*F*) Note erythema in medial canthus (arrow) 1 month after radiation. (*G*) Note lack of erythema 6 months after treatment.

teum from the underlying bone. This dissection is carried out in a temporal direction until the anterior lacrimal crest and finally the entire lacrimal fossa are exposed (Plate 7-1). A 0–0 Bowman probe is inserted into the upper canaliculus through the common internal punctum in order to tent the central portion of the medial aspect of the acrimal sac. The sac wall is incised with a No. 11 blade until the inside of the lacrimal sac is exposed and examined.

Intraoperative biopsy with frozen sections of the lacrimal sac wall should be performed whenever tumor is suspected. An osteotomy is fashioned only after the lacrimal sac has been explored and the surgeon is assured that no tumor is present. If there is any question of tumor, frozen sections should be obtained. Epithelial lesions tend to have a gelatinous appearance similar to pattern is grossly evident; a fine vascular frond in each papillary projection may be present. The differentiation of a benign and malignant epithelial lesions on clinical grounds is impossible. Even on evaulation of permanent sections, it may be quite difficult to determine whether an epithelial lesion is benign or malignant.

As stated above, frozen sections may be helpful in confirming the presence of a lacrimal sac tumor. In addition, frozen section control of tumor margins is extremely worthwhile. Frozen sections cannot be done on bone because decalcification is required prior to processing.

The necessity for complete removal of the tumor cannot be overemphasized. When clinical examination or frozen sections show that the tumor extends into the nasolacrimal duct, lateral rhinostomy is imperative for complete excision. Tumors that are clearly malignant on permanent sections may require radical surgery; even then prognosis is guarded.[7] Radical surgery may include exenteration, local lymph node dissection, and paranasal sinus resection. The CO_2 laser may be helpful for complete extirpation of epithelial tumors. ENT evaluation is essential in tumors likely to metastasize to distant sites; a medical work-up by an oncologist is recommended before such heroic surgery is performed.

Postoperative radiation of incompletely excised papillomas and carcinomas may be of little value.[17,18] Malignant transformation of a benign papilloma may be induced by radiation.[3] CT scan and preoperative photograph are helpful to the radiation therapist. If the pathologist cannot confirm the benign nature of the lesion or if the surgeon is not assured that an entirely benign epithelial lesion is totally excised, additional surgery should be considered.

The patient should have periodic ophthalmologic evaluations during the period of radiation therapy because of the possibility of corneal drying, erosion, and ulceration. Artificial tears and lubricating ointment should be administered for comfort, and, at times, local steroids

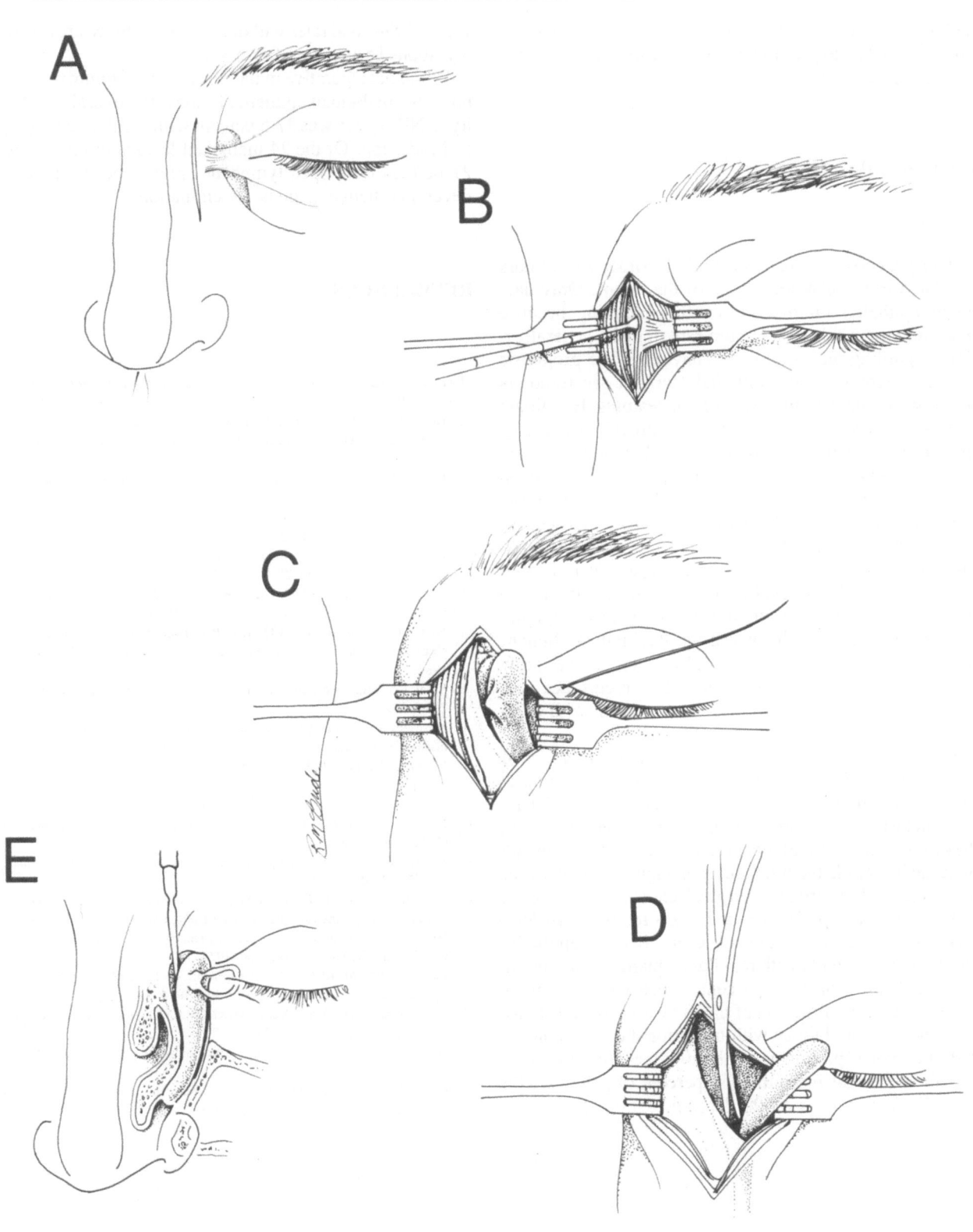

Plate 7-1. (*A*) The initial incision is on the side of the nose midway between the medial canthus and the bridge of the nose. (*B*) The periosteum is incised and the lacrimal sac reflected laterally and exposed (*C*). (*D* & *E*) The sac and duct are isolated and excised.

and frequent observation are necessary. Treatment of nonepithelial lesions of the lacrimal sac must be governed by the type of tumor.

PROGNOSIS

The prognosis of patients with lacrimal sac tumors is related to the histologic type of the tumor. Only data about epithelial tumors are worth examining because other tumors in this area are too rare to make generalizations regarding their biologic behavior.[18] The prognosis of the patient with an epithelial lacrimal sac tumor is roughly correlated with the histologic features. Histologic evaluation of such tumors is at best difficult because of their rarity and the lack of clear-cut histologic criteria for differentiating benign from malignant tumors. Aston et al. feel that papillomas arising in the lacrimal sac are probably malignant from the beginning.[18] The confusion about prognosis relates to the fact that expert pathologists may disagree about whether the lesion is benign or malignant. As a result, the literatue is difficult to interpret. In general, epithelial tumors with endophytic growth, that is, growth toward the lacrimal sac lumen, have a worse prognosis than exophytic tumors that grow away for the lumen of the sac.[4] The recurrence rate within a 5-year period approaches 50 percent with combined surgery and radiation.

In Ryan and Font's series of epithelial tumors, 2 of 27 patients died as a result of local invasion by tumor.[4] Local lymph node metastases have been reported.[19] Distant metastases are rare but have been reported, and they may occur without local recurrence.[7] Sites of distant metastasis include the lung and esophagus and may occur 5–17 years after primary surgical excision. Long-term follow-up of the patients is therefore required. In Ni's series of 82 cases, there were no benign epithelial papillomas.[7] Patients with papillary squamous carcinoma had a mortality of 13.6 percent, those with squamous carcinoma with infiltration of the sac wall had a mortality of 50 percent, and those with transitional cell carcinoma had the worst prognosis with 100 percent mortality. Spaeth stated that more than 50 percent of patients with epithelial carcinomas of the lacrimal sac died within 5 years.[13] Survival rates without prior recurrence are probably about 85 percent after 5 years.

While postoperative radiation appears to improve prognosis for malignant epithelial lesions, the overall mortality in Ni's series was 37.5 percent with combined surgery and radiation. Of the 74 malignant lesions in this series, 27 percent developed lymphatic spread and 9.1 percent developed hematogenous dissemination.[7]

REFERENCES

1. Flanagan JC, Stokes DP: Lacrimal sac tumors. *Ophthalmology* 85:1282–1287, 1978.
2. Hornblass A, Jakobiec FA, Bosniak S, Flanagan JC: The diagnosis and management of epithelial tumors of the lacrimal sac. *Ophthalmology* 87:476–490, 1980.
3. Radnot M, Gall J: Tumoren des Tranensackes. *Ophthalmologica* 151:1, 1966.
4. Ryan SJ, Font RL: Primary epithelial neoplasms of the lacrimal sac. *Am J Ophthalmol* 76:73–88, 1973.
5. Bambirra EA, Dairton M, Rayes A: Mucoepidermoid tumor of the lacrimal sac. *Arch Ophthalmol* 99:2149–2150, 1981.
6. Marback RL, Kincaid MC, Green WR, Iliff WJ: Fibrous histiocytoma of the lacrimal sac. *Am J Ophthalmol* 93:511–517, 1982.
7. Ni C, D'Amico DJ, Fan CQ, Kuo PK: Tumors of the lacrimal sac: A clinicopathological analysis of 82 cases. *Int Ophthalmol Clin* 22:121–140, 1982.
8. Spratt CN: Primary carcinoma of the lacrimal sac. *Arch Ophthalmol* 18:267–273, 1937.
9. Mauriello JA, Stabile CS: Acute dacryocystitis associated with Kawasaki's disease. *J Ophthalm Plast Reconstruct Surg* 2:209–211, 1987.
10. Mauriello JA, Fiore P, Kotch M: Dacryocystitis: Late complication of orbital floor fracture repair with silicone implant. *Ophthalmology* 94:248–250, 1987.
11. Jones IS: Tumors of the lacrimal sac. *Am J Ophthalmol* 42:561–566, 1956.
12. Milder B, Smith ME: Carcinoma of the lacrimal sac. *Am J Ophthalmol* 65:782–784, 1968.
13. Spaeth EB: A surgical technique for lacrimal sac malignancy. *Arch Ophthalmol* 57:351–354, 1957.
14. Kohn R, Nofsinger K, Freedman SI: Rapid recurrence of papillary squamous cell carcinoma of the canaliculus. *Am J Ophthalmol* 92:363–367, 1981.
15. Hyams VJ: Papillomas of the nasal cavity and paranasal sinuses. *Ann Otolaryngol Rhinol Laryngol* 80:192–206, 1971.
16. Flanagan JC, Mauriello JA: Management of lacrimal sac tumors. *Adv Ophthalmol Plast Reconstruct Surg* 3:399, 1984.
17. Stokes DP, Flanagan JC: Dacryocystectomy for tumors of the lacrimal sac. *Ophthalmic Surg* 8:85–90, 1977.
18. Ashton N, Choyce DP, Fison LG: Carcinoma. *Br J Ophthalmol* 35:366–376, 1951.
19. Khalil MK, Lorenzetti D: Epidermoid carcinoma of the lacrimal sac: A clinicopathological case report. *Can J Ophthalmol* 15:40–43, 1980.

8

Tumors and Inflammations of the Lids

Joseph A. Mauriello, Jr.
Joseph C. Flanagan

INTRODUCTION

In their daily practices, physicians commonly encounter tumors and inflammations of the lid. As in other areas of the orbit, physicians must decide whether they are dealing with a tumor or an inflammation (see Chapter 1). In most cases, this differential is more simple than in the orbit; rarely, a trial of antibiotics is necessary. In this chapter, tumors will be discussed before inflammations.

When confronted with a tumor, physicians must next decide whether the tumor is benign, and therefore only a cosmetic problem, or a possible malignant lesion that warrants biopsy and proper management. A rational approach to the management of eyelid tumors can more easily be accomplished by employing a working histologic classification and differential diagnosis.

This chapter provides the physician with a practical approach to all eyelid tumors including decision to biopsy and method of biopsy. Surgical reconstructive techniques are considered at the end of the chapter. Unfortunately, this chapter cannot be an all-encompassing dermatologic text of all tumors and inflammations. It is intended, however, to be a detailed practical approach to virtually any tumor encountered on the eyelids. Other textbooks and papers may be consulted for more obscure lesions.

The indications and roles of frozen sections are considered. The authors' method of obtaining frozen sections in the operating room is also presented. The role of radiotherapy and cryotherapy in managing eyelid tumors is also evaluated. Special problems peculiar to ophthalmic pathology that are less frequently encountered by the general pathologist are emphasized. Lastly, the management after biopsy is considered.

ANATOMY OF THE LIDS

A basic knowledge of the anatomy and microanatomy of the eyelids is necessary for an understanding of lid tumors. More detailed descriptions may be obtained elsewhere.[1]

Gross Anatomy

The four layers of the lid at the level of the tarsus from anterior to posterior include: (1) skin, (2) muscle, (3) tarsus, and (4) conjunctiva. In the upper lid, the levator aponeurosis and orbital septum fuse 6–8 mm from the upper border of the tarsus. Above this point, the preaponeurotic fat pad separates the orbital septum anteriorly from the levator aponeurosis, Muller's muscle, and conjunctiva posteriorly (Plate 8-1, Fig. 8-1). Muller's muscle and levator are the retractors of the upper lid. The lower lid anatomy is similar to the upper lid at the level of the tarsus. The analogous structure to the levator aponeurosis of the upper lid is the capsulopalpebral head of the inferior rectus muscle of the lower lid; Muller's muscle of the upper lid is analogous to the inferior tarsal muscle of the lower lid. Muller's muscle inserts at the upper border of the tarsus and expands approximately

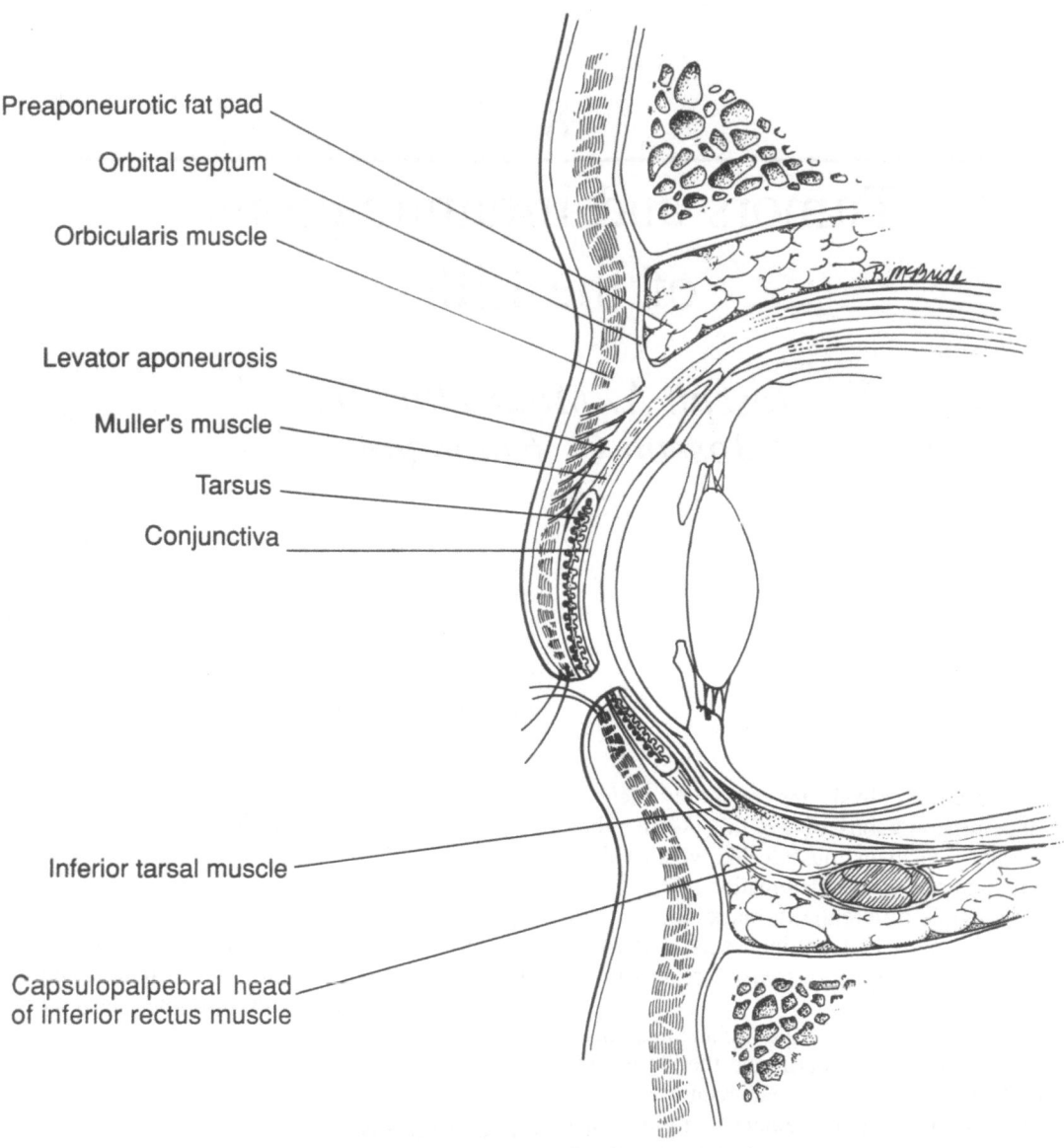

Preaponeurotic fat pad

Orbital septum

Orbicularis muscle

Levator aponeurosis

Muller's muscle

Tarsus

Conjunctiva

Inferior tarsal muscle

Capsulopalpebral head of inferior rectus muscle

Plate 8-1. Schematic drawing of lid anatomy.

10 mm in a vertical direction just anterior to the conjunctiva. The layers from anterior to posterior in the upper lid are (1) skin, (2) orbicularis muscle, (3) orbital septum, (4) preaponeurotic fat, (5) levator aponeurosis, (6) Muller's muscle, and (7) conjunctiva. In the lower lid the layers are (1) skin, (2) orbicularis muscle, (3) orbital septum, (4) fat, (5) capsulopalpebral fascia, (6) inferior tarsal muscle, and (7) conjunctiva (Table 8-1). Classic textbooks state that capsulopalpebral fascia and orbital septum do not fuse in the lower lid, while a more recent study suggests that they do fuse and the anatomy is therefore entirely analogous to the upper lid.[1,2]

The nerves are located under the orbicularis muscle; therefore, local infiltrative anesthesia must be directed at this level. Lymphatics at the temporal aspect of the lids drain into the parotid and preauricular nodes, while lymphatics from the medial aspect of the lids drain into the submaxillary nodes. The parotid, preauricular, and submaxillary nodes then drain to the deep cervical nodes. These nodes should be palpated and examined when evaluating patients with tumors of the lids that have the potential for local metastases.

Microanatomy of the Lid

Two types of cells constitute the epidermis: (1) keratinocytes and (2) clear (dendritic) cells that are predominately melanocytes (Table 8-2).[3]

The keratinocytes of the epidermis possess intercellular bridges and ample eosinophilic cytoplasm. The outermost

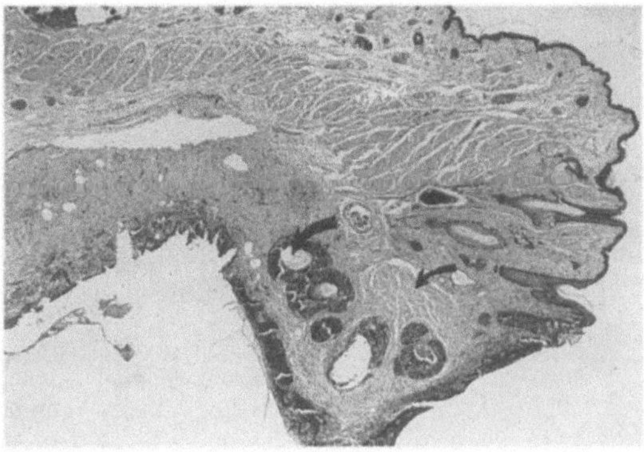

Fig. 8-1. Microscopic section of lid showing skin, orbicularis muscle, tarsus composed of dense collagen with associated meibomian glands, and conjunctiva adherent to tarsus. Note muscle of Riolan (solid arrow), which is histologic counterpart of clinical "gray" line. Note lid thickening near lid margin to replacement of sebaceous units in tarsus by basophilic cells of meibomian gland carcinoma. Some meibomian glands away from the margin are normal but adjacent conjunctival epithelium is replaced by tumor with central necrosis (open arrow). (Courtesy AFIP, Washington, DC.)

layer of the skin is coverd by keratinized stratified squamous epithelium. The epidermis of the eyelids consists of four layers from deep to superficial. (1) The basal cell layer (stratum germinativum) or germinative layer often contains a few mitoses. (2) The prickle cell or squamous cell layer (stratum spinosum) contains intercellular spinous processes (desmosomes) that may be seen on light microscopy. Intracellular cytoplasmic tonofilaments are the precursors of keratin and are eosinophilic. (3) The granular cell layer (stratum granulosum) is composed of cells that contain round, basophilic keratohyalin granules and tonofilaments. (4) At the keratin layer (stratum corneum), the basal cells of the epidermis are basophilic and produce all the cells of the epidermis; the cells become eosinophilic or squamoid as they mature and produce keratin. The principle role of the epidermis

Table 8-1
Anatomy of the Upper and Lower Eyelids*

Upper Lid	Lower Lid
Skin	Skin
Orbicularis muscle	Orbicularis muscle
Orbital septum	Orbital septum
Orbital fat (preaponeurotic fat)	Orbital fat
Levator aponeurosis	Capsulopalpebral fascia
Muller's muscle	Inferior tarsal muscle
Conjunctiva	Conjunctiva

*Above and below the tarsus 10mm, respectively, from anterior to posterior.

Table 8-2
Cells of the Epidermis

Keratinocytes
Clear cells
   Dendritic
      melanocytes (lower epidermis)
      Langerhans' cells (upper epidermis)
   Nondendritic
      Merkel's cell (lower epidermis)

is to provide a regenerative, protective keratinizing surface.[3]

The term *stratum malpighii* is most often used to describe the lower three nucleated layers of the epidermis, but some use the term to refer to the stratum spinosum.

The clear or dendritic cells in the epidermis include (1) the melanocytes, (2) Langerhans' cell, (3) Merkel's cell, and (4) an undetermined dendritic-type cell. The melanocytes have a small dark-staining nucleus and may appear "clear" due to their clear cytoplasm and shrinkage. The melanocytes are wedged between the basal cells of the epidermis. The melanocytes have dendritic processes that can be recognized only with special melanin stains. Silver stains indicate the presence of melanin that is both argyrophilic (impregnatable with silver nitrates, stains black) and argentaffin (stains brown with Masson and Fontana).[4] Silver nitrate is not specific for melanin but also stains nerve fibers and reticulum fibers. Bleaching of melanin by strong oxidizing agents such as hydrogen peroxide or potassium permanganates is specific for melanin. Melanin in melanocytes is transfered by means of dendritic processes to the basal keratinocytes where the melanin is stored and later degraded. About 10 percent of the cells in the basal layer are melanocytes. Light skin individuals have melanin in only the basal layers. Darker skin individuals and blacks have melanin predominantly in the basal layer but also throughout the epidermis and in some cases in macrophages (melanophages) in the upper dermis.[3]

The Langerhans' cell, like the melanocyte, is a clear cell and is also dendritic. Langerhans' cells are in the upper epidermis and contain the cytoplasmic disk-shaped Langerhans' granules. Histocytic processes contain Langerhans' or Birbeck granules as well. The histocytosis X group of tumors, unifocal and multifocal eosinophilic granuloma, originate from this cell.

The Merkel's cell is a nondendritic, nonkeratinocytic epithelial clear cell that is in or near the basal layer of the epidermis. On electron microscopy, these cells contain characteristic cytoplasmic neurosecretory granules that belie their neurocrest origin. The Merkel's cell functions as a slowly adapting mechanoreceptor that mediates the sense of touch.

The dermis contains the various skin appendages including pilar and sebaceous units and eccrine sweat glands. Sebaceous glands are holocrine glands and, therefore, secrete by releasing the entire sebaceous cell into the lumen (Fig. 8-2). The glands of Zeis are the sebaceous glands associated with the hair follicles at the lid margin. There are also sebaceous glands associated with tiny cilia over the skin surface of the lid. The sebaceous glands in the tarsus are not normally associated with hair follicles. Under certain pathologic circumstances, the hair follicles may generate from the basal epithelium of these sebaceous glands.

Secretion of eccrine glands such as sweat glands does not involve loss of any part of the secreting cell. Moll's glands are often described as modified sweat glands and are considered apocrine glands. The hallmark of apocrine glands is decapitation secretion.

Dermal pathology terms are worth reviewing.

Acanthosis is thickening of the squamous or prickle cell layers due to an increased number of cells (Fig. 8-3).

Hyperkeratosis is a thickening of the keratin layer. The increased keratin may be due to defective shedding

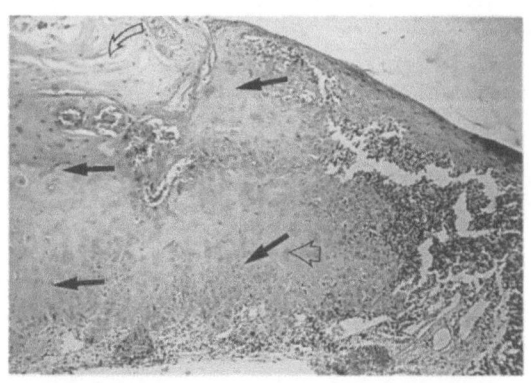

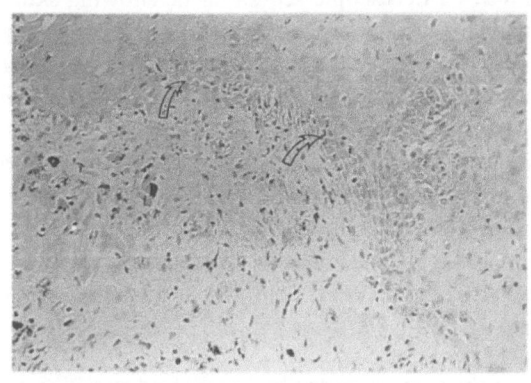

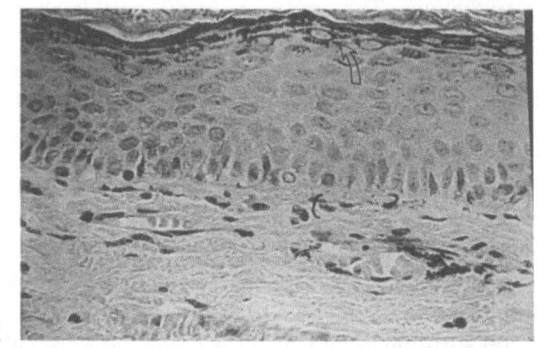

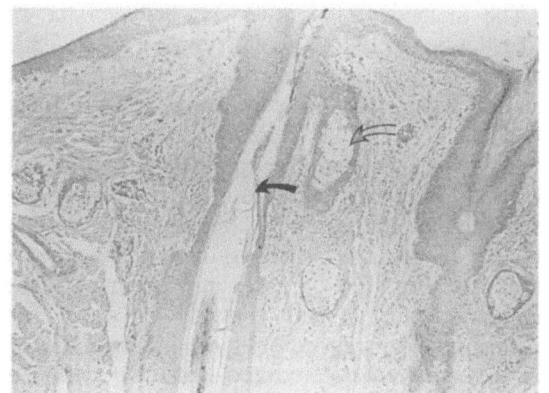

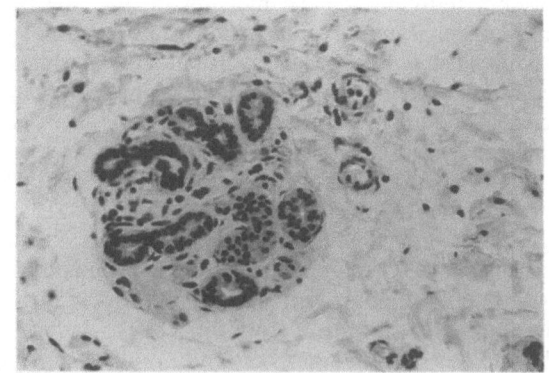

Fig. 8-2. (*A*) Microscopic section of eyelid skin showing pilar unit (solid arrow) with associated sebaceous gland (open arrow) (AFIP ACC #1124370). (*B*) Sweat gland is composed of lighter staining secretory portion of cuboidal cells and flattened myoepithelial cells and darker staining ducts composed of a double layer of cuboidal epithelium (AFIP ACC #1267112).

Fig. 8-3. (*A*) Acanthosis or thickening of prickle cell layer between solid arrows that is more marked on right side than left side of photograph. Note parakeratosis (retained nuclei of keratinocytes) involving 8–10 layers. Note dyskeratosis (large open arrow) with individual cell keratinization before cells reaches surface. (*B*) Basal epithelial layer (open arrows) with chronic inflammatory cells in upper dermis. (*C*) Note hyperkeratosis with preservation of the granular cell layer (arrow) in a Bitot spot of the conjunctiva (AFIP ACC #1155312).

of keratin, in which case there is no thickening of the granular layer and/or increased production of keratin and so there is a prominent granular cell layer.

Parakeratosis is abnormal maturation of the epidermis such that there is retention of nuclei in the keratin layers and an absence of the granular layer.

Acantholysis is a loss of cohesion between epidermis cells resulting in clefts, vesicles, and bullae.

Dyskeratosis has two definitions. We use the term to refer to keratinization of the individual epidermal cells before they reach the surface. This particular feature may occur in malignant as well as reactive proliferative lesions. Dyskeratosis may also be used to refer to atypical changes such as an enlargement of nuclei and nucleoli with loss of cell polarity and increased mitotic activity in premalignant conditions. We prefer the term *dysplasia* to signify atypia. If the atypia is full thickness, the lesion represents a *carcinoma in situ*. Atypia that invades the underlying basement membrane of the basal layer is technically invasive carcinoma. In general, normal maturation involves a change from a basophilic rounded umbrella cells at the basement membrane to squamoid eosinophilic cells that flatten as they mature and produce keratin.

HISTORY

The differentiation of tumors versus inflammation is more clear-cut in the eyelid than in the orbit. Pain, rapid onset, and redness suggest inflammation. In general, inflammations of the lids, other than acute meibomitis, acute hordeolum, bacterial infections, and allergic conditions, are rare. Allergic dermatitis secondary to a contact blepharitis or insect bites are common office practice entities.

In the orbit, a tumor that necroses may present with inflammation; lid tumors are so signficantly large that their presence is well known by the time they undergo necrosis. In addition, while idiopathic orbital pseudotumor may mimic an orbital cellulitis, "pseudotumor of the lid" is almost always a spillover from the orbital component of pseudotumor. With two main exceptions, lid tumors rarely masquerade as inflammation; the first exception includes tumors that invade the tarsus, obstruct the meibomian glands, and cause a secondary inflammation of the meibomian glands and chalazion. In all such cases, antecedent history of a preexisting tumor should point to the appropriate diagnosis. Second, meibomian gland carcinomas also classically may present as chronic blepharitis. Blepharitis, however, is usually a bilateral condition, while meibomian gland carcinoma would be reportable if present bilaterally.

When approaching any patient with a lid lesion, certain questions should always be asked (Fig. 8-4). Specifically, the duration that the lesion has been present and its rate of growth are of prime importance. A rapidly growing umbilicated lesion is most likely a keratoacanthoma, while a lesion that has been present for 3 years and has not grown is unlikely to be a malignancy. In general, basal cell carcinomas grow over months, tend to ulcerate

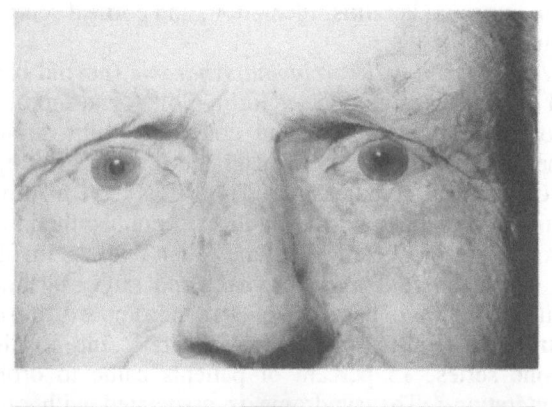

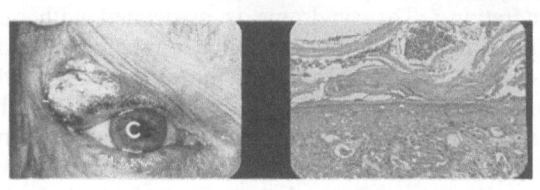

Fig. 8-4. (*A*) 66-year-old patient with history of psoriasis treated with radiation 20 years ago. Now patient has multiple actinic keratoses. (*B*) Patient with single, inflamed actinic keratosis of the left upper lid. Histologically, there is marked parakeratosis with inflammatory cells present.

or bleed, scab, and rebleed by history, and occasionally are pigmented. Pigmented lesions should always raise suspicion of a melanoma or a vascular lesion.

A history of sun exposure predisposes patients to certain tumors: actinic keratosis (solar keratosis), squamous cell carcinoma (SCC), basal cell carcinoma (BCC), and malignant melanoma. In addition, patients with fair complexions because of their lack of melanin to block the damaging effects of ultraviolet light are more prone to such tumors.

A history of inherited disorders such as xeroderma pigmentosum, basal cell nevus syndrome, and dysplastic nevus syndrome should be obtained. It is worthwhile to consider these three rare but characteristic entities.

Xeroderma pigmentosum is inherited in an autosomal-recessive or, rarely, a sex-linked recessive fashion. In this rare, premalignant dermatosis, DNA repair is genetically defective. In general, the disease starts between the ages of 6 months and 2 years in 75 percent of patients with increased dryness and freckling on the skin areas with greatest light exposure. Skin tumors present in these affected areas usually before 20 years of age. There is an increased risk of many skin tumors, most commonly BCC and SCC but also melanoma, angiosarcoma, and fibrosarcoma. Death as early as 3 years of age may occur. There is also a great predisposition to SCC of the conjunctiva. In addition to multiple malignancies, patients with xeroderma pigmentosa typically have atrophy of the lower eyelid that starts at the lid margin and eventually involves the entire lower lid. Symblepharon, exposure keratitis, ulceration, and corneal scarring ensue.[4-6]

Nevoid basal cell carcinoma syndrome (nevoid basal cell epithelioma syndrome, Gorlin-Goltz syndrome), an autosomal-dominant inherited condition with variable penetrance, has several characteristic features. Multiple BCCs occur at a young age.[7] The BCCs have a similar clinical presentation to multiple trichoepitheliomas (Brooke's tumor); however, the latter tend to involve the nasolabial fold, remain small, and rarely ulcerate, while the lesions of basal cell nevus syndrome are difusely distributed, tend to enlarge, may ulcerate, and invade.[8] In one series, 15 percent of patients came to orbital exenteration.[9] The syndrome is associated with other benign skin lesions such as milia, epithelial inclusion cysts, lipoma, and fibromas of the entire body. Other features include: a characteristic dyskeratosis of the palms and soles due to absent keratin that presents as erythematous pits or holes of 1–2 mm; jaw (mandibular) cysts and maxillary cysts; bony abnormalities of the ribs including bifid ribs, rib synostosis and agenesis, and rudimentary cervical ribs; other bone and dental abnormalities including spina bifida in up to 20 percent of patients, shortening of the fourth metacarpal, and misshapen carious teeth; neurologic findings including mental retardation, dural calcifications, seizures, agenesis of the corpus callosum, and ectopic calcifications, especially of the falx cerebri, which is almost a constant finding; and sexual anomalies including infantile genitalia in males and increased incidence of ovarian fibromas in females.[10]

The basal cells are multiple but tend to be superficial and invade later than the garden variety of BCC (Fig. 8-5). Other than the fact that foci of osteoid may be present within the tumors, the BCCs are not histologially distinctive from other BCCs.

Other ophthalmologic findings include frontal bossing with hypertelorism, squint, and medullated nerve fibers in the retina.[11]

The *dysplastic nervus syndrome* (DNS) (K-K Mole syndrome) is characterized by familial incidence of cutaneous melanoma, often with multiple primaries, and atypical nevi that vary in size, outline, and color. The syndrome is felt to be inherited as autosomal-dominant. There is also a sporadic type. On examination, a single prototypic dysplastic nevus is greater than 5 mm in diameter, irregular in outline, and a mixture of tan, brown, black, and pink. There is often a small palpable dermal component despite a macular appearance on inspection. These atypical nevi are probably histogenic precursors to primary malignant melanoma in a greater number of instances than common acquired melanocytic nevi. The number of nevi in the syndrome may vary from less than 10 to greater than 100.[12] The lesions are generally most numerous on the "horse collar" area of the trunk and upper extremities. In patients with a large number of nevi, the scalp and buttock may be involved; these are unusual sites for common nevi. Unlike the garden variety of nevi, dysplastic nevi continue to appear

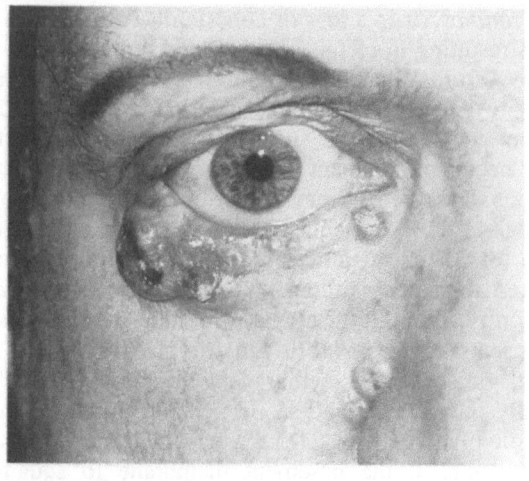

A

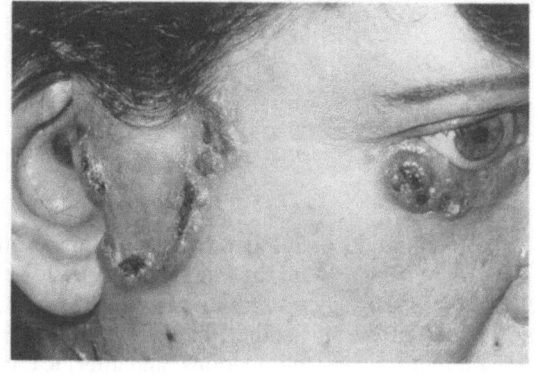

B

Fig. 8-5. (*A,B*) 32-year-old female with multiple nodulo-ulcerative basal cell carcinomas of the face. Patient also had palmar pits and other findings consistent with nevoid basal cell carcinoma syndrome.

throughout adult life even in the sixth and seventh decades.[13]

Simultaneous cutaneous and choroidal melanomas have been reported in association with the syndrome in greater proportion than in the general population. In addition, nevi of the conjunctivia, iris, and choroid occur disproportionately more frequently in such patients.[13-14]

Histologically, the dysplastic nevi shows melanocytic dysplasia, lymphocytic infiltration, fibrosis, and neovascularization. There are two histopathologic subtypes. In the epithelioid cell melanocytic dysplasia, the intraepidermal component is arranged in nests of horizontally oriented epithelioid melanocytes. In the lentiginous melanocytic dysplasia, there is an irregular basal proliferation of pleomorphic, hyperchromatic melanocytes.

In all patients with a suspected lid malignancy, a history of radiation exposure should be obtained. Radiation may predispose to BCC, SCC, malignant melanoma, and sebaceous gland carcinoma. In addition, a number of soft tissue tumors may be induced by radiation; these tumors may present in the orbit or in skin of the lids.

Patients may have been exposed to radiation therapy in their childhood for benign conditions such as acne or hirsutism.

Immunosuppressed transplant patients are predisposed to SCCs of the lids more commonly than BCC. SCCs may be bilateral. In addition, B-cell lymphomas of the lids may occur in such patients.

Family history may be helpful in establishing the diagnosis of neurofibromatosis, familial hypercholesterolemia, and trichoepithelioma. The latter condition, when mulitple, is often inherited as an autosomal-dominant disease.[15] A geographic history is useful in establishing unusual skin lesions due to infectious agents such as coccidioidomycosis and blastomycosis. In addition, a drug history should be taken because the presence of other skin lesions may be due to a drug reaction.

In the appropriate clinical setting, recurrent lesions suggest a certain diagnosis, particularly where the pathologic diagnosis may not be readily apparent. For example, a recurrent chalazion should arouse suspicion of a sebaceous gland carcinoma. A recurrent SCC might represent a halogen drug toxicity or fungal infection.[16]

Previous studies from pathologic laboratories have recorded the incidence of eyelids tumors.[17–20] The results of these studies do not reflect the true incidence of such tumors but at least give an indication of the incidence of those tumors that are excised and sent for pathologic examination. In three studies[17,18,20] epithelial inclusion cyst, chalazion, and BCC were frequently found pathologically. Papilloma and seborrheic keratosis were common in two of the three studies,[17,20] and nevus in one of the studies.[17]

A working histologic classification of tumors is necessary when approaching the individual patient with an eyelid tumor. The histologic origin of the tumors often provides insight into the clinical presentation of certain tumors. For example, epithelial tumors originate from the surface, while adnexal tumors begin deep to the surface and usually do not ulcerate. BCC originates from the epithelium and often ulcerates, while sebaceous gland carcinoma arises from the sebaceous glands of the ocular adnexae and rarely if ever ulcerates.

A histologic classification is also helpful because it is important when considering the spectrum of possible tumors to realize that any structure in the skin can give rise to malignancy. For example, while there are many tumors of pilar origin, we have chosen to design a simplified working classification (Table 8-3). Unlike the histologic classification of lid tumors, the classification of inflammatory lid lesions is based on clinical presentation.

Table 8-3
Working Histologic Classification of Lid Tumors

Epithelial—Benign
    Seborrheic keratosis (SK)
    Inverted follicular keratosis (IFK)
    Epidermal inclusion cyst (EIC)
    Keratoacanthoma (KA)
    Pseudoepitheliomatous hyperplasis (PEH)
    ''Benign keratosis''
    Viral infections that present as tumors
        molluscum contagiosum
        verruca vulgaris
Epithelial—Premalignant
    Actinic keratosis (AK)
    Bowen's disease
    Radiation dermatosis
    Xeroderma pigmentosum
    Nevoid basal cell carcinoma syndrome
    Dysplastic nevus syndrome
Epithelial—Malignant
    Basal cell carcinoma (BCC)
    Squamous cell carcinoma (SCC)
Adnexal—Pilar
    Trichoepithelioma
    Trichofolliculoma
    Pilomatrixoma (benign calcifying tumor of Malherbe)
    Tricholemmoma

Table 8-3 (Continued)

Pilar (sebaceous) cysts
Milia
Adnexal—Sebaceous
  Sebaceous gland hyperplasia
  Sebaceous adenoma
  Sebaceous gland carcinoma
Adnexal—Sweat Gland
  Eccrine
    eccrine hydrocystoma
    syringoma
    eccrine acrospiroma
    adenocarcinoma of eccrine sweat glands (infiltrating signet ring
      carcinoma)
  Aprocrine
    adenoma of apocrine Moll's glands
    adenocarcinoma of apocrine Moll's glands
  Uncertain origin
    pleomorphic adenoma
    mucinous sweat gland carcinoma
Soft Tissue—Neurogenic
  Neurofibroma
  Schwannoma
Soft Tissue—Vascular
  Capillary hemangioma
  Pyogenic granuloma
  Lymphangioma
  Cavernous hemangioma
  Hemangiopericytoma
  Glomus tumor
  Kaposi's sarcoma
  Angiolymphoid hyperplasia with eosinophilia (Kimura's disease)
  Angiosarcoma
Soft Tissue—Fibrous
  Fibroma
  Dermatofibroma
  Juvenile fibromatosis
  Fibrosarcoma
  Atypical fibroxanthoma
  Nodular fasciitis
  Fibrous histiocytoma
Soft Tissue—Histiocytic
  Xanthoma
  Juvenile xanthogranuloma
  Xanthelasma
  Necrobiotic xanthogranuloma
  Eosinophilic granuloma
  Letterer-Siwe disease
  Hand-Schüller-Christian disease
  Erdheim-Chester disease
  Myxoma
  Malakoplakia

Table 8-3 (Continued)

Miscellaneous
  Depositions in the lid
    amyloidosis
    ligneous conjunctivitis (fibrin deposition)
    lipoid proteinosis
  Tumors metastatic to the lid
    breast (most common)
    lung
  Phakomatous choristomas
Neural Crest (Melanocytic)
  Freckle
  Lentigo senilis
  Melanotic macule of Albright's syndrome
  Café-au-lait spot of neurofibromatosis
  Nevus
    junctional
    dermal
    compound
    balloon cell
    halo
    spindle and epitheloid (Spitz nevus, benign juvenile melanoma)
    blue
  Precancerous Melanosis—Lentigo Maligna (Hutchinson's Freckle)
  Malignant Melanoma—Origins
    De novo (nodular)
    Superficial spreading
    Arising in lentigo maligna
  Congenital oculodermal melanocytosis (nevus of Ota)
  Merkel's cell tumor (trabecular cell carcinoma)

CLINICAL APPROACH TO EXAMINATION OF THE PATIENT BASED ON WORKING HISTOLOGIC CLASSIFICATION

In general, the physician should attempt to assess whether the primary process is an inflammation or a tumor. As in the orbit, lesions that have inflammatory signs such as pain, redness or swelling should be treated with local or systemic antibiotics as deemed appropriate (Fig. 8-6).

Many patients, however, will have obvious tumors. The physician should in these patients try to determine whether the lesion appears to arise superficially from the epidermis or more deeply from the soft tissues of the lid. Adnexal tumors may have a superficial or deep component. By utilizing the histologic classification, a differential diagnosis can be be established.

Every structure in the skin is the possible origin of an eyelid tumor: (1) epidermis; (2) skin adnexae, including the pilar apparatus, sebaceous, and sweat glands; (3) soft tissue, including peripheral nerves, blood vessels, fibroblasts, histiocytes; and (4) melanocytic cells and Merkel's cells of neural crest origin.

Loss of Cilia

The cilia adjacent to the tumor should be carefully examined. Focal loss of cilia occurs with BCC, sebaceous gland carcinomas, SCC, and Merkel's cell tumor.[21] However, benign tumors such as primary localized amyloidosis and trichoepithelioma may cause loss of cilia also.[22-23] Rarely, mucoepidermoid carcinoma of the conjunctiva may present as a red, thickened, and indurated ulceration on the lid margin.[24] Telangiectasia is noted on the palpebral conjunctiva. As stated above, ulceration of the lid border often accompanies BC, while sebaceous gland carcinomas rarely ulcerate. With sebaceous gland carcinoma, there is usually lid thickening with an orange-yellow appearance of the lesion due to the presence of lipid. In some cases, thickening may be minimal, yet the meibomian orifices will be scarred. In one such case, the patient was treated for 18 months for superior limbic

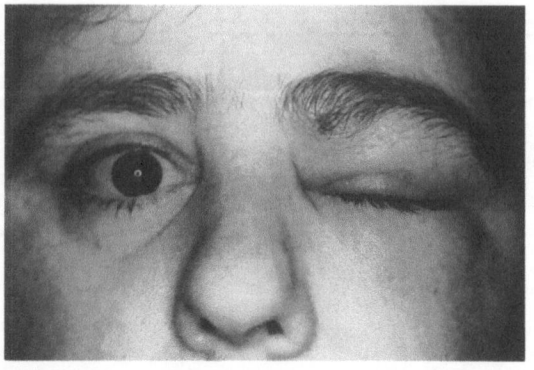

Fig. 8-6. 36-year-old female with 1-day history of pruritic, slightly painful swelling of left upper lid with necrotic center, possibly secondary to insect bite. Patient was treated symptomatically with oral antibiotics and local cool compresses with complete resolution of process. (Patient referred by Joseph Landolfi, M.D., Belleville, NJ)

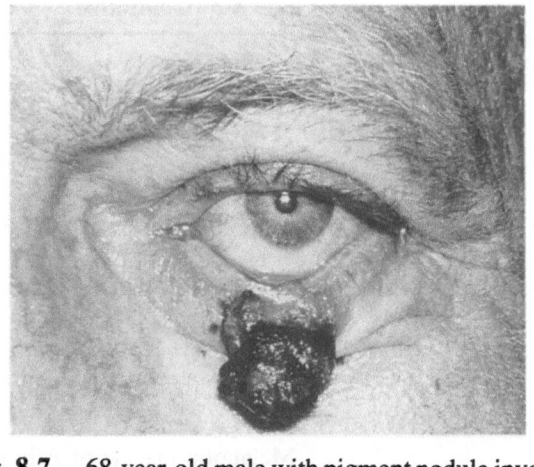

Fig. 8-7. 68-year-old male with pigment nodule involving left lower lid. Incisional biopsy showed malignant melanoma arising in the lid. Treatment consisted of wide surgical excision without recurrence.

keratoconjunctivitis, before a full-thickness lid biopsy showed diffuse intraepithelial sebaceous gland carcinoma.[25] Inflammatory disease of the lid including blepharitis and chalazion may also cause focal loss of lashes. Fungal infections such as blastomycosis and bacterial infections such as anthrax may cause lid ulcerations with loss of cilia, although these processes tend to spare the lid margin with its excellent blood supply.

Pigmented Tumors

The presence of pigment in a lesion should always arouse suspicion of malignant melanoma of the eyelid. Pigment in the lid skin generally arises from two sources: melanocytes or blood. Any brown, black or slate-gray lesion may represent melanin. Melanin in superficial layers of the skin (epidermis and upper dermis) will appear brown in color. A high concentration of melanocytes or pigment in the indivdual melanocytes or a large number of melanophages will give the lesion a darker brown or black color. Melanin in the lower dermis or episclera will appear slate-gray.

Melanocytic lesions with irregular borders, variegated color, and history of growth are suggestive of malignant melanoma (Fig. 8-7). In addition, a brown lesion that has been present for months to years and develops a focal nodule strongly suggests that a superficial spreading melanoma has changed from its radial growth to a vertical growth phase. A new pigmented lid lesion that occurs in a patient over 25 years of age should be biopsied. In general, pigmented lesions will darken and possibly enlarge at puberty or during pregnancy. Any enlarging pigmented lesion should be biopsied. Aside from truly melanocytic lesions, other pigmented lesions include se-

borrheic keratosis, Bowen's disease, actinic keratosis, and BCC (Fig. 8-8).

The other main source of pigment or color present in lid lesions is blood (Fig. 8-9). Blood may occur in vascular tumors and in tumors that have associated hemorrhage (eccrine acrospiroma, dermatofibroma, Kaposi's sarcoma). A vascular tumor that appears bluish gray will rarely be confused with a deep melanocytic lesion such as a blue nevus, because the latter is flat while a vascular tumor will be raised (Fig. 8-10). A vascular tumor such as hemangioma, Kaposi's sarcoma, or any lid tumor with associated hemorrhage will appear red, blue or purple. Lymphangiomas of the lid may not appear colored until hemorrhage occurs into the tumor.

In addition, depositions such as lipid in histiocytic lesions (juvenile xanthogranuloma) or in sebaceous tumors will appear orange, yellow, or red (Fig. 8-11). Amyloid appears yellow, orange, or red due to its deposition about blood vessels and associated hemorrhage. Pilomatrixoma may appear red. Pyogenic granuloma due to the presence of fibrous tissue, vessels, and subacute inflammation may also appear red. Cylindromas are pink to blue dome-shaped (apocrine and eccrine sweat gland) tumors that occur in multiple form and are transmitted as an autosomal-dominant trait. Solitary cylindromas are nonhereditary. The inherited form may be associated with multiple trichoepitheliomas. Cylindromas may cover the entire scalp like a turban, hence the term *turban tumor*.

Both dacryops and canaliculops (dilated canaliculus) may appear blue in color.[26] In addition, lipofuscins in apocrine secretions may impart a bluish hue to apocrine hydrocystomas (apocrine cystadenomas).[27] Merkel's cell tumors have a red or blue color and may present as a rapidly growing protuberant upper lid tumor with intact overlying skin in elderly patients. Leukemia may present as single multiple red-to-brown subcutaneous nodules.[28]

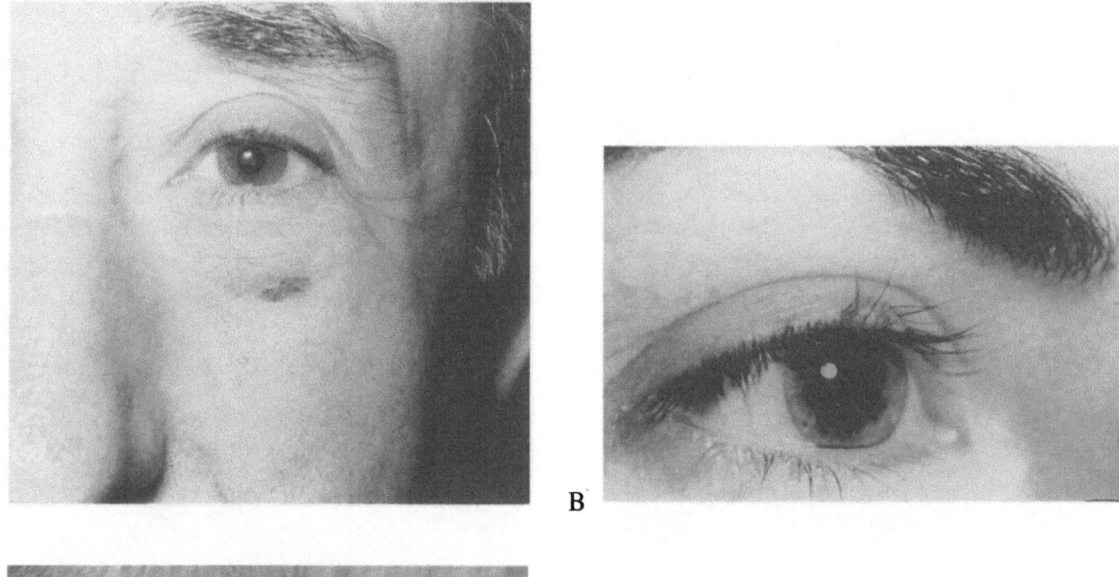

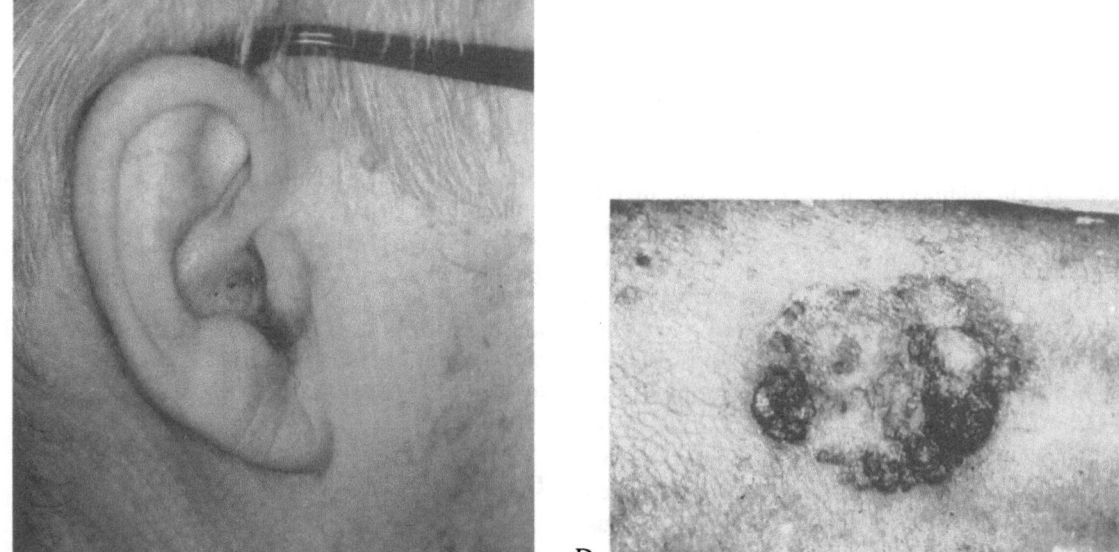

Fig. 8-8. 66-year-old male with light brown pigmented mass resembling seborrheic keratosis. Excisional biopsy with frozen sections of main mass and margins showed pigmented basal cell carcinoma, completely excised. (*B*) Patient with seborrheic keratosis of lid margin that may be clinically mistaken for a nevus. (*C*) While Bowen's disease of the skin most often presents with a scaling erythematous base, (*D*) the lesion may show significant pigmentation. (*B–D* courtesy AFIP, Washington, DC.)

Multiple Tumors

Any patient with multiple skin tumors should be suspected of xeroderma pigmentosa, basal cell nevus syndrome, or dysplastic nevus syndrome (see discussion above). Other tumors that tend to be multiple include apocrine or eccrine hydrocystoma, milia, syringoma (as in young females and in Down's syndrome), trichoepithelioma, actinic keratosis, xanthogranuloma, verruca vulgaris, molluscum contagiosum, glomus tumor of the face, pseudorheumatoid nodules, multiple neurofibroma in patients with von Recklinghausen's disease, metastatic disease, and multiple cylindromas. Multiple sebaceous gland adenomas should always make the ophthalmologist consider the diagnosis of Torre's (Rulon-Helwig) syndrome in which multiple sebaceous gland adenomas are associated with low-grade visceral carcinomas usually of the colon. Other squamous proliferative lesions of the skin may occur: epidermal hyperplasia, keratoacanthomas, and SCC (Fig. 8-12).[29,30] Multiple epidermal inclusion cysts may be encountered with Gardner's syn-

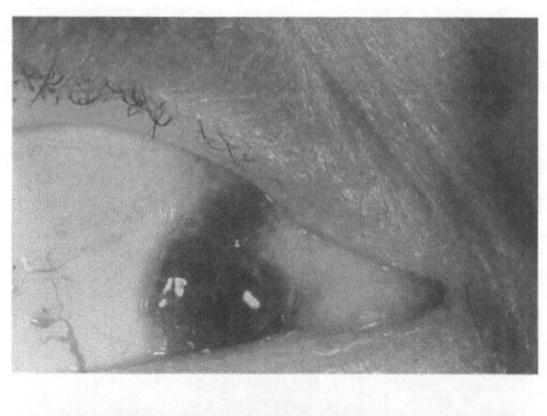

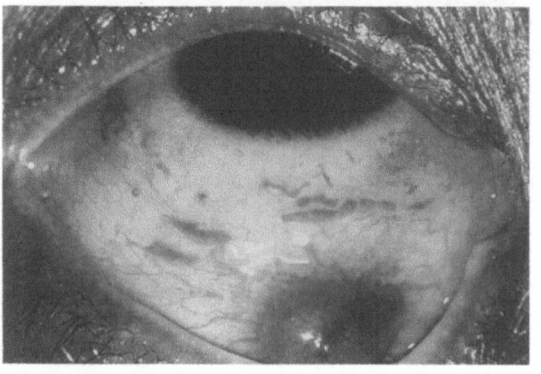

Fig. 8-9. (*A*) In addition to melanin, pigment may be due to blood as in the bright red tumor present on the plica semilunaris in the right eye of a 70-year-old white female. The lesion had been present for more than 60 years but recently enlarged. Biopsy showed a hemangioma that apparently bled spontaneously, possibly due to the aspirin that she took regularly for arthritis. (Courtesy of Dr. Andrew Ferry, Richmond, VA.) (*B*) A 51-year-old black male presented with a subconjunctival hemorrhage that did not resolve. Biopsy was consistent with Kaposi's sarcoma. This diagnosis should be suspected in any patient who has a subconjunctival hemorrhage that does not resolve. (Courtesy of Dr. George Kurz, Flemington, NJ.)

drome, including multiple intestinal polyposis, multiple oesteomas of the facial bones, and fibromas of the abdominal wall, mesentery, and breast.[31] In Cowden's disease, an autosomal-dominant condition, multiple flesh-colored papules and verucoid lesions involve the face and lids, oral mucosa, and acral portions of the upper extremities.[32] Histologically, these lesions may be trichilemmomas or nonspecific keratoses.[32] Cutaneous harmartomas of the skin, oral mucosa, and larynx include fibbromas, angiomas, and lipomas. There may be associated malignancies of the thyroid and breast. Kaposi's sarcoma of the lids, conjunctiva, or elsewhere in the body when multiple may be found in AIDS patients.[33,34]

Other tumors that tend to occur in the same patient

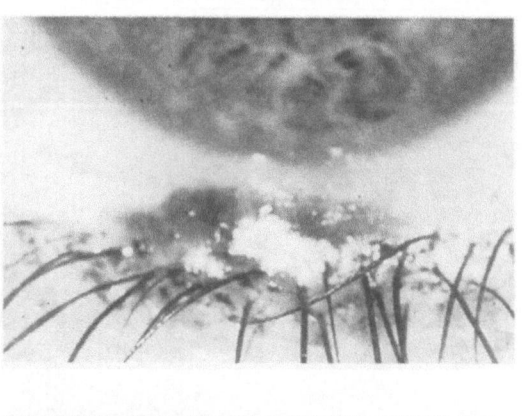

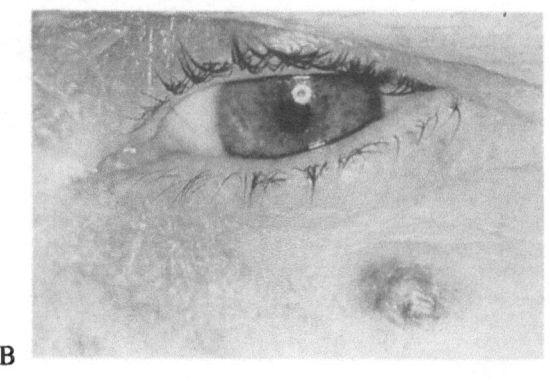

Fig. 8-10. (*A*) Melanin that is deep in the dermis will appear blue in color, blue nevus of lid border, (AFIP ACC #981781) while (*B*) venous blood will also appear blue (right, varix, AFIP ACC #1083556)

are premalignant epithelial and malignant epithelial lesions such as actinic keratosis, Bowen's disease, BCC, and SCC (Fig. 8-13).[35,36]

Umbilicated Tumors

Umbilicated tumors include molluscum contagiosum and keratoacanthoma (KA) (Fig. 8-14). These tumors

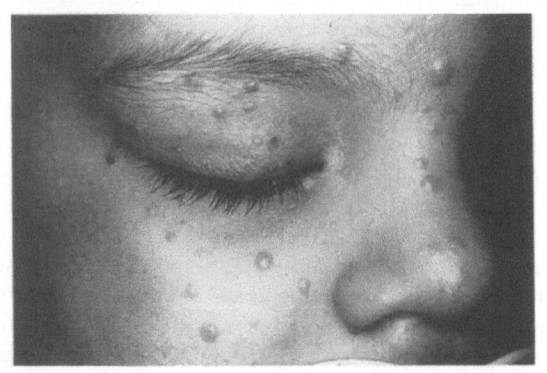

Fig. 8-11. Child with multiple xanthogranuloma that are reddish-orange, dome-shaped papules. (Courtesy AFIP, Washington, DC.)

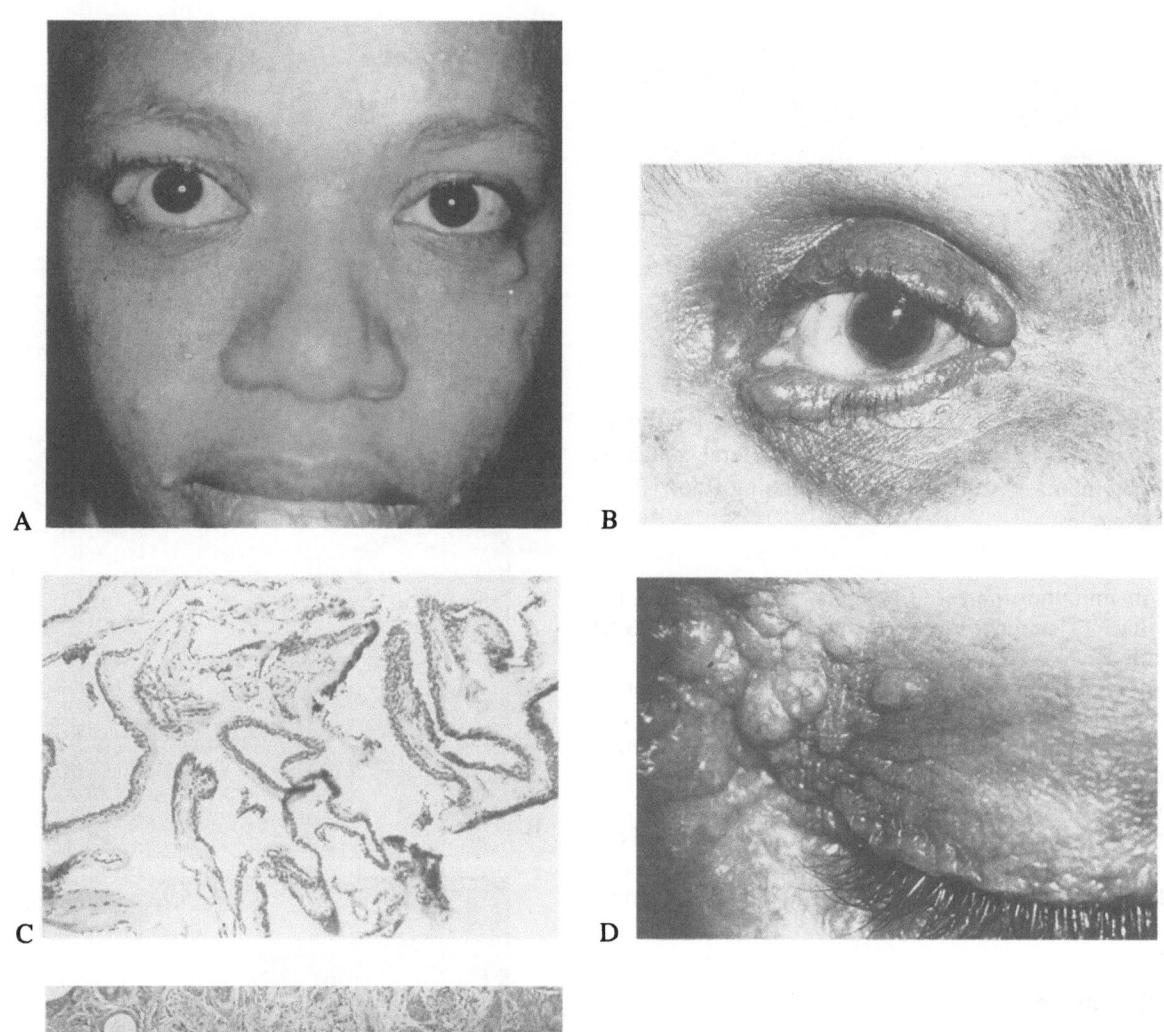

Fig. 8-12. (*A*) 15-year-old female with known neurofibromatosis and multiple neurofibroma. (*B*) Patient with multiple eccrine sweat gland cysts. (*C*) Biopsy shows cysts lined by double layer of cuboidal epithelium consistent with eccrine hydrocystoma. (*D*) Multiple trichoepithelioma are inherited in autosomal-dominant pattern. (*E*) Biopsy shows typical horn cysts.

have regular cup-shaped configuration, but KA usually has a necrotic center while molluscum contagiosum usually does not have a necrotic center. Other umbilicated tumors include BCC, which usually has an irregular border with or without necrosis, eccrine acrospiroma, a sweat gland tumor that may resemble KA, and pleomorphic ademona of sweat gland origin that appears to arise deep from the dermis (sweat gland origin) and has a central small orifice.

Tumors That Ulcerate

There are a number of lesions that may ulcerate; these include (1) a number of epithelial lesions of which BCC is the most common cause, (2) adnexal tumors including trichilemmoma, eccrine sweat gland carcinoma, and trichoepithelioma (Fig. 8-15), (3) soft tissue tumors such as atypical fibroxanthoma, (4) B-cell lymphomas of the

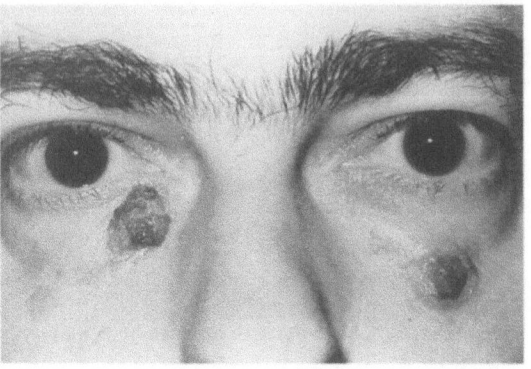

Fig. 8-13. 41-year-old on immunosuppressive therapy for renal transplantation developed bilateral squamous cell carcinomas. (Courtesy of Dr. Narsing Rao, USC—Los Angeles.)

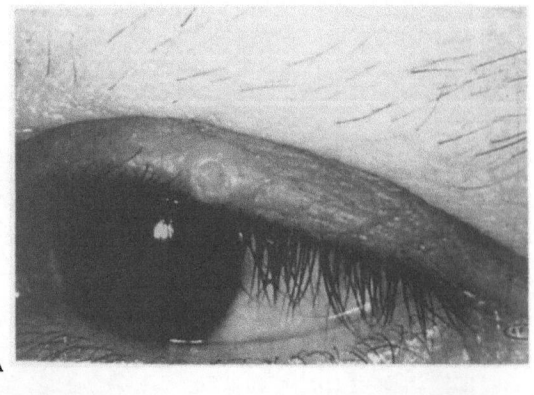

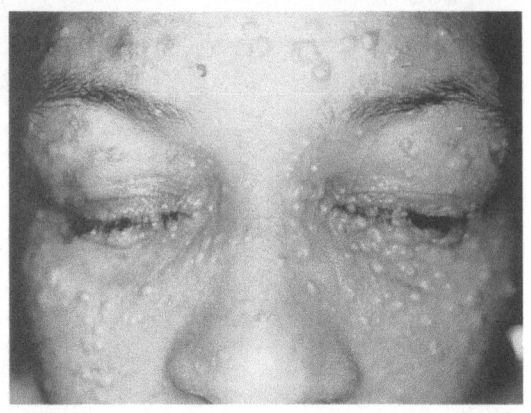

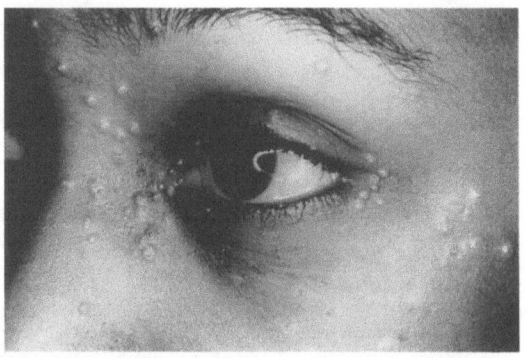

Fig. 8-14. (*A*) Patient with umbilicated molluscum contagiosum (AFIP ACC #733646). Note lack of necrotic plug present in keratoacanthoma. (*B*) 21-year-old known drug addict with AIDS and multiple molluscum contagiosum. (*C*) 16-year-old female with multiple molluscum with no evidence of immunosuppression.

lids in immunosuppressed patients with associated loss of cilia,[37–40] and (5) rarely, metastatic carcinoma to the eyelid.

Another helpful diagnostic point is the location of the tumor. For example, the differential diagnosis of a mass in the upper temporal lid should include dermoid cyst, eosinophilic granuloma, and pilomatrixoma.

In any patient with a suspected malignant tumor, the regional lymph nodes including the preauricular and cervical nodes should be palpated. Any suspicious lymph node should be reexamined and biopsied by the appropriate specialist.

Cystic Tumors

Cystic tumors are listed in the Table 8-4. Milia are follicular cysts caused by obstruction of the orifices of the pilosebaceous units. Prior radiation predisposes the patient to the formation of milia. They may also be associated with bullous disease. Clinically, a small central depression corresponds to the occluded orifice. Histologically, a dilated hair follicle is filled with laminated masses of keratin. Sebaceous (pilar) cysts are clinically indistinguishable from epidermal inclusion cysts except for the fact that pilar cysts are less common and occur in areas containing multiple, large hair follicles such as in the brow region and scalp. Histologically, the lining epithelial cells show distinct peripheral palisading. There is abrupt keratinization without formation of a granular layer; this type of keratinization is typical of hair follicles. Calcification of the keratin occurs frequently. Some cystic BCCs may show a dark blue color due to the presence of blood in the lumen of the central cavity surrounded by the islands of tumor. Eccrine acrospiromas may appear as bluish-red cysts due to hemorrhage. Rarely, mucinous sweat gland carcinoma may present as a rapidly growing, cystic-appearing lesion on the lid border.[41] In general, sweat gland tumors have a superficial appearance. Moll's

gland cyst may also occur. Yellowish material present at the apex of cysts might represent cellular membrane debris that has a high lipid content from decapitation secretion in apocrine tumor.[27] Dacryops is a dilated duct from lacrimal tissue, while canaliculops has recently been described as a blue-tinged ectasia of the canaliculus without inflammatory signs.[26]

A subcutaneous tumor in the lateral aspect of the upper lid or orbit includes cystic tumors such as dacryops origi-

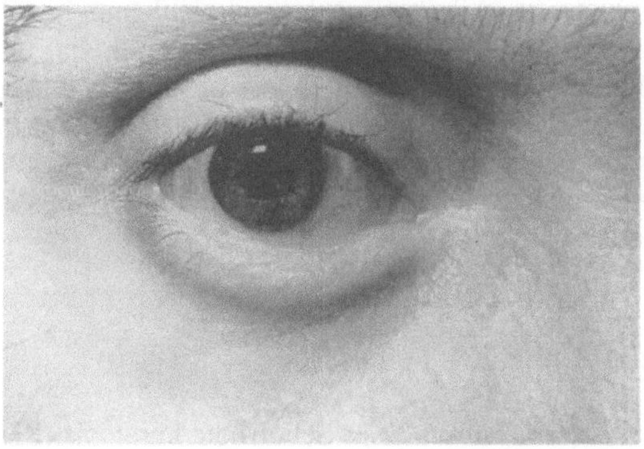

Fig. 8-15. 35-year-old male with ulcerating tumor with focal loss of lashes found to have trichoepithelioma.

Table 8-4
Clinical Appearance of Tumors of the Eyelids

Loss of Cilia
  Tumors
    sebaceous gland carcinoma
    basal cell carcinoma
    mucoepidermoid carcinoma of the palpebral conjunctiva
    lymphoma
    trichoepithelioma
    amyloidosis
    Merkel's cell tumor
  Inflammation
    chalazion
    infections—fungal
      acute or chronic blepharitis
      anthrax
Colored Lesions (Red, Blue, or Brown)
  Vascular tumor
    capillary hemangioma
    cavernous hemangioma
    venous angioma
    hemangiopericytoma
    glomus tumor
    angiolymphoid hyperplasia with eosinophilia
    Kaposi's sarcoma
    angiosarcoma
    pyogenic granuloma
  Melanocytic tumor
  Merkel's cell tumor
  Seborrheic keratosis
  Bowen's disease
  Actinic keratosis
  Basal cell carcinoma
  Eccrine acrospiroma
  Apocrine hydrocystoma
  Pilomatrixoma

  Dermatofibroma
  Dacryops or canaliculops
  Cylindroma, "turban tumor"
Multiple Tumors of Same Type in Same Patient
  Nevoid basal cell carcinoma syndrome
  Xeroderma pigmentosa
  Dysplastic nevus syndrome
  Apocrine or eccrine hydrocystoma
  Milia
  Syringoma
  Trichoepithelioma
  Actinic keratosis
  Xanthogranuloma
  Molluscum contagiosum
  Glomus tumor (as autosomal-dominant condition)
  Dermatofibroma
  Pseudorheumatoid nodules
  Sebaceous gland adenomas (Rulon-Helwig syndrome)
  Epidermal inclusion cyst (Gardner's syndrome)
  Verruca vulgaris, trichilemmoma (Cowden's syndrome)
  Kaposi's sarcoma (in AIDS patient)
  Neurofibromas (in von Recklinghausen's disease)
  Squamous cell carcinoma (bilateral in immunosuppressed patient)
  Metastatic disease
  Cylindroma ("turban tumor")
Multiple Tumors of Different Type in the Same Patient
  Actinic keratosis
  Bowen's disease
  BCC
  SCC
Cutaneous Horn
  Actinic keratosis
  Bowen's disease
  Inverted follicular keratosis
  Verruca vulgaris
  Squamous cell carcinoma
  Sebaceous gland carcinoma
Umbilicated Appearance
  Molluscum contagiosum
  Keratoacanthoma
  Basal cell carcinoma
  Trichofolliculoma
  Eccrine acrospiroma
  Pleomorphic adenoma of the sweat gland
Cystic Lesions
  Hydrocystomas (apocrine, eccrine)
  Eccrine sweat gland carcinoma (may ulcerate)
  Epidermal inclusion cysts
  Milia
  Sebaceous (pilar) cysts
  Epidermal inclusion cyst

Table 8-4 (Continued)

    Dermoid cysts
    Pilomatrixoma
    Eccrine acrospiroma
    Basal cell carcinoma
    Dacryops
    Canaliculops
Lesions That Ulcerate
    Epidermal (BCC most commonly)
    Adnexal
        trichilemmoma
        eccrine sweat gland carcinoma (may be cystic)
    Soft tissue
        atypical fibroxanthoma
    Necrobiotic axanthogranuloma (not garden variety
        xanthelasma)
    Metastatic cancer to the lid
    B-cell lymphoma of lid in immunosuppressed patient
Subcutaneous Tumor Temporal Aspect of Upper Lid
    (Orbit)
    Eosinophilic granuloma
    Pseudorheumatoid nodules
    Pilomatrixoma
    Dacryops
    Dermoid cyst
    Pilar cyst
Immunosuppression Predisposes To:
    Squamous cell carcinoma more than basal cell carci-
        noma
    B-cell lymphoma of lid

nating in the accessory lacrimal gland or in the palpebral lobe of the main lacrimal gland, dermoid cyst, pilar cyst, pilmatrixoma, eosinophilic granuloma, and pseudorheumatoid nodule. All are cystic except the latter two entities. Eosinophilic granuloma and dermoid cyst are oribital tumors.

CLINICAL AND HISTOLOGIC FEATURES OF SPECIFIC ENTITIES

Epithelial Tumors

Epithelial tumors may be broken down into benign, premalignant, and malignant tumors including seborrheic keratosis, inverted follicular keratosis, epidermal inclusion cyst, keratoacanthoma, pseudoepitheliomatous hyperplasia, benign keratosis, and viral infections such as molluscum contagiosum and verrucous vulgaris.

It is worthwhile to consider clinical and histologic features at the same time. In general, epithelial tumors tend to arise superficially with loss of the skin markings. In tumors arising from dermal appendages, the skin markings are generally preserved unless there is a histologic connection between the epidermis and underlying dermal tumor.

Benign Epithelial Tumors

Seborrheic Keratosis.   Seborrheic keratosis (SK) often occurs in elderly patients and is the most common tumor involving the eyelids. The tumors are characteristically well-circumscribed and have a stuck-on appearance and occur anywhere on the skin surface. The pattern may be nodular, papillary, or verrucous and may be confused with a wart or papilloma (Fig. 8-16). A *papilloma,* by definition, has a fibrovascular core while the

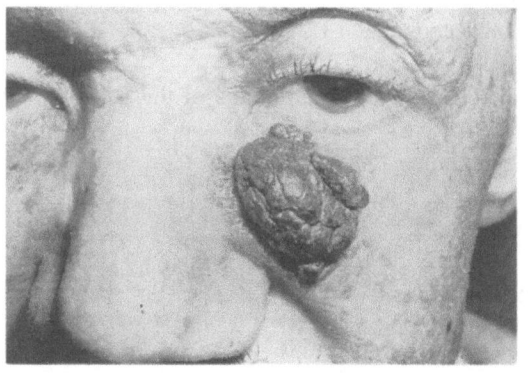

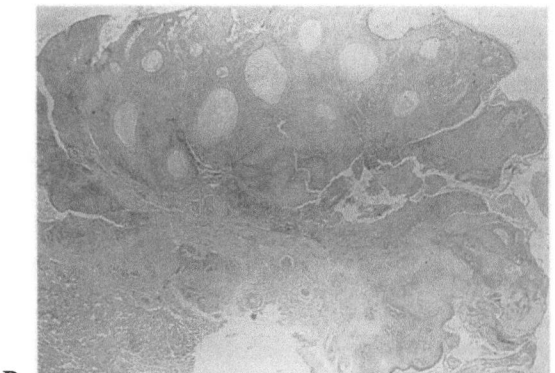

Fig. 8-16.   (*A*) Large seborrheic keratosis causing mechanical ectropion has the clinical appearance of a button on the skin. Removal and reconstruction with full-thickness skin graft was necessary in order to avoid postoperative cicatricial ectropion. (*B*) Histologic features of a basaloid proliferation of epidermal cells with "pseudohorn cysts" that are due to tangential cuts across the papillary fronds of proliferating cells (AFIP ACC #866115).

term *papillary* is due to folds of epithelium without a fibrovascular core.[3]

Because SKs are light tan in color, they may be confused clinically with a nevus or malignant melanoma; histologic confusion is rarely, if ever, a problem.

As the clinical appearance suggests, the lesion is elevated above the level of the adjacent epidermis and its hallmark is a uniform proliferation of basaloid cells. As stated above, the presence of fibrovascular cores regularly spaced within the epidermal proliferation gives the papillomatous pattern. Keratin cysts are another characteristic histologic feature of SK. The "cysts" are invaginated surface keratin that is cut in cross-section.

The histologic differential diagnosis includes SCC. However, unlike SCC, there is no atypia of the proliferat-

ing epithelium. The lack of peripheral palisading of the islands of basaloid cells is helpful in ruling out the diagnosis of BCC. *Irritated seborrheic keratosis* is another name for inverted follicular keratosis.

Inverted Follicular Keratosis. Inverted follicular keratosis (IFK) occurs mainly on the face and may be a solitary nodule, papilloma, verruca, and occasionally a cutaneous horn. The tumors are usually small (Fig. 8-17).

Histologically, the lesion may have a cup-shaped configuration and pathologically may be confused with a keratoacanthoma.[35,36] Invaginating bands or folds of epithelium are present. The characteristic histologic feature of the lesion is the presence of squamous eddies. Squa-

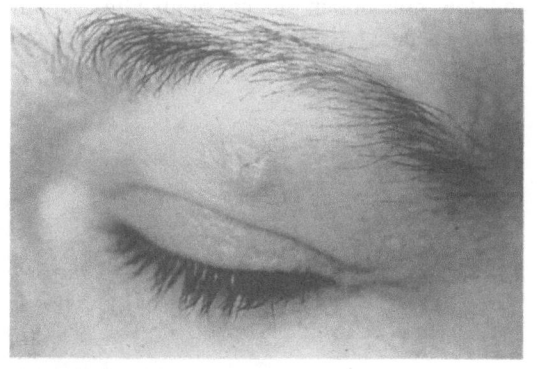

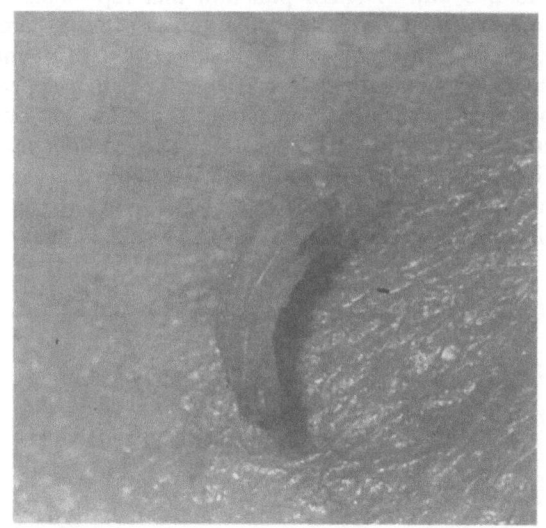

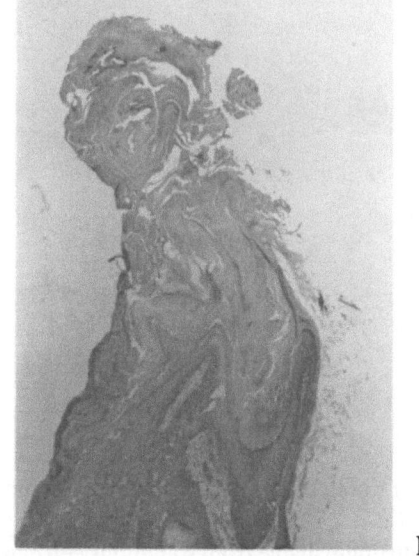

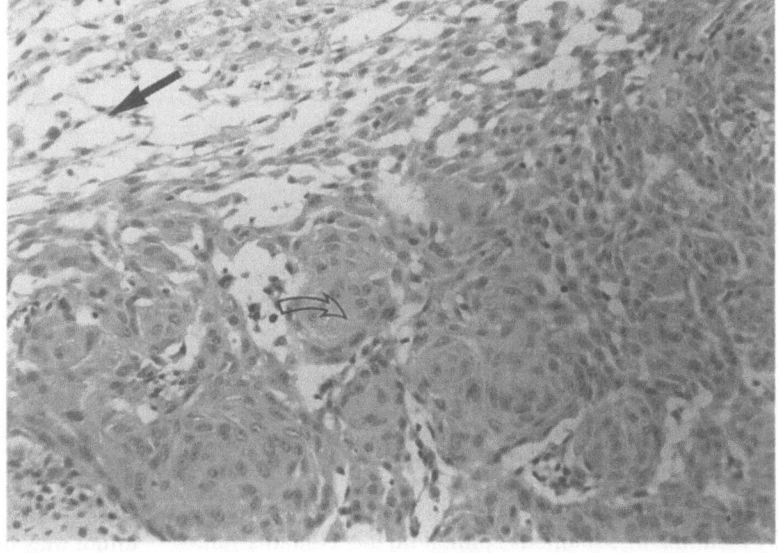

Fig. 8-17. (*A,B*) Inverted follicular keratosis may present as an umbilicated tumor (*A*) or a cutaneous horn (*B,C*). (*D*) Histologically, the tumor is composed of squamous eddies (open arrow) with acantholysis (solid arrow). (Courtesy AFIP, Washington, DC.)

mous eddies are present between the basaloid cells in the deep layers of epithelium and the squamoid cells in the superficial layers. At the junction of these cell groups, there is acantholysis, intercellular edema, and nests of uniform squamous cells known as squamous eddies. Acantholysis is classically present adjacent to the squamous eddies.

Most pathologists do not consider IFK a distinct entity but categorize IFK as an irritated variant of seborrheic keratosis. The histologic features of IFK have been induced in seborrheic keratosis. The lesion is benign and should not be confused with SCC.

Epidermal Inclusion Cyst.　　Clinically, these lesions may be single or multiple and appear as yellowish-white well-demarcated growths. They range in size from 1 mm to 2–3 cm. A small punctum that represents the site of invagination of the epithelium is often apparent (Fig. 8-18). An epidermal inclusion cyst (EICs) may be confused with xanthelasma, but the latter appears deeper in the skin and is generally not round or well-circumscribed. When EICs are multiple, the diagnosis of Gardner's syndrome and Torre's syndrome should be considered.

Histologically, the tumor forms because the epidermis invaginates in order to form a cyst. Keratin that is produced by normal maturation of the keratinizing epidermis expands the cyst.

Keratoacanthoma.　　This tumor is often clinically and histologically confused with SCC. The tumor tends to affect the elderly and most commonly involves the sun-exposed areas of the body including the face, forearm, and head. Usually, the lesion is single (Fig. 8-19). The history of rapid growth over a few weeks to months is the single most helpful means of differentiating this lesion from SCC, which usually has a slower rate of growth. The lesions are large, round, and elevated with an umbilicated center. The center may appear crusted. Spontaneous regression may occur.

A cup-shaped configuration is classic, but this pattern may not be recognized if the biopsy does not include the center of the lesion or if a representative section is not cut in the pathology laboratory. There is often acanthosis and hyperkeratosis in the center of the lesion, while the lateral margins are composed of normal epidermis. The epidermis at the base of the lesion is smooth and does not contain tongues of invading squamous cells that are characteristic of SCC. There is often a chronic

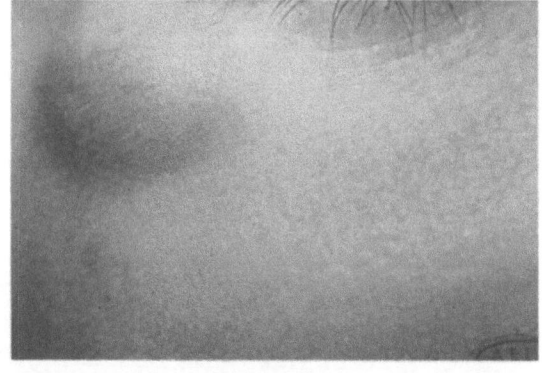

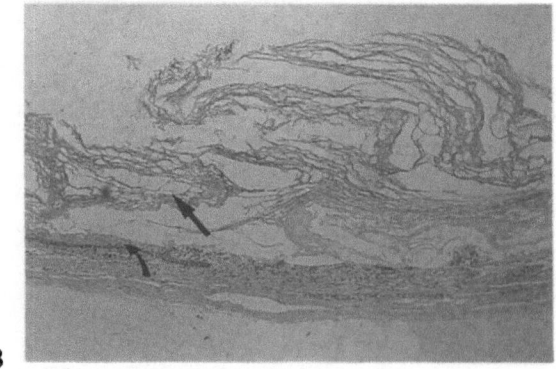

Fig. 8-18. (*A*) Epidermal inclusion cyst is a cyst lined by keratinizing squamous epithelium that contains yellow keratin. (*B*) Note keratin (straight arrow) above epithelium (curved arrow) on histologic section. (Courtesy AFIP, Washington, DC.)

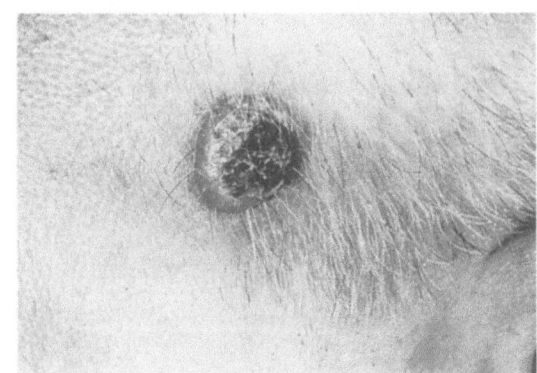

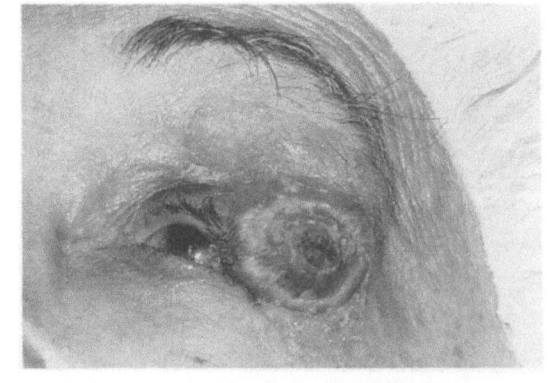

Fig. 8-19. (*A,B*) Keratoacanthoma typically has umbilicated edges with a necrotic center. Histologically, the tumor may be indistinguishable from squamous cell carcinoma. Compare with umbilicated mulluscum contagiosum without necrotic center (Fig. 8-14) and IFK (Fig. 8-17*A*).

inflammatory cell infiltrate in the dermis under the lesion. Perineural invasion has been reported at the base of the lesion. This invasion does not adversely affect the biologic behavior and prognosis.[42-44] This pattern was observed in 18 cases: one involved the cheek, two the forehead, and four the nose.

Unfortunately, the histologic criteria alone are not always satisfactory in determining the biologic behavior of some keratoacanthomas. About 30 percent of keratoacanthomas may not be cytologically distinguished from SCC. The term *carcinoma-like keratoacanthoma* has been applied to lesions with histologic features intermediate between keratoacanthoma and SCC.

Extensive tissue destruction and rapid growth over weeks associated with some growths and the possibility of recurrence favors definitive surgical therapy in large periocular keratoacathomas.

Pseudoepitheliomatous (Pseudocarcinomatous) Hyperplasia.
Pseudoepitheliomatous hyperplasia (PEH) is a descriptive histopathologic term that refers to invasion of the dermis by proliferating bands of squamous epithelium. PEH is not a tumor.

Underlying causes of PEH include local skin tumors or inflammatory processes including granulomatous inflammation from insect bites, drugs (hypersensitivity reaction to halides including iodides, fluoride, and bromides), and infectious agents, particularly fungus infections.[16] An adjacent tumor such as a granular cell tumor, BCC, or dermatofibroma may be accompanied by PEH. The rapid proliferation of epidermis may be associated with hyperkeratosis and crusting.

Histologically, SCC may be confused with PEH, but the presence of microabscesses in the epidermis and foreign body giants cells and a chronic inflammatory cell infiltrate in the dermis are findings tha mitigate against the diagnosis of SCC and favor PEH due to a drug effect or infection (Fig. 8-20).[45]

Benign Keratosis.
A number of tumors are found to arise in the epidermis pathologically and have clearly benign features. These lesions cannot all be pigeonholed into one of the possible diagnostic categories and are therefore conveniently termed *benign keratosis*.

Papilloma.
Papilloma is a clinical term that refers to a variety of lesions such as seborrheic keratosis or verruca vulgaris. *Papilloma* is a descriptive pathologic term that defines an epithelial lesion with a fibrovascular core. The papilloma may be sessile or pedunculated. Sessile papillomas are raised from the adjacent epidermis, while pedunculated polyps contain a connective tissue stalk.

Viral Lesions—Molluscum Contagiosum and Verruca Vulgaris.
Molluscum contagiosum is a mildly contagious autoinoculable disease of the skin caused by a pox virus. The lesions may be pinhead to pea-sized, waxy, firm, button-like, pruritic papules. They develop slowly over a period of weeks and may remain indefinitely

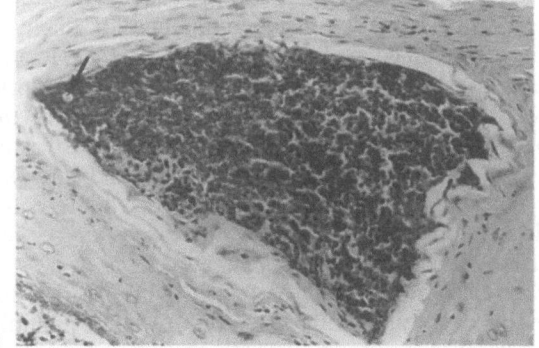

Fig. 8-20. (*A*) 35-year-old with biopsy interpreted as "squamous cell carinoma." A second biopsy showed microabscesses (*B*) in the epidermis and foreign body giant cells (solid arrow) adjacent to proliferating tongues of epidermis (large open arrows) in the dermis. (*C*) Budding yeasts (arrow) characteristic of North American blastomycosis were found in the microabscesses (*B*). The patient underwent work-up for systemic fungal disease and was treated with systemic antifungal agents (AFIP ACC #1797037).

without therapy. We have seen multiple facial lesions associated with AIDS.

Histologically, there is a bulbous downgrowth of epithelium with an umbilicated configuration. The molluscum bodies are the pathognomonic feature and consist of homogeneously smooth, brightly eosinophilic cytoplasmic structures involving the lower cells of the malpighian layer that contains the virus. The nucleus is flattened to one side of the cell.[45]

Verruca vulgaris is the common papillary wart.

Histologically, the verruca vulgaris is characterized by a papillary acanthosis with overlying friable hyperkeratosis. Basophilic intranuclear inclusions with a clear halo are present in the upper malpighian and granular layers. These layers contain groups of large vacuolated cells due to the virus; these infected cells contain few or no keratohyaline granules. This DNA virus belongs to the papova group. Intranuclear eosinophilic material is related to the keratin.[45]

Decision to Biopsy

The decision to biopsy is determined by whether, based on history and clinical examination, the tumor is benign or suspected of representing a malignancy.

Management of Presumed Benign Tumors

Lesions such as seborrheic keratosis should be excised on the basis of cosmetic considerations since the diagnosis in most cases can be made without biopsy. Full-thickness lid resections are generally not indicated without prior biopsy. Benign tumors with evidence of growth that are on the lid border should be initially shaved if small (less than 3 mm). Should they enlarge and encroach posterior to the gray line, full-thickness lid resection should be considered for cosmetic reasons or because the lesion mechanically irritates the eye.

Recurrent verrucae may be treated with excision followed by cautery, cryotherapy, or CO_2 laser. Intralesional injections with dinitrochlorobenzene have been advocated in order to stimulate an immunologic response.[46] For multiple recurrences, intralesional injection of bleomycin has been used for conjunctival papillomas with encouraging results.[47]

Epithelial—Premalignant (Precancerous Dermatoses) Conditions

Actinic Keratosis (Solar Keratosis, Senile Keratosis). Actinic keratosis develops in older patients with a history of sun exposure. Arsenic, oils, tar, and radiation are also predisposing causes (Fig. 8-4). The extreme rarity of the lesion in children except in cases of radiation or xeroderma pigmentosum and lack of occupational exposure highlights the importance of years of actinic damage as the main underlying cause. The face is frequently involved. The lesions are multiple, scaling, and erythematous. They may present as cutaneous horns, as may Bowen's disease, verruca vulgaris, benign keratosis, inverted follicular keratosis, SCC, and sebaceous gland carcinoma.

It has been estimated that SCC infrequently arises from actinic keratosis (in 0.5% of cases) and from Bowen's disease in 5 percent of cases.[48,49]

Histologically, the hallmarks of the lesion are the epidermal proliferations, cellular pleomorphism, and mitotic figures confined to the basal layers. The irregular buds of atypical keratinocytes extend into the papillary dermis. The superficial layers appear squamoid and eosinophilic and contain acanthosis, hyperkeratosis, and parakeratosis. The upper dermis shows moderate-to-severe basophilic "elastotic" degeneration with a moderate lymphoplasmacytic infiltrate. The material is "elastotic" and not true elastic tissue in that the degenerated collagen stains with elastic stains, but pretreatment of the slide with elastase does not affect the staining of the collagen.

Bowen's Disease. Bowen's disease appears as an erythematous pigmented scaling plaque sharply demarcated from the surrounding skin (Fig. 8-8). The lesion is most common in elderly white patients and is single in most cases, but may be multiple. The disease is associated with cancers of internal organs in 28 of 35 patients.[48,50] Bowen's disease should not be diagnosed in the conjunctiva.

Histologically, the lesion shows a plaque-like involvement with acanthosis, hyperkeratosis, and parakeratosis. The epidermal cells show full-thickness atypia, unlike actinic keratosis where the atypia is confined to the basal epidermis.

Radiation Dermatosis. Generally, doses of 800–12,000 rad cause severe if not permanent damage to the lid structures. In one study, scarring of the tarsus with total obliteration of the meibomian glands and their ducts occurred.[51] Diffuse lacrimal gland atrophy also occurs. Thirty-six of 368 patients who received radiation therapy developed skin cancer of the head and neck with a median interval of 21 years after the treatment. Two-thirds of the tumors were BCC. SCC occurred much less frequently but showed a significantly greater chance of metastases than the garden variety of SCC.[52]

Xeroderma Pigmentosum, Nevoid Basal Cell Carcinoma Syndrome, Dysplastic Nevus Syndrome. See discussion above.

Epithelial Malignant Conditions

Basal Cell Carcinoma. Basal cell carcinoma is the most common malignant tumor of the eyelids. The tumor is associated with sun and radiation exposure and inherited conditions such as nevoid basal cell carcinoma syndrome and xeroderma pigmentosum.

Clinically, there are several variants. First, the noduloulcerative type begins as a firm, raised, pearly nodule that may have fine telangiectatic vessels over its surface. The pearly edge typically loses its skin lines. The noduloulcerative type develops a central area of ulceration (rodent ulcer) that crusts, bleeds, scabs, and rebleeds. Second, the pigmented type is similar to the nodular or noduloulcerative type except for the presence of brown pigment. The pigmented BCC may be confused with seborrheic keratosis, nevus, or melanoma. Third, the morphea or sclerosing type of basal cell is a pale indurated plaque with an ill-defined border. Fourth, superficial basal cells may rise in the eyelid but are more common in the trunk. They appear as erythematous scaling patches and often have a fine pearly border. They may ulcerate and crust. Fifth, nevoid basal cell carcinoma syndrome may affect the lids. Other types not found on the face include fibroepithelioma, linear basal cell nevus, and generalized follicular basal cell nevus (Fig. 8-21.)[7–11] The tumor is more common in the lower than the upper lid where SCC is more common.

Histologically, the undifferentiated tumor is composed of solid masses of uniform basaloid cells with scanty cytoplasm. There is often a desmoplastic stroma and artifactitious clefts between the basaloid proliferations and the fibrous stroma (Fig. 8-22).

There are three types of differentiation that may be present in any one tumor and all are due to differentiation toward cutaneous appendages: (1) keratotic differentiation shows features of hair structures, (2) cystic differentiation shows characteristics resembling sebaceous glands and clinically may be confused with an epidermal inclusion cyst, and (3) adenoid differentiation shows differentiation toward apocrine and eccrine structures.

In general, the pigmented, morphea, and superficial types of BCC show little or no differentiation, while the noduloulcerative type often shows differentiation.

In addition, there are several types of growth patterns; the main variants are (1) nodular, (2) ulcerative, (3) fibrosing or morpheaform, and (4) multicentric. The various histologic types are of no prognostic significance except for the morpheaform BCC.[53] The morphea variant contains dense fibrous stroma that contains narrow epithelial strands of cells one to two cell layers wide. A worse prognosis is associated with this type of BCC than with the other forms of BCC.

Other tumors with features of a true invading SCC along with features of a BCC (basosquamous cell carcinoma, metatypical BCC) have the prognosis of the more aggressive lesion, the SCC.[54]

Management of Biopsied BCC. Prevention including protective clothing and pharmacologic sun-blocking agents including paraaminobenzoic acid are necessary in patients prone to develop precancerous dermatosis.

BCCs of the lid areas should be excised with frozen section control since one study showed that only 50 percent of lesions were completely excised without frozen section control.[55] We do not believe that all patients with BCC should have Mohs microsurgery. Rather, we rely on wide excision with frozen section control. There are two main indications for the Mohs technique. First, a medial canthal mass that occurs in a young individual (less than 40 years of age) may benefit from Mohs microsurgery. Medial canthal tumors tend to be worrisome because of their adjacency and, therefore, propensity for bone and subsequent sinus invasion. Such tumors should be at least treated more aggressively in terms of wider excision than lateral canthal tumors. Second, recurrent BCC in the lid area should be an indication for Mohs microsurgery (see Chapter 5).

Frozen section control or Mohs microsurgery is less precise when the tumor extends into the orbital fat and is impossible in the examination of bones.

Topical chemotherapy using 5-fluorouracil cream has been used in the treatment of SCC in situ, actinic and arsenical keratoses, and Bowen's disease. Local chemotherapy is not advocated in the routine treatment of invasive SCC.[56–57]

Radiation therapy has been utilized more effectively in the treatment of BCC than SCC.[58] It may be less efficacious with tumors of the morphea type[57] Because SCC is relatively radioresistant, greater amounts of radiation are needed, for example, a total dose of 5440 rad versus 3400 rad in BCC. With shielding, 57 rad is below the minimum cataractogenic dose.[58] Complications of radiation include erythema and edema of the treated skin, canalicular occlusion due to keratinization, ectropion with exposure keratitis due to fibrosis, and dry eye due to atrophy of the meibomian and main and accessory lacrimal glands.

Cryotherapy has been utilized in the treatment of SCC and BCC. Complications include recurrence of tumor and lacrimal obstruction (see Treatment of Eyelid Tumors).

Squamous Cell Carinoma. In one study, SCC accounted for about 9.2 percent of all eyelid malignancies.[41] Other studies of eyelid SCC show a range from 2.9 to 30.2 percent.[48] SCC tends to occur in the sun-exposed portions of the body, particularly the face and hands; actinic damage is the most common predisposing cause. Other inciting factors include soot in chimney sweeps, which also predisposes to scrotal carcinoma and hydrocarbon exposure. Forrest reported a case of SCC following radiation for retinoblastoma.[59]

A review of material in the Registry of Ophthalmic Pathology showed that SCC of the eyelid is 39 times

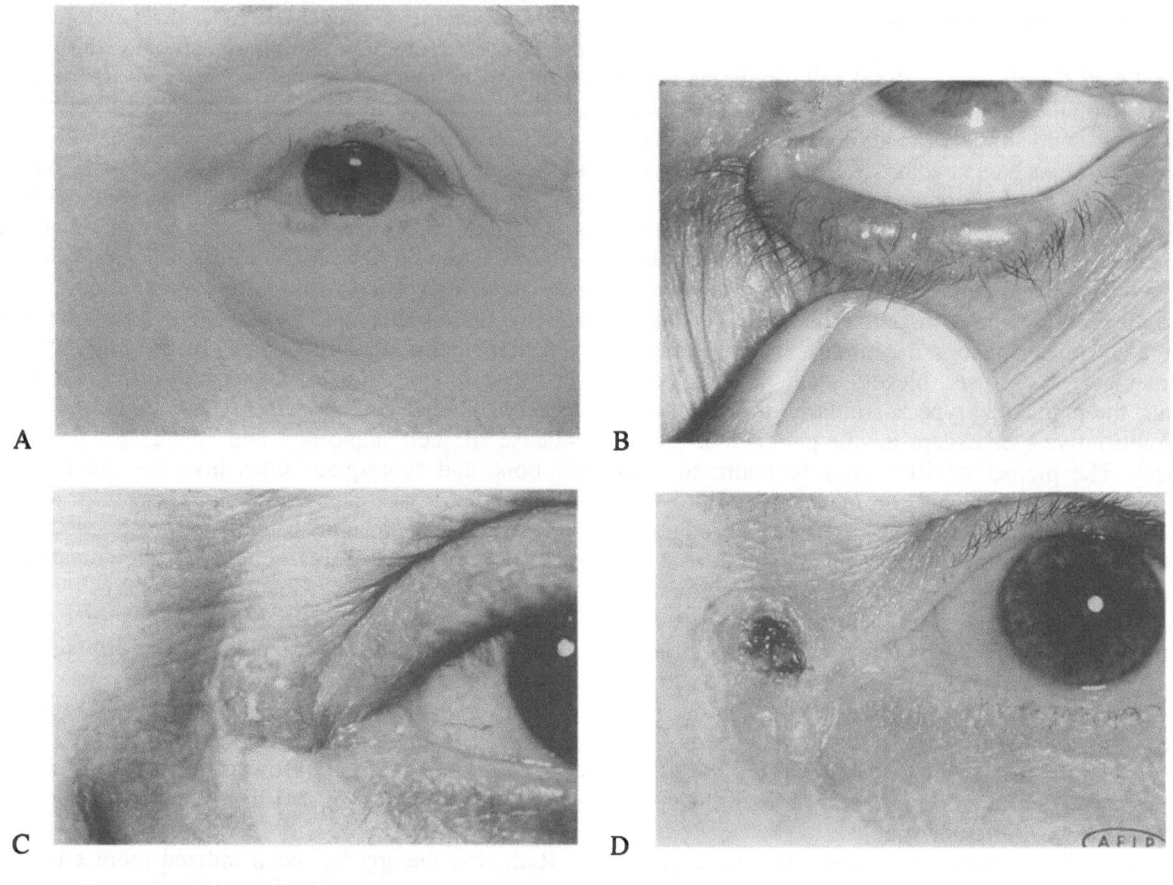

A

B

C

D

E

Fig. 8-21. (A) 58-year-old female with slow-growing mass associated with loss of lashes, foacl lid retraction, and chronic mucous discharge in left eye. Biopsy showed basal cell carcinoma. (B) Solid pink, multicentric basal cell carcinoma of lid margin. (C) Polypoid basal cell carcinoma of medial canthus (AFIP ACC #990758). (D) Nodular ulcerative basal cell carcinoma of medial canthus. (E) 68-year-old male with BCC in area traumatized by glasses.

less frequent than BCC.[19] SCC tends to arise in actinic keratosis, Bowen's disease, xeroderma pigmentosum, and after radiation or arsenic exposure. The tumor is less malignant when it arises in AK than when it arises in chronic ulcers, burn scars, radiation dermatitis, arsenic deposition, Bowen's disease, or de novo.

While BCC is more common in the lower lid, SCC is more common in the upper lid (Fig. 8-23). As discussed above, immunosuppressed patients who are recipients of organ transplants may develop bilateral SCC of the lower lids rather than the upper lids as in other patients with SCC of the lids.

In addition, patients who are the recipients of organ

transplants with therapeutic suppression of their immunologic systems are at a greater risk of developing SCC than the general population.[37–40] Skin cancers constituted 39 percent and lymphoid 27 percent of the cases in a tumor registry study of transplant patients. SCC outnumbers BCC in this subpopulation of patients at risk. Patients with long-term immunosuppressive therapy after renal transplantation developed bilateral lower lid SCC. Such patients usually have other tumors elsewhere in the skin. There is a predilection for lower lid involvement, particularly at the lid margin, in contrast to upper lid involvement if de novo.

In summary, SCC may arise from a precancerous der-

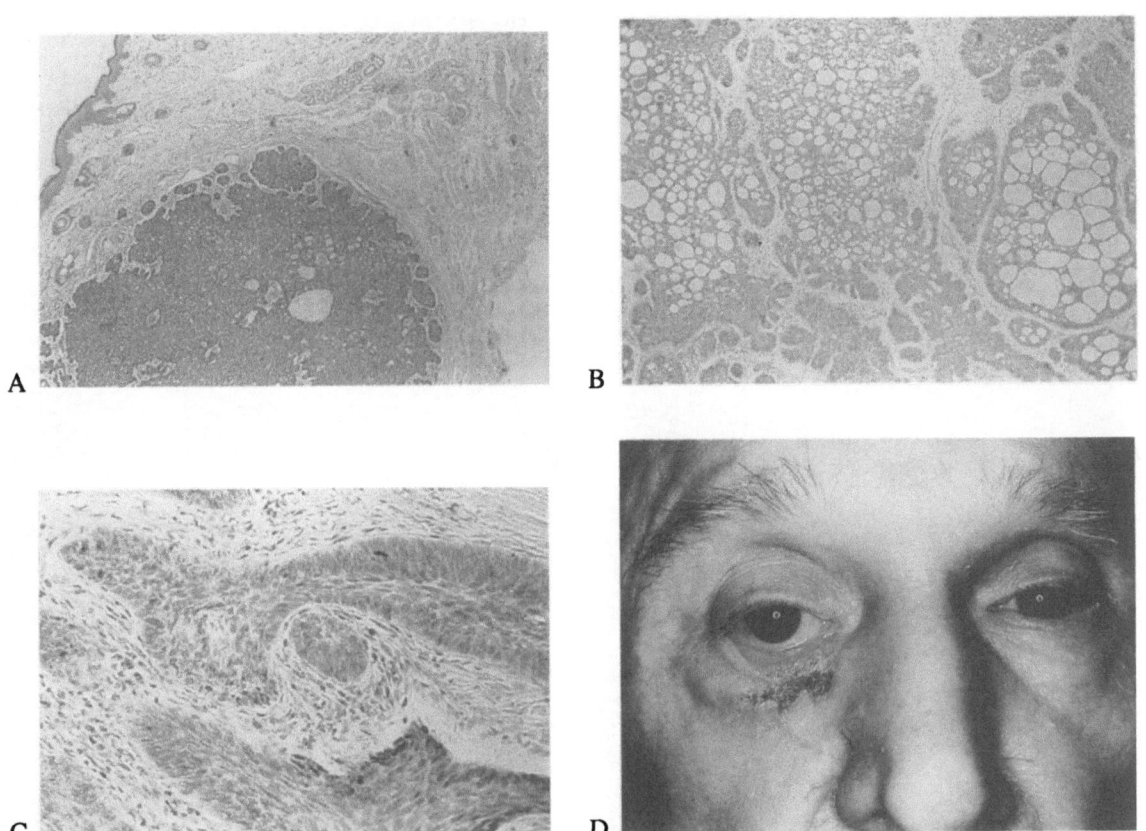

Fig. 8-22. (*A*) Nodule of basal cell carcinoma composed of basaloid cells. Note islands of tumor cells adjacent to main tumor mass. (*B*) Cystic variant of basal cell carcinoma with multiple cysts. (*C*) Higher power magnification shows hallmarks of basal cell carcinoma: basaloid cells and peripheral palisading of tumor cells. (*D*) Patient with basal cell carcinoma of lower lid causing ectropion. (*A–C* courtesy AFIP, Washington, DC.)

matosis such as Bowen's disease, actinic keratosis, in immunosuppressed patients, or de novo.

Clinically, the lesions appear as roughened scaly patches that may develop crusting, erosion, and fissures over a period of months. After crusting occurs, the central portion of the tumor may ulcerate. The base appears red and sharply defined. The borders are indurated and elevated. Ulcerations generally occur more quickly than in BCC.[48,60] Other clinical presentations include papillomatous growth, rounded nodular or cyst-like lesion, or a cutaneous horn. BCC and SCC may present virtually identically. However, keratin, appearing as crusting, may be more evident in SCC.

In general, the lymphatic spread of tumors of the upper lids and lateral canthus is toward the preauricular nodes and tumors of the lower lid and medial canthus is toward the submaxillary nodes. Rates of metastasis vary from 1 in 79 cases to 3 in 14 cases.[60,61] Orbital invasion is much more common with SCC than with BCC. SCC that involves the orbit is significantly more likely to arise in the paranasal sinuses than the periorbital skin. Mortality ranges from 0–40 percent.

Histologically, the pattern is dependent on the degree of differentiation. In general, SCC shows irregular nests of epidermal cells that have infiltrated the basement membrane and invaded the dermis. In well-differentiated tumors, the nests of squamous cells that invade the dermis may have intercellular spines (desmosomes) keratin. In some cases of highly anaplastic SCC, differentiation may be lacking. Spindle cell carcinoma often follows radiation and shows no differentiation. Such tumors tend to have a greater propensity for metastasis.[45] Immunoperoxidase studies for keratin may be helpful in such cases.

Adenoid squamous cell carcinoma (adenoacanthoma, pseudoglandular SCC, is a histologic variant of SCC characterized by acantholysis that gives the appearance of glandular structures. Adenoid SCC is associated with a better prognosis than other forms of SCC.[62]

SCC that arises in AK has a significantly lower rate of metastasis (0.25%) than SCC that arises de novo (approximately 2% rate of metastases). SCC that is secondary to a burn scar, radiation dermatitis, or osteomyelitis of the sinus bone carries a significantly higher (10–30%) rate of metastasis. In addition, mucocutaneous SCC has a high (11%) rate of metastasis.

Management of SCC. Management is similar to that of BCC. We tend to excise SCC more widely than BCC

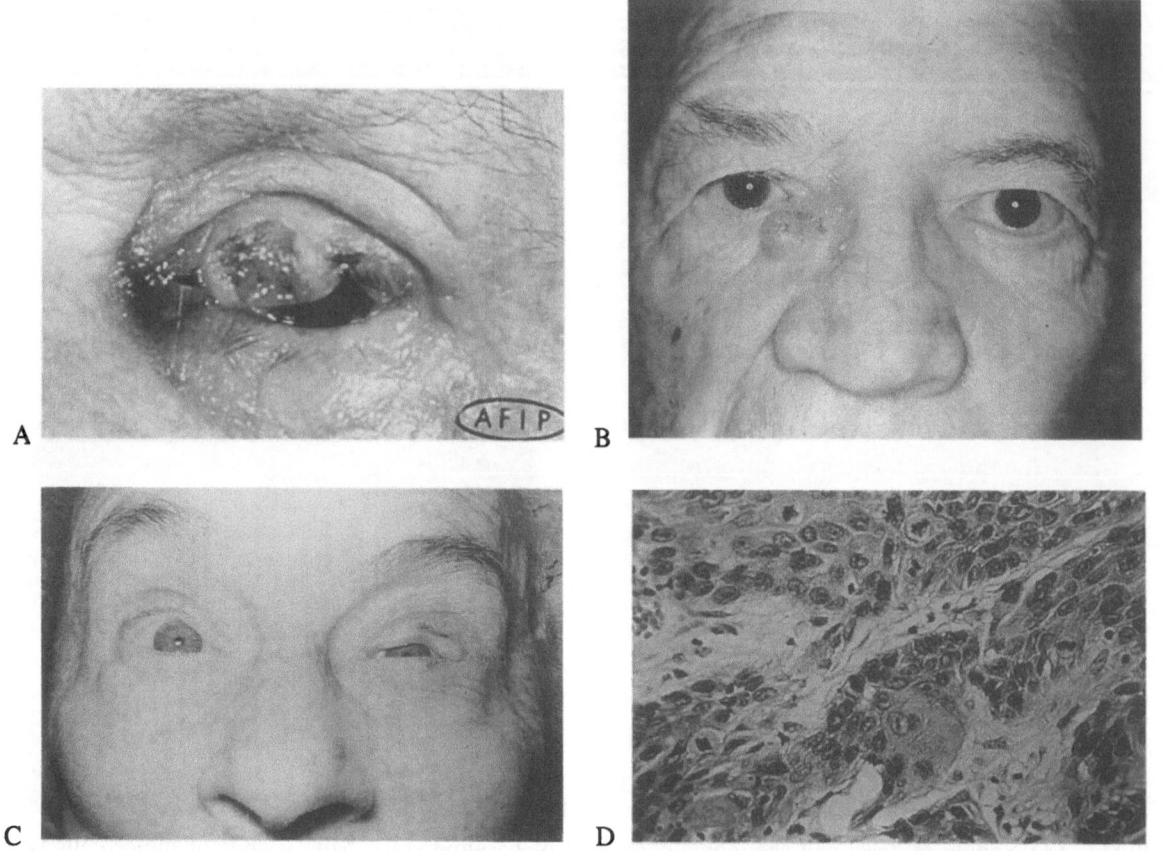

Fig. 8-23. (*A*) Ulcerated squamous cell carcinoma of upper lid is indistinguishable from basal cell carcinoma (AFIP ACC #1046857). (*B*) Squamous cell carcinoma of medial canthus that was thought to represent a BCC. (*C*) 72-year-old female with squamous cell carcinoma of left upper lid. (*D*) Note malignant squamous cells invading the dermis.

because of its greater tendency to metastasize (see Treatment of Eyelid Tumors).

Adnexal—Pilar

In general, pilar tumors appear to clinically arise from the dermal structures rather than from the superficial epidermis. The exceptions include trichofolliculoma, with its central umbilication containing a white hair, and pilar cyst, which may appear identical to an epidermal inclusion cyst. Trichilemmomas may ulcerate and resemble a noduloulcerative BCC.

Trichoepithelioma. Trichoepithelioma (Brooke's tumor, epithelioma adenoides cysticum, multiple benign cystic epithelioma, Brooke's tumor), when multiple, is inherited as an autosomal-dominant condition. Multiple smooth, flesh-colored papules rarely ulcerate and involve the face and chest (Fig. 8-12*D, E*). This lack of ulceration is helpful in distinguishing this condition from basal cell nevus syndrome.[15] Patients with hereditary trichoepithelioma should be observed for ulcerated lesions that

might indicate transformation of a benign trichoepithelioma into a BCC.[63]

Histologically, the hallmarks of this tumor are horn cysts and basaloid proliferations. The horn cysts have a keratin core demarcated by a layer of basal cells. The epidermis is intact. The histologic differential diagnosis includes keratotic BCC and nevoid basal cell carcinoma syndrome when the tumors are multiple.

Trichofolliculoma. Trichofolliculoma is a hamartoma that is the most differentiated pilar tumor. Clinically it is a solitary, slightly elevated nodule of 4–5 mm with a central area of umbilication representing the opening of a keratin-filled dilated follicle. Small white hairs often grow from the central pore.

Histologically, it is a cystic structure that consists of a dilated hair follicle filled with keratin (Fig. 8-24). The cyst is surrounded by basaloid cells showing variable degrees of abortive pilar formation (secondary "immature" hair structures).

Pilomatrixomas (Benign Calcifying Tumor of Malherbe). Pilomatrixoma may be a solid or cystic tumor

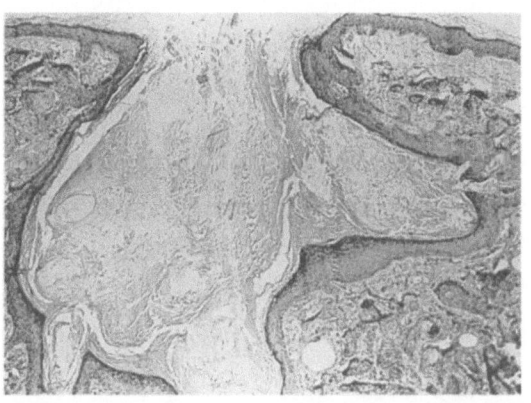

Fig. 8-24. Biopsy shows cystic structure consisting of dilated hair follicle surrounded by immature hair structures, consistent with trichofolliculoma (AFIP ACC #1354541).

that arises from the hair matrix cells. It is a solitary, freely moveable subcutaneous nodule that has a definite predilection for the upper lid and brow areas (Fig. 8-25). The lesion is pink to purple in color. Sixty percent occur in patients 20 years of age or younger.[64,65] A typical case report is that of a 51-year-old who presents with a corneal ulceration due to a white, calcified pilomatrixoma that eroded through the superior tarsal conjunctiva. The tumor presumably arose from a congenitally ectopic hair follicle tumor.

Histologically, a well-demarcated nodule involving the lower dermis is composed of islands of basophilic cells and shadow cells. The basophilic cells are located at the periphery of the islands and the shadow cells at the center. Calcium is deposited in older tumors that show increased number of shadow cells as the tumor ages. Calcified shadow cells often elicit a foreign body giant bell reaction.

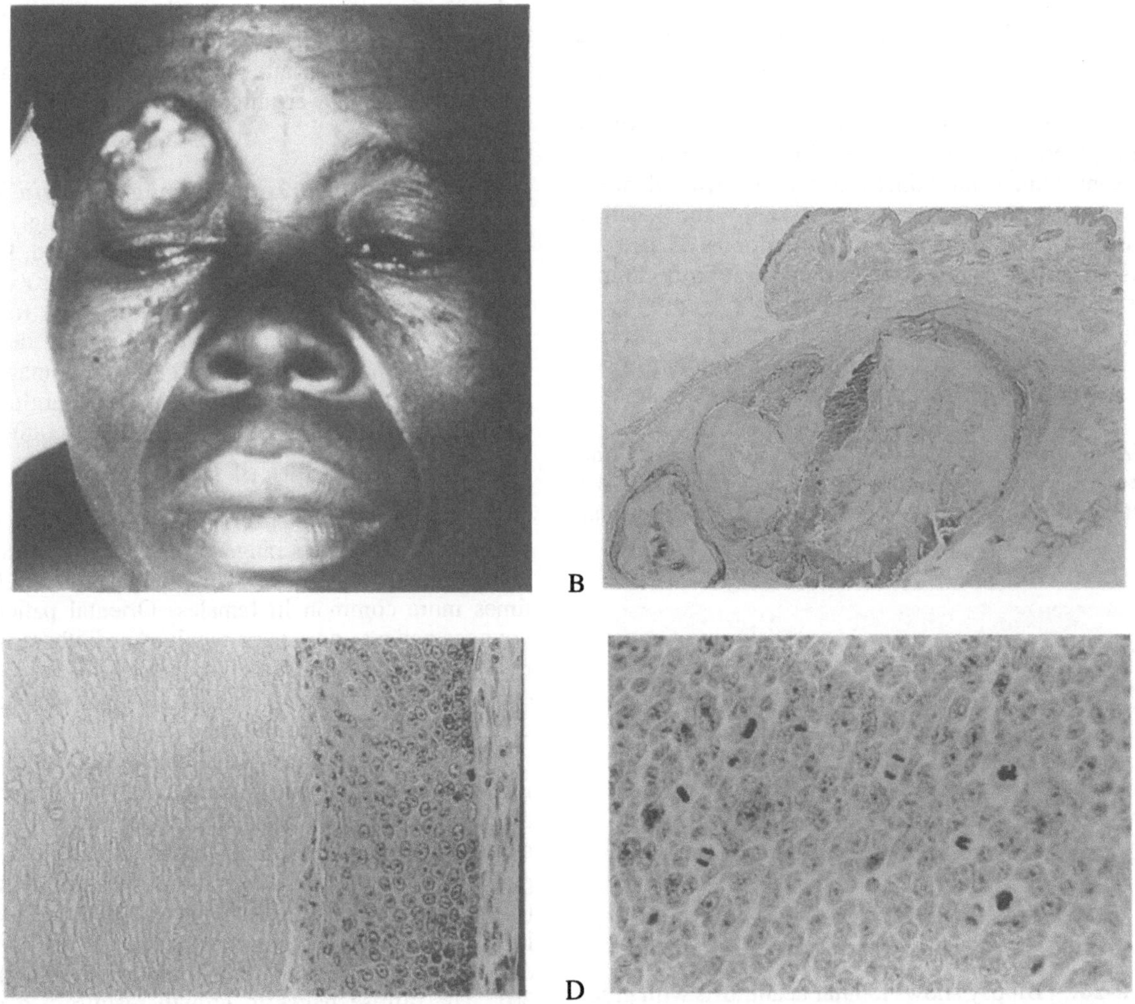

Fig. 8-25. (A) 50-year-old African woman with neglected pilomatrixoma (Courtesy of Ralph C. Eagle, Jr., M.D., Wills Eye Hospital, Philadelphia, PA.) (B) Histology from a similar case shows a subcutaneous tumor that (C) on higher power magnification has "shadow cells" and (D) basophilic cells with many mitotic figures (AFIP ACC #808810 and 814184).

Trichilemmoma. This benign tumor arises from the outer hair sheath that contains glycogen-rich clear cells. The tumors are single, small, and asymptomatic papules or nodules with irregular, rough surfaces that may ulcerate. The latter clinical presentation is due to the tumor's connection with the overlying epidermis.

Histologically, the tumor shows lobular acanthosis of glycogen-rich cells (Fig. 8-26). The periphery of the tumor lobules show palisading of columnar cells with a distinct basement membrane. The center of the lesion often shows epithelial islands with squamoid differentiation. The tumor may be confused pathologically with BCC.[67]

Milia. See discussion of multiple lid tumors.

Pilar Cyst. See discussion of multiple lid tumors.

Adnexal—Sebaceous

Sebaceous Gland Hyperplasia and Adenoma. Sebaceous gland hyperplasia is an overgrowth and multiplication of sebaceous glands that produce a lesion resembling a neoplasm. True adenomas show a loss of the normal glandular pattern (Fig. 8-27). Acinar organization is present, but a central duct is absent in a true adenoma. The adjacent tissues are compressed by the localized tumors but no invasion occurs. Hamartomas of the sebaceous gland (adenoma sebaceum) occur at birth in tuberous sclerosis.

Multiple sebaceous adenomas have been associated with low-grade visceral carcinomas of the colon. In general, the visceral lesions precede the skin lesions.

Management of Possible Benign and Premalignant Tumors. When evaluation of tumor is not clear-cut, a history of recent growth would influence the physician

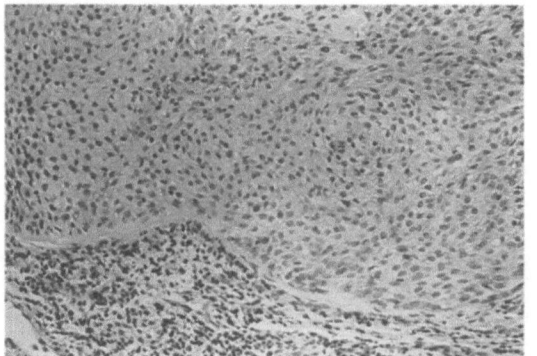

Fig. 8-26. Biopsy shows lobular acanthosis with glycogen-rich cells. The edge of the tumor shows a distinct basement membrane on which columnar cells rest (AFIP ACC #1467417).

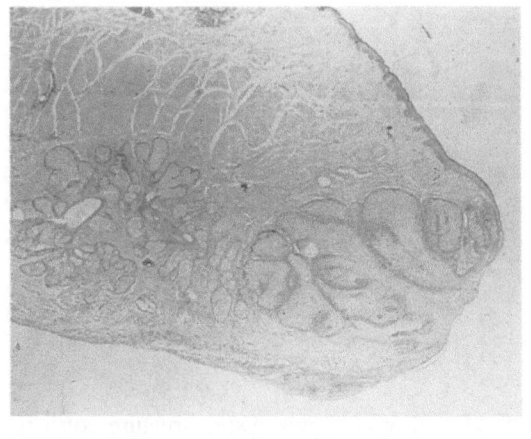

Fig. 8-27. Sebaceous gland adenoma of lid margin (AFIP ACC #942326) in which there is a proliferation of the ductal elements of the sebaceous glands.

to biopsy the lesion. A premalignant tumor such as Bowen's disease or actinic keratosis warrants excisional biopsy if possible. A shave biopsy with a No. 11 blade is often most appropriate. In general, full-thickness lid resections are not warranted for benign tumors or premalignant tumors.

Management of Presumed Malignant Skin Tumor. In cases where malignancy is possible or strongly considered, an incisional biopsy should be performed. Depending on the size of the tumor, an incisional or excisional biopsy is indicated. Tumors on or adjacent to the lid order require a shave biopsy to confirm the diagnosis. Malignant tumors such as basal cell carcinomas require a full-thickness lid resection with 2–3 mm margins. Sebaceous gland and squamous cell tumors require wider excision.

Sebaceous Gland Carcinoma. In a series of 104 patients,[68] the patients ranged in age from 13 to 89 years with a median age of 65. The condition is 1.5 to 2.75 times more common in females. Oriental patients and younger patients who have received radiotherapy are at risk. The upper lid is involved more than twice as frequently as the lower lid. In 6 of 104 patients, both lids on the same side were involved.[68]

Clinically, sebaceous gland carcinoma causes a yellowish-orange thickening of the lid (Fig. 8-27). While there is often loss of cilia, the lesions are not papillary and rarely ulcerate; this latter feature is helpful in distinguishing sebaceous gland carcinoma from SCC and BCC (Figs. 8-28–29). The lesions may be nodular and well-localized but often are multicentric. Moreover, the tumor can spread by pagetoid intraepithelial growth (Fig. 8-30). The diffuse pagetoid growth results in a clinical presentation that mimics several other conditions including conjunctivitis, blepharitis, keratitis, and even superior limbic keratoconjunctivitis.[68,69] In such cases, the clinical

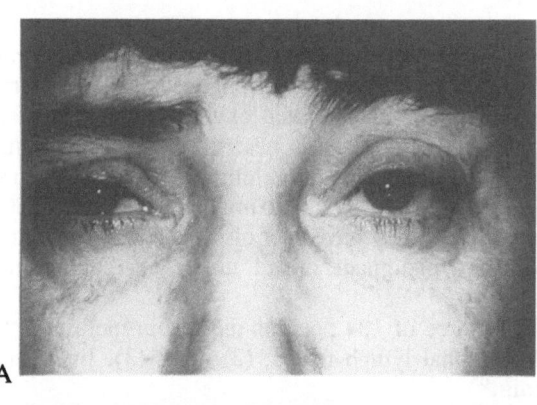

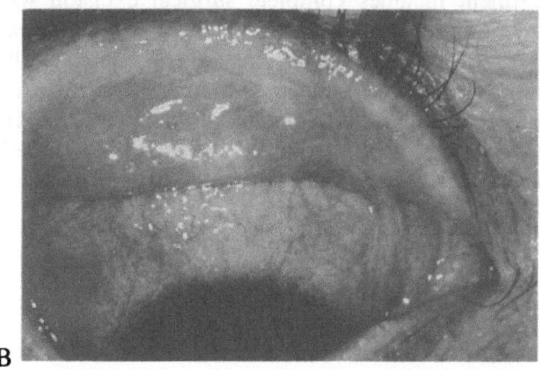

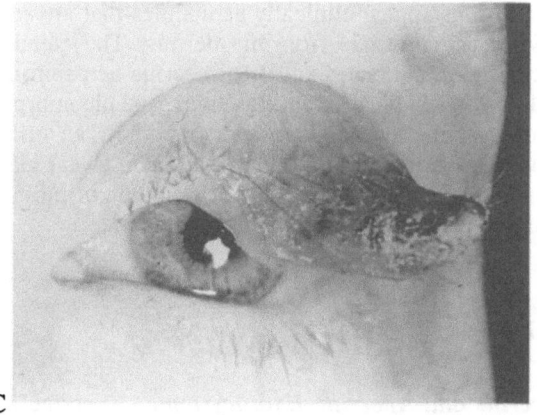

Fig. 8-28. (A) 47-year-old woman with diagnosed superior limbic keratoconjunctivitis in the eye that was treated for 7 years. (B) Finally, because of persistent chronic inflammation and suspicion of tumor, a full-thickness lid biopsy of the thickened right upper lid was performed. The biopsy showed basal cell carcinoma (Courtesy of Dr. Seymour Brownstein, Montreal). (C) Sebaceous gland carcinoma presenting as cutaneous horn (AFIP ACC #1032614).

appearance of conjunctival follicles and erythema should be interpreted as tumor until proven otherwise. Pagetoid spread also occurs with malignant melanoma of the skin and conjunctiva. Recurrence rate after excision may be as high as 32 percent.[68]

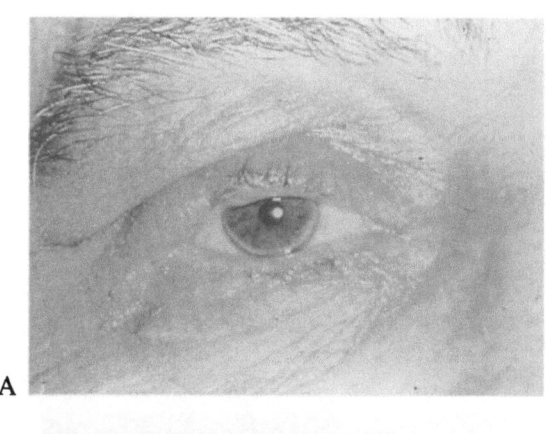

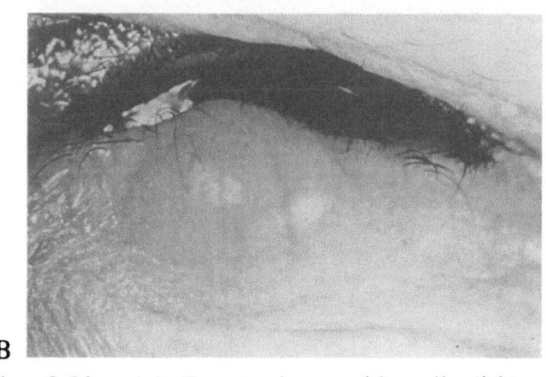

Fig. 8-29. (A) Two patients with yellowish-orange thickening of right upper lid (AFIP ACC #1079561) and (B) right lower lid (AFIP ACC #546724). There is focal loss of lashes without ulceration in both cases.

Sebaceous gland carcinoma may originate from the meibomian glands, gland of Zeis, sebaceous gland of the caruncle, or the sebaceous glands associated with the hair follicles of the brow or the lids away from the lid margin.

Prognosis is worsened by four factors: (1) vascular invasion, (2) lymphatic invasion, (3) upper and lower lid involvement, and (4) orbital invasion. In addition, multicentric tumors, that is, those associated with meibomian and glands of Zeis, had a 58 percent mortality in one series.[68] No mortality has been reported with lower lid tumors or with tumors that measured less than 6 mm by the pathologist.

Sebaceous gland carcinomas that originate in sebaceous glands away from the lids are much less malignant than sebaceous gland carcinomas of the lids.[29]

As stated above, the tumor may rarely present as a cutaneous horn. In addition, there may be an associated chalazion due to secondary obstruction of the sebaceous gland duct. In these cases, the lid involvement is greater than in the garden variety chalazion.

Histologically, the tumor is composed of large anaplastic basophilic cells with open vesicular nuclei and prominent nucleoli with a foamy or frothy cytoplasm. The appearance of the cytoplasm is due to the presence of

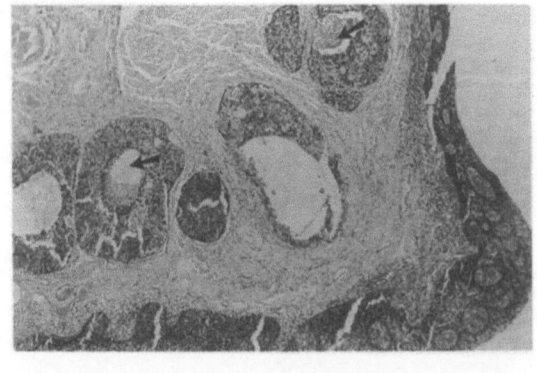

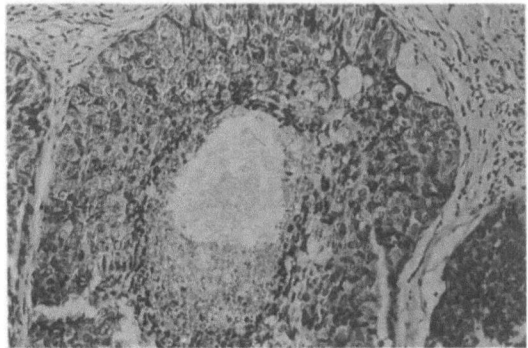

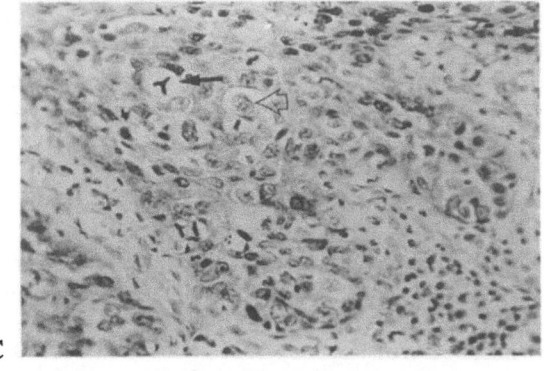

Fig. 8-30. (*A*) Full-thickness biopsy shows a proliferation of basaloid cells with large nuclei and scanty cytoplasm in the distribution of the meibomian glands (AFIP ACC #1267112). There are focal areas of necrosis (arrow) (comedocarcinoma) and pagetoid spread. (*B*) shows higher power. (*C*) Single cell intraepithelial spread with tripolar mitotic figure (straight arrow) and tumor cells with clear cytoplasm dissolved in processing (open arrow).

lipid vacuoles. The lipid in these vacuoles is dissolved by alcohol in the processing of tissues; therefore, frozen sections stained with a fat stain such as oil red O are helpful in making the diagnosis. Tissue fixed in formalin and then processed in the usual manner may not show the lipid vacuoles. Unlike BCC, sebaceous gland carcinoma may have large nuclear forms including multinucleated tumors giant cells (Fig. 8-30).

Normal sebaceous glands show differentiation with the formation of increasing amounts of cytoplasmic lipid toward the center of the lobule as opposed to its periphery. Normal meibomian gland ducts exhibit squamous differentiation with keratinization near the lid margin. Some sebaceous gland carcinomas exhibit distinct foci of keratinization. These tumors should not be mistaken for SCC. Similarly, BCC may have foci of sebaceous differentiation as may malignant mixed tumor of the lacrimal gland.[68–72]

Twenty-three of 104 patients died from metastasis to the (1) regional lymph nodes, (2) lung, (3) liver, and (4) brain.[68]

Treatment includes complete surgical excision with wide margins of 5–6 mm.[73] "Conjunctival map biopsies" have been advocated to determine pagetoid spread. This technique utilizes 16 conjunctival biopsy specimens from the palpebral and bulbar cnjunctiva to delineate the area of tumor involvement. The results of such biopsies help determine which cases may be treated by full-thickness lid resection and orbital exenteration.

Adnexal—Sweat Gland

Various adnexal sweat gland tumors occur on the lids. These lesions appear clinically as nodules that are solid or cystic and protrude from the dermis. They tend to spare the skin surface, except for eccrine acrospiroma, which may resemble a keratoacanthoma and pleomorphic adenoma of the sweat gland and may show an orifice on the skin surface. In addition, malignant sweat gland carcinomas (not the eccrine adenocarcinoma or infiltrating signet ring adenocarcinoma) may ulcerate.

Eccrine

Eccrine and Apocrine Hydrocystoma. Eccrine and apocrine hydrocystoma occur on the face and lids as translucent cystic bluish nodules. They may occur as single or multiple lesions and contain a clear or milky fluid.[3,45]

Histologically, eccrine hydrocystoma consists of cystic spaces in the dermis lined by two rows of small cuboidal epithelial cells; only one layer may be present (Fig. 8-12*B*). Apocrine hydrocystoma differs in that papillary projections may be present and in that the inner row of columnar cells have characteristic bulbous expansions typical of cells undergoing decapitation secretion. In addition, unlike eccrine hydrocystoma, myoepithelial cells may be present.

Syringoma. Syringoma occurs most commonly in young females and are multiple yellow irregular nodules 2 mm in size that, apart from their distribution, irregular shape, and pattern that matches the surrounding skin, may be confused with milia (Fig. 8-31).[74] They typically involve the lower lids, but may involve the cheeks, upper lids, and forehead. Multiple syringoma often occurs in patients with Down's syndrome. Excision, curettage and cauterization of multiple tumors often lead to recurrence; CO_2 laser vaporization has been suggested.

Two malignant syringoma of the eyelids have been reported.[75] They presented as painless nodular masses. Both patients had no recurrence after local excision.

Histologically, the tumor consists of ducts lined by two rows of epithelial cells embedded in a fibrous stroma. Myoepithelial cells are absent. Keratin may appear in some of the dilated ducts.[3] The tumors probably arise from eccrine glands. The features that help to distinguish malignant from benign syringoma are the larger size, solitary nature, and subcutaneous muscular and perineural invasion. In addition, malignant syringoma are generally well-differentiated. For sweat gland carcinomas, in general, the most important histologic factor indicating prognosis is the degree of cellular atypia. Anaplastic sweat gland carcinomas elsewhere in the body are associated with metastases.

Eccrine Acrospiroma (Clear Cell Hidradenoma, Clear Cell Myepithelioma, Porosyringoma).

This tumor is a single nodule that may be solid or cystic and may resemble a keratoacanthoma.[76] The overlying skin may have superficial hemorrhage and appear reddish-blue. Rarely, the tumor is verrucous. The median size is 1 cm.

Histologically, the tumor consists of lobules of epithelial cells or as cysts that contains serous or hemorrhagic fluid. Two cell types are present: a round-to-polyhedral cell with eosinophilic cytoplasm and a clear cell that contains glycogen. When the latter clear cell predominates, the term *clear cell hidradenoma* is often employed. The epithelial elements may connect to the overlying

acanthotic epidermis. Structures resembling eccrine sweat ducts may be present. These ductal elements are lined by an eosinophilic cuticle.

Malignant Eccrine Sweat Gland Tumors.

Malignant eccrine sweat gland tumors are quite rare.[77-78] These tumors may ulcerate.

Pathologically, the tumors show a broad spectrum of cellular patterns: solid nests of cells, interlacing cords, mucin-secreting elements, and acinar, ductal, cylindromatous, papillary, clear-cell hidradenomatous, and mixed patterns. The degree of anaplasia, invasion, and the development of regional lymph node metastasis determine the primary route of spread. Hematogenous spread to bone and viscera is a later event.

Optimal treatment is the wide surgical excision. Irradiation as a primary form of therapy has little or no value in the management of these tumors, although control of recurrent tumor by radiation has been reported.[77]

Adenocarcinoma of Eccrine Sweat Glands (Infiltrating Signet Ring Carcinoma).

This tumor is very rare, yet has characteristic clinical and pathologic features. It tends to initially involve the lower lid and extends to the inner canthus as a nodular indurated mass with diffuse infiltrating margins. The overlying skin may appear erythematous. Recurrences with orbital invasion tend to follow incomplete excision.[79-80]

Histologically, the tumor appears identical to the histiocytoid mammary carcinoma metastatic to the eyelid described by Hood et al. (Fig. 8-32).[80] The histogenesis of the tumor, whether of eccrine as first thought or apocrine, remains uncertain.[81] The tumor shows cords of atypical histiocytoid cells in single rows in so-called Indian-file pattern. The cytoplasm has a foamy or vacuolated appearance that stains positively with Alcian blue, mucicarmine, and PAS. The cells interdigitate between

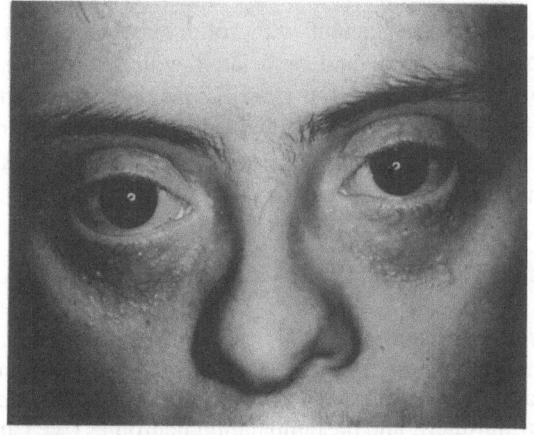

Fig. 8-31. Patient with Down's syndrome and multiple flesh-colored papules (syringoma). (Courtesy AFIP, Washington, DC.)

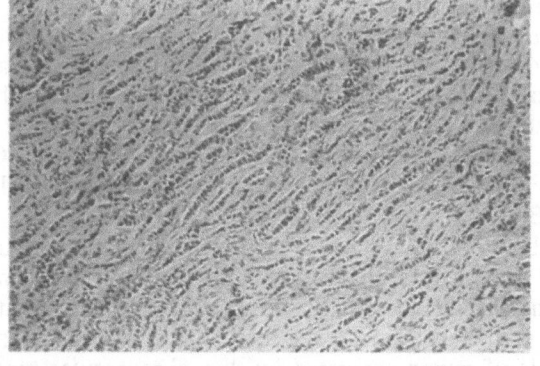

Fig. 8-32. Adenocarcinoma of eccrine sweat glands is histologically identical to the metastatic breast cancer to the eyelid. Medical evaluation for primary breast cancer is essential in all patients. Histologically, the tumor in either case is composed of atypical histiocytoid cells that line up in an "Indian-file" pattern.

individual collagen fibers of the collagen and skeletal muscle of the lid.

Because of the histologic confusion, a complete clinical evaluation for primary breast carcinoma should be made in patients with such eyelid lesions.

Apocrine

Adenoma (Adenocarcinoma) of Moll's Glands. An adenoma of Moll's glands is extremely rare. By definition, such tumors are located near the lid margin.[45,82]

Histologically, the tumor is composed of cuboidal cells with an eosinophilic cytoplasm. Decapitation secretion is the hallmark. Malignant variants have been reported.[82]

Adnexal Tumors of Uncertain Origin

Pleomorphic Adenoma (Mixed Tumor of the Skin, Chondroid Syringoma). Clinically, these tumors are intradermal and multilobulated and range from 0.5–3 cm.[83]

Histologically, they are identical to the pleomorphic adenomas (benign mixed tumors) that arise in the lacrimal gland (see "Lacrimal Gland Tumors"). For this reason, tumors that arise in the lateral aspect of the lid may originate from the sweat glands or lacrimal tissue. The histologic presence of adjacent lacrimal gland tissue may imply that the particular tumor arose from lacrimal gland tissue.

Mucinous Sweat Gland Carcinoma (Mucinous Adenocarcinoma, Colloid Carcinoma, Gelatinous Carcinoma, "Adenocystic" Carcinoma). A series of 21 cases of mucinous sweat gland adenocarcinoma of the eyelid have been reported.[84] The tumor occurs in middle-aged adults with a median age of 60 years and has a predilection for males. The eyelids appear to be involved in almost half of the cases of this tumor.

Clinically, the lesions may be confused with BCC, papilloma, chalazion, keratoacanthoma, and a cyst (Fig. 8-33).

Histologically, there is a mixed population of light and dark secretory cells within the tumor lobules. Small gland-like or ductal structures may be observed within the epithelial islands. The epithelial cells float in large pools of mucin separated by thin fibrovascular septae.

The tumor has a low potential for widespread metastatic disease. Only 4 of 21 cases developed metastasis to the regional lymph nodes and only one tumor has spread beyond the regional lymph nodes to the systemic circulation.

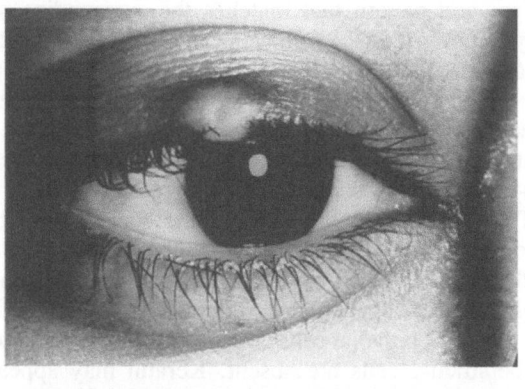

A

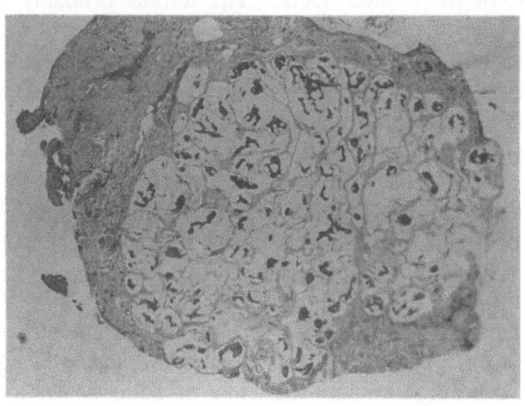

B

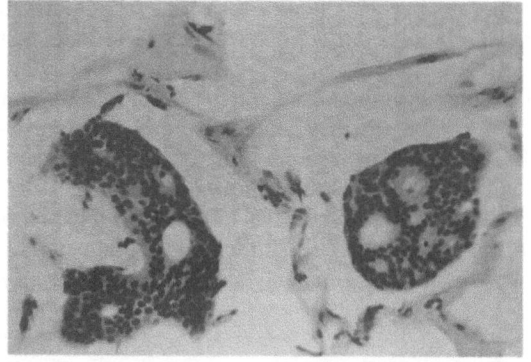

C

Fig. 8-33. (*A*) Patient with solid mass at lid border without ulceration and associated with loss of lashes (AFIP ACC #1398204). (*B,C*) Biopsy shows a dermal tumor composed of basophilic bland secretory cells floating in a sea of mucin consistent with mucinous sweat gland carcinoma (AFIP ACC #1833903).

Soft Tissue—Neurogenic

Neurofibroma. Several types of neurofibromas occur in the lids and orbit: diffuse and localized neurofibromas, isolated and circumscribed neurofibromas, plexiform neurofibromas, and postamputation neuromas (see Chapter 3 for discussion of isolated neurofibromas and postamputation neuroma). All such tumors present as subcutaneous mass. The plexiform neurofibroma is considered pathognomonic of neurofibromatosis.

Clinically, the tumor appears during the first decade of life and often presents as a lid mass that pervades the lid and orbital structures. The characteristic s-shaped deformity of the upper lid confirms the diagnosis (Figs. 8-34–8-36).

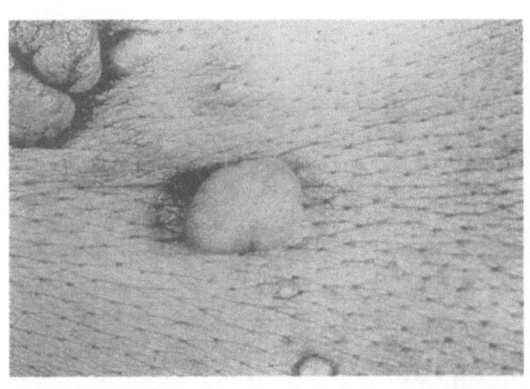

A

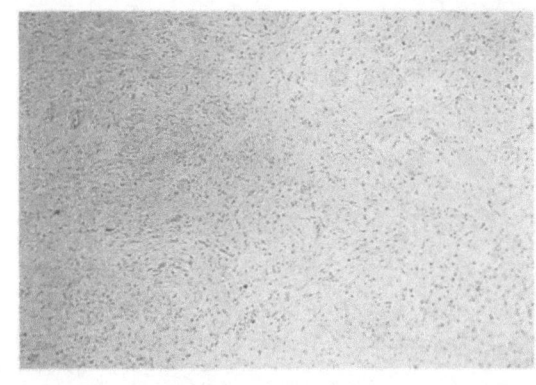

B

Fig. 8-35. (A) Localized neurofibroma contains (B) dense compact neuronal elements (AFIP ACC #1192377).

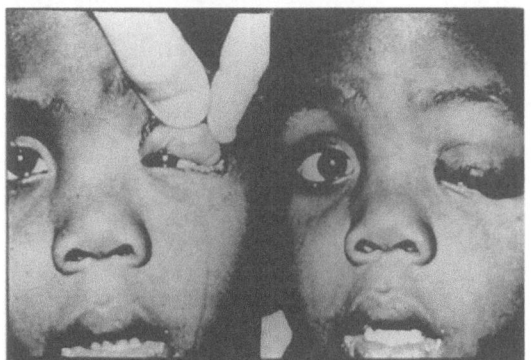

A

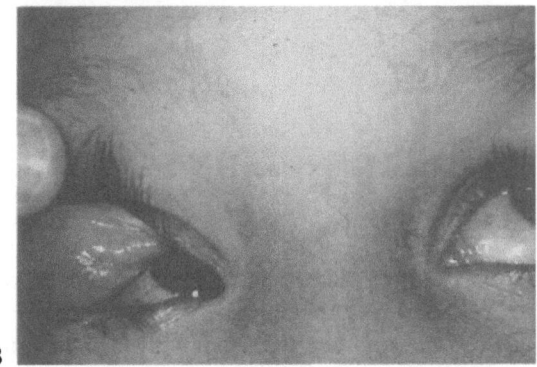

B

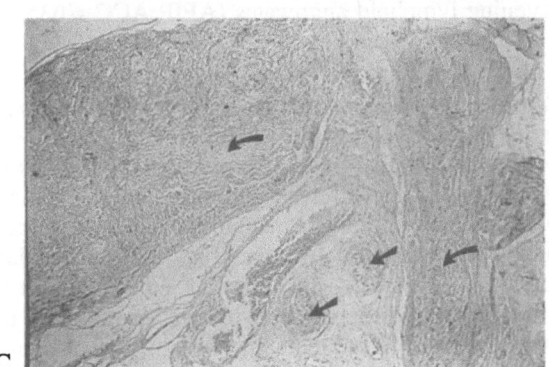

C

Fig. 8-34. (A,B) Children with "s-shaped" lid typical of plexiform neurofibroma, which is pathognomonic of neurofibromatosis (AFIP ACC #1148044). (C) Excisional biopsy shows dilated nerve sheaths (cut in longitudinal section, straight arrows, and at cross-section, straight arrows) filled with peripheral neuronal elements including axons, fibrous tissue, and schwann cell. Interstitial tissue stains Alcian-blue positive.

The tumor has the consistency of a "bag of worms" and has no attachment to the deep tissues. Associated defects of the sphenoid bone may be present and lead to pulsating exophthalmos. Patients with plexiform neurofibromas of the lid have an increased incidence of unilateral glaucoma on the involved side.

Histologically, plexiform neurofibroma is composed of multiple tumor units surrounded by a perineurium. The individual units consist of axons, peripheral nerve sheath cells that have eel-shaped nuclei, endoneural fibroblasts, and hyaluronic acid deposited in the stroma.[45] The Bodian stain will demonstrate the individual axons. These tumors tend to bleed during excision due to their vascularity. For this reason, the CO_2 or contact YAG laser is recommended. Recurrence is common and is more likely to occur in adolescent and younger patients than in older patients. En-bloc surgical excision has been recommended rather than the classical surgical treatment of dissection of the tumor with the preservation of normal lid structures.[85]

Schwannomas of the eyelid are rare. They may occur as a solid tumor on the eyelid margin, and they have a yellow appearance and resemble a chalazion.[86]

Histologically, they resemble their orbital counterparts (see orbit).

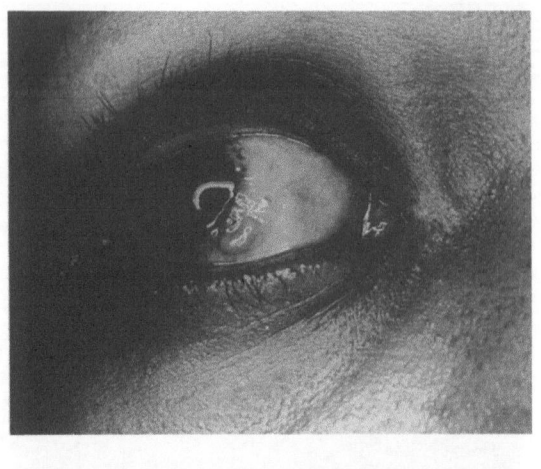

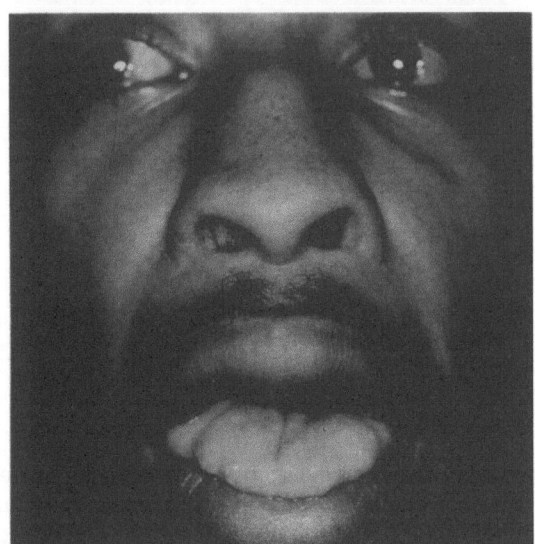

Fig. 8-36. 22-year-old male with multiple endocrine adenomatosis with neurofibroma of conjunctiva (*A*) and multiple mucosal neuromas (*B*).

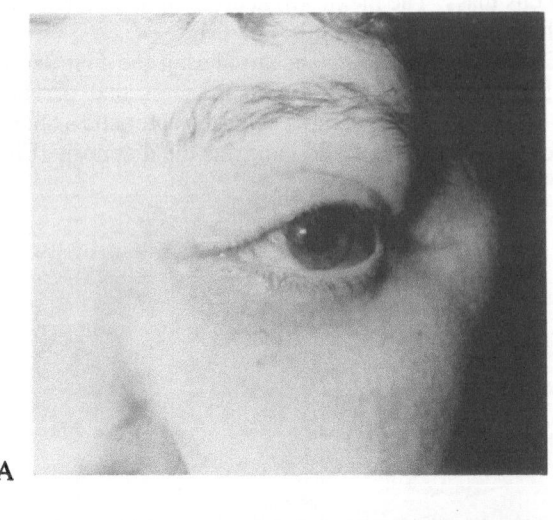

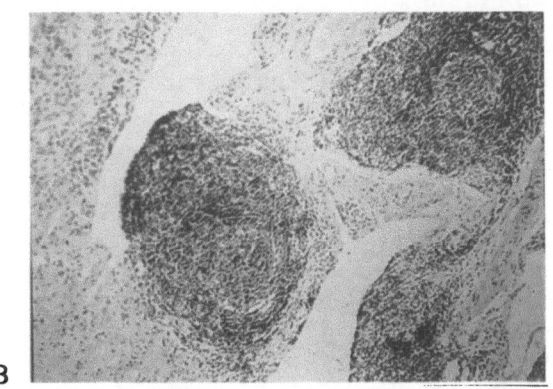

Fig. 8-37. (*A*) 36-year-old female who presented with subconjunctival hemorrhage. Patient had had prior surgery for a lymphangioma. (*B*) Histologically, the tumor is composed of endothelial-lined lymph channels with intervening lymphoid aggregates (AFIP ACC #63566).

Soft Tissue Vascular. All vascular tumors generally show either red or blue blood vessels that belie their cell or origin. In addition, several types may be multiple: Kaposi's sarcoma when associated with AIDS, glomus tumor, and angiosarcoma in the scalp region.

Lymphangioma. The differential diagnosis of capillary hemangioma and lymphangioma are discussed in Chapter 4. Lid and orbital lymphangioma tend to be congenital, while lymphangiomas confined to the conjunctiva tend to have an adult onset (Fig. 8-37).[87,88] These lesions may present as focal tumors with or without coloration. After hemorrhage into the tumor, lymphangiomas become red or bluish in color. The differential diagnosis includes capillary, cavernous, or venous angiomas and Kaposi's sarcoma. The latter tumors should have a long-standing reddish-blue hue.[88]

Capillary Hemangioma (Strawberry Hemangioma, Juvenile Hemangioma, Strawberry Nevus, Nevus Vasculosus, Benign Hemangioendothelioma of Childhood) (Fig. 8-38). The differential diagnosis of pyogenic granuloma and capillary hemangioma is based on both clinical and pathologic features (Fig. 8-39). Capillary hemangioma occurs as a congenital lid tumor during the first year of life, while pyogenic granulomas are acquired later in life and there may be a history of trauma or inflammatory process such as a chalazion. Generally, pyogenic granuloma has a shorter duration of growth than capillary hemangioma.

Histologically, both tumors are composed of a polypoid fibroblastic proliferation with many capillaries. The polypoid configuration and diffuse inflammatory infiltrate composed of both acute and chronic nongranulomatous inflammation is characteristic of pyogenic granuloma.

Nevus Flammeus (Port Wine Stain). Nevus flammeus often associated with Sturge-Weber syndrome is

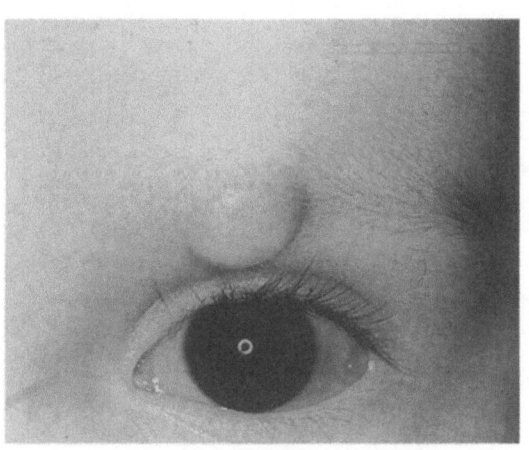

Fig. 8-38. Capillary hemangioma with focal fibrosis that occurs with regression of tumor.

a congenital hamartoma that should be easily distinguished from capillary hemangioma on clinical grounds. While capillary hemangiomas is a raised lesion, nevus flammeus is a macule. Nevus flammeus has a deeper hue than capillary hemangioma, and it does not blanch, enlarge, or deepen in color with Valsalva's maneuver

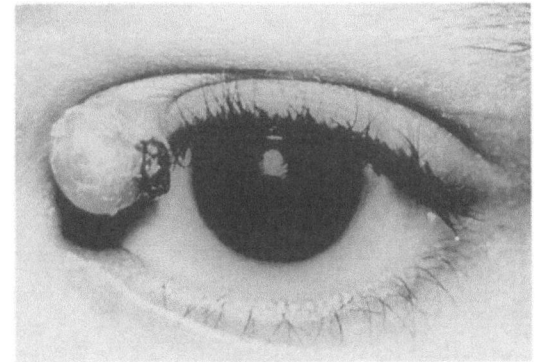

A

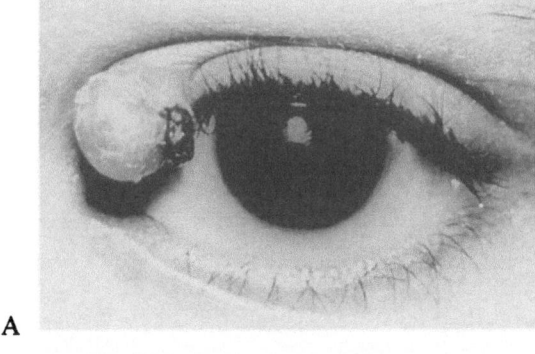

B

Fig. 8-39. (*A*) Pyogenic granuloma appears as a pedunculated mass with a collarette at the base (AFIP ACC #1083558). (*B*) Histologically, it is composed of fibrous tissue and capillaries with a mixed inflammatory cell infiltrate (AFIP ACC #1540377).

or crying. This lesion does not resolve spontaneously and grows proportionately with the patient (see Figs. 4-3 and 4-4). Pathologically, nevus flammeus is characterized by the presence of large dilated capillaries in the dermis.[3]

Cavernous Hemangioma and Hemangiopericytoma (See Chapter 3)

Glomus Tumor (Glomangioma). This benign vascular hamartoma is related to the special vascular smooth muscle structure, the glomus, that is concerned with temperature regulation via its arterial and venous segments.

Clinically, the tumor may be solitary or multiple, reddish-purple nodules that are often tender and small (1–3 mm). Solitary tumors occur in young adults and involve the nail beds with no pattern of inheritance. Multiple tumors occur in the face, palate, eyelid, and conjunctiva, spare the nails, and tend to be inherited as an autosomal-dominant condition.

Histologically, multiple glomus tumors resemble cavernous hemangioma except that a narrow rim of 1–3 layers of glomus cells surround the vascular spaces. Solitary glomus tumors are circumscribed, are more cellular, and have a prominent perivascular mantle (Fig. 8-40).[89]

Angiolymphoid Hyperplasia with Eosinophilia (Kimura's Disease, Eosinophilic Granuloma, Eosinophilic Folliculosis). This tumor, described in both the lid and orbit, may have a similar clinical appearance to Kaposi's sarcoma or angiosarcoma.[90] The lesions may be multiple, especially in Asian patients, and tend to involve the head and neck regions; an associated eosinophilia of the peripheral blood may occur. Patients may have bronchial asthma, increased levels of serum IgE, and IgE in the glomeruli.

Histologically, the caliber of vessels is large, unlike

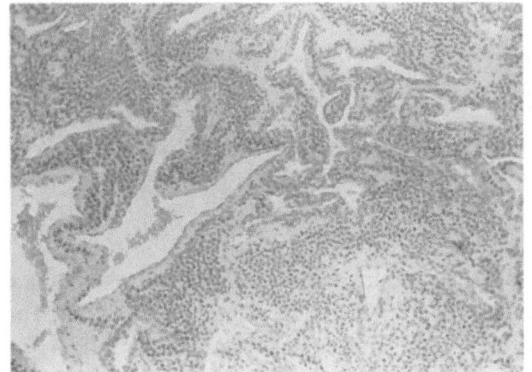

Fig. 8-40. Clinically, lesions appear as solitary or multiple red to purple nodules. Biopsy shows glomus cells surrounding vascular spaces (AFIP ACC #320982).

angiosarcoma. There is a striking endothelial proliferation. Unlike angiosarcoma, there are no anastomoses between the vessels (Fig. 8-41). There are no areas that resemble Kaposi's sarcoma. Kaposi's sarcoma and angiosarcoma lack the eosinophilic inflammatory infiltrate.

Kaposi's Sarcoma. Kaposi's sarcoma of the lid presents as a localized red papule. Prior to the development of AIDS in the United States, the tumor was most commonly reported in eastern Europeans and Africans. There may be surrounding hemorrhage (Fig. 8-42). On the conjunctiva, the lesion may appear only as a subtle subconjunctival hemorrhage. Such tumors may be multicentric and bilateral in patients with AIDS.

Histologically, the tumor is composed of spindle cells, with cleft spaces that often contain extravasated red blood cells. Hemosiderin is usually found. Silver stains in Kaposi's sarcoma show that the tumor cells are entrapped by reticulin fibers.

Surgical excision for diagnostic purposes in a patient with known AIDS is unnecessary. Cosmetically unacceptable lesions are amenable to surgical excision or CO_2 ablation (after dissection from the overlying conjunctiva).

Angiosarcoma. Angiosarcoma characteristically involves the scalp but may also involve the face. The tumor affects elderly patients, is multiple in 60 percent of cases, and presents as a bluish or violaceous plaque or nodule. There may be a peripheral erythematous ring or satellite nodules as well as intratumoral hemorrhage resembling "blood blisters." The tumors tend to spread locally, and approximately one-third eventually give rise to distant metastases.

Histologically, the angiomatous areas consist of freely anastamosing channels linked by atypical endothelial

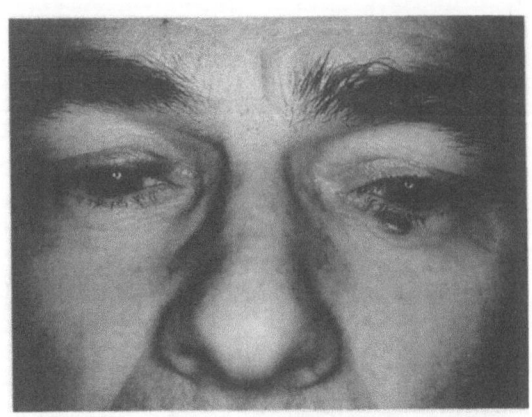

A

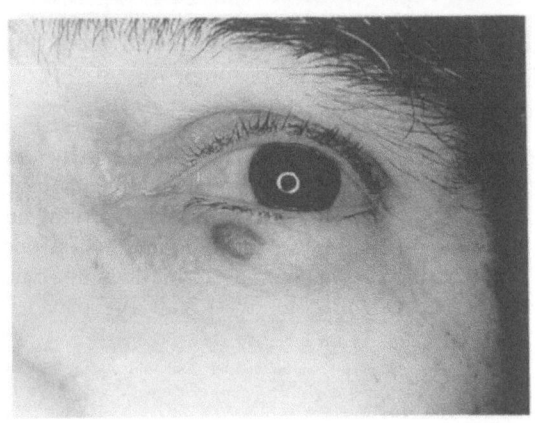

B

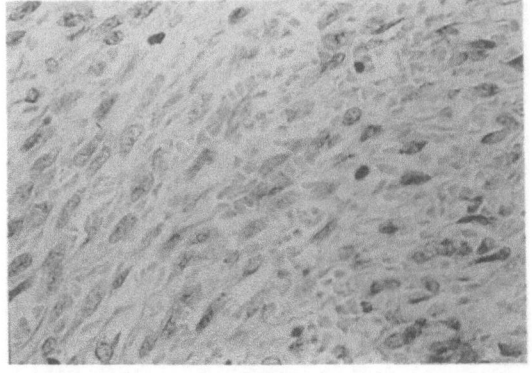

C

Fig. 8-42. (*A,B*) 54-year-old homosexual with AIDS and bilateral Kaposi's sarcoma. (*C*) Tumor is composed of spindle cells with extravasated red blood cells (AFIP ACC #990268).

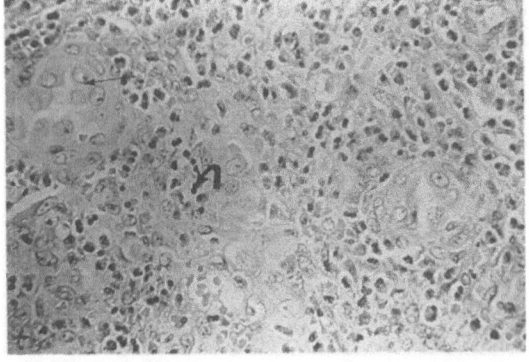

Fig. 8-41. Kimura's disease, Kaposi's sarcoma, and angiosarcoma may be clinically indistinguishable. Biopsy of patient with Kimura's disease shows characteristic large proliferating endothelial cells (straight arrow). Note the prominent eosinophilic infiltrate (curved arrow) lacking in Kaposi's sarcoma and angiosarcoma (AFIP ACC #1405464).

cells that alternate with Kaposi-like spindle cell areas (Fig. 8-43). The epidermis is spared. The well-developed freely anastomasing vascular channels lined by recognizable endothelium found in angiosarcoma are not a feature of Kaposi's sarcoma.[92-93]

Angiosarcoma may be confused with intravascular atypical endothelial proliferations. In the latter condition, papillary-like projections of organizing thrombus material may lead to confusion with an angiosarcoma. The

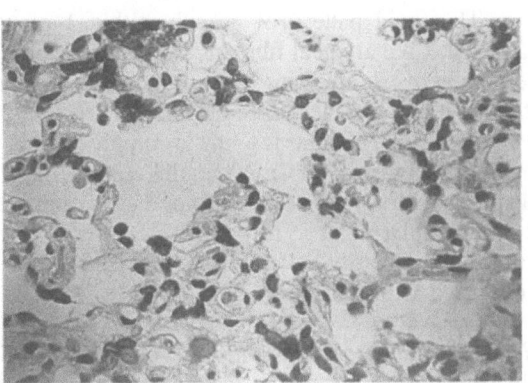

Fig. 8-43. Biopsy of 80-year-old male with slow-growing tumor of right temple. Biopsy shows low-grade angiosarcoma. Note the tumor cells constitute the wall of the vessels (AFIP ACC #1316240).

solid endothelial proliferations, however, occur inside one or several large veins.[94,95]

Treatment of single, well-circumscribed angiosarcomas is surgical. In multiple lesions that have ill-defined margins, radiation has been suggested.

Soft Tissue—Fibrous. As in the orbit, the differentiation of reactive fibroblastic process from a true neoplasm is often difficult. Reactive processes such as a nodular fasciitis, sclerosing of a periosteal hematoma, or fibrosis about a retained foreign body or a tumor that undergoes secondary sclerosis like a ruptured dermoid or sclerosing hemangioma, or idiopathic pseudotumor may all present as ''fibrous'' tumors. Such conditions are sometimes distinguished by careful history and pathologic examination.

True fibrous tumors include the fibroma, fibrosarcoma, and fibromatosis. A fibromatosis is a condition of intermediate aggressiveness between a true fibroma and a fibrosarcoma. Histologically, a fibroma is composed of well-differentiated fibroblasts that produce substantial amounts of intercellular collagen. There is no atypia or mitotic activity to suggest malignancy. Stout[96] classified a fibrosarcoma as a fibroblastic tumor composed of cells and fibers arranged in interlaced bands in which collagen and reticulin are evident. A herringbone pattern of fibroblasts is evident. He distinguished fibrosarcoma from fibromatosis on the basis of the marked degree of cellularity of fibrosarcomas compared with fibromatoses. In addition, fibromatoses have rare mitoses and absence of necrosis (see Chapter 3).

Of the fibrous tumors, all present clinically as subcutaneous masses with two exceptions. Atypical fibroxanthoma may ulcerate and resemble a BCC and nodular fasciitis; a reactive proliferation of fibroblasts and blood vessels may also ulcerate and appear as a keratoacanthoma.

Dermatofibroma. Clinically, these tumors occur in the skin of adults as firm, single, or multiple nodules.

They are most common on the extremities. Most lesions have a reddish color but may be reddish-brown because of the hyperpigmentation of the overlying skin. Rarely, they are bluish-black because of the presence of large amounts of hemosiderin within the tumor. In the latter case, the lesion may resemble a malignant melanoma.

Histologically, the tumor is composed of varying amounts of fibrous tissue and fibroblasts. Both hemosiderin and lipid deposits may be found. In some instances, multinucleated giant cells that resemble Touton giant cells are present. Hyperplasia of the overlying epidermis often occurs.[3]

Juvenile Fibromatosis. Six cases of juvenile fibromatosis of the periorbital region and eyelid have been described in patients with a median age of 8 years.[97] The lesions has a predilection for involvement of the infraorbital region and lower eyelid. The tumor is slow-growing and usually painless. Bone invasion is rare (Fig. 8-44).

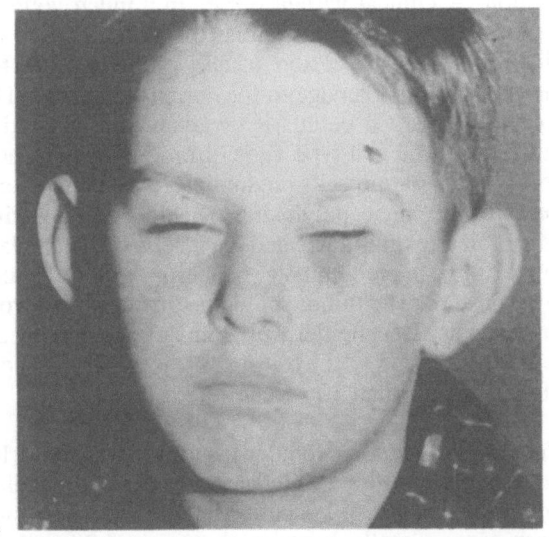

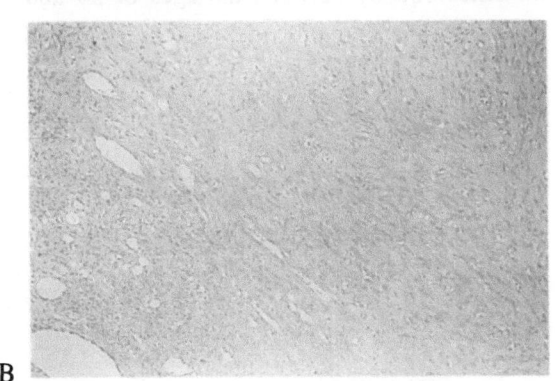

Fig. 8-44. (*A*) Child with slow-growing tumor of left lower lid and orbit. (*B*) Biopsy shows thick collagenous matrix of tumor consistent with juvenile fibromatosis (AFIP ACC #1037215) (Courtesy of Dr. Ahmed Hidayat, Washington, DC).

Histologically, the tumor is composed of interlacing fascicles of spindle-shaped fibroblasts embedded in a collagenous background matrix containing reticulum fibers that surround the individual tumor cells.

Treatment involves surgical excision. When the lesions recur after surgical excision, it is difficult to distinguish recurrence from postoperative scar tissue. Radiation has been advocated but the fibrous tumors are generally radioresistant. We do not advocate radiation for the treatment of young patients with this condition because of the possibility of secondary, radiation-induced soft tissue tumors.

Atypical Fibroxanthoma. Atypical fibroxanthoma occurs in the head and neck of older patients, especially males. The tumor is rare in blacks and affects patients with fair complexion with a history of sun exposure (Fig. 8-45).

The tumor may present clinically as a single firm nodule or ulcer. The ulceration suggests an epithelial malignancy and is unusual for a fibrous tumor. Pain is the exception. A clinical variant occurs in a much younger age group on the unexposed areas of the body.

Histologically, the lesion usually closely abuts the epidermis. Actinic damage to the dermis is present. The lesion has a marked cellularity without any distinctive organization. The cell type varies from tumor to tumor. In some cases, plump cells predominate, while in others, large pleomorphic, polyhedral, histiocytic-appearing cells and bizarre multinucleated giant cells with abundant foamy cytoplasm predominate. Numerous mitotic figures may be present. The tumor should be distinguished from a fibromatosis. Despite the worrisome cytologic appearance, the tumor rarely if ever metastasizes. Recurrences are found in less than 10 percent of cases.[98]

Nodular Fasciitis. Nodular fasciitis is a reactive localized lesion of the subcutaneous tissue. Preceding trauma may explain its occurrence. The tumor occurs in both sexes equally between the ages of 20 and 35 years. The rapid pattern of growth within 1 month is distinctive. Like atypical fibroxanthoma, the lesion may ulcerate the overlying skin.[99] The tumor may be present in the orbit and episclera (see Chapter 3).

Histologically, nodular fasciitis is composed of benign spindle cells arranged in wavy bundles. Intercellular slits and spaces with extravasated red blood cells, and a myxoid intercellular matrix is present. Scattered foci of chronic inflammatory cells are present. The tumor may be confused with a fibrosarcoma.

Juvenile Fibrosarcoma and Fibrosarcoma. Clinically, juvenile fibrosarcoma may occur at birth and is a painless subcutaneous mass of the periorbital region. The tumor may also involve the orbit.

Histologically, juvenile fibrosarcoma may be confused with rhabdomyosarcoma. Electron micrographic studies and special stains such as PAS, PTAH, and Masson's trichrome to look for cross-striations may be helpful in difficult cases.[100,101]

Management of Soft Tissue Tumors

Benign tumors are treated by biopsy followed by judicious local excision to improve function and cosmesis as in debulking a lymphangioma or diffuse neurofibroma. In many cases, a frozen section only is necessary to establish the diagnosis in typical cases.

Management of malignant soft tissue tumors of the lids are considered in Chapter 3 and require permanent section biopsy results before radical surgery is recommended.

Fibrous Histiocytoma (See Chapter 3)

Soft Tissue—Histiocytic. Xanthelasma palpebrae appear as yellowish-tan, soft plaques on clinical examination. They begin at the inner canthus and involve the medial portions of the upper or lower lids in an arc distribution. Systemically induced eruptive xanthomas develop in areas of trauma such as elbows or knees (Fig. 8-46). It has been proposed that the trauma of blinking may induce increased vascular leaking over time in such patients.[102] Treatment of a hyperlipidemia that is associated with xanthelasma, Types II, III, IV, and V, may cause regression of the xanthoma.

Histologically, the lesion consists of an accumulation of lipid-laden histiocytes in the dermis around capillaries in the upper reticular and papillary dermis. Fibrosis may occur in old lesions.

Unfortunately, all forms of surgical excision lead to recurrence. Too aggressive removal of skin in the lids may lead to cicatricial ectropion and lagophthalmos. CO_2 laser ablation has been suggested.

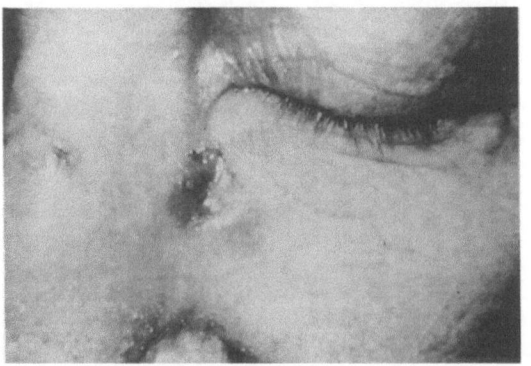

Fig. 8-45. Atypical fibroxanthoma presenting as a nodule with central ulceration that thus mimics a basal cell carcinoma (AFIP ACC #1038094).

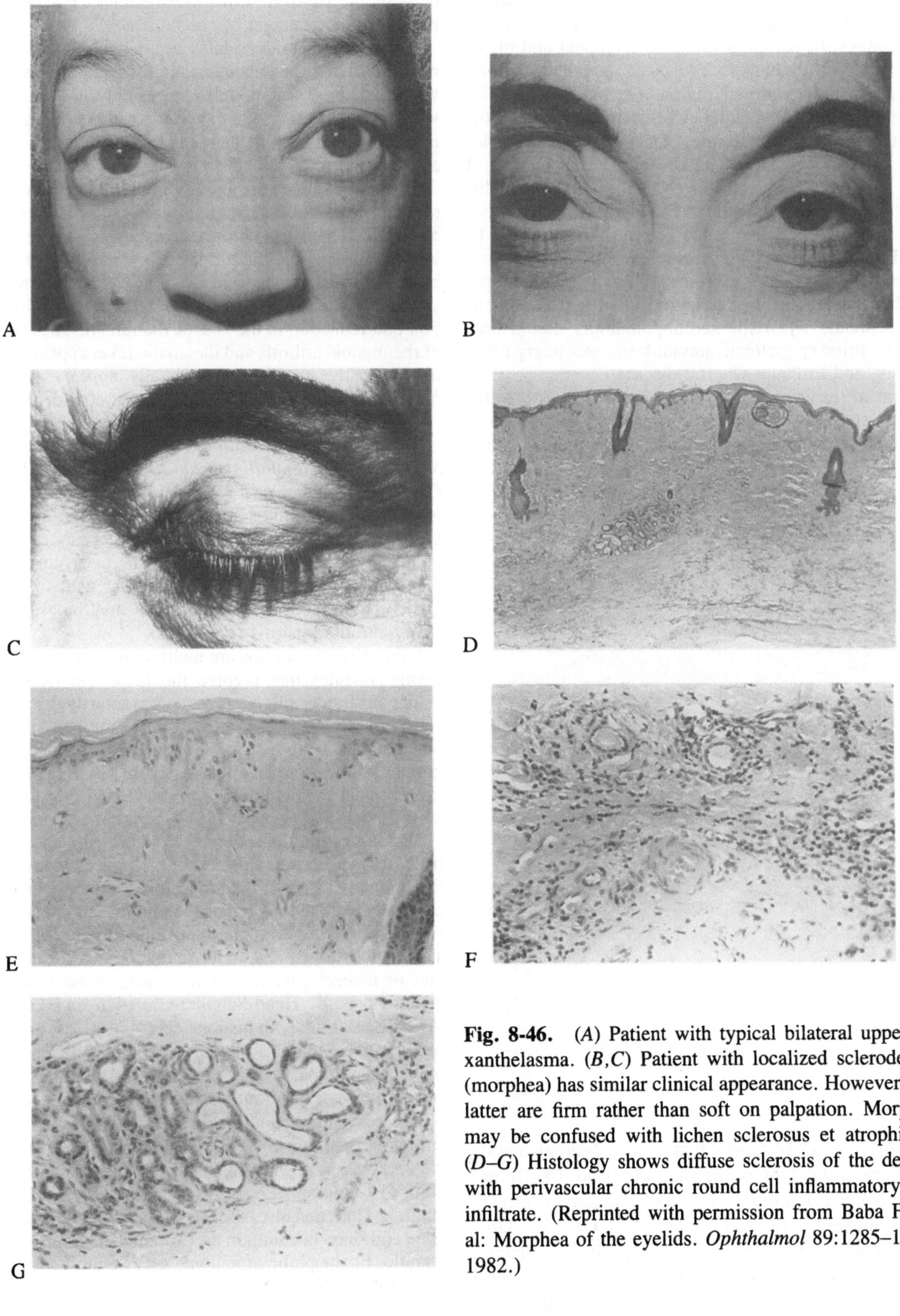

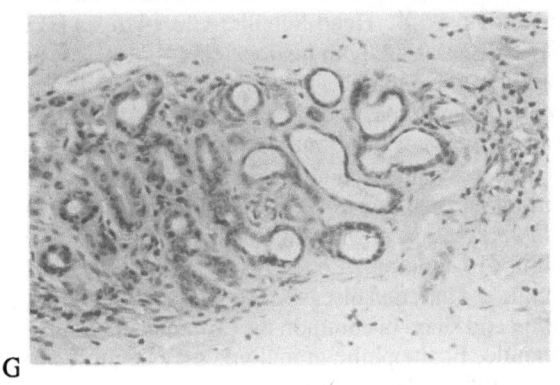

Fig. 8-46. (*A*) Patient with typical bilateral upper lid xanthelasma. (*B,C*) Patient with localized scleroderma (morphea) has similar clinical appearance. However, the latter are firm rather than soft on palpation. Morphea may be confused with lichen sclerosus et atrophicus. (*D–G*) Histology shows diffuse sclerosis of the dermis with perivascular chronic round cell inflammatory cell infiltrate. (Reprinted with permission from Baba FE et al: Morphea of the eyelids. *Ophthalmol* 89:1285–1288, 1982.)

***Necrobiotic Xanthogranuloma with Paraproteinemia
and Pseudorheumatoid Nodules.*** Necrobiotic xanthogranuloma with paraproteinemia is a clinical and histopathologic entity characterized by (1) xanthelasma-like
lesions of the periorbital region, (2) paraproteinemia,
(3) leukopenia, (4) anemia, (5) cryoglobulinemia, (6)
elevated sedimentation rate, and (7) low complement. Multiple myeloma has been reported in several
cases.[102–106] Unlike xanthelasma, the lesions of necrobiotic xanthoma are almost always indurated and may become inflamed and then superficially ulcerate (Fig. 8-
47). The differential diagnosis includes sarcoidosis, chalazion, xanthelasma, necrobiosis lipoidica, granuloma
annulare, subcutaneous rheumatoid nodules, pseudorheumatoid nodules, juvenile xanthogranuloma, lipoid proteinosis, primary systemic amyloidosis, secondary amyloidosis, and Erdheim-Chester disease.

Surgical excision may result in recurrence. Intralesional steroid injections have given transient results.
However, the best treatment consists of alkylating agents
or systemic steroids. Low-dose radiation has been reported in the treatment of one patient.[105]

Pseudorheumatoid nodules are necrobiotic granulomata involving the subcutaneous tissue in children and
young adults. These nodules are usually not associated
with any collagen or other systemic disease. They occur
most commonly in the lateral aspect of the upper eyelid
and respond to local excision.

Histologically, necrobiotic granulomata are surrounded by a palisade of fibroblasts and histiocytes in
a zonal pattern. The innermost layer consists of the necrobiotic collagen, the middle layer is composed of fibroblasts and histiocytes, and the outer zone is a row of
sclerotic vessels with marked endothelial cell proliferation and reduction in the size of the lumen. The nodules
of rheumatoid arthritis and rheumatic fever appear similar
histologically, yet the latter usually appears after the
clinical manifestations of the disease are evident.[107,108]

***Juvenile Xanthogranuloma (JXG) and Unifocal and
Multifocal Eosinophilic Granuloma (Hand-Schüller-
Christian Disease, and Letterer-Siwe Disease).*** JXG
is benign, self-limited histiocytic proliferation of unknown etiology that occurs in infants 2 years of age or
younger. The tumor involves the lid, uvea, and rarely
the orbit. Recurrent hyphema, uveitis, and secondary
glaucoma may occur. The condition may be associated
with neurofibromatosis (Fig. 8-11).[109]

Clinically, the lesions are multiple or solitary reddish-
orange nodules that involve the head and neck. The
cutaneous lesions often regress spontaneously; by adolescence all the lesions tend to subside. Zimmerman found
that patients with JXG of the skin within the first 17
months of life were significantly more apt to have uveal
involvement than children who developed lid lesions at
an older age.[110]

Histologically, the lesion consists of histiocytes, lymphocytes, and eosinophils. Touton giant cells are more
likely to be present in mature lesions. Touton giant cells
have a wreath of nuclei that encircle a homogeneous
eosinophilic cytoplasm; lipid surrounds the ring of nuclei.
The histiocytes of JXG do not contain Langerhans' granules or Birbeck granules characteristic of the lesions of
histiocytosis X. Hand-Schüller-Christian and Letterer-
Siwe diseases are both histiocytosis X diseases, and they
rarely involve the lid. The other histiocytosis X, eosinophilic granuloma, has associated deep nodules in the
superotemporal quadrant and is discussed in Chapter 3.

JXG responds well to systemic steroids. In some recalcitrant lesions, low doses of radiation are also necessary.

All diseases known as histiocytosis X including eosinophilic granuloma, Letterer-Siwe disease, and Hand-
Schüller-Christian disease are termed *eosinophilic granuloma* and share in common the presence of a Langerhans'
granule. Eosinophilic granuloma may be unifocal (local)
or multifocal (systemic).

Erdheim-Chester Disease. This disease is a systemic
lipoid granulomatosis or xanthogranulomatosis that may

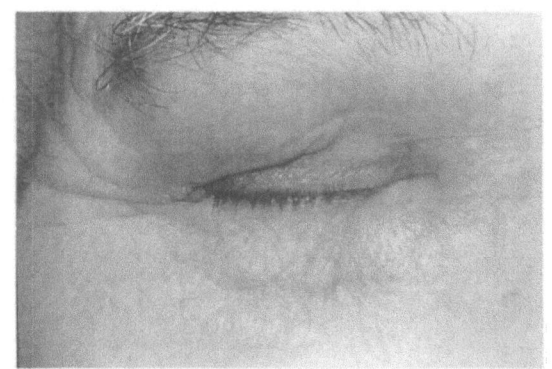

A

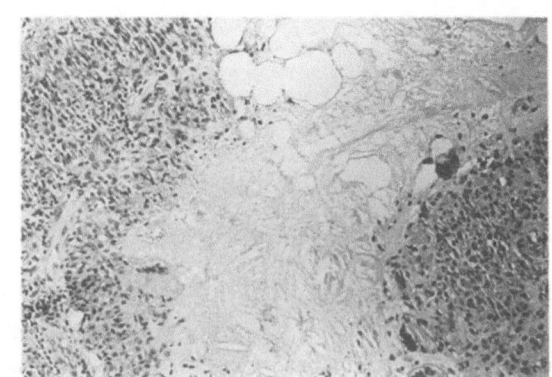

B

Fig. 8-47. (*A*) 83-year-old female with 2-month history
of redness and itching of the right upper lid. (*B*) Biopsy
shows a dermal infiltrate composed predominantly of
epithelioid cells with giant cells present. There is a large
area of necrosis with cholesterol clefts. Protein electrophoresis showed a monoclonal IgG-lambda protein spike
that confirmed the diagnosis of necrobiotic xanthogranuloma with paraproteinemia (Courtesy of John Weiner,
M.D., Melbourne).

affect the eyelids or orbit. Lipoid granulomatosis causes xanthelasma-type lesions of the lid and orbit, causing bilateral exophthalmos and ophthalmoplegia with optic nerve swelling or atrophy (Fig. 8-48). Elevated blood lipids may also be present. The disease results in excessive amounts of lipids, particularly cholesterol, being imbided and not properly metabolized by the histiocyte.

Long tubular bones are often symmetrically involved by the characteristic infiltration of large xanthomatous histiocytes, multinucleated giant cells, often of the Touton type, and secondary fibrosis. There is an accompanying mononuclear mixed cell infiltrate of lymphocytes and plasma cells. The bone disease may lead to sinus tract discharge. Visceral involvement includes the heart, lungs, and kidney. The disease is probably distinct from the histiocytosis X group of diseases.[111,112]

After biopsy is performed to establish the diagnosis, systemic steroids are of benefit in controlling the disease.

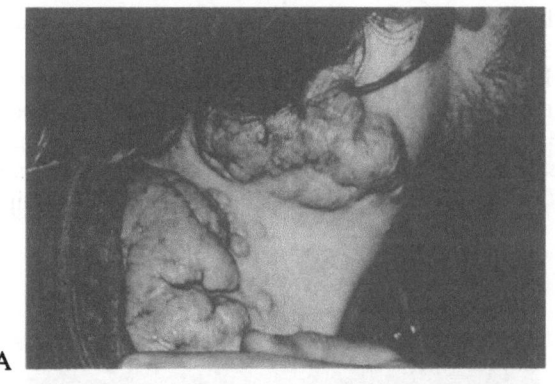

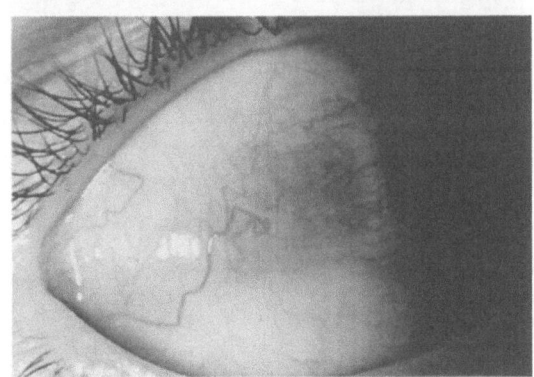

Fig. 8-48. (*A*) 33-year-old white male with chronic pleural and pericardial effusions since age 20. He first developed migratory bone pain in the arms and legs and skin nodules. He since developed carious teeth. (*B*) He developed bilateral conjunctival nodules over the lateral rectus muscles. The symmetric bone findings, xanthomatous masses of the neck, shoulders, and thorax, and conjunctiva combined with multiple biopsies showing histiocytes with variable fibrosis are most compatible with Erdheim-Chester disease. As in this case, the serum lipids are characteristically normal (Courtesy of David G. Cogan, M.D., Bethesda, MD).

Myxoma. Myxomas are rare, painless growths that may involve the lids, orbit, conjunctiva, or even the caruncle. Myxomas of the eyelids have been associated with a syndrome of pigmented lesions of the bulbar conjunctiva, caruncle and facial skin, and cardiac myxoma.[113]

Histologically, a myxoma is rather hypocellular but contains stellate and spindle cells that have mild hyperchromatic and slightly pleomorphic nuclei and mast cells, embedded in a loose collagenous matrix and mucoid stroma. They are well-circumscribed and contain hyaluronidase-sensitive mucopolysaccharides. The tumor cells may contain intranuclear and intracytoplasmic vacuoles. The tumors have little vascularity, which is helpful in differentiating myxoma from richly myxoid malignant neoplasms such as myxoid liposarcoma, botryoid-type rhabdomyosarcoma, myxoid malignant fibrous histiocytoma, and myxoid chondrosarcoma. In addition to a rich vascularity, these other tumors have the associated malignant lipoblast, rhabdomyoblast, fibroblast, histiocyte, and chondroblast, respectively.[114]

Myxomas are treated by local excision.

Malakoplakia. Malakoplakia is a rare disorder in which tumor-like masses of characteristic histiocytes (von Hansemann histiocytes) are present. The histiocytes contain inclusions known as Michaelis-Gutmann bodies that are intracytoplasmic lamellar calcospherules that are pathognomonic for the disease. The histiocytes occur subjacent to an epithelial surface. Malakoplakia may be due to a histiocytic response to chronic infection.[115]

The disease affects the genitourinary tract and less commonly the gastrointestinal (GI) tract. There is one reported eyelid case that presented as an orange-red mass that recurred after local excision. The patient died of chronic renal failure complications.

The histologic differential diagnosis includes JXG and Whipple's disease. Unlike JXG, malakoplakia contains no Touton giant cells. Whipple's disease occurs in the GI tract and is characterized by histiocytic lesions in which the cytoplasmic inclusions are amorphous debris.

Depositions in the Lid Tissues

Amyloidosis. (See Chapter 3). Typically, the tumor occurs as discrete or confluent bilateral, small, smooth papules or nodules that appear as waxy yellowish-orange or purple and hemorrhagic. Amyloidosis of the conjunctiva is usually not associated with a systemic disease, while amyloidosis of the lid usually is. Amyloidosis may occur as a nodular recurrent growth of the lid margin.[22] Loss of cilia in association with amyloid deposition has been reported. There is a thickening of the lid border with ulceration. Treatment of this particular case involved excision with reconstruction of the full-thickness lid involved (Fig. 8-49).

Work-up for systemic amyloidosis should include a

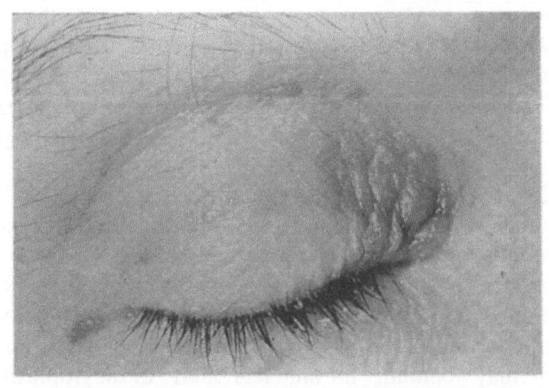

A

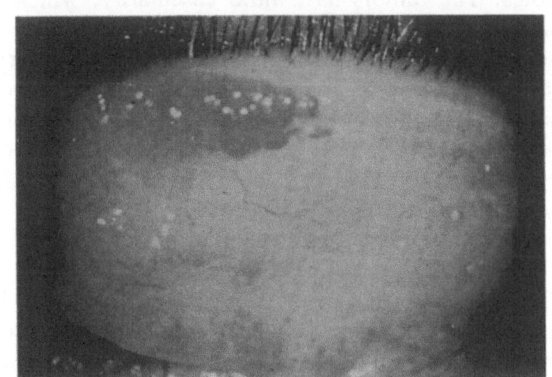

B

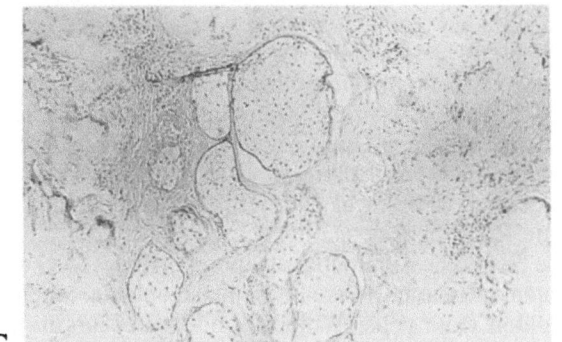

C

Fig. 8-49. (*A*) Purpuric appearance of lid in amyloidosis may be confused with Kaposi's sarcoma on lid (AFIP ACC #1404254). (*B*) In conjunctiva, amyloid, because of its tendency to cause hemorrhage, may be confused with Kaposi's sarcoma as well (AFIP ACC #1501414). (*C*) Amyloidosis of the tarsal conjunctiva appears more eosinophilic than surrounding collagen of tarsus (AFIP ACC #1076097).

familial history of amyloidosis and a physical examination, blood count, and routine urinalysis and 24-hour urine protein levels.

Ligneous Conjunctivitis. Ligneous conjunctivitis is a rare form of chronic membranous conjunctivitis that usually affects young girls. The disease is occasionally

familial and causes a marked thickening of the lid that may be mistaken for a tumor (Fig. 8-50).

Histologically, the membrane is a thick amorphous plaque of acellular eosinophilic material with associated granulation tissue. It has recently been demonstrated that the major component of the woody pseudomembrane is fibrin.[116]

Lipoid Proteinosis (Hyalinosis Cutis et Mucosae, Urbach Wiethe Syndrome). Lipoid proteinosis is a rare condition of the skin of the face, elbows, knees, and mucous membranes including the lip, mouth, pharynx, and larynx. It has an autosomal-recessive inheritance pattern.

Clinically, it is characterized by multiple, waxy, pearly nodules that cover all four lid margins similar to a row of beads. The number of cilia are fairly preserved, although they are distorted. The skin of the face has a "pigskin leather" appearance (Fig. 8-51). The mucous membranes may show leukoplakic lesions or submucosal infiltration. Laryngeal involvement may cause hoarseness.

Histologically, there are large dermal collections of an amorphous, homogeneous, eosinophilic, PAS-positive hyaline material that tends to surround blood vessels, sweat glands, and hair follicles. The material stains mildly with Congo-red stain and inconsistently with lipid

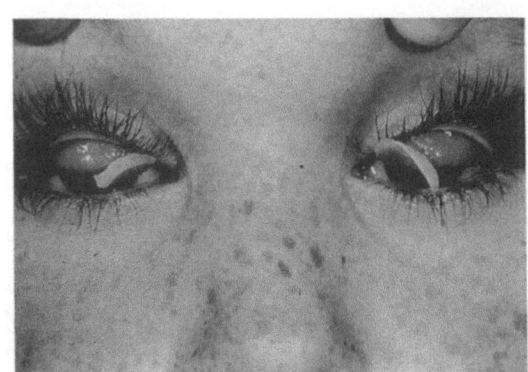

A

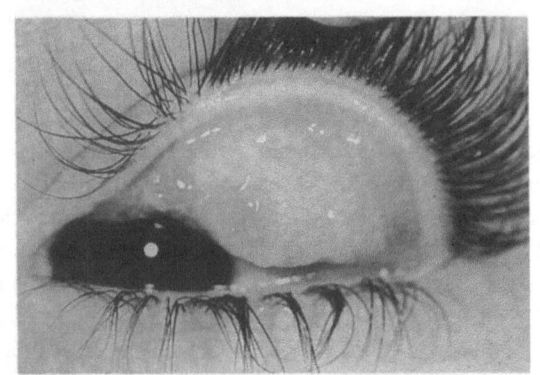

B

Fig. 8-50. (*A,B*) Bilateral thickening of lids due to ligneous conjunctivitis. The woody membrane is probably fibrin (AFIP ACC #1274282).

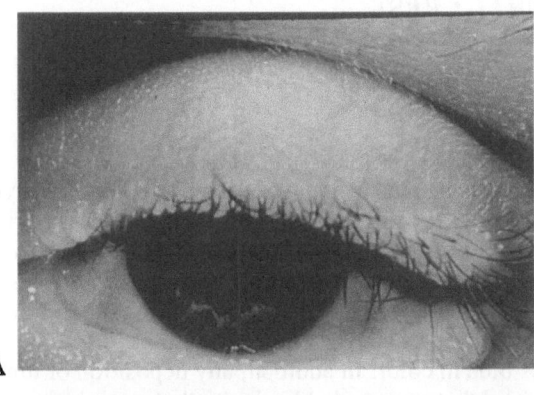

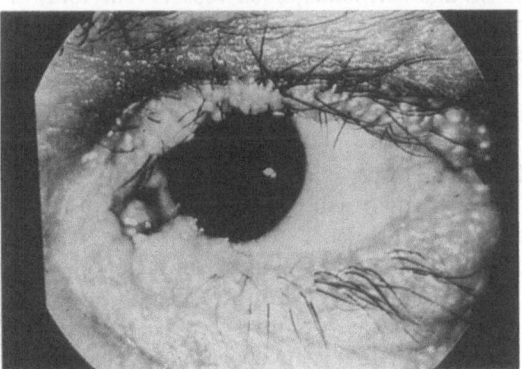

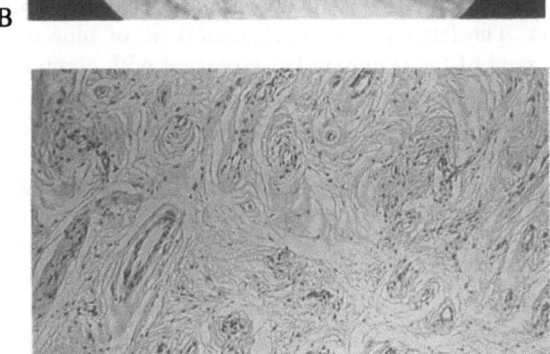

Fig. 8-51. (*A,B*) Patients with lipoid proteinosis typically show small pearly nodules (AFIP ACC #229747 and 1309455). (*C*) Histologically, the material has some of the characteristics of amyloid (AFIP ACC #221698).

stains. Mucopolysaccharide stains show that the substance is mainly hyaluronic acid. The material is not amyloid but is similar to the material observed in porphyrias.[3,45,117]

There is no known treatment. Local excision of the lid tumors would probably result in recurrence.

Tumors Metastatic to the Lid

Metastatic carcinoma to the lids is rare. In Aurora and Blodi's series, only 3 of 214 malignant lid lesions

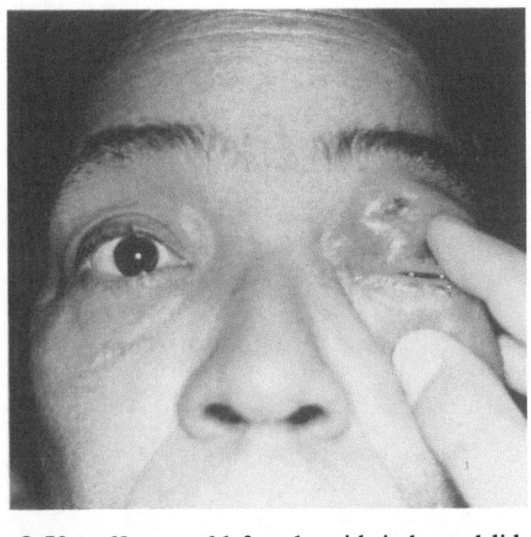

Fig. 8-52. 62-year-old female with indurated lid secondary to metastatic breast carcinoma. Orbital tumor seen on CT scan with focal bone erosion was recalcitrant to radiation. In view of progression of disease, no further treatment was recommended.

were metastatic carcinoma.[18] In a review of 2023 eyelid biopsy specimens, only three cases of metastatic eyelid carcinoma were identified.[118] A recent clinicopathologic study of 31 cases reviewed at the AFIP showed that the most common primary site was breast in 32 percent of cases. Lungs rarely metastasize to the lids, while they commonly metastasize to the orbit.[118,119]

There are four main clinical presentations: (1) most commonly as a solitary, painless, mobile nodule; (2) as a painless, diffuse swelling and induration of the lids, especially in metastatic breast cancer; (3) as an ulcerated lesion that may mimic a primary epithelial carcinoma; and (4) as a lesion that simulates a chalazion as an acutely painful nodule (Figs. 8-52 and 8-53).[120] Histologically, the pattern of metastatic carcinoma of the breast has been coined "histocytoid carcinoma" by Zimmerman.[80] The cells appear bland and uniform and have abundant cytoplasm that often contains small or large vacuoles of mucin resistant to hyaluronidase digestion; the nuclei are small. The tumor cells are arranged in columns one cell wide, the so-called "Indian file" pattern. Histologically, the pattern of metastatic breast carcinoma is indistinguishable from infiltrating signet ring carcinoma (adenocarcinoma of eccrine sweat glands).

Treatment includes excisional biopsy for localized lesions, while diffuse lid involvement usually seen with breast primaries responds well to radiation.

Phakomatous Choristoma of the Lid. A phakomatous choristoma is a congenital lid tumor that occurs at the inner aspect of the lower lid and may appear cystic or purplish. Only three cases have been reported. The tumor is believed to be derived from a lenticular anlage.

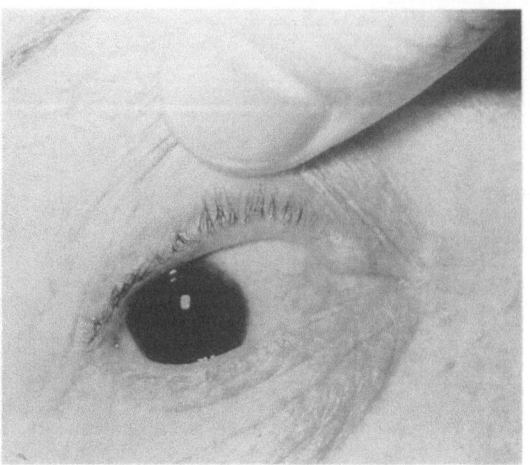

A

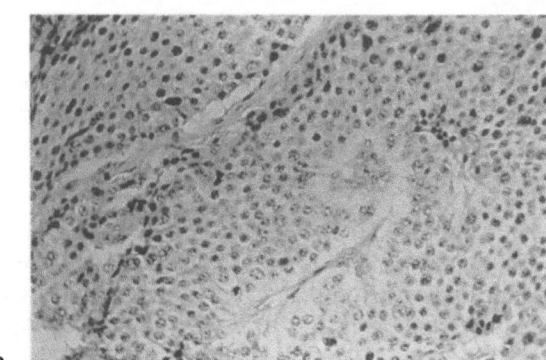

B

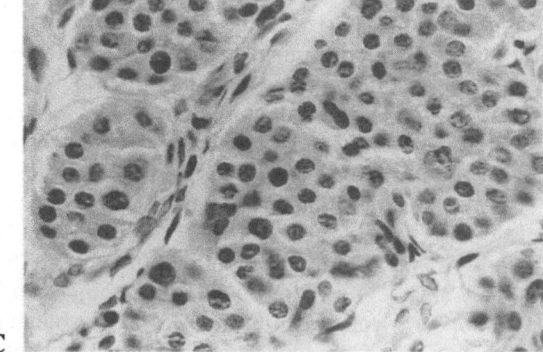

C

Fig. 8-53. (*A*) Patient with carcinoid metastatic to lid (AFIP ACC #1353373). (*B*) Biopsy shows organoid pattern with fine fibrovascular septae between the compartments of cells. (*C*) There are two cell types: cells with dark-staining nuclei and other cells with light-staining nuclei; both cells have large cytoplasm and small bland nuclei (AFIP ACC #178185).

Surgical excision is the treatment.

Histologically, the tumor is composed of solid cords or tubules consisting of a single layer of cuboidal cells resting on a basement membrane with virtually no lumen.[121]

NEURAL CREST

Introduction

Appropriate management of a pigmented, melanocytic lesion of the eyelid or conjunctiva requires appropriate knowledge of the clinicopathologic features of such lesions. Basically, any brown, black, or slate-gray lesion may represent melanin in a potentially malignant tumor of skin or conjunctiva. Vascular lesions often appear red or blue in color. In addition, any deposition or tumor in the lid that surrounds blood vessels (amyloid) or that is prone to have associated hemorrhage (eccrine acrospiroma, dermatofibroma, Kaposi's sarcoma) will appear red, blue, or purple. Finally, lipid in histiocytic lesions or in sebaceous tumors will appear orange, yellow, or red.

Melanin in superficial layers of the skin (epidermis and upper dermis) will appear brown in color. A high concentration of melanocytes or pigment in the individual melanocytes or a large number of melanophages will give the lesion a darker brown or black color. Melanin in the lower dermis or episclera will appear slate-gray and in addition will usually appear flatter than a vascular lesion. The latter pattern is characteristic of blue nevi. Blue nevi of the skin may be associated with compound nevi ("combined nevus"), and in such cases they will not appear flat clinically. Rarely, they may be associated with melanoma.

Epithelial lesions that contain pigment are listed in Table 8-4. These lesions include seborrheic keratosis, actinic keratosis, Bowen's disease, and BCC. Scaling erythematous lesions are likely to be epithelial. Such lesions as AK and Bowen's disease should be biopsied and removed. Seborrheic keratosis as stated above does not need to be biopsied.

A clinicopathologic classification is listed in Table 8-5.

Table 8-5
Configuration of Types of Nevocellular Nevi

Junctional
tend to be flat
Compound
minimally elevated
may be papillomatous
Intradermal
dome-shaped*
pedunculated*
papillomatous

* May not be pigmented

Pigmented Presumed Melanocytic Skin Lesions—Which Should Be Biopsied?

In general, any pigmented lesion on the lid that appears to be nonepithelial and is acquired in an adult should be biopsied. Certain conditions listed below that are clearly macules and represent only an increased concentration of melanin or an increased number of melanocytes and do not require biopsy.

Lesions That Are Brown Macules Due to Increased Pigmentation or Number of Nontumorous Dendritic Melanocytes.   All conditions listed in this section are macules and do not require biopsy. Junctional nevi tend to appear flat and are in a different histologic category (see below).

Freckles.   Freckles or ephelides (ephelis, singular) are small, brown macules scattered over skin exposed to the sun. In contrast to lentigo simplex, the sun exposure deepens the pigmented freckles.[3]

Lentigo Senilis.   Lentigo senilis occurs in multiple lesions in areas exposed to the sun and increase with age in elderly patients. They possess a uniform dark brown color and an irregular outline. Malignant degeneration does not occur.

Albright's Syndrome.   Albright's syndrome consists of fibrous dysplasia of bone, precocious puberty in females, and melanotic patches that are usually large in size, few in number, and are present in the midline but are observed on only one side of the midline. Unlike neurofibromatosis that has a smooth "coast of California" configuration to its café-au-lait patches, the patches of Albright's syndrome have a jagged, irregular "coast of Maine" appearance.

Histopathology

Freckles.   Freckles are hyperpigmentation of the basal cell layer of the epidermis. The melanocytes may

Table 8-6
McGovern Prognosis of Cutaneous Melanomas

Level I—malignant cells confined to epidermis

Level II—confined to papillary dermis, 72–92 percent 5-year survival

Level III—invades to level of subpapillary levels but not into reticular dermis, 46–56 percent 5-year survival

Level IV—invasion of reticular dermis, 31–54 percent survival

Level V—invasion to subcutaneous fat, 12–48 percent survival

Table 8-7
Conditions Associated with Increased Pigmentation or Increased Number of (Nontumorous) Dendritic Melanocytes

Freckle
Lentigo senilis
Melanotic macule of Albright's syndrome
Café-au-lait spot of neurofibromatosis

actually be less in number than normal but those melanocytes present are larger and show more numerous and longer dendritic processes than ordinary melanocytes (Table 8-7).

Lentigo Senilis.   Elongated rete ridges show considerable hyperpigmentation and a markedly increased number of the melanocytes in the basal layer.

Albright's Syndrome.   Biopsy shows hyperpigmentation of the basal layer.

Café au Lait of Neurofibromatosis.   This condition is characterized by increased melanin in the melanocytes and keratinocytes and may contain "giant" melanosomes in both the melanocytes and basal cells.

Lesions That Are Brown (Associated with Nevus Cells).   Clearly the clinical problem is distinguishing benign nevi from melanoma (Table 8-8). Nevi tend to grow at puberty and pregnancy and do not tend to be acquired later in life (Fig. 8-54). Therefore, any pigmented lesion that shows growth, has irregular margins, or a variegated color should be excised. Incisional biopsies are indicated only for large lesions.

Nevocellular Nevus.   Clinically, nevi may appear (1) flat, (2) slightly elevated, (3) papillomatous, (4) dome-

Table 8-8
Conditions Associated with Nevus (Nondendritic Melanocytes) Cells

Clinically Appear Brown:
  junctional
  dermal
  compound
  balloon cell
  halo
  spindle and epithelioid (Spitz' nevus, benign juvenile melanoma) (appears red in color)

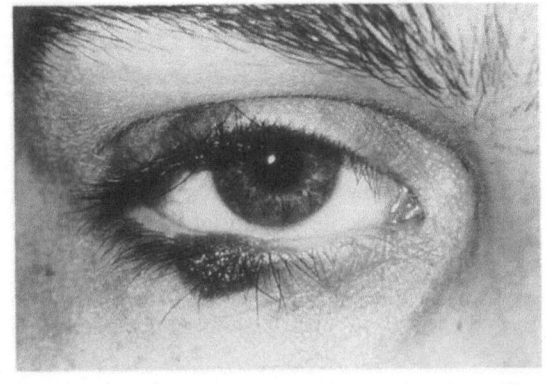

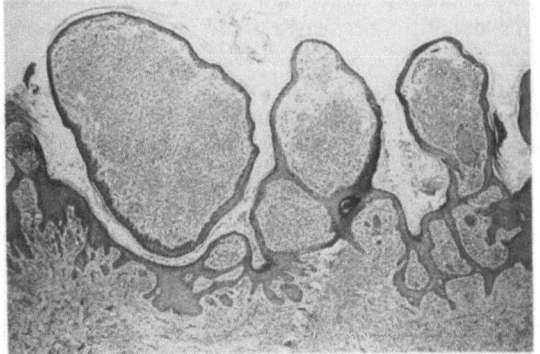

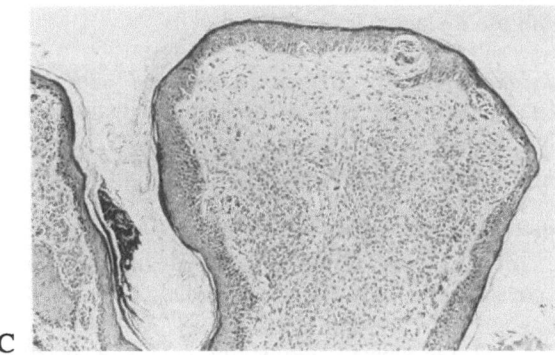

Fig. 8-54. (*A*) Congenital kissing nevus nevus with papillary clinical pattern. (*B,C*) Biopsy shows papillary pattern with dermal nevus cells with some junctional component typical of a compound nevus.

shaped, or (5) pedunculated.[3] While all five clinical presentations may be pigmented, dome-shaped lesions and pedunculated lesions may not be pigmented. *Junctional* lesions tend to appear flat. Minimally elevated lesions and some of the papillomatous lesions are *compound* nevi. Most papillomatous pigmented masses and nearly all dome-shaped and pedunculated are *intradermal* nevi. Therefore, a nonpigmented dome-shaped or pedunculated lesion may represent an intradermal nevus (Table 8-5).

Balloon cell nevi are not clinically distinguishable from other nevi. Usually they are slightly elevated, soft, and light brown in color.

A *halo nevus* is a pigmented nevus that is surrounded by a depigmented zone or halo. The area of depigmentation shows no clinical signs of inflammation, and it may persist for many months or even years. The halo nevus is undergoing involution. A halo may also be associated with a blue nevus or a melanoma may be located around the metastases of a melanoma.

While a *spindle* and *epithelioid nevus* is usually red in color rather than brown, on pathologic examination, it may be confused with melanoma.

The spindle and epithelioid nevus arises predominantly in children but also in adolescents and adults in about 15 percent of cases.[122] They are usually solitary and involve the face and extremities most commonly. They have a characteristic reddish color and appear as a dome-shaped, hairless small nodule. They may occur as a group. In addition, they usually grow rapidly over a few months. The main difficulty with these lesions is that the pathologist may confuse them with melanomas.

Biopsy Results

Nevi. Nevi are composed of cluster or nests of nevus cells that do not contain dendritic processes. Nevus cells show variation in size and shape and may be a spindle cell. Rather than specific cellular characteristics, their most diagnostic feature is their formation of clusters or nests. Cellular features of nevus cells are often determined by their location in the dermis. For example, nevus cells in the lower epidermis and upper dermis often resemble epithelioid cells and are cuboidal or oval in shape with a distinct outline, homogeneous cytoplasm, and a large round or oval nucleus. These cells not infrequently contain melanin. Nevus cells in the mid-dermis are small and resemble lymphoid cells. They rarely contain melanin. Nevus cells in the lower dermis are elongated and spindle-shaped like fibroblasts. The nevus cells become more mature or "spindly" as they penetrate the dermis. A nevus that lacks "maturation" would make the pathologist consider a diagnosis of melanoma.

Junctional Nevus. Nevus cells are present as well-circumscribed nests in the lower epidermis. Nests of cells may lie beneath the epidermis but are still in contact with it. There may be nests in the upper dermis.

Intradermal Nevus. The upper dermis shows nests and cords of nevus cells with only a slight or no junctional component or activity. In multinucleated nevus cells, small nuclei lie in a rosette-like pattern. Giant cells are found only in mature nevi. Spindle-shaped nevus cells in the mid- and lower dermis tend to lack melanin. The cells are embedded in a loose, pale, collagenous matrix and appear as "neuroid tubes." A concentric arrangement of nevus cells form nevus corpuscles that resemble Meissner's tactile bodies. Neural nevi contain only nevus cells in the deep dermis and may be impossible to distinguish from a solitary neurofibroma.

Compound Nevus. Compound nevus has features of both a junctional and an intradermal nevus.

Balloon Cell Nevus. Balloon cell nevus may form only a part of an intradermal or compound nevus (Fig. 8-55). The balloon cells are larger than ordinary nevus cells and contain finely granular or empty cytoplasm and a central nucleus. Multinucleated balloon cells may be present. Stains for lipid, glycogen, and mucopolysaccharides are negative. Balloon cells may also be associated with melanomas.

Halo Nevus. A halo nevus may be a dermal or compound nevus that has an accompanying infiltrate of lymphoid cells and melanophages.

Spindle and Epithelioid Nevus (Spitz Nevus). This lesion is a compound nevus. The pleomorphism of the cells and the presence of inflammation make this lesion easily confused with a nodular melanoma. Considerable junctional activity is present with a downward proliferation of the epidermis in irregular strands. The cells may be spindle-shaped or epithelioid and are usually arranged in nests. Multinucleated epithelioid cells and bizarre giant cells may be present. Mitoses, uncommon in nevi, in general, are frequently seen in spindle and epithelioid nevi.

The clinicopathologic presentation of a red dome-shaped lesion in a child confirms the diagnosis. Histologic parameters alone may cause the pathologist to confuse this benign lesion with a melanoma.

Lesions That Are Brown and Grow and That Predispose to Melanoma. *Lentigo Maligna* (melanotic freckle of Hutchinson, lentigo maligna melanoma) begins as an unevenly pigmented macule several centimeters in size that gradually enlarges peripherally while other areas

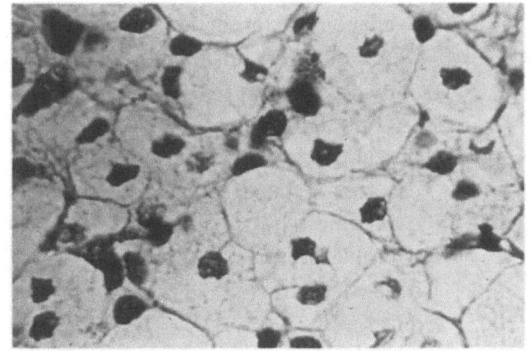

Fig. 8-55. Balloon cell nevus (AFIP ACC #1367550) showing cells with abundant cytoplasm and small benign nuclei.

spontaneously regress. The borders are irregular and show no induration. The color varies from light brown to brown with minute dark brown to black flecks. In essence, the lesions change shape and size and may also change in color from tan to brown to black. They are nonpalpable.[123] The lesion occurs in older individuals in sun-exposed areas of the body.

Clinically, development into an invasive melanoma is indicated by the presence of one or several intradermal bluish-black nodules. However, invasion may occur without any obvious clinical change. Invasion may take years to occur. Approximately one-third of all lentigo maligna lesions will become the invasive lesion of lentigo maligna melanoma. Since these tumors grow slowly and metastasize late, biopsy is not indicated when the lesion is a macule. Metastases tend to be limited to the regional lymph nodes. The 5-year survival rate is between 80 and 90 percent.[124]

Superficial spreading melanoma (pagetoid melanoma) usually occurs on nonexposed skin and is rare on the eyelids. It is an acquired lesion that usually appears in middle-aged people. The lesions are palpable from the outset and most frequently are circular with small protrusions and indentations along its borders. The lesions rarely measure more than 2.5 cm. Superficial spreading melanomas may present as a pigmented skin tag. The color is similar to that of lentigo maligna, characteristically a rose hue. Development into an invasive melanoma is indicated by ulceration, bleeding, and an increase in the induration of the lesion. Late in the disease, nodules may appear. The 5-year survival rate is about 70 percent.[124]

Histopathology

Lentigo Maligna. The melanocytes at the base of the epidermis are markedly increased in number and appear elongated, spindle-shaped, and pleomorphic. Normal-appearing melanocytes are found next to large, bizarre melanocytes. The difference between lentigo maligna and lentigo maligna melanoma is invasion beyond the basement membrane of the epidermis. Nests of cells are not usually seen until invasion into the dermis develops. Spindle cells are most frequently seen in the invasive areas. The melanocytes retain their dendritic processes. The dermis shows numerous melanophages and a band-like chronic inflammatory cell infiltrate.

Superficial Spreading Melanoma. The epidermis shows a striking pagetoid pattern of rather uniformly round, large melanocytes with uniform nucleus and prominent nucleoli. Unlike the cells of spindle and epithelioid nevus, the abundant cytoplasm of the tumor's cells in superficial spreading melanoma is dusted with pigmentation. In addition, nests of such cells lie in the lower epidermis. The cells contain varying amounts of melanin;

superficial spreading melanoma will show a radial growth phase usually in multiple foci. The cells in these areas are more bizarre than those seen in lentigo maligna melanoma and frequently are of the epithelioid type. There are almost no dendritic melanocytes. Dermal melanophages and a dermal infiltrate are usually present.

Nodular Melanomas. Nodular melanomas arise de novo, that is, without an antecedent lesion. Clinically, an elevated, usually deeply pigmented "blueberry"-like nodule increases in size rapidly and then undergoes ulceration. The uniform color varies from blue-black in one lesion to rose-gray in another. These tumors occur most commonly in the fifth decade and are twice as common in men as in women. The 5-year survival rate is between 50 and 60 percent.[124]

Pathologically, nodular melanomas have no intraepidermal growth phase without a concomitant dermal invasion.[125] This feature helps explain their poor prognosis.

A rare variant of melanoma is the desmoplastic malignant melanoma or spindle cell melanoma, which has a high rate of recurrence and mortality. In one case report is the ophthalmic literature, the lesion arose in the palpebral conjunctiva. Pathologically, the spindle cell tumor may be confused with a fibrous or neural tumor, but the atypical cells in the junctional area are diagnostic.[126]

No matter what the origin of the malignant melanoma, whether from a lentigo maligna, superficial spreading, or nodular, there are certain characteristic histopathologic features. In a typical malignant melanoma, there is considerable irregular junctional activity with downward streaming of anaplastic tumor cells from the epidermis into the dermis. The epidermis may show irregular proliferation of its rete ridges. Tumor cell migration upward into the epidermis leads to ulceration of the epidermis. The tumor's cells in the dermis show great pleomorphism. The cells are of two basic types: (1) spindle, associated with lentigo maligna, and (2) epithelioid, associated with superficial spreading and de novo melanomas. Depth of invasion is the most important prognostic factor and varies from level I, in which tumor cells are confined to the epidermis, to level V where tumor cells invade the subcutaneous fat (Table 8-6).[124]

Like conjunctival melanomas, metastases occur to the local lymph nodes rather than to the blood. Choroidal melanomas spread hematogenously to the liver most commonly.[125]

Nevi That Appear Blue (Dendritic Melanocytic Tumors). Nevus of Ota is a bluish macule of the skin with an ipsilateral slate-gray patch on the sclera. The condition is rarely bilateral.

It may present at birth or later in childhood or adolescence. The lesions tend to gradually enlarge with age. Malignant degeneration of the skin or epibulbar lesions rarely occur. However, a nevus of Ota that shows a

Table 8-9
Melanocytic Lesions That Clinically May Appear Blue

Blue nevus
Congenital oculodermal melanocytosis (nevus of Ota)
Precancerous Melanosis—lentigo maligna (Hutchinson's freckle)
Malignant melanoma—Origins
   de novo (nodular)
   superficial spreading
   arising in lentigo maligna

nodule should probably be biopsied. Histologically, the skin lesion is a blue nevus. Nevus of Ito, involving the supraclavicular, scapular, or deltoid regions, may occur alone or in association with nevus of Ota.[3] While more common in blacks and Orientals, nevus of Ota is associated with an increased incidence of melanoma of the choroid, especially in white patients.

Blue nevi occur as two types: (1) the common blue nevus and (2) the cellular blue nevus (Tables 8-9 and 8-10).

The common blue nevus is a small, well-circumscribed, dome-shaped nodule of slate-blue or bluish-black color. They are usually solitary. Malignant degeneration is not associated with the common blue nevus. When a common blue nevus is associated with an overlying compound nevus, it is termed a *combined nevus.*

The cellular blue nevus is a large bluish nodule or plaque that extends deeply into the subcutaneous tissue (Fig. 8-56). Its surface may be smooth or irregular. They are most commonly located over the buttocks in the sacrococcygeal region. Rarely, malignant degeneration of a cellular blue nevus may occur.

Table 8-10
Pigmented Tumors

Vascular tumor
Melanocytic tumor
Seborrheic keratosis
Bowen's disease
Actinic keratosis
Basal cell carcinoma
Eccrine acrospiroma[*]
Apocrine hydrocystoma
Dermatofibroma[*]
Kaposi's sarcoma[*]
Dacryops
Canaliculops

[*] Pigment due to associated hemorrhage.

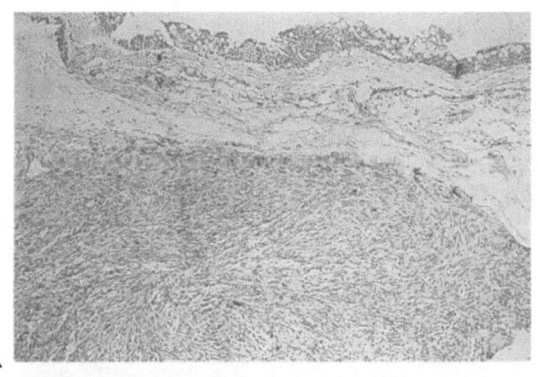

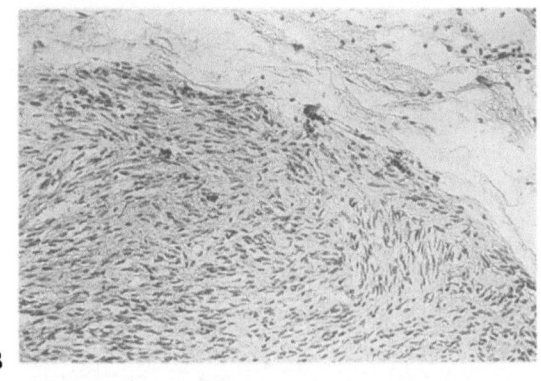

Fig. 8-56. (*A*) Cellular blue nevus of caruncle composed of dendritic melanocytes and fibroblasts (AFIP ACC #1428334) (*B*) Note that the lesion is deep to the epithelium. Because of its marked cellularity, this lesion is termed a *cellular* blue nevus rather than a blue nevus.

Biopsy Results

Nevus of Ota. The lower dermis shows greatly elongated, slender, often slightly wavy dendritic cells containing melanin granules lying between collagen fibers. The cells are dendritic and bipolar.

Blue Nevus. Blue nevus has same histology as nevus of Ota but the blue nevus is more cellular than the nevus of Ota.

Cellular Blue Nevus. In addition to dendritic melanocytes, the cellular blue nevus has islands composed of closely aggregated, rather large, spindle-shaped cells with ovoid nuclei and abundant pale cytoplasm with little or no melanin. Cellular blue nevi may undergo malignant degeneration into a malignant cellular blue nevus or a melanoma. Invasion of the subcutaneous fat, necrosis, and mitotic figures favor the malignant diagnosis.[126]

Miscellaneous Tumors of Neural Crest Origin. Merkel's cell tumors occur in elderly patients. They are usually hard, smooth-surfaced, painless lesions measuring 1–3 cm and are more common in the upper lid. The tumors often are red or blue in color with an overlying telangiectasia.[127] The tumor often appears protuberant with intact skin overlying the tumor. The clinical differential diagnosis includes amelanotic melanoma, a primary cutaneous lymphoma, and a cutaneous metastasis of a lymphoma or carcinoma.

Biopsy shows an unencapsulated dermal neoplasm that extends into the subcutaneous tissue. The cells grow in interconnecting sheaths and cords in a trabecular pattern, hence the previous designation as trabecular cell carcinoma. The cells are round, with scanty cytoplasm and uniform size and shape. The nuclei are large overall and have prominent nucleoli. Mitotic figures are abundant. The histologic differential diagnosis includes lymphoma, leukemic infiltrate, and metastatic (particularly oat cell) carcinoma.[127,128] In general, electron microscopy is necessary to make the diagnosis. The characteristic finding is scattered membrane-bound, round, dense-core neurosecretory granules 100–250 nm in diameter. Positive staining for neuron-specific enolase is strongly suggestive of this tumor.

The important clinical point is that the tumor behaves aggressively and should be treated with wide local excision and regional lymph node dissection. Distant metastases and death occur in approximately 20 percent of patients.[127,128]

LESIONS OF THE CARUNCLE

The common tumors of the caruncle are listed in Table 8-11. All of these entities have been discussed elsewhere with the exception of adenochrome pigment.

Chronic use of epinephrine compounds in the treatment of glaucoma lead to the deposition of the oxidized form of epinephrine in the cornea, conjunctiva, and caruncle as brownish-black masses. The oxidized epinephrine compound has properties similar to melanin (Figs. 8-57–8-60).

Histologically, this compound appears as an amorphous pink material that stains black with silver stains and bleaches with hydrogen peridoxide.[129,130]

INFLAMMATIONS OF THE LIDS

Inflammations of the lids may have several clinical presentations such as (1) diffuse edema with pain, (2) diffuse edema without pain, (3) chronic blepharitis, (4)

Table 8-11
Lesions of the Caruncle

Pigmented Lesions
    Nevi
    Melanoma
    Freckle
    Oxidized epinephrine pigment
Epithelial Lesions
    Papilloma
    Actinic keratosis
    Seborrheic keratosis
Nonepithelial Tumors
    Sebaceous gland hyperplasia
    Granular cell tumor (granular cell myoblastoma)
    Dermatofibroma
    Sebaceous gland carcinoma
    Ectopic lacrimal
Cystic Lesions
    Oncocytoma (see lacrimal gland section)
    Epidermal inclusion cyst
    Dermoid cyst
    Apocrine hydrocystoma
    Pilar cyst
Vascular Lesions
    Pyogenic granuloma
    Capillary hemangioma
    Cavernous hemangioma

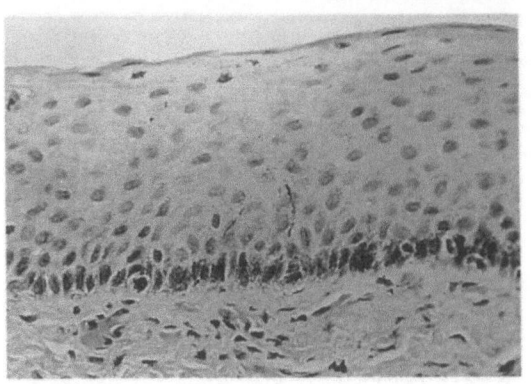

A

B

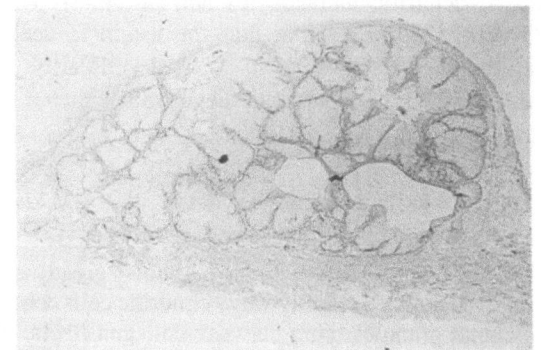

C

Fig. 8-57. (*A*) Ephelis of caruncle (AFIP ACC #1376253). (*B*) See melanin in basal epithelial cells. (*C*) Sebaceous gland adenoma of the caruncle (AFIP ACC #638761). Note that sebaceous glands are a normal component of the caruncle, and therefore sebaceous gland carcinomas may also arise here.

focal inflammatory nodules of the lids, and (5) ulceration and destruction of the lid due to infections and inflammations.

As in the orbit, tumors may cause local necrosis of lid tissues. A thickened necrotic lid may be due to an inflammation such as anthrax, but may also be due to a lid tumor such as lymphoma with or without secondary infection.[37,131] For example, a case report involved a 39-year-old woman who had undergone renal transplantation. Nine years later, she developed an inflammatory yellow lesion on her left lower eyelid. Gradually, the palpebral conjunctiva thickened and ulcerated, and the same process involved the adjacent skin surface of the left lower eyelid with complete loss of lashes. Over the 2-month course, she developed multiple ulcerations of the lid skin, upper lip, and hard palate. The biopsy showed a polymorphic B-cell lymphoma. Thus, in addition to inflammatory lesions, a B-cell lymphoma should be considered in immunosuppressed patients with necrotizing eyelid and conjunctival lesions.[37]

lid edema and pain without ulceration or loss of cilia (Table 8-12). The underlying cause may be orbital pseudotumor or bacterial orbital cellulitis.

Diffuse Edema with Pain

As in patients with presumed bacterial orbital cellulitis, a trial of antibiotics may be necessary in patients with

Diffuse Edema without Pain

There are multiple causes of edema of the eyelid without pain (Table 8-12).

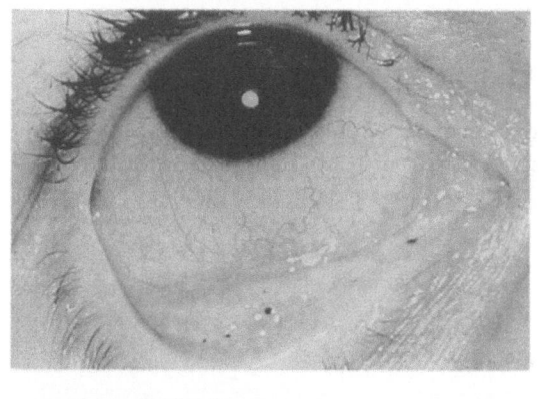

A

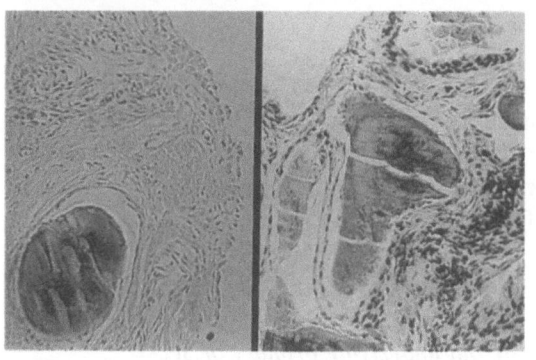

B

Fig. 8-58. (*A*) Epinephrine deposits of the conjunctive are (*B*) subepithelial (AFIP ACC #1096690).

Allergic Blepharitis. Allergic blepharitis may be due to contact dermatitis or an insect bite. There is usually a strong pruritic component. The skin is edematous, and there is a diffuse erythema with oozing and crusting. Vesicles may be present. In the chronic forms, scaling and lichenification (exaggerated skin markings) predominate (Fig. 8-61). A history of cosmetics, locally applied atropine, and epinephrine may be the cause. In addition, patients with angioneurotic edema may have episodes of recurrent eyelid edema (Fig. 8-62). They often have

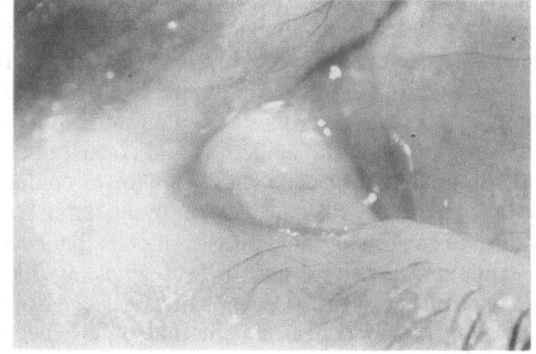

Fig. 8-59. Epithelial inclusion cyst of the caruncle (Courtesy of Dr. Louis Karp, Philadelphia, PA).

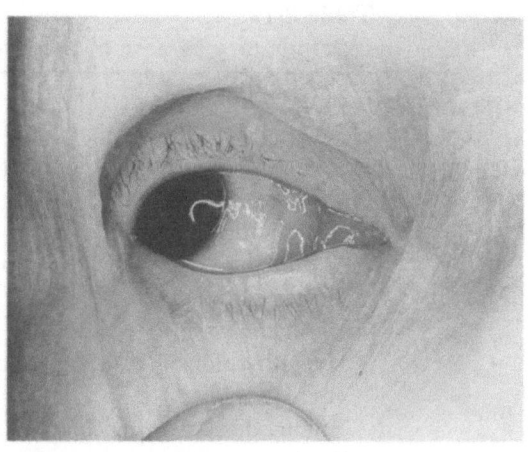

Fig. 8-60. Lymphoid infiltrate of caruncle. Biopsy showed reactive lymphoid hyperplasia.

atrophy of the nasal fat pad. Atopic dermatitis may also have lid involvement.

Systemic conditions such as hypothyroidism, hyperthyroidism, renal disease, trichinosis, and dermatomyositis should be considered. The latter three conditions present with edema.

Trichinosis. Trichinosis results from the ingestion of raw or insufficiently cooked pork that contains *Trichinella* cysts. The larvae encyst in the patient's duodenum and develop into adults. After fertilization, the female deposits larvae that invade the intestinal lymphatics and venules. Within 2 weeks, larvae are migrating throughout the body. By the third week encystment in striated muscle is in progress. Infectious disease consultation is indicated. Eosinophilia, periorbital edema, and splinter nail hemorrhages are characteristic.

Biopsy shows muscle fiber atrophy, edema, and degeneration. The encysted larvae of *Trichinella spiralis* may be present.[3]

Dermatomyositis. Dermatomyositis causes erythematous to purplish patches that show slight edema. The face, chest, and arms are commonly involved; the myositis component results in pain, weakening, and later atrophy of the muscles.[3]

Mycosis Fungoides. Mycosis fungoides may also cause diffuse eyelid edema without pain. This disease has three clinical and histologic stages: the erythematous stage, the plaque stage, and the tumor stage. The three stages may overlap and all be present in one patient at the same time.

In the erythematous stage, scattered erythematous scaling patches have an irregular but fairly sharp demarcation. In the plaque stage, the slightly indurated plaques are irregularly shaped and well-demarcated. In the tumor

Table 8-12
Inflammatory Disease of the Eyelid

Edema with Pain
    Rule out bacterial orbital cellulitis with lid component or preseptal orbital
        cellulitis versus pseudotumor (see Chapter 3)
Lid Edema without Pain
    Allergic blepharitis
        Rule out contact blepharitis insect bite
    Angioneurotic edema
    Dermatomyositis
    Hyperthyroidism (pain only if corneal exposure)
    Hypothyroidism
    Kidney disease
    Trichinosis
    Tumor masquerading as inflammation
        mycosis fungoides, meibomian carcinoma
        metastatic carcinoma
Chronic Blepharitis Presentation with Minimal Loss of Cilia (always consider
    tumor—see "Eyelid Tumors with Loss of Cilia")
    Hordeolum
    Internal hordeolum—acute meibomitis
    External hordeolum—acute inflammation of Zeis' gland
    Chronic meibomitis (chalazion)—*always rule out underlying primary or sec-*
        ondary lid tumor
    Chronic blepharitis (Staphlococcus)
    Parasitic
    Phthiriasis palpebrum
    Demodex blepharitis
Focal Nodules of the Lid with Pain
    Myiasis
    Subcutaneous *Dirofilariasis*
    Cysticercosis (usually minimal pain)
    Metastatic carcinoma

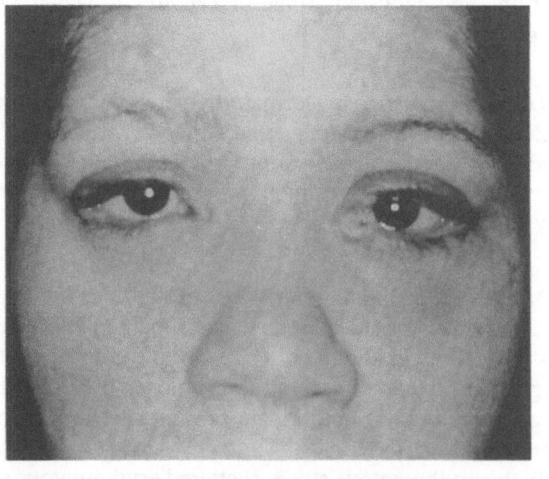

Fig. 8-61. 28-year-old female with history of atopic dermatitis has thickened eyelids, especially around medial canthal area.

stage, round or irregularly shaped, raised brownish-red tumors are present.

On biopsy, the erythematous stage shows an inflammatory infiltrate composed mainly of histiocytes, lymphoid cells, eosinophils, and plasma cells. Some neutrophils and fibroblasts are often present. In the papillary and subpapillary dermis, suspicious scattered mononuclear cells with hyperchromatic, irregularly shaped nuclei, mycosis cells, are diagnostic. The plaque stage has a high percentage of such mycosis cells. Pautrier's microabscesses are present in the epidermis and consist of small groups of mononuclear cells within the lower epidermis surrounded by a halo-like clear space. In the tumor stage, the infiltrate consists of large masses of cells that occupy the dermis and penetrate into the subcutaneous tissue. Superficial ulceration may occur. In late stages of the disease, the lymph nodes and internal organs become involved.[3]

Management of such patients should involve a dermatologist and oncologist.

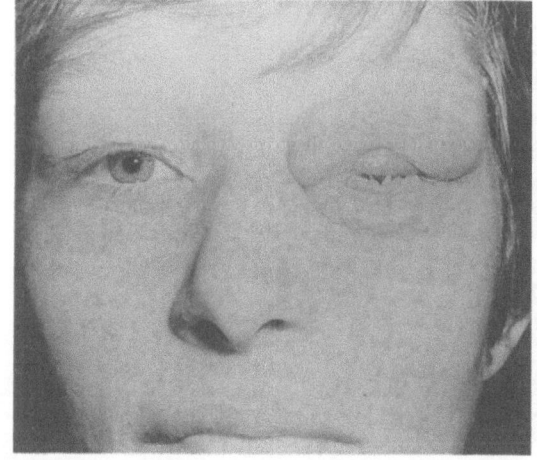

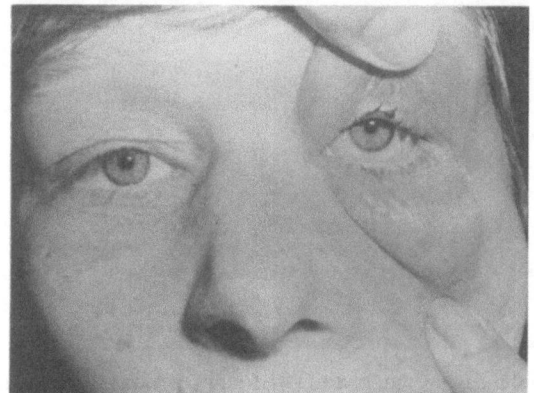

Fig. 8-62. 35-year-old female with recurrent episodes of angioneurotic edema refractory to any therapy.

Chronic Blepharitis with Minimal Loss of Cilia

Chronic staphylococcal blepharitis will result in loss of cilia and, in some cases, distichiasis (an extra row of lashes posteriorly) (Table 8-12). The sebaceous glands of the lids are the only site in the body with unassociated pilar units. However, the basal cells of the meibomian glands are pluripotential, and certain conditions such as chronic inflammation will cause these cells to differentiate into hair follicles (Figs. 8-63 and 8-64).

An internal hordeolum is due to an acute inflammation of the meibomian glands. An external hordeolum is a purulent folliculitis that involves the glands of Zeis and Moll or the glands of Zeis alone. A chronic lipogranulomatous inflammation affecting meibomian or Zeis glands produces a chalazion and rarely leads to loss of lashes (Fig. 8-64).

Many patients with chalazion have a chronic staphylococcal blepharitis with scaling along the lid margin.

Lid hygiene, topical antibiotics, and systemic tetracycline may be necessary to treat recurrent large or multiple chalazion. Incision of the chalazion wall may be neces-

sary. A chalazion that has multiple recurrences should have a full-thickness lid biopsy to rule out a sebaceous gland carcinoma.

Phthiriasis Palpebrum (Crab Lice)

The pubic louse (*Phthirus pubis*) normally infests the pubic hair and inguinal areas but may involve the eyelashes as well. The condition is usually transmitted sexually to the eyelids and is associated with poor personal hygiene. Pruritis with conjunctivitis, preauricular lymphadenopathy, and secondary infection occurs. The nits (eggs) and feces from the lice are reddish-brown granules located at the bases of the lashes (Fig. 8-65). The crab louse may sometimes be observed on the lid margin.

Treatment includes mechanical removal of the lice and nits; eserine ophthalmic ointment or any ophthalmic ointment applied to the lashes asphyxiates the louse. Local application of a pediculicide to the pubic area combined with proper hygiene are also necessary.[45] In addition, treatment with one or two drops of fresh 20% fluorescein on the lid margin is reported to be effective. The lice and nits are removed with forceps and a wet cotton swab if necessary. The fluorescein may be reapplied on the tenth day to remove any nits if reinfestation has occurred.[132]

Demodex Blepharitis

Demodectic mites infest the pilosebaceous structures of the lids. Two species of mites have different sites of

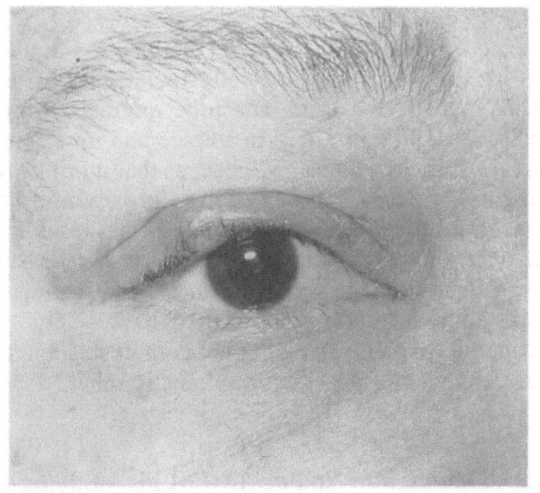

Fig. 8-63. 64-year-old female with 2-month history of growth of the right upper lid. Clinical diagnosis was that of chalazion, although there was focal loss of lashes suggesting a meibomian gland carcinoma.

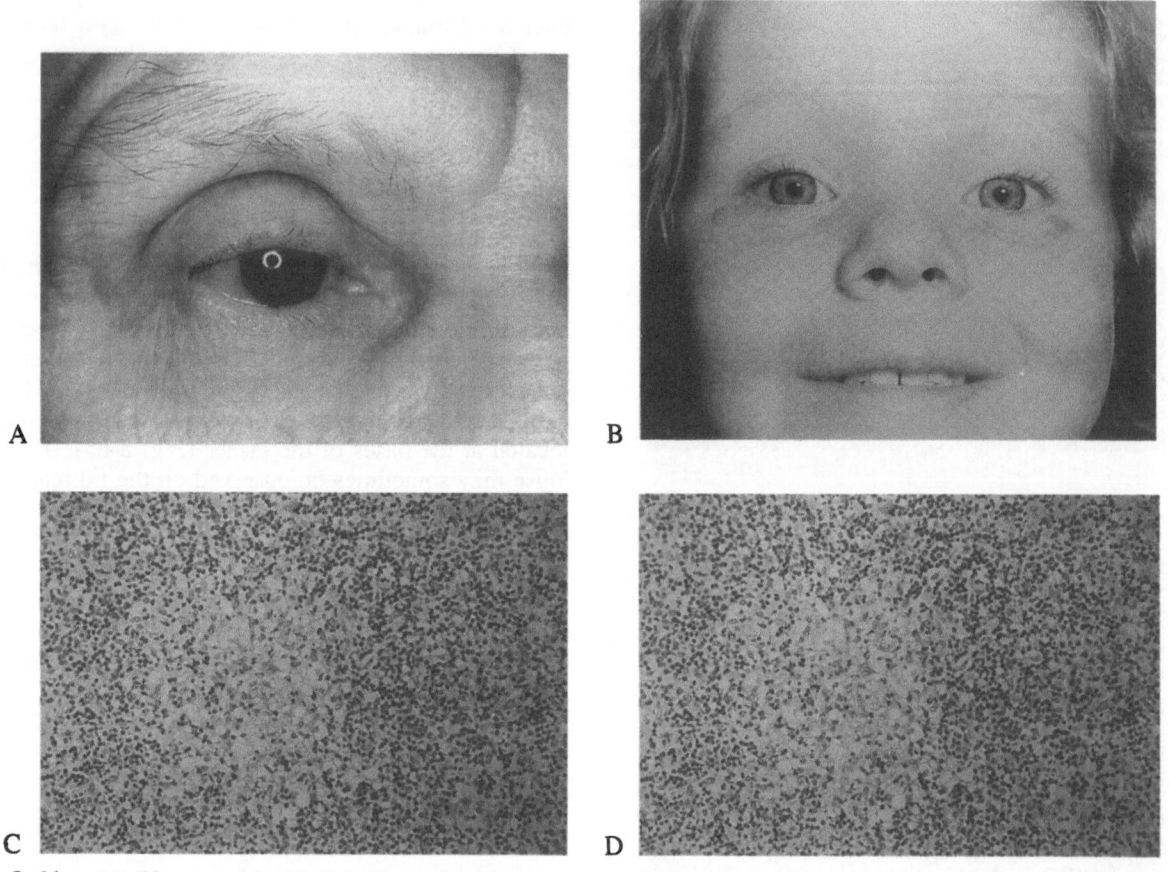

Fig. 8-64. (A) 68-year-old with "chalazion" refractory to medical management and two local currettage procedures. Full-thickness lid biopsy showed no evidence of sebaceous gland carcinoma. (B) 4-year-old child had chalazion that had been treated with local injection of steroids. Note displacement of the lipid into the lower lid and cheek with consequent (C,D) lipogranulomatous inflammation.

predilection. *D. folliculorum* is found in small hair follicles, and *D. brevis* is present in the sebaceous glands of small hairs of the eyelid skin, in sebaceous glands associated with the cilia of the lid margin, and in mebomian glands. The mite is usually found near or at the bulb of the epilated lash. The mite migrates from the follicles at night onto the skin surface and may actually infect the follicle with staphylococcus that it brings from the night's sojourn. Fine waxy debris forms a transparent collar of mite feces that surround the lashes for 1–2 mm. In severe cases, the mite may be observed. Symptoms include burning, itching, redness, and scaling with pigmentation about the roots of the cilia.

Proper lid hygiene including hot compresses and topical antibiotics will provide symptomatic relief.[45]

Focal Inflammatory Nodules of the Lids—Edema with Pain

Focal inflammatory nodules with lids that present without pain are listed in Table 8-12.

Myiasis. Myiasis is an infestation of vertebrates with insect larvae belonging to the order *Diptera*. The condition is rare in the United States, but it does occur in international travelers. External ophthalmomyiasis refers to infestation of the lid and conjunctiva, while internal ophthalmiasis refers to the penetration of the larvae into the conjunctiva, sclera, and subretinal space. The third form, orbital myiasis, is the least common form. Certain preexisting conditions predispose to infestation; these include gonococcal conjunctivitis in children and periocular ulcerated skin cancers in adults.

Clinically, the cutaneous lesion is similar to a furuncle. The lesions usually have serosanguineous discharge and may be mildly tender or pruritic unless secondarily infected. In the latter case, a preseptal cellulitis occurs.[133]

Treatment includes removing all invading organisms and controlling the almost inevitable secondary infection. In external myiasis, the larvae can be readily removed following their paralysis through topical application of cocaine. A layer of petroleum jelly suffocates the larvae.[134] The deeply imbedded larvae in cases of orbital myiasis are more difficult to remove. Turpentine packing drives larvae from the wound. Ether irrigation has been

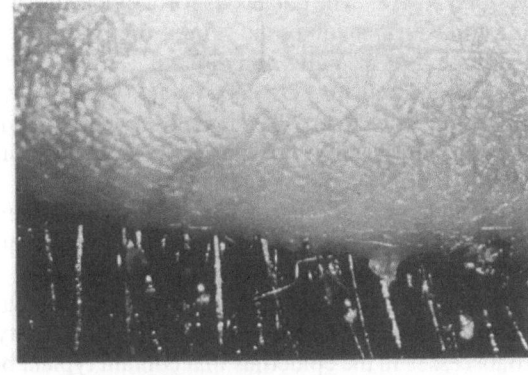

A

B

Fig. 8-65. (*A*) Note nits around lashes. (*B*) Louse is seen.

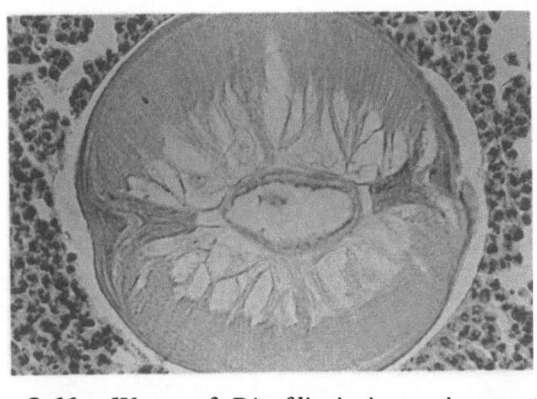

Fig. 8-66. Worm of *Dirofilariasis tenuis* nematode surrounded by suppurative inflammation in the subcutaneous lid tissue (AFIP ACC #1500480).

proposed for patients who cannot tolerate turpentine packing. Ether may be used carefully; an adequate airway must be obtained because of the anesthetic effect of ether.[135]

Subcutaneous Dirofilariasis. *Dirofilaria tenuis* is a nematode that may invade the eyelid, periorbital skin, and rarely the conjunctiva.[136] *Dirofilaria tenuis,* a natural parasite of the raccoon, is the most common species in the United States, particularly in the southeastern region such as in Florida. The nodules are often painful and tender; they may be pruritic and often appear inflamed.

Histologically, the lesion shows a mixed granulomatous and suppurative reaction with prominent eosinophilia (Fig. 8-66). Subcutaneous dirofilarial infection is caused by a single worm, located within an abscess in the center of the nodule.

Surgical excision of the nodule is the treatment of choice.

Cysticercosis. *Cysticercus,* the larval form of *Taenia solium,* is rare in the western world. Cysticercosis most commonly involves the retina and vitreous, especially the subretinal space in the macular region. Rarely, the organism lodges in the orbit or lids and the death of the organism leads to a severe inflammatory reaction.[137]

The lids usually show minimal inflammatory signs. A subcutaneous cyst develops. Central nervous system (CNS) involvement should be ruled out in such cases. Autoinfection occurs through fecal contamination and reinfection by family members.

Histologically, the inflammatory reaction of the wall of the cyst is composed of three distinct layers. The outer wall is dense, chronically inflamed, fibrovascular connective tissue, the middle layer consists of histiocytic cells with some fibroblasts, and the inner layer contains many polymorphonuclear leukocytes. The central structure contains the organism, *C. cellulosae,* with identifying morphologic features including the scolex with suckers and hooklet (Fig. 8-67).

Local treatment includes surgical excision of the cystic mass.

Infections with Ulceration and Destruction of the Lid and Loss of Celia

Several infections may be necrotizing and include untreated bacterial infections, especially anthrax, fungal infections, and protozoan infestations by *Leishmania* (Table 8-13).

Anthrax. Anthrax (malignant pustule, woolsorter's disease) is an infection of workers in tanneries and wool-scouring mills who handle imported animal hides. Most lesions appear on the face and hands; lid involvement is uncommon. *Bacillus anthracis* is a large, spore-forming, aerobic, nonmotile, gram-positive rod that infects traumatized skin.

The lesion starts as a papule that enlarges, becomes ulcerated, and later is covered by a typical black eschar.

Histologically, the epidermis is ulcerated and covered by necrotic tissue. Large gram-positive rods with square ends are demonstrated.[45]

Infectious disease consultation is recommended.

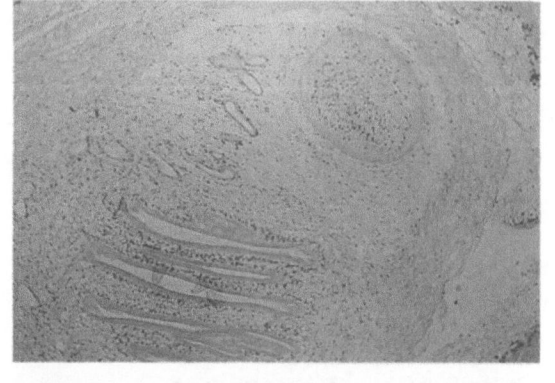

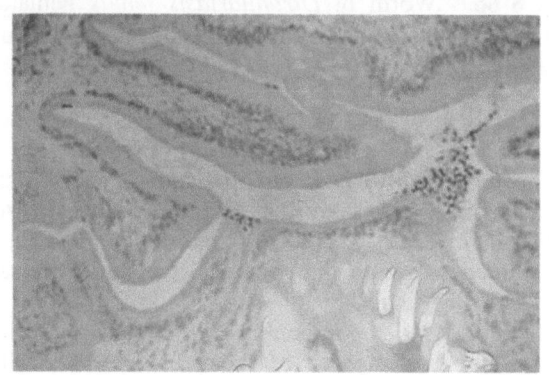

Fig. 8-67. (*A*) Cysticercus organism, larval form of *Teania solium,* present in subcutaneous lid tissue. (*B*) Note hooklets (AFIP ACC #1558619).

Table 8-13
Infections and Inflammations with Ulceration and Destruction of Lid with Loss of Cilia

Infections
    Bacterial skin infection
    Anthrax
    Fungal infection
    Blastomycosis
    Coccidioidomycosis
    Cryptococcus
    Protozoa
    Leishmaniasis
Inflammations
    Idiopathic midline destructive disease (IMDD) lethal
      midline granuloma
    Radiation necrosis
Discoid Lupus Erythematosis (may present as chronic
blepharitis)
    Factitious ulceration of eyelids
    Necrosis of primary eyelid tumor
    Chalazion
    Metastatic eyelid tumor
    Brown recluse spider bite
    Pyoderma gangrenosum

Blastomycosis. The cutaneous form of North American blastomycosis involves the skin of the face and lids. This disease is especially common in Kentucky.[138] It tends to affect patients 50 years of age or older, who are farmers or who are involved in outdoor work. Primary infection usually involves the lung (see "Pseudoepitheliomatous Hyperplasia of the Lid") (Fig. 8-68).

Lid involvement is characterized by hyperkeratotic verrucous plaques and nodules that become confluent, ulcerated, and crust.

Histologically, the pseudoepitheliomatous hyperplasia may be mistaken for an SCC or for halogen toxicity.[16] Microabscesses in the epidermis that contain typical budding yeast forms as well as giant cells and epithelioid cells in the dermis confirm the diagnosis.

The disease may be self-limited or mildly progressive. Amphotericin B is recommended to eradicate both the visceral and cutaneous lesions. A low dose is started and increased daily to a level of 0.6–1.0 mg/kg until a total of 2 g has been given.

Coccidioidomycosis. Endemic in the southwestern United States, this infection probably is acquired by inhalation of the infectious arthrospores of *Coccidioides immitis.* Its hallmark is the granuloma. Clinically, the lesion appears indurated with areas of ulceration and crusting of the lids, periorbital region, and conjunctiva as a manifestation of disseminated disease.

Histologically, a mixed suppurative and granulomatous inflammation is present with multinucleated giant cells that contain the spherules of *Coccidioides immitis.*

Treatment requires infectious disease consultation.[139]

Cryptococcus. Cutaneous *Cryptococcus* may be part of a disseminated disease or a localized process.

Clinically, the lesions appear as papules, pustules, nodules, plaques, subcutaneous abscesses, or ulcerations. They may occasionally resemble keratoacanthomas.

Histologically, lesions may exhibit a gelatinous or granulomatous pattern. In the gelatinous type, minimal inflammatory infiltrate is present, but many budding

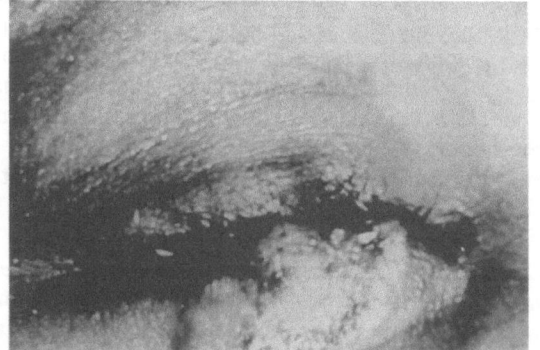

Fig. 8-68. North American blastomycosis causes destruction of all involved lid tissue.

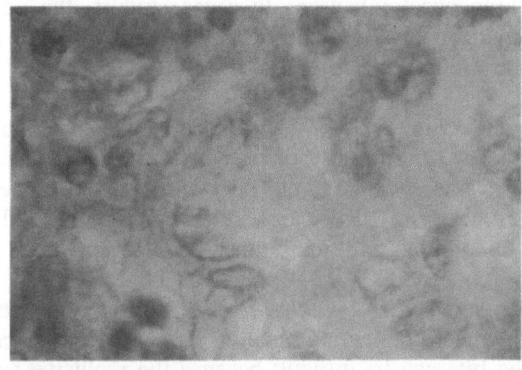

Fig. 8-69. Acute leishmaniasis is seen as an ulcerating papule or nodule. The organisms are found predominantly in macrophages but are also extracellular protozoa. (Courtesy AFIP, Washington, DC.)

forms separated by a clear halo that represents the mucopolysaccharide capsule are found. In the granulomatous type, significant chronic granulomatous inflammation is present, but fewer organisms are demonstrated.[45]

Leishmaniasis. Leishmaniasis often presents as a small, erythematous, reddish-purple plaque that is usually painless. The lesion forms a nodule 1–2 cm in diameter, and over weeks to months, central dry scaling ulceration develops. Satellite lesions may be present. The lesion heals gradually leaving a depressed scar.[45]

Biopsy shows subcutaneous nodules with lymphocytes and a preponderance of plasma cells (Fig. 8-69).

TREATMENT

Treatment of all the above involves infectious disease consultation and appropriate work-up for systemic disease.

Inflammations Causing Ulceration and Destruction of the Lid

Idiopathic Midline Destructive Disease. Idiopathic midline destructive disease (IMDD) often causes central facial necrosis. In addition, one patient with known IMDD had undergone 5000 rad of radiation treatment of the central face and developed subcutaneous nodules in the lids and brow.

Histology of the nodules showed sclerosis, loss of cellularity, and zones of fibrinoid necrosis adjacent to vessels. No organisms could be identified with special stains for bacteria and fungi or on electron microscopy.[140]

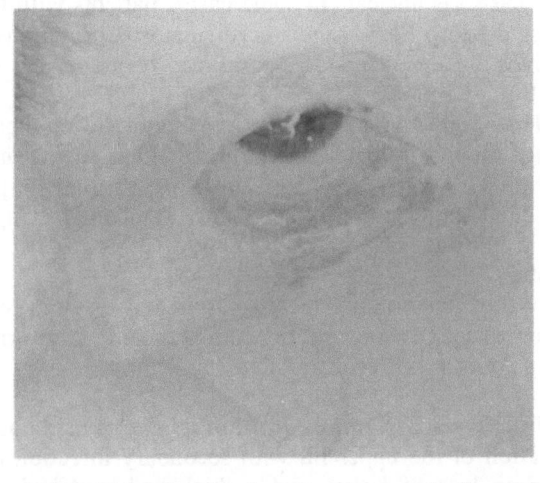

Fig. 8-70. 55-year-old female who had had radiation for a basal cell carcinoma of the right lower lid. Five years after radiation, patient has symblepharon and severe dry eye.

Radiation Necrosis. Radiation necrosis results in loss of cilia and atrophy of the lid structures. Telangiectasis is often present. Symblepharon and dry eye with corneal vascularization also occur (Fig. 8-70). Cicatricial ectropion and punctal and canalicular stenosis are often present.[45]

Discoid Lupus Erythematosus. Discoid lupus erythematosus (DLE) is a chronic disease of the skin that predominantly affects patients between the ages of 20 and 40 and has a definite predilection for women. The typical skin lesion is well-circumscribed, slightly raised, and erythematous. Minimal scaling may be present. Scarring with loss of lashes causes deformities of the lid margin and tear film irregularly (Fig. 8-71).

The relationship of DLE to systemic lupus erythemato-

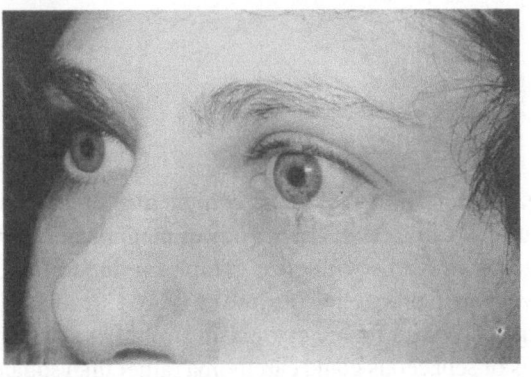

Fig. 8-71. 38-year-old female with discoid lupus involving left lower lid. Note loss of lashes with thickened inflamed mucosa. Patient was treated with excision and reconstruction without complication (Patient referred by James Fleishman, MD, Iselin, NJ).

sus (SLE) is unclear. In some cases, patients with DLE later develop SLE. Lupus erythematosus profundus involves the subcutaneous fat and may be associated with SLE.

Histologically, the mildly hyperkeratotic epithelium plugs the hair follicles. Focal intracellular edema of the basal cell layers is often present. A dense, patchy, perivascular and periappendageal, predominantly lymphocytic infiltrate may cause atrophy of the pilosebaceous units.

Marked distortion of the lid margin may result in symptoms related to exposure. In addition, cosmetic deformity may warrant lid reconstruction.[141]

Factitious Ulceration of the Eyelids.   Factitious ulceration of the upper lid with secondary infection may lead to loss of lashes and a thickened, notched, and ectropic lid despite treatment of the secondary bacterial

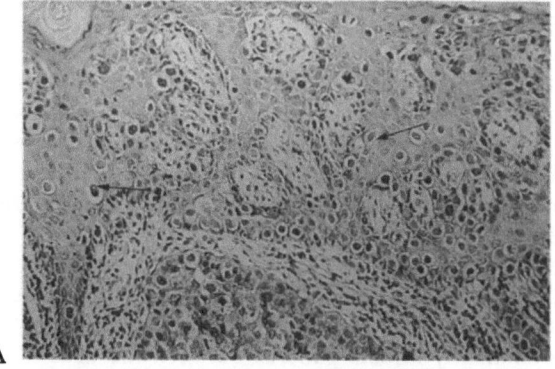

A

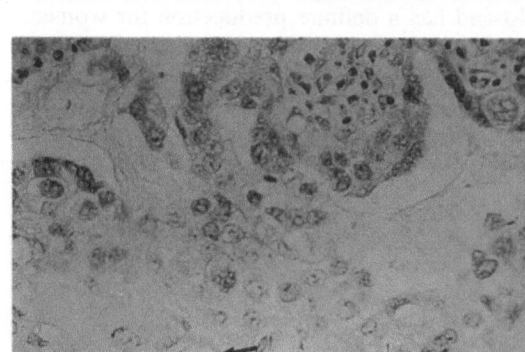

B

Fig. 8-72.   Biopsy of tarsal conjunctiva suggests squamous cell carcinoma. Higher power magnification shows large bizarre cells with clear cytoplasm due to lipid dissolved out in processing (arrow) (AIFP ACC #1274133). Large cells with foamy cytoplasm strongly suggest diagnosis of sebaceous gland carcinoma rather than squamous cell carcinoma. Because of the multifocal nature of sebaceous gland carcinoma, map biopsies help determine the areas of of involvement. Definitive wider excision of the involved areas than with squamous cell carcinoma is necessary.

staphylococcal infection. In a case report, the patient traumatized her lids with a handkerchief that she used to constantly wipe her lids.[142]

Lid Necrosis Due to Tumor.   Lid necrosis may occur secondary to a primary or metastatic tumor. Generally, there is an associated tumor thickening that accompanies such ulceration. Ulcerations are common with basal cell and uncommon with meibomian carcinoma (Fig. 8-72).

Brown Recluse Spider Bite.   This presents as an enlarging necrotizing inflammation of the lid. Confirmation of the bite can be difficult because the reclusive spider typically strikes when cornered in a darkened garage or abandoned building. Deaths may result rarely from systemic reactions that include red cell hemolysis and renal failure from the polymorphonuclear leukocyte infiltration and concomitant complement activation that causes tissue necrosis.[143]

Pathologically, there is a polymorphonuclear leukocyte infiltration with intravascular thrombosis and platelet aggression.

Treatment includes debridement, antihistamines, steroids, antibiotics, and heparin with little effect on the ultimate outcome of the lesion. Oral dapsone, a nonsteroidal antiinflammatory agent that is administered at a dose of 50 mg orally twice daily for 10 days, helps to inhibit the polymorphonuclear leukocyte infiltration and leads to resolution of process.

Pyoderma Gangrenosum.   There has been one report of pyoderma gangrenosum involving the lid. The lesions present as one of many pustules throughout the body that rapidly progress to an ulceration with elevated violaceous borders and excavated purulent bases. The lesions are associated in 50 percent of cases with ulcerative colitis, Crohn's disease, rheumatoid arthritis, myeloproliferative disease, chronic active hepatitis, and other diseases.

Pathologic findings are nonspecific and include abscess formation with later ulceration of the epidermis.

Treatments include intralesional and systemic steroids, azathioprine, chlorambucil, cyclophosphamide, dapsone, and clofazimine.[144]

MANAGEMENT OF EYELID TUMORS

After an eyelid tumor has been biopsied, the appropriate management in the case of primary malignant tumors consists of complete surgical excision under frozen section control with reconstruction. Other treatment modalities including radiation, cryotherapy, and CO_2 and contact YAG laser treatment will be discussed in this section.

Possible Pathologic Pitfalls

Before treatment, the physician must first ascertain whether the pathologic diagnosis conforms to the clinical differential diagnosis. Because ophthalmic pathology is somewhat specialized, the community hospital patholo gist may not encounter and, therefore, have difficulty making certain diagnoses.

The main problem has been in two areas: (1) the diagnosis of sebaceous gland carcinoma, (2) the misinterpretation of squamous lesions, and (3) failure to review prior biopsies from other hospitals.

Diagnosis of Sebaceous Gland Carcinoma

As discussed above, if there is strong clinical suspicion of a sebaceous gland carcinoma, a full-thickness lid biopsy should be performed. Permanent sections are necessary, frozen section analysis is not adequate from a diagnostic viewpoint but is relied on for surgical margins at the time of definitive excision. The intraepithelial pagetoid spread of tumor requires that a close scrutiny of the epithelium be performed in order to identify individual malignant sebaceous cells in the epithelium.

Ideally, the material should be formalin-fixed and followed by frozen sections with fat stains so that the solvent in the tissue processor does not dissolve the lipid. Intracytoplasmic lipid in malignant cells is diagnostic. However, this method is often impractical and diagnosis should be made on permanent, nonfrozen sections. The pathologist should be told in advance of the possibility of the diagnosis. The material can always be sent for pathologic consultation.

Epithelial Tumors

Many epithelial tumors may be misdiagnosed. For example, the pathologist may have difficulty in differentiating squamous cell carcinoma and keratoacanthoma. Because the latter benign tumor appears to infiltrate the underlying orbicularis muscle and also cutaneous nerves, it is sometimes misinterpreted as an invading squamous cell carcinoma by the pathologist.[35,36] The cup-shaped nodular-elevation, thickened epidermis with its central mass of keratin is helpful in making the diagnosis. Epithelial microabscesses are typically present.

Pseudoepitheliomatous (pseudocarcinomatous) hyperplasia may also be misdiagnosed as squamous cell carcinoma. Whenever acanthotic proliferating bands of epithelial cells are noted, the pathologist should examine the dermis and search for giant cells that along with microabscesses would point toward a fungal infection or halogen toxicity.[16]

Lymphoid Tumors

Lymphomas of the skin are rare. Whenever there is round-cell monotonous infiltrate of the dermis, the diagnosis of Merkel's cell (trabecular) carcinoma should be considered. The presence of neurosecretory granules on electron microscopic study is diagnostic. Immunohistochemical studies may be helpful in making the diagnosis.[128]

TREATMENT OF EYELID TUMORS

Frozen Section Control, Mohs Microsurgery

In removing a diagnosed basal cell carcinoma, we allow clinically free margins of 3–4 mm on all sides of the tumor. With sebaceous gland carcinoma or squamous cell carcinoma, we allow for margins of 5 mm and 4 mm, respectively.

In general, we excise the main tumor and place a 4–0 silk suture at the medial or lateral lid margin. We then obtain frozen section margins in a clockwise fashion and include 2 mm of full-thickness lid including skin, muscle, tarsus, and conjunctiva on the medial and lateral border of the tumors assuming the tumor involves the lid border. Inferiorly, a thin 2-mm segment of skin is sent and a corresponding "deep" section of orbicularis muscle, orbital septum, and lower lid retractors is sent. If the tumor extends beyond the tarsus to the medial or lateral canthus, both superficial skin and deep muscle sections are sent from the respective canthus. In some hospitals, the frozen sections are taken by the pathologist from the main specimen. We prefer to take our own frozen sections because in this way, we have satisfied ourselves that the appropriate margins have been studied. Furthermore, we are assured that not only are the margins free on the main tumor but the frozen sections are free as well.

Many studies have shown that (1) without frozen section control, about 50 percent of lesions are incompletely excised,[55,145] (2) relative to the number of incomplete excisions, the rate of recurrence is relatively low,[146] (3) frozen section control offers an extremely low rate of recurrence,[147,148] and (4) Mohs microsurgery offers the lowest rate of recurrence of any modality.[149] Unfortunately, Mohs chemosurgery may require 50 or more histologic sections. For this reason, we favor Mohs microsurgery for patients 40 years or younger with medial canthal tumors and for recurrent tumors in any age group. The technique is of limited usefulness in orbital fat and cannot be utilized if the tumor extends into bone.

Role of Radiation Therapy

In general, we reserve radiation treatment for patients who are not candidates for surgical excision of basal cell carcinoma or squamous cell carcinoma because of medical reasons. In addition, it should be kept in mind that young patients who will be exposed to further actinic damage have a greater risk of later radiation changes.

The most common complication of radiation is a dry eye that may progress to corneal vascularization. In addition, telangiectasia, atrophy, and ulceration of the skin with punctal stenosis may occur with cicatricial ectropion. We advocate insertion of a lacrimal stent such as a Johnson wire or silicone tube when the medial canthal area is radiated. The wire may be inserted just after radiation to avoid any interference from the metal stent in administering radiation. Alternatively, a silicone tube can be passed into the sac without a probe. In the latter cases, only the canaliculi and not the nasolacrimal duct are protected from stenosis. This office technique avoids the outpatient hospitalization necessary to insert silicone tubes.

Other complications include cataract, retinal neovascularization, and optic neuropathy. Shielding of the lens is imperative, and avoidance of the treatment of central lid lesions will minimize complications. Radiation causes atrophy of the meibomian glands, lacrimal gland, and keratinization of the canaliculi as observed in radiated exenterated specimens.[51]

Radiation is ineffective in eradicating tumors that have invaded bone. Because of the recurrence of sebaceous gland carcinoma of the lid after radiation as the primary treatment modality, we reserve radiation for recurrent sebaceous gland carcinoma in patients who refuse surgery or who are at medical risk to undergo a surgical procedure.[150] One study reports good results in three patients. However, one of the patients died of an unrelated disease 10 months after radiation treatment, and the second patient had recurrence 10 years later with a parotid metastasis that required exenteration and radical neck dissection. The third patient was free of tumor 25 months after radiation.[151] The usual doses of radiation for treatment of basal cell carcinoma and squamous cell carcinoma of the lids is 5000 rad in 5 weeks given five times a week in 200-rad fractions. The convenience of surgical excision versus multiple sessions required for radiation are a practical consideration in determining the modality of treatment for any given patient. The lack of ability to ensure that the lesion is excised is another drawback to radiation, as is the treatment of recurrences. Recurrences often occur deep and become clinically apparent at a late stage. In addition, radiation-induced atrophy of the surrounding tissues makes reconstruction and reexcision more difficult. Grafts do notoriously poorly on an irradiated bed, while tissue flaps are not always available.[152]

Cryotherapy

We have little practical experience with cryotherapy. This modality has achieved wider acceptance among dermatologists. The main disadvantage of the technique is that there is no assurance that the tumor is completely excised. Patients with tumors of thicknesses greater than 5 mm, tumors invading the fornices, medial canthal tumors, and morpheaform lesions are not candidates for cryosurgery. Patients with modular BCC involving the lid margin and close to the punctae may be candidates since cryotherapy does not damage the canaliculus.[148] Good results have been reported in the treatment of eyelid BCCs.[153,154]

Technique. The clinical extent of the tumor is outlined with a marking pen. A second outline is made 4 mm beyond the first. In diffuse lesions, the second mark is made 6 mm beyond the tumor. Local anesthetic with epinephrine is infiltrated with a corneal protector in place. Thermocouple needles are placed in the peripheral mark. The ice ball forms in all directions until the temperature at the peripherial mark reaches -30° C. The area is allowed to thaw slowly until the temperature register is at least −25° C. The tumor is then refrozen. The eye is pressure-patched for 1 day and cool compresses are begun in 24 hours. There is marked postoperative edema that subsides in 1 week. Blisters form and break, and an eschar develops and heals slowly over a 4–10-week period depending on the size of the lesion treated. Persistent redness may occur for several months. Elevated areas that correspond to pseudoepitheliomatous hyperplasia may appear 3–6 months after treatment. Suspected recurrence requires biopsy before further cryotherapy.

In general, treatment involves two freeze-thaw cycles with a nitrous oxide cryo unit to -30°C. Premalignant conditions that cover large areas of the periorbital skin such as actinic comedonal plaques may be treated with cryosurgery.[155] Overtreatment may lead to distortion and scarring of the lid with entropion. Animal studies show that minimal clinical or histologic evidence of canalicular obstruction occurs after cryotherapy.[156] Clinical reports show that occlusion of the superior or inferior punctum or canaliculi may occur. Permanent loss of lashes and dipigmentation are common sequellae of treatment, and therefore we do not recommend cryotherapy in darkly pigmented tumors or in any darkly pigmented patient with a lid tumor.[157]

CO$_2$ Laser

At the present time, the CO$_2$ has its greatest application in the treatment of eyelid and orbital tumors in patients with blood dyscrasias of vascular tumors or in patients with diffuse neurofibromas where loss of blood may be a problem.

The CO_2 laser produces energy with a wavelength in the infrared region of the electromagnetic spectrum. The energy is invisible to the eye; therefore, a low-energy helium-neon laser is used as a visible aiming beam. The energy from the laser is absorbed by cellular water and is converted to heat at 100°C with vaporization known as the laser plume. The effectiveness of the laser in destroying any tissue is directly related to its water content. However, with the appropriate power adjustment, the laser cuts through all tissues including bone. The laser causes a necrosis limited to 0.1 mm at the wound edge and seals blood vessels and lymphatics up to 0.5 mm in diameter as a "hemostatic scalpel." Large vessels need to be clamped. Postoperative pain is reduced because the laser also damages the nerves. Because of the heat induced, the laser theoretically creates a sterile wound.

In general, a 1-mm spot size is practical since the smaller the spot size, the more focal the tissue damage induced by the laser. Small 200-micron spots are more difficult to focus. Most CO_2 lasers operate in a continuous wave mode that produces a zone of tissue damage surrounding the incision. A pulsed or gated laser delivers bursts of energy over short periods of time and decreases thermal damage by allowing cooling of the tissue. Rapid superpulsed lasers produce higher energy outputs for more brief periods of time than the pulsed or gated lasers.

The power density is a measure of laser energy and is determined by the spot size and the energy output. The rate at which the laser is moved across the tissue will affect tissue damage. Slow movement will result in greater tissue contact time. Tension on the edges of the wound speeds the incision by separating the tissue that has already been lased. Power may vary from 5–15 watts. Protective goggles are worn. An opaque contact lens is used to protect the cornea. Moistened surgical drapes are used and all flammable articles are removed from the operative field. Cottonoids are helpful. The patient's eye is protected by a plastic eye shield.

A large eschar is produced when debulking large, diffuse orbital tumors, and the operative time is long. By debulking the tumor with a scissor and lasering the bleeding vessels, surgical and anesthesis time may be reduced.

Argon Laser

The argon laser emits energy in the visible spectrum that is readily absorbed by hemoglobin and melanin. A handpiece with a fiberoptic cable from a standard ophthalmic laser is preferable to a slit-lamp delivery system. A spot size of 1 mm is usually adequate. The instrument is held perpendicular to the skin source 2–4 inches from the skin. Power settings are adjusted from 1–3 watts. The pulsed duration may be set from 0.2–0.4 seconds. The surgeon wears protective goggles. The endpoint of treatment is blanching of the treated tissue. The technique cannot be used in black patients. The argon laser penetrates only a few millimeters into a vascular tumor before it is absorbed. In such tumors a CO_2 laser may be indicated. The contact neodymium: YAG laser may be of value as well. The laser energy is absorbed by hemoglobin and paravascular tissue leading to vessel wall damage and tumor obliteration.

Hematoporphyrin-Derivative Photoradiation Therapy in Managing Basal Cell Nevus Syndrome

Hematoporphyrin derivative is a photodynamically active dye that is preferentially retained by malignant tissue. The dye initiates a cytotoxic reaction when exposed to red light. Normal tissue retains the dye to a lesser degree and is thus spared damage from the light-induced reaction. The tumors become inapparent within 4–6 weeks without clinical damage to the surrounding skin. This experimental treatment may be helpful in the management of difficult patients.[158]

Intralesional Steroids

Triamcinolone, 10 mg/ml, has been utilized to treat chalazion and sarcoid granuloma of the lid. In the treatment of chalazion, 0.2–1 ml is injected into the lesion. In treating sarcoid, a 1-ml test dose is used in order to check for hypopigmentation.[159,160] Caution must be utilized in the intralesional injection of steroids in the face and periocular region. Occlusion of the retinal and choroidal vasculature has rarely been reported after injections of the nasal turbinates, tonsillar pillars, scalp, lids, and retrobulbar space.[161] This occurrence is probably due to anastamoses between the ophthalmic artery and facial arteries. Insoluble, crystalline "depot forms" appear to be more likely to cause microembolization. Preinjection aspiration should always be performed, and the lesion itself should be injected rather than the surrounding tissue.

Reconstruction of Eyelids

In the operating room, after the surgeon has removed the tumor under frozen section control, his or her next goal is to reconstruct the defect. The reconstructions can be divided into those that spare the lid margin and those that involve the lid margin. This section will be

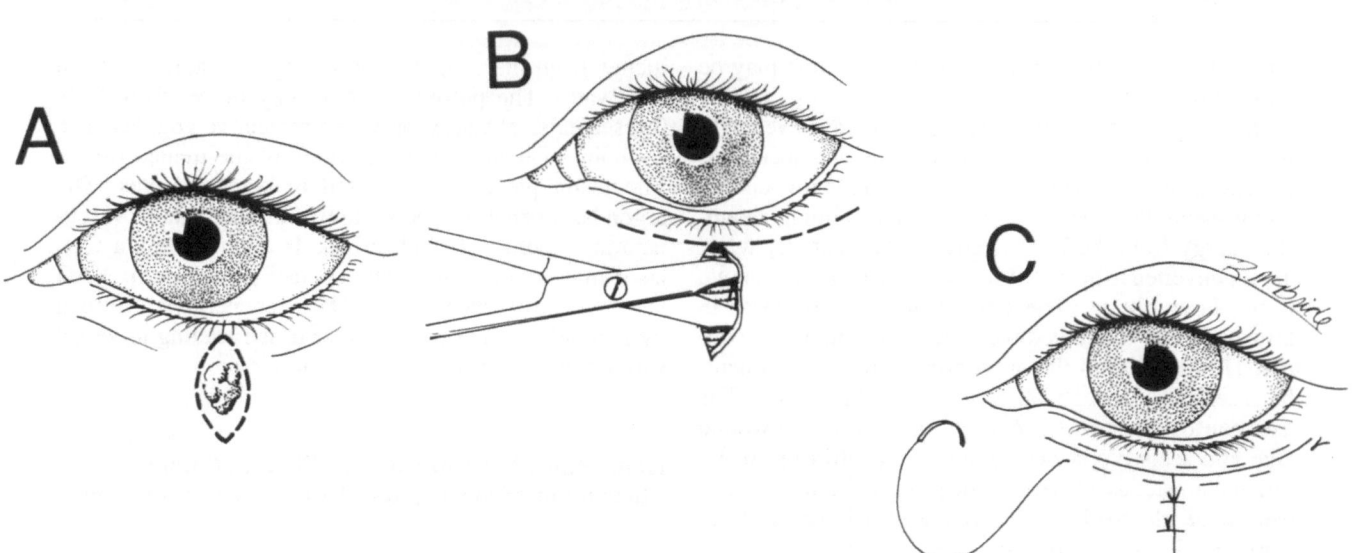

Plate 8-2. (*A–C*) Tumors sparing the lid margin may be excised using a vertical ellipse and are reconstructed with skin muscle advancement flaps.

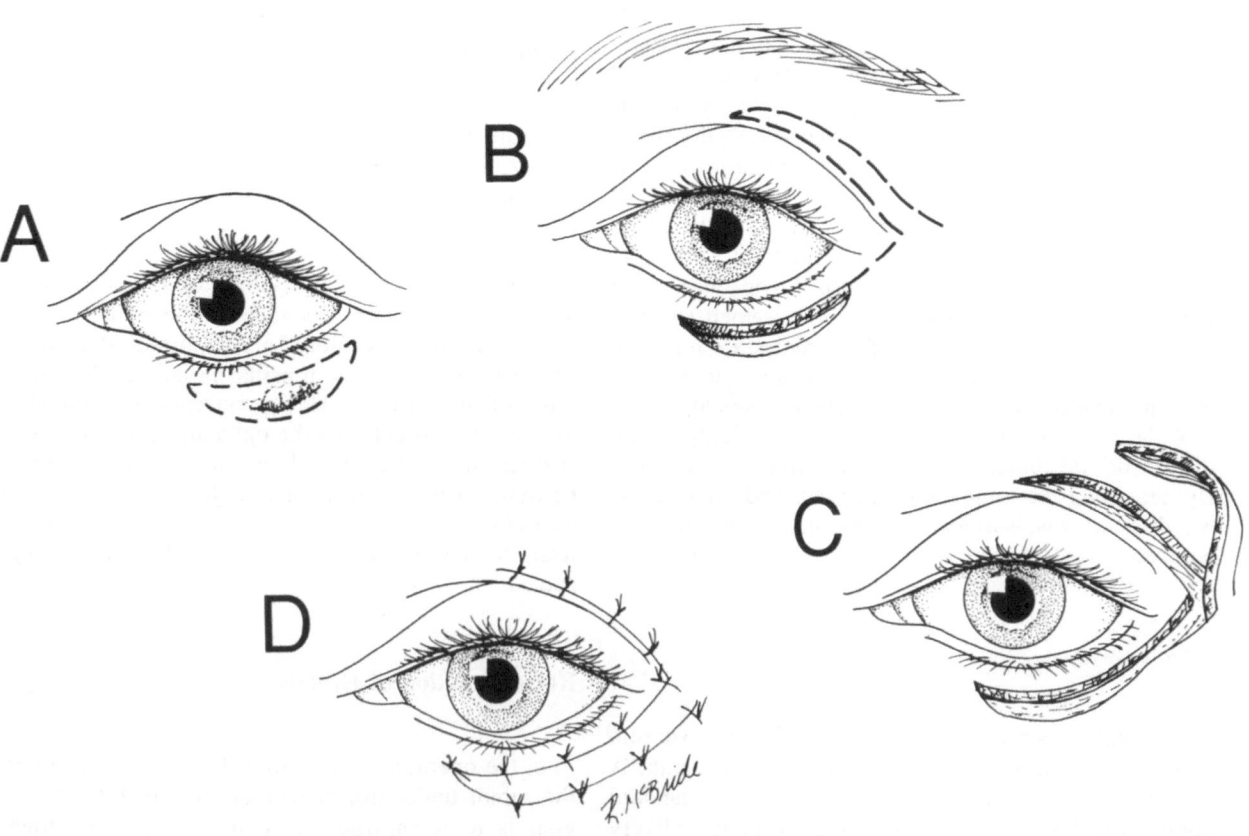

Plate 8-3. (*A–D*) Use of skin graft may be avoided by transposition of upper lid skin muscle flap for lateral lower lid defect.

divided into reconstructions that are based on the size of the defect of upper lid, lower lid, and canthal areas. While this chapter describes our favorite techniques of reconstruction, we hope to provide surgeons with techniques they can apply to their patients. Other texts and publications should be consulted for a complete summary of eyelid reconstruction.

Tumors Sparing the Lid Margin. Because of the laxity of the lid skin, especially in elderly patients, many small defects can be repaired with simple undermining. In some cases, a subciliary incision is used after a vertical elliptical excision of a benign tumor when horizontal closure would result in ectropion (Plate 8-2). The lesions should be excised parallel to the relaxed skin lines of the lids and face. In all cases, vertical excision of the anterior lamella will prevent the complications of cicatricial ectropion of the upper or lower lid and legophthalmos. A winged V-plasty is helpful in reconstructing the lid defect without resorting to a full-thickness skin graft.

For lower lid, a lateral canthal defect, a skin muscle rotation flap from the upper lid may be hinged at the lateral canthal area and place into the lower lid defect (Plate 8-3). A sliding advancement flap from the redundant lateral canthal tissues may also be used. This flap can be thought of as a modified semicircular flap that does not involve the lid border (Plate 8-3).[162–165] If a skin graft is necessary, the retroauricular skin is best for the lower lid. The underside of the upper arm and supraclavicular areas may also be used. For upper lid reconstruction, upper lid skin is optimal. Retroauricular skin that is thinned out also works well. We prefer upper lid skin to reconstruct the medial canthus.

The graft of appropriate size is outlined with a marking pen (Plate 8-4). The graft is obtained by infiltrating the donor site with lidocaine and epinephrine, then is outlined with a No. 15 blade, and is harvested using the blade. Upper lid grafts are harvested with a Westcott scissor after outlining the graft with the No. 15 blade. Next, the graft is thinned with a Westcott scissor. The graft is sutured into the donor site, taking bites from the graft to the recipient site. The graft should be slightly larger in a vertical dimension than the defect since all grafts shrink. The donor site is closed with a running horizontal mattress 3–0 or 4–0 nylon suture.

Transmarginal traction sutures of 4–0 silk help to keep the lid on stretch, so that a vertically undersized graft is not used. The sutures apply traction while the graft heals under a moderately tight pressure-patch for 5 days. 6–0 and 5–0 silk sutures are used to suture the graft in place. Multiple arms of the 5–0 silk sutures are left long on the upper and lower aspects of the graft. Cuts

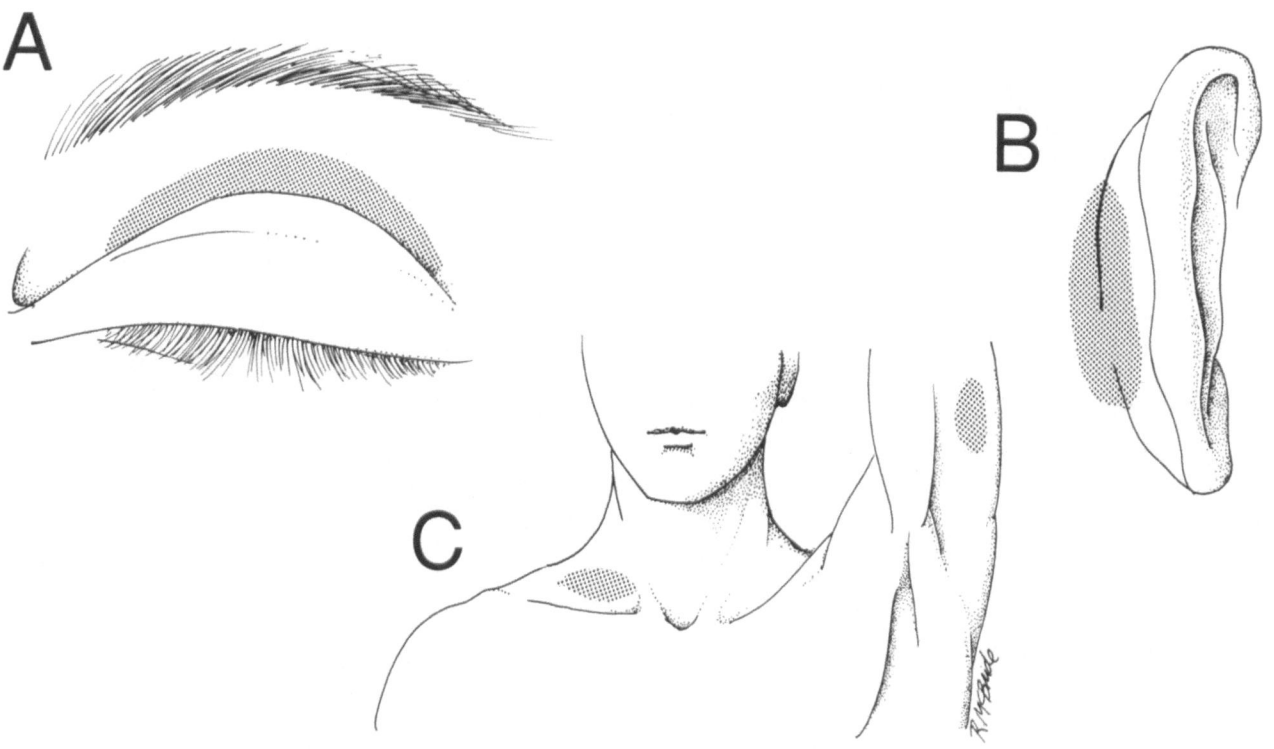

Plate 8-4. (*A*) Upper lid donor skin is optimal for upper lid defects but (*B*) retroauricular skin may be used. Lower lid defects are best repaired with retroauricular skin. (*C*) Skin from arm or supraclavicular area may be used in the upper or lower lid. Medial canthal tissue is best replaced with thin upper lid skin rather than relatively thick retroauricular skin.

are made into the graft to allow egress of fluid. A telfa dressing that fits inside the sutures is placed, and 5–0 silk sutures are tied to themselves over a wet cotton bolster that is molded to conform to the configuration of the lid (Plate 8-5). Telfa is applied over the cotton bolster so that the dressing consisting of two patches and fluff does not stick to the cotton when the dressing is removed. Alternatively, the graft may be supported by bites of 4–0 nylon through skin on either side of the graft; the 4–0 nylon is tied over a bolster. In this way, the edges of the graft remain flat.

Medial Canthal Reconstruction

As stated above, the medial canthal area when grafted is best reconstructed with thin upper lid skin and a flap from the upper lid. Median forehead flaps are good for reconstructions for tumors involving the side of the nose and the thick skin of the brow, and rarely when no other technique is possible for upper lid reconstruction. In the latter instance, a mucous membrane lining is needed for the undersurface of the flap.

The median forehead flap is hinged in the glabellar area and sutured with deep 3–0 and 4–0 chromic sutures and 4–0 and 5–0 nylon skin sutures (Plate 8-6). In general, any flap's length should be no more than 5 times more than its width in order to ensure vascularity of the flap. The flap should be gently handled with skin hooks, and cautery should be avoided. Median forehead flaps occasionally will need secondary revision 8 weeks later. The flap may be bilobed for large defects. The base of the flap is separated and replaced into the donor glabellar area to prevent narrowing of the eyebrows and improve cosmesis. Where recurrence of tumor is a strong clinical

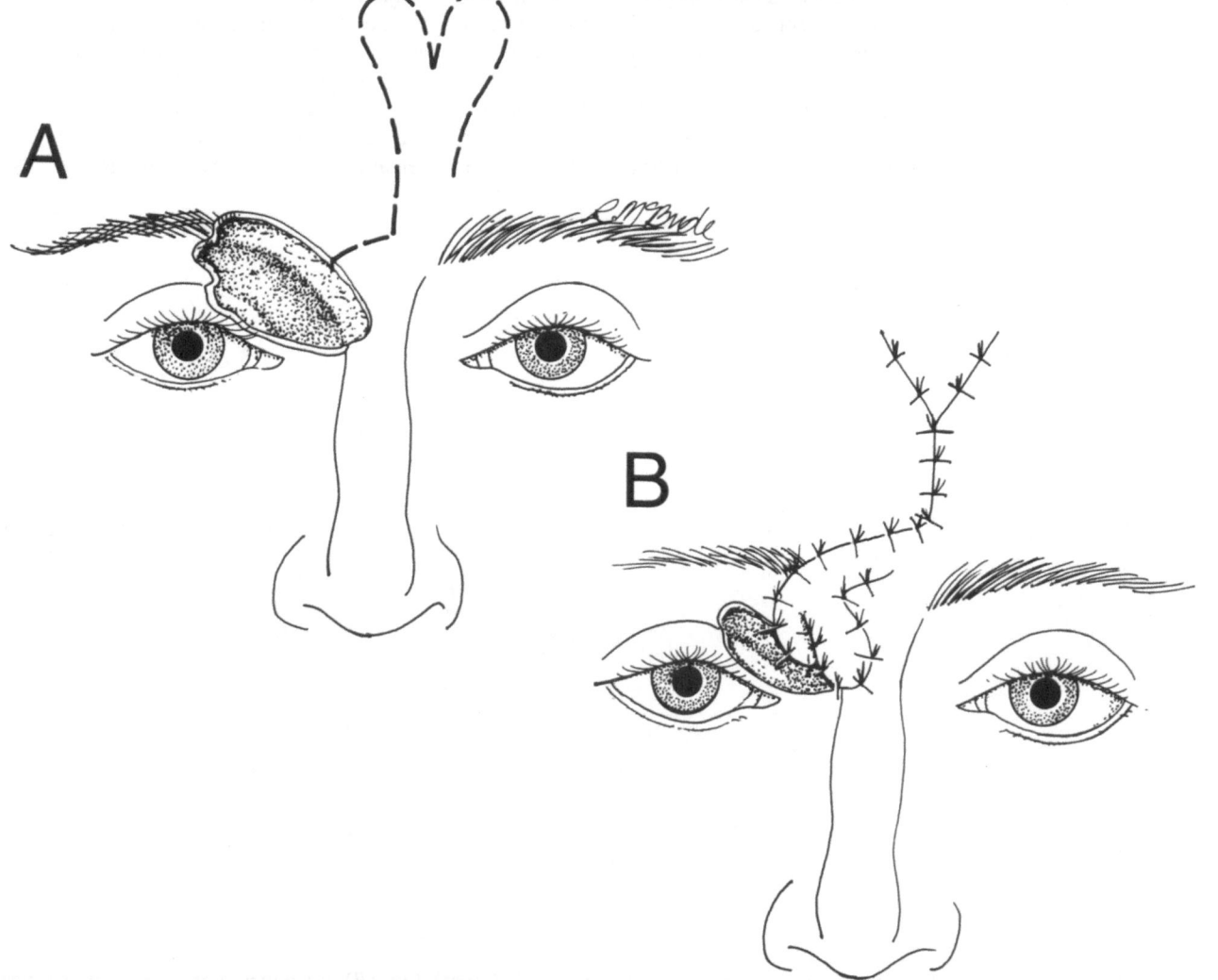

Plate 8-5. Forehead pedicle advancement flaps may be single (not shown) or bilobed (A) in order to fill defect of (B) nose, brow, and upper lid. Remainder of upper lid may be repaired with skin graft.

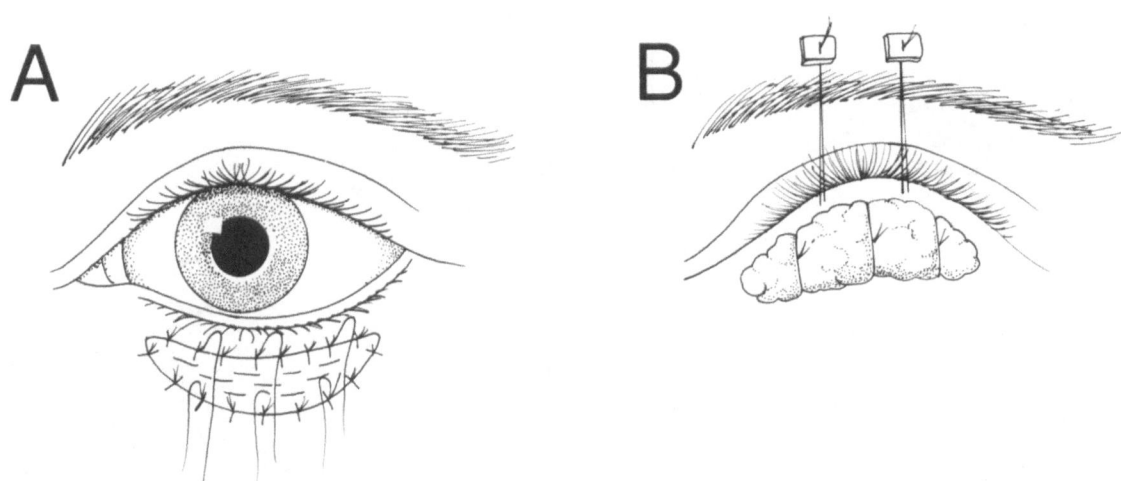

Plate 8-6. (*A*) Skin graft has been sutured into lower lid defect. Lower lid traction sutured is used to close eye. (*B*) Cotton pledget ensures adequate contact between graft and host.

possibility, immediate reconstruction with a median forehead flap is not advised because the thick flap may mask recurrent tumors.

Alternatively, a laissez-faire technique can be utilized. The medial edge of the upper and lower lids are sutured together. The lids are then sutured to the posterior aspect of the medial canthal tendon at the level of the posterior lacrimal crest. Granulation occurs over a period of weeks. Ophthalmic ointment and telfa dressings are applied. The area is observed for recurrence.[163] Secondary surgery may be required depending on the scarring and distortion that takes place.

Where there is sufficient lid laxity, the remnant of medial lid, whether of the upper or lower lid, should be sutured deep to the medial canthal tendon so that (1) the upper and lower lids hug the globe and (2) the upper and lower lids touch one another medially.

A 4–0 PDS (polydioxanone) suture works well in this situation and in lateral canthal reconstructions as well (Plate 8-7). For upper lid medial canthal reconstruction, a bite is taken through the upper aspect of the tarsus parallel to the lid border, from medial to lateral, and from anterior tarsus to conjunctival edge, and is brought out. The same needle is then brought through the edge of tarsus at its upper aspect and out through the edge of lower tarsus near the lid margin. The same arm is then brought from lateral to medial through the conjunctival edge of tarsus and out on its anterior surface. In this manner, there is an intarsal bite with the two arms of the suture on the anterior aspect of the tarsus. The latter allows for deep placement of the tarsus and lid. The arms are brought deep into the medial canthal tissues and tied to themselves or may be brought through the skin and tied over cotton pledgets. A lacrimal stent such as a Johnson wire may be placed in the canalicular system (Plate 8-7). In the case of lateral canthal reconstructions, the needles must take a bite of the lateral orbital tubercle

area on the inside of the lateral orbital rim. The surgeon must remember that the lateral canthus is approximately 2 mm higher than the medial canthus (Plate 8-8).

Z-plasties of the entire medial and lateral canthi may be utilized to elevate or lower the canthus. In the case of medial canthoplasties, transnasal wiring is helpful, and in lateral canthoplasties 30-gauge wire is brought through osteotomies. An 18-gauge needle may be passed transnasally as a conduit for 28-gauge transnasal wires (Plate 8-9). An awl may also be used. An incision is made in the other medial canthal area. The periosteum is lifted from the underlying bone and the lacrimal gland is reflected. The optimum site is in the superior aspect of the posterior lacrimal crest. The 28-gauge wire is doubled over and passed singly or in two steps. A 4–0 PDS suture is used to secure the deep medial canthal tissues. A hemostat placed in the medial canthus helps to define the tissue that is best secured with the suture. Bites of the upper and lower aspect of the deep medial canthal tissues provide good support. The 4–0 PDS suture is then looped around and tied securely to the loop of wire that has been passed transnasally. Two additional 28- or 30-gauge wires are passed through the same or another transnasal osteotomy site. The 28-gauge wire attached to the medial canthus is then tightened as the assistant uses an Adson forceps to push the medial canthus medially. Additional deep sutures of 4–0 PDS may be used to further secure and align the medial canthus. The skin is closed with interrupted 5–0 nylon sutures. The other two wires are brought through the wound and through silicone orbital floor implants and tied to themselves to prevent webbing of the medial canthal tissues. These wires are removed in the office 10–14 days after surgery.

Repair of Defects Involving Lid Margin. Defects of less than 25 percent of the lid are closed primarily.

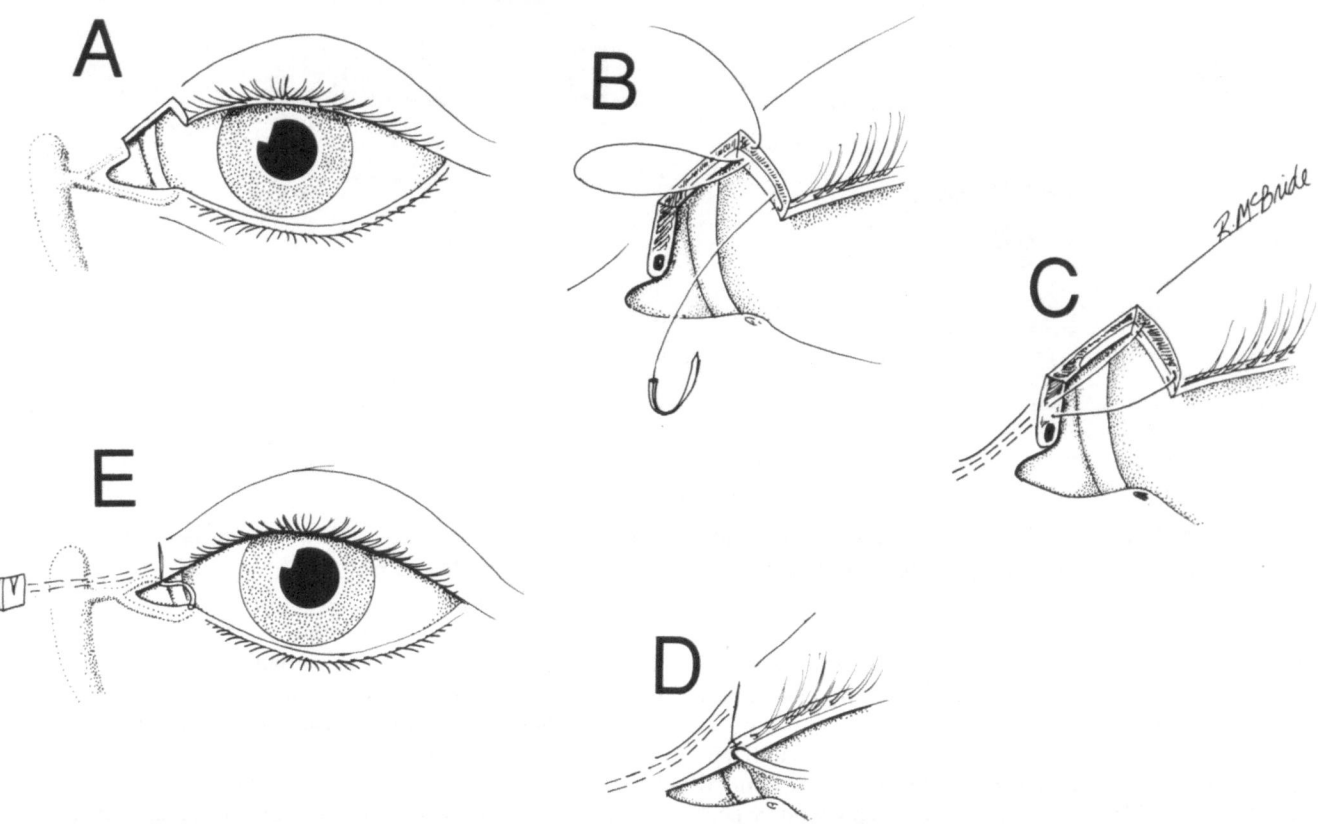

Plate 8-7. Repair of medial canthal defect (*A*) requires fixation of tarsal plate of lower lid to medial canthal tendon area with a buried 4–0 PDS suture (*B, C*). Each arm of the suture is brought through the deep medial canthal tissues just inferior to the canaliculi and tied to itself over a cotton pledget that is removed in 14 days. Alternatively, the suture may be buried under a skin muscle flap (not shown). We prefer the former method. A lacrimal stent may be inserted to insure integrity of the canalicular system (*D, E*).

The degree of laxity of the lid increases with age. The tumor should always be excised perpendicular to the lid margin to create a pentagonal resection rather than a v-shaped resection. In this way, the tension across the wound is equal and not exaggerated at the lid margin. Tension on wounds creates thick scars, dehiscences, and possibly notching. It is also imperative that the surgeon complete the incision through the entire vertical height of tarsus, especially in the upper lid, to prevent unequal tension across the wound. The lid margin is reapposed with a preplaced 5–0 vicryl or silk suture at the gray line at a distance and depth of 2 meibomian orifices from the edge of the wound. Two 6–0 silk sutures are placed within a millimeter of the central 5–0 vicryl suture with a slightly shorter bite (1½ meibomian orifices). The 5–0 vicryl suture is useful because its purple color helps to identify the suture.

Two 5–0 chromic or vicryl sutures are passed parallel to the lid margin through the anterior surface of the tarsus and out at the midtarsal thickness to avoid corneal irritation, especially in upper lid reconstructions (Plate 8-10). The bites are relatively longer than the lid margin bites to prevent cheese-wiring of the suture through the

tarsus. The lid tissues are delicate and the surgeon is allowed two, possibly three, passes before the tissues start to become disrupted. The tarsal bites are taken at the base of the tarsus and 2–3 mm above the lower tarsal bite. In the upper lid, the tarsus measures 10 mm in vertical height as compared with 5 mm or less in the lower lid. Three tarsal bites are needed in the upper tarsus compared to two sutures in the lower tarsus. The lid border is then tied first to align the lid border; the tarsal sutures are then tied. Additional sutures are then placed inferior to the tarsus through lower lid retractors and orbital septum. These bites are again parallel to the lid border. Next, the skin muscle layers are undermined laterally, medially, and inferiorly. Burrow's triangles are excised to create an inverted "T." The skin muscle layer is closed with 5–0 and mostly 6–0 silk sutures. The disadvantage of nylon is that it cheese-wires through tissue and it may abrade the cornea.

The marginal sutures are incorporated into one of the silk sutures on the skin. There should be no tension on the lid margin sutures to prevent eversion of the lid margin. In order to prevent skin necrosis, two throws are taken before the six ends from the lid margin sutures

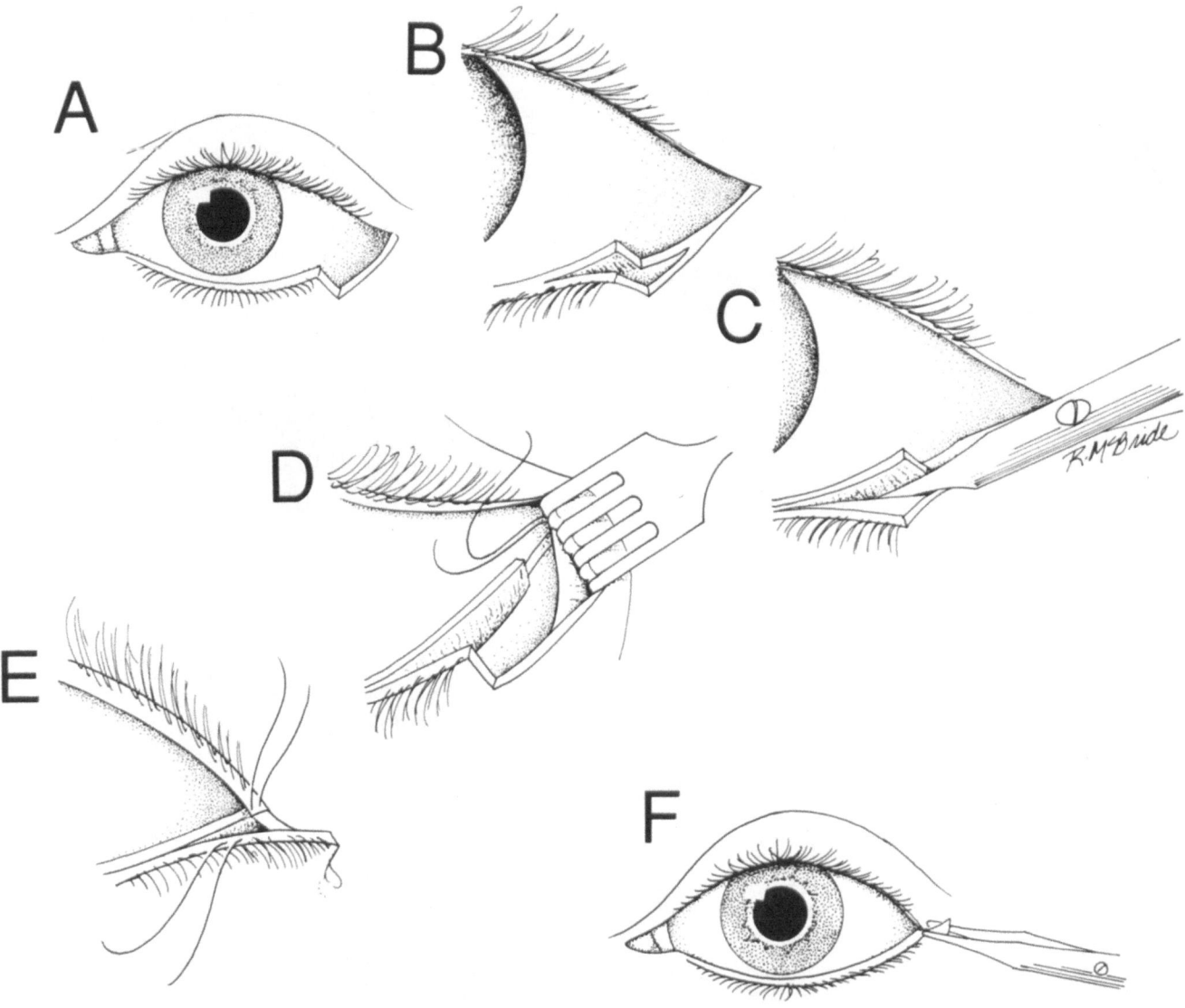

Plate 8-8. Lateral canthal reconstruction (A) consists of a lid-splitting procedure into a skin muscle flap anteriorly and a tarsal conjunctival strip posteriorly (B). The lower lid retractors may be severed from their attachment to the inferior tarsal border laterally (C). A 4–0 PDS suture fixates the tarsal strip to the lateral canthal tendon (D, E). Excess skin is excised laterally (F).

are incorporated. The patient should be instructed not to rub his or her eye to avoid a corneal abrasion from the posterior lid margin suture. Light dressings are used. The skin sutures are removed in 5–7 days and the lid margin sutures in 10–14 days. Ice packs are continuously applied in all lid and orbital surgery for 3–4 days, almost continuously for the first 48 hours, and 4 times a day for 10–15 minutes thereafter. Prolonged use of ice decreases the risk of postoperative hemorrhage and avoids a lot of calls from panicked patients. Patients are instructed not to take any aspirin products or antiinflammatory drugs for arthritis for 2 weeks before or after surgery.

Heparin, coumadin, and persantine are discontinued in conjunction with the internist.

Hot compresses from the tap, rewarmed every 1–2 minutes, for 10–15 minutes are utilized on the fifth day and continued indefinitely until all edema resolves. The hot packs serve to cleanse the wound, promote healing, and lessen the itching that occurs with healing.

Defects of 50 Percent of the Lid. The size of the defect is assessed intraoperatively by the degree of tension on the wound as the wound is gently pulled together with two forceps. A lateral canthotomy with cantholysis

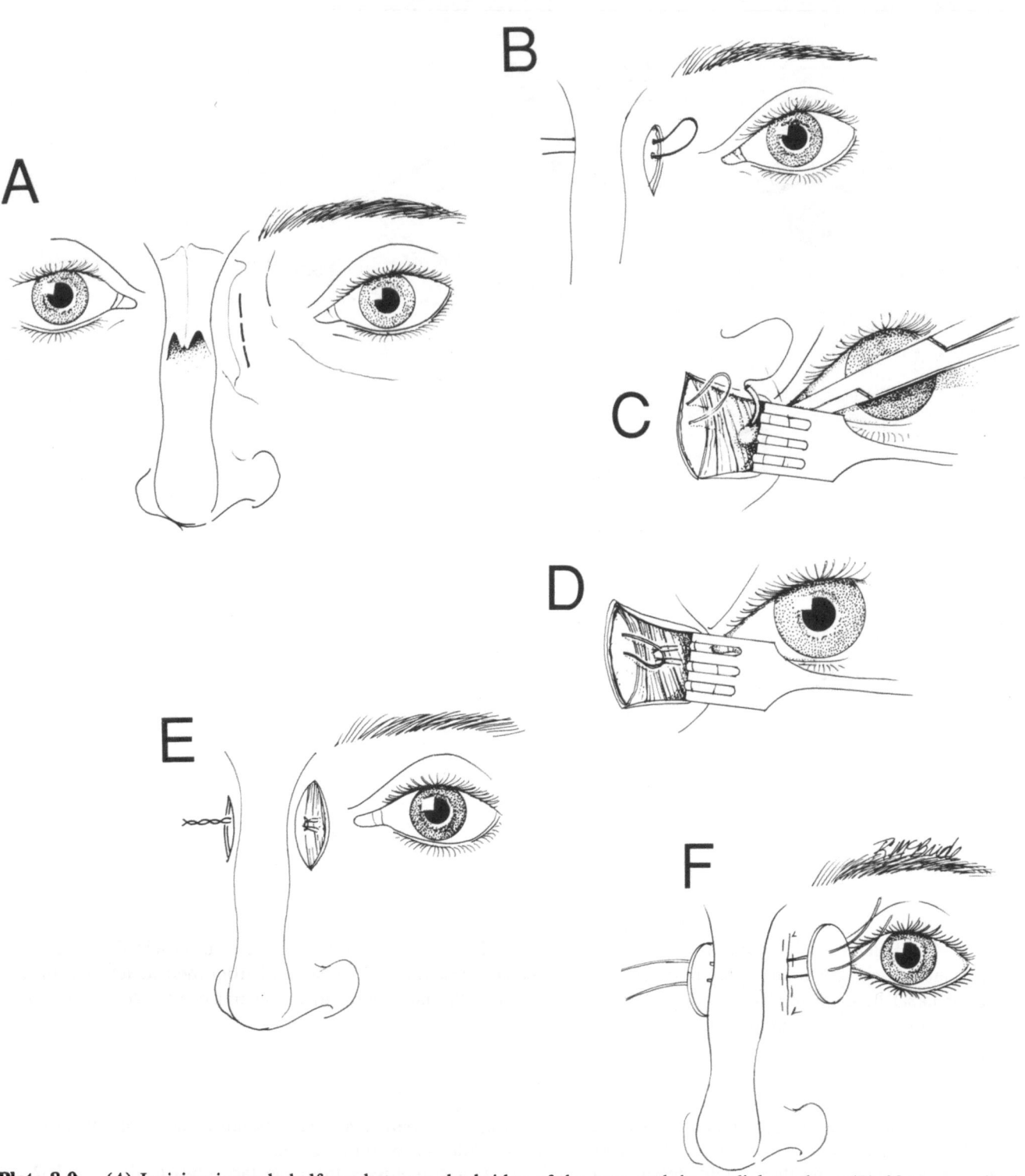

Plate 8-9. (*A*) Incision is made halfway between the bridge of the nose and the medial canthus. (*B*) 28-gauge wire is passed through a 16- or 18-gauge needle through two separate holes. A dental drill, awl, or large-bore needle, 16- or 18-gauge needle that is "tapped" across the nose with a mallet may be used to make the initial opening (not shown). (*C, D*) The tissues of the medial canthus are sutured to the wire loop that has been passed transnasally. A 4–0 PDS suture is suitable. A hemostat placed beneath the caruncle and plica is helpful in exposing the tissues for the medial canthal bite. (*E*) The two 28-gauge wires are twisted to themselves. (*F*) Two other 28-gauge wires are brought through the wound and tied to themselves over silicone implants after the skin edges are apposed with vertical mattress sutures. The purpose of the latter two wires is to keep firm apposition of the medial canthal tissues to the underlying bone and prevent webbing of the soft tissues and skin.

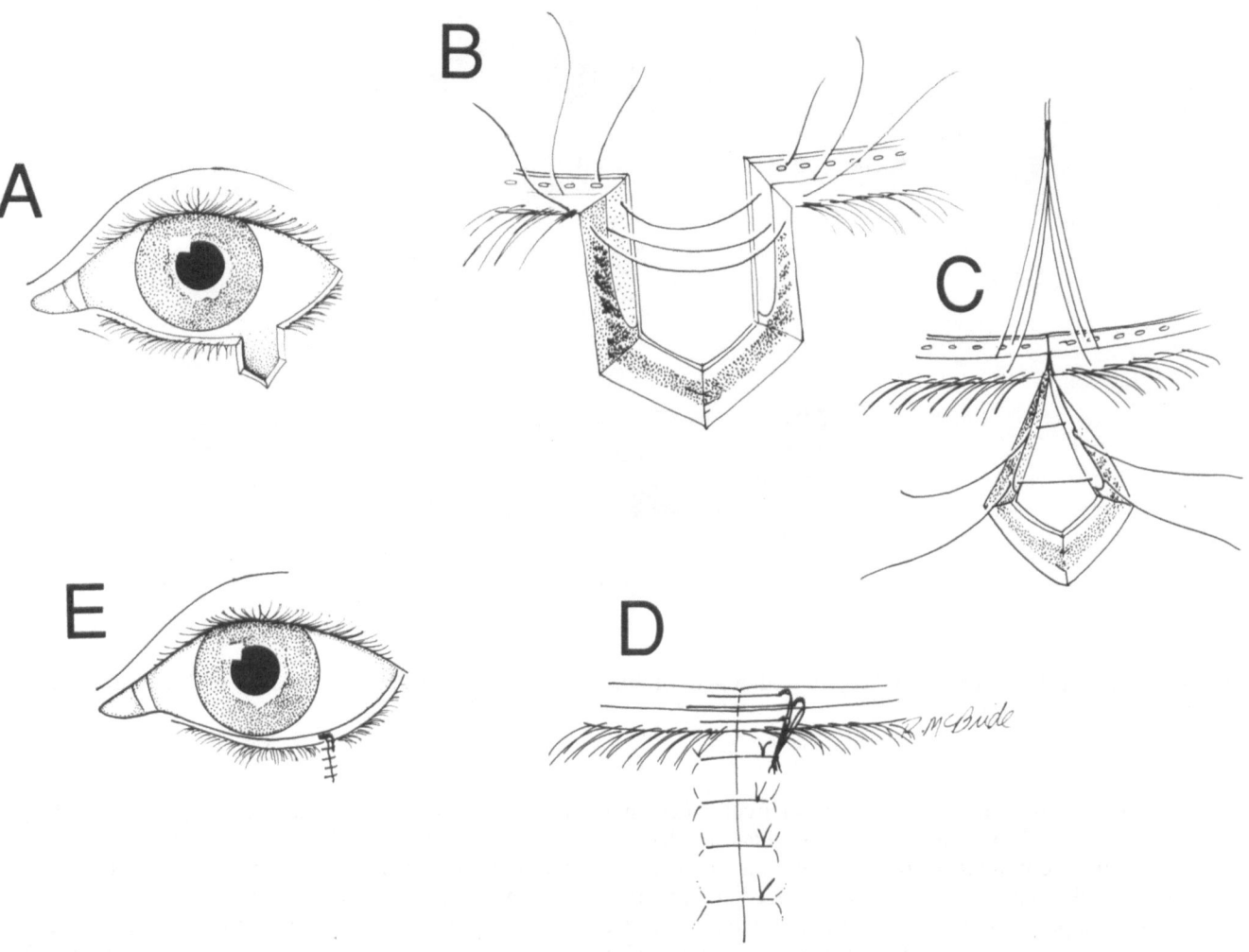

Plate 8-10. *(A–E)* Repair of full-thickness defect lower lid (or upper lid) involves separate closure of the tarsus and lower lid retractors and skin.

of the inferior crus (lower lid reconstruction) and superior crus (upper lid reconstruction) is utilized to obtain additional tissue. The canthotomy is performed slightly above the midline at the lateral canthus for lower lid reconstruction and slightly above the midline for upper lid reconstruction (Plate 8-11). In either case, the canthotomy is started where the upper and lower lids meet. The cantholysis is performed by inserting the Westcott or Stevens scissors with one blade under the conjunctiva and one blade inside the wound and outside the orbicular muscle. A small lateral canthotomy incision need not be closed.

Isolated medial or lateral defects of the upper lid may be closed by horizontally sliding a section of tarsus from the remaining lid segment into the defect and covering the anterior lamella with a skin graft. The lid is everted over a Desmarres retractor. A horizontal incision is made in the tarsal plate with a No. 15 blade 4 mm above the lid margin for the approximate width of the defect. An

additional relaxing incision is then made vertically in the tarsus to the superior border of the tarsus and into the upper fornix. The flap of tarsus and conjunctiva is mobilized horizontally into the defect. The one edge is sutured to the appropriate canthus. A full-thickness skin graft is obtained and sutured in place as described above.

Defects of 50 Percent or More. The canthotomy may be extended in the form of a Tenzel semicircular flap.[164] A semicircular skin muscle flap is outlined. The lower lid retractors and inferior orbital septum are disinserted from their attachment to the lower tarsal border to amplify the effect of the rotation. In this manner, defects of 60 percent or greater can be closed.[165] The flap should be anchored to the periosteum of the lateral orbital rim under some tension (Plate 8-12). The lateral canthus is restored with a vertical mattress suture from the skin muscle flap to the lateral aspect of the upper

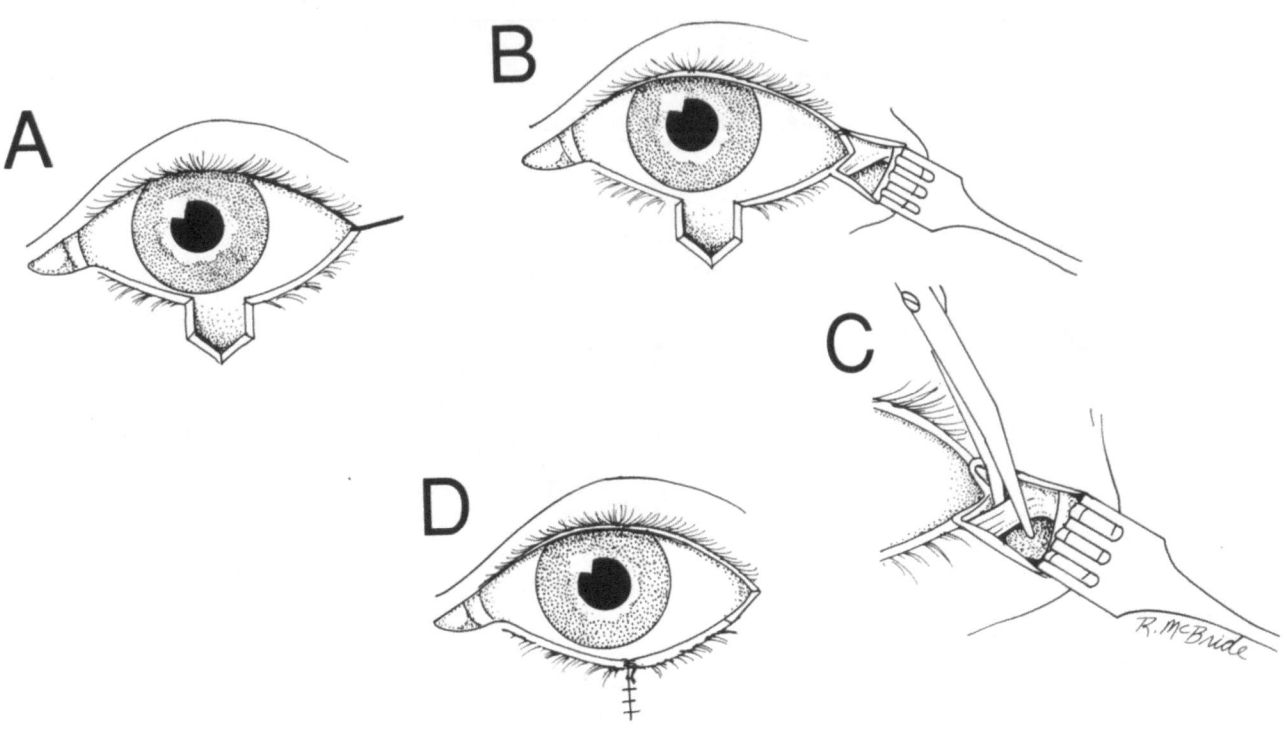

Plate 8-11. (*A–D*) Lateral cantholysis and repair of full-thickness lid defect after removal of lid lesion involving 25–50 percent of the lid.

lid margin. An "upside-down" semicircular flap may also be utilized for upper lid defects. (Plate 8-12.)

Alternatively, a tarsal rotational flap may be used for upper eyelid reconstruction. In this procedure, a vertical strip of upper lid tarsus adjacent to the defect is rotated horizontally and sutured to the lateral canthal tendon area. The anterior lamella is repaired with a skin graft or a skin muscle flap.[166] A tarsal conjunctival pedicle flap may be used in the lower lid as well.

Alternatively, a tarsal pedicle flap may be utilized for lower eyelid reconstruction at the lateral aspect of the lower lid.[167] This technique utilizes a pedicle flap of tarsus from the upper lid to reconstruct lower lid. The upper lid is everted and the lateral 2.5–3.0 mm of upper lid is split to the superior tarsal border. The horizontal length of the upper tarsus necessary to fill the defect is outlined 2 mm parallel from the lid margin. The incision is directed vertically 4 mm then back horizontally to the lateral canthus. The flap is similar to a "T" on its side. The flap of tarsus must be dissected superiorly so that it fills the lower lid defect. A skin muscle lateral canthal rotation creates the anterior lamella.

Free Nasal Chondromucosal Graft (Free Tarsal Conjunctival Graft) with Nasal-Based Skin-Muscle Pedicle and Skin Graft. Moderate or large defects of the upper or lower lids that do not extend vertically may be reconstructed with a nasal chondromusocal graft covered by a nasal-based, horizontal skin muscle flap. The defect

left by the muscle advancement flap is covered by a skin graft. Alternatively, sclera may be used, but then a mucous membrane graft is also required. The mucous membrane graft may not survive.[168]

A free tarsal conjunctival graft may be harvested from the upper lid. The donor upper lid is everted on a Desmarres lid retractor and a free tarsal-conjunctival graft 4 mm wide and of the same length as the lid defect is outlined on the tarsus with a No. 15 Bard-Parker blade (Plate 8-13). The graft is harvested with a Westcott scissors and left unsutured. At least 3 mm of normal tarsus is left adjacent to the lid border.

The graft is sutured in place with interrupted sutures of 6–0 chromic so that the graft slightly overcorrects the lid border. The graft should be sutured against the globe. The conjunctiva should be undermined inferiorly to prevent lower lid retraction. The skin muscle below the defect forms a pedicle flap based nasally that is slightly larger in size than the defect. Alternatively, a bipedicle flap with its greater blood supply than a single pedicle flap is mobilized inferiorly. The skin and tarsal-conjunctival graft are sutured with 6–0 silk to form the new lid margin. A free skin graft of postauricular skin is sutured in place.

Defects of 75 Percent or More. The mainstay of defects of 75 percent or more in the lower lid is the Hughes procedure, and in the upper lid is the Cutler Beard procedure (Plate 8-14). The other technique for

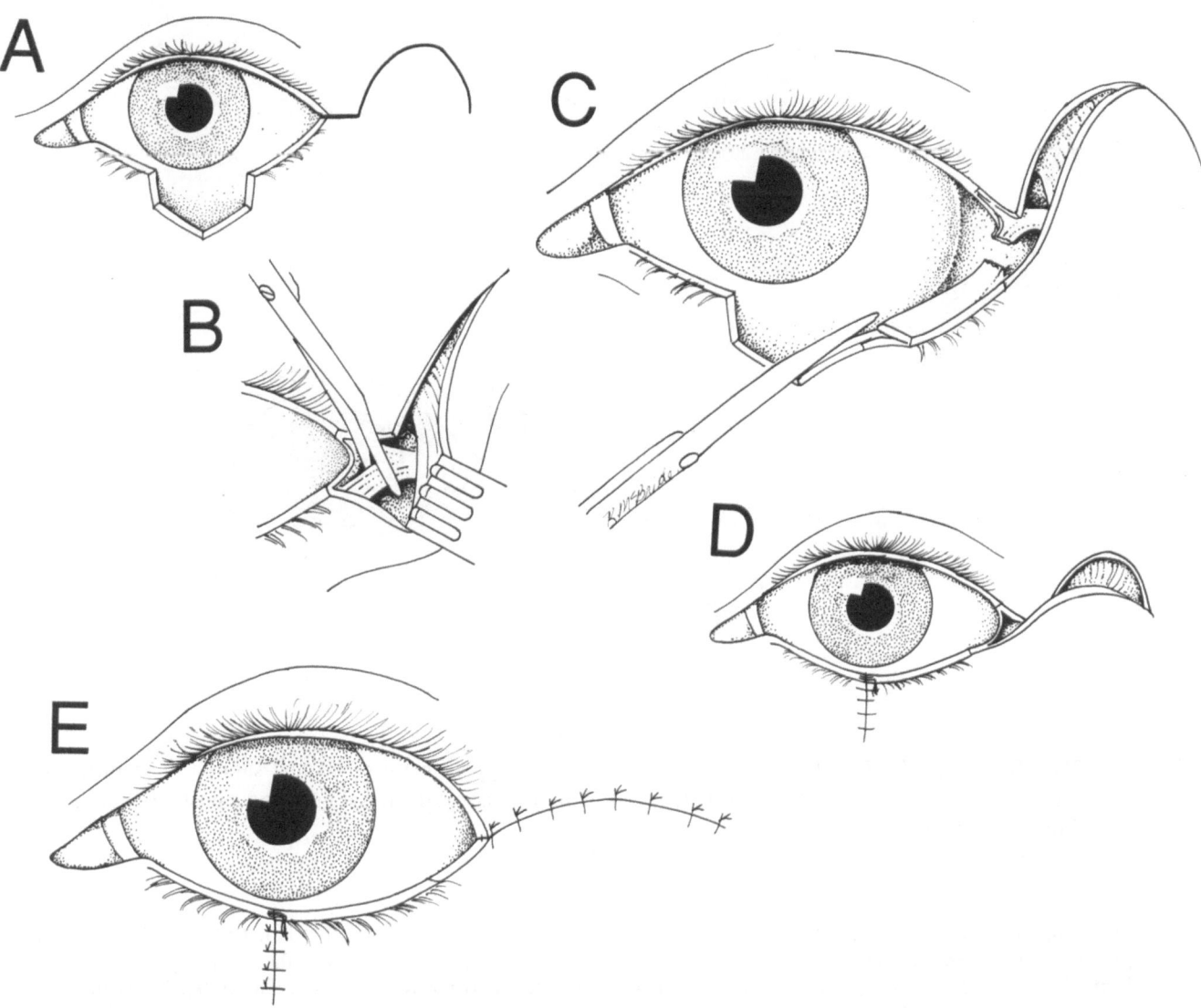

Plate 8-12. (*A*) For defects involving more than 50 percent of the lid, a semicircular flap of Tenzel may be necessary. (*B*) A cantholysis is first performed and the inferior crus of the lateral canthal tendon is severed. (*C*) The lower lid retractors are detached from the inferior tarsal border to assist in mobilizing the lateral lid tissues. One blade of the Westcott scissors is placed in the suborbicularis space and the other outside the conjunctiva. (*D*) The lid margin is reapposed. (*E*) The lateral canthus is reconstructed with a horizontal mattress 4–0 silk suture.

lower lid reconstruction is the Mustarde flap. We prefer not to utilize Mustarde-type cheek flaps because of their heaviness and tendency to pull the lateral canthus and lower lid down.

Hughes and Modified Hughes Procedure. In the modified Hughes procedure, a 4–0 silk transmarginal traction suture is utilized to evert the upper lid on a Desmarres lid retractor.[169] A horizontal incision is made 4 mm above the lid margin. If the incision is closer than 4 mm, an unstable retracted lid may result. In addition, cicatricial entropion with trichiasis of the upper

lids may develop. The incision is slightly shorter horizontally than the defect in the lower lid to prevent ectropion of the lower lid. Vertical incisions are made through the full thickness of the tarsus and conjunctiva at both ends of the tarsal incisions (Plate 8-15). It is better to first lightly outline the tarsal incision with a No. 15 blade and then gradually extend the incision through full-thickness tarsus. A dissection plane is identified in the pretarsal space. By blunt dissection, the tarsus and conjunctiva are freed from Muller's muscle and levator aponeurosis. The dissection should be high into the cul-de-sac so that there is no arching of the upper lid at

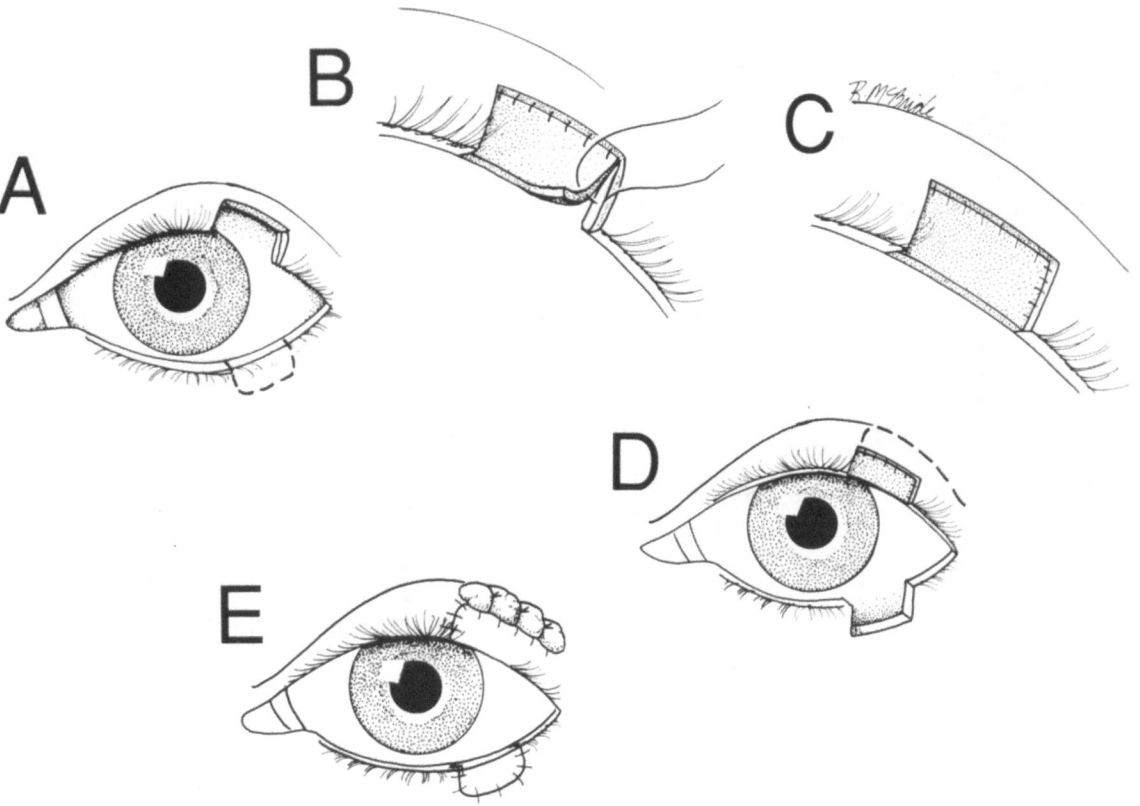

Plate 8-13. *(A–E)* Tarsal free graft is harvested from apposing lower lid and sutured to reconstruct posterior lamella defect. A skin muscle flap is mobilized to cover the tarsal graft and a posterior auricular skin graft fills the skin defect in the lower lid.

the completion of the second stage.[170] Muller's muscle may be included in the flap since it provides graft vascularity.[171] Orbicularis muscle may be mobilized into the recipient skin graft bed in order to increase the viability of the graft and enhance eyelid motility.[172] Next, the remaining normal tarsus is split into anterior and posterior lamellae for 1–2 mm. The upper lid flap is then brought into the defect. A 4–0 double-armed silk suture is passed first through the tarsus of the remaining lid, out through the incision, through the edge of the tarsal flap, and then through the skin muscle flap and tied to itself. A cotton pledget may be used. Alternatively, tarsus is sutured to tarsus without bringing the ends through the skin. The horizontal cut edge of tarsus is sutured to the conjunctive and lower lid retractors with a running 5–0 chromic suture. The anterior lamella is reconstructed by advancing a skin muscle flap from the lower lid and cheek, excising Burrow's triangle as necessary or with a skin graft. The skin graft should not be from the upper lid of the same eye to avoid vertical contraction of the donor lid. Four to six weeks later, the new lower lid is reconstructed by incising the graft with its donor skin parallel to the remaining lid with Westcott scissors. A grooved director may be used to protect the eye and

the flap is incised with a No. 15 blade. The conjunctival edge must extend over the skin edge to prevent skin from irritating the globe. The upper lid is then everted and the residual flap is excised flush with the upper lid. Curretting of the upper lid removes any keratinized epithelium that may irritate the cornea. Any advanced Muller's muscle must be tenotomized. Local infiltrative anesthesia is used for the lower lid and a frontal nerve block for the upper lid.

This same technique may be utilized for marginal defects in the upper lid. For larger vertical defects in the upper lid, apposing tarsal conjunctival flaps from the upper and lower lids may be conjoined.[173] A skin graft is used to create the anterior lamellae of the upper lid.

Mustardé Flap for Reconstruction of Lower Lid. This flap has several distinct disadvantages, and therefore we prefer not to use it. First, it results in a long surgical scar on the face. Second, a triangle of normal tissue has to be excised and discarded. Third, the result leads to a thick cheek flap that has little motion and tends to cause ectropion and lateral canthal downward displacement. The technique is briefly described.[174] A large, nasal-superior triangle with the medial edge in the nasola-

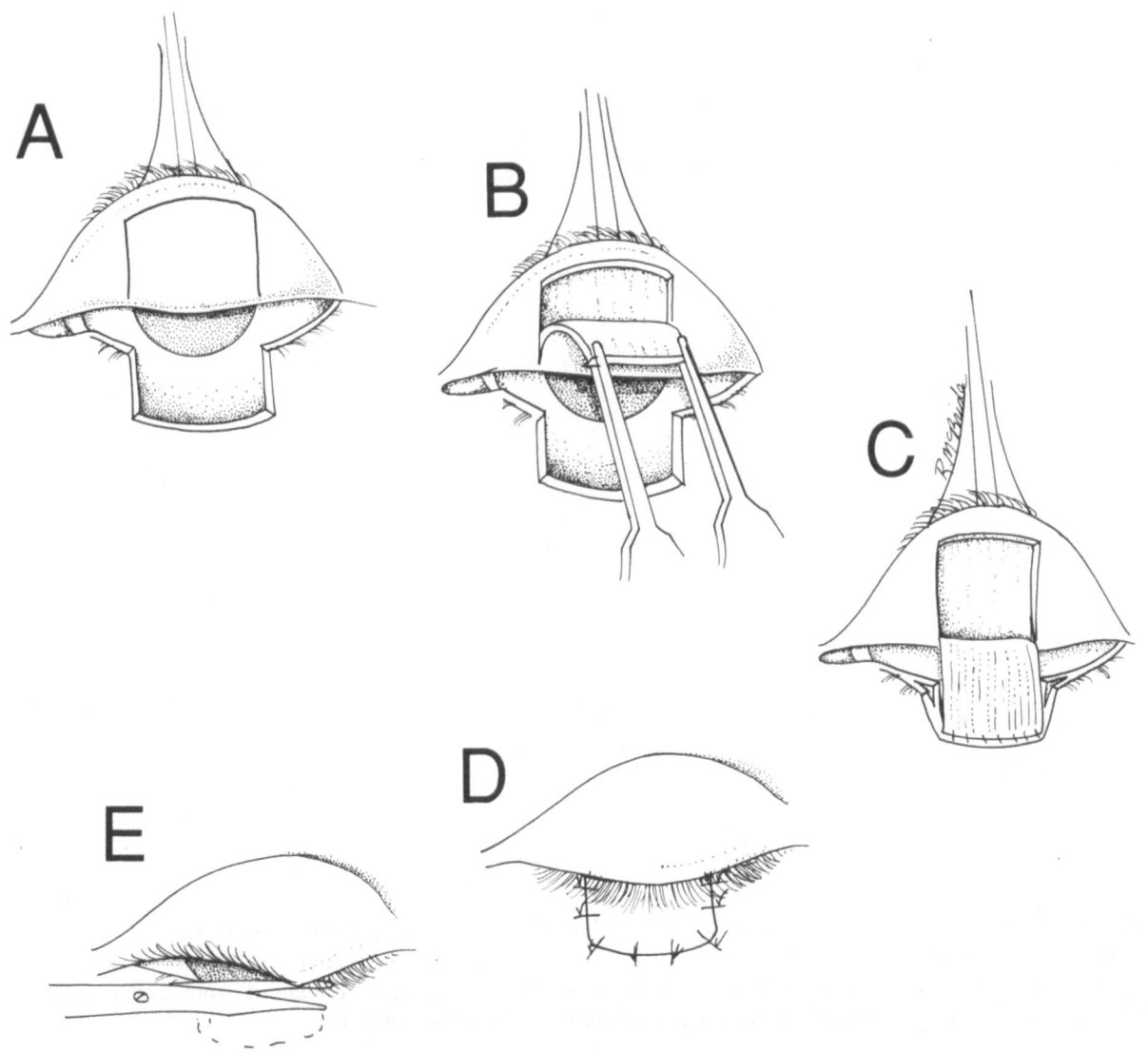

Plate 8-14. (*A–C*) Hughes procedure for reconstruction of large, low, lid defects involves reconstruction of posterior lamella with tarsoconjunctival flap mobilized from upper lid and sutured to tarsus and lower lid retractors of recipient lid. (*D*) Skin graft is utilized to form anterior lamella. (*E*) Lid tissues heal for 4–8 weeks and are then opened using Westcott scissors.

bial fold is outlined. For this reason, this technique is most suited for medial lid defects. The flap begins at the lateral canthus and extends as a semicircle just anterior to the tragus of the ear. Most importantly, the superior limit of the semicircle must extend at least to the level of the brow or higher since the height of the flap will help to counteract postoperative sagging of the reconstructed lower lid. A skin muscle flap is undermined. Branches of the facial nerve are avoided. Next, a chondromucosal graft is obtained and sutured into lid defect from canthus to canthus. The nasal septum contains cartilage as well as a mucosal surface (Plate 8-16).

A 4–0 silk retention suture is placed through the nasal ala and a relaxing incision is made through the nasal

ala. A rectangular strip of nasal mucosa and cartilage is outlined 10 × 5 mm parallel to the turbinates. The opposite nasal muscosa is not violated. The nasal ala is resutured, and the naris is packed with petroleum jelly-impregnated gauze. The rotation cheek flap is then mobilized nasally to fill the nasal triangular defect. The cheek flap is sutured to the medial canthal tendon and to the lateral canthus. Additional 4–0 PDS sutures are used to apply upward traction at the apex of the flap. The eyelids are sutured together to ensure upward traction on the flap. These are left in place 5–7 days.

Cutler Beard and Modified Cutler Beard Bridge Flap. The Cutler Beard bridge flap borrows a full-thick-

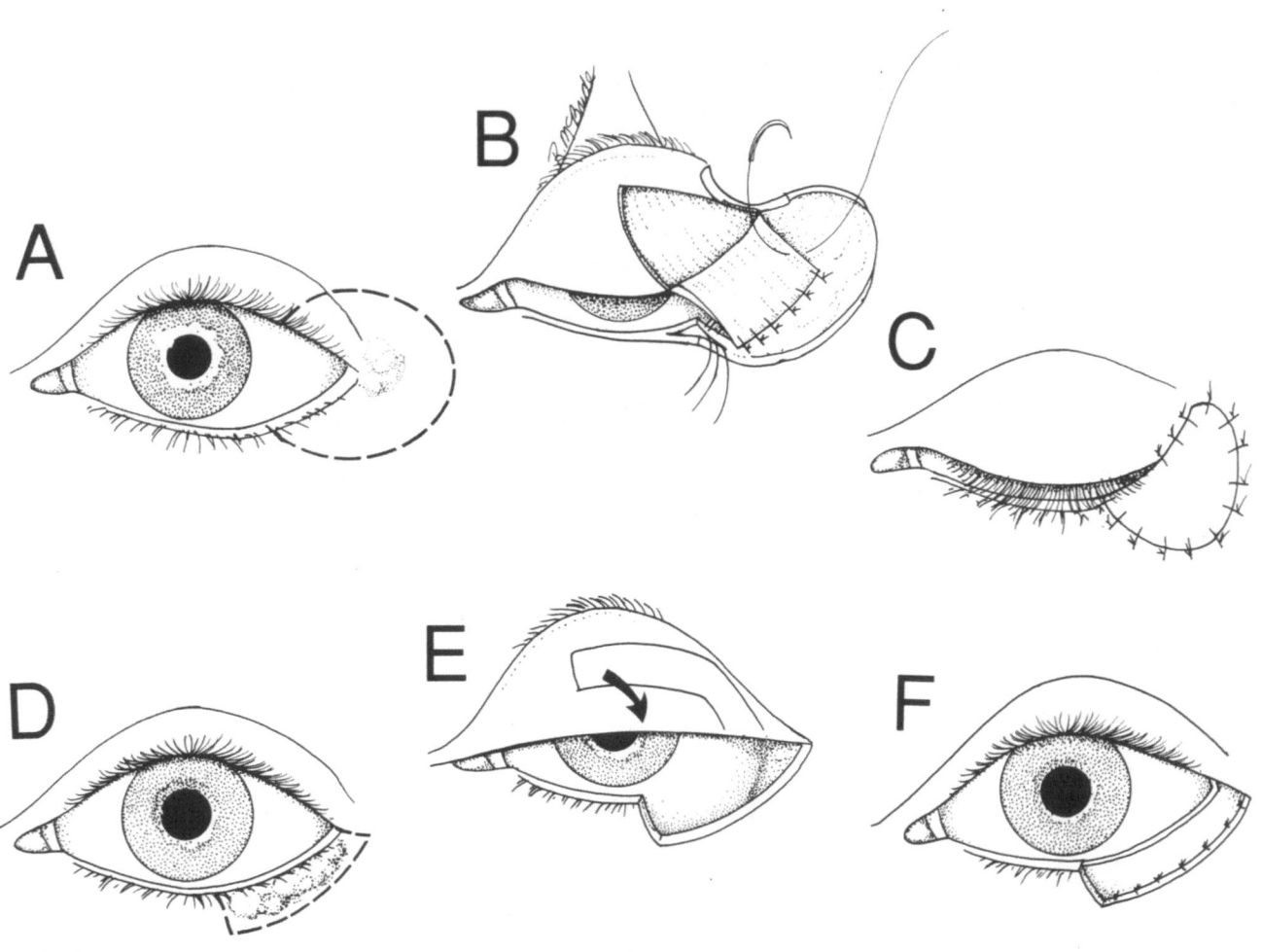

Plate 8-15. (*A–F*) The Hughes' method can be applied to lateral canthal reconstruction as well. (*B*) Tarsoconjunctival flap from upper lid forms posterior lamella of left lower lid defect. Lower lid defect is reconstructed using modified tarsal strip procedure. Skin graft forms anterior lamella. Lids are later severed. (Modified from Leone CR: Tarsal pedicle flap for lower eyelid reconstruction. *Arch Ophthalmol* 95:1423–1424, 1977.)

ness flap from the opposing normal lower lid. The incision is made 4–5 mm below the lower lid margin to preserve the lower lid blood supply (Plate 8-17). A modified Cutler Beard procedure involves the use of donor sclera as a tarsal replacement, which may be used to reconstruct the upper lid since the lower lid flap contains little tarsus.[175] The rectangular flap is designed to exactly fit into the rectangular defect in the upper lid. The donor flap is outlined with a No. 15 blade with the scleral lens in place. A skin muscle flap is undermined to the orbital rim. The conjunctival layer is then dissected from the skin muscle flap and sutured to the conjunctival edge of the upper lid defect with a running 6–0 plain suture. Donor sclera is then sutured to the tarsal remnants or medial or lateral canthal tendon and superiorly to the cut edge of the levator aponeurosis or the levator muscle

itself with interrupted 7–0 silk sutures. Finally, the skin muscle flap from the lower lid is advanced under the bridge of the lid margin and sutured with interrupted 6–0 silk sutures. Thus, the sclera is between the donor conjunctiva and skin muscle flap.

The flap is separated 8 weeks later by cutting the flap 2 mm below the proposed new upper lid margin. The 1–2 mm of keratinized skin is excised and the conjunctiva is rotated anteriorly over the lid margin. The lower lid skin edges are sutured and Burrow's triangles excised as necessary. The lower lid conjunctiva is not closed. Full-thickness mattress sutures of 4–0 silk can be used to form an upper lid fold at the time the bridge flap is separated. All sutures are removed in 1 week.

A shortened upper lid with lagophthalmos is prevented by suturing the upper lid remnants as far down on the

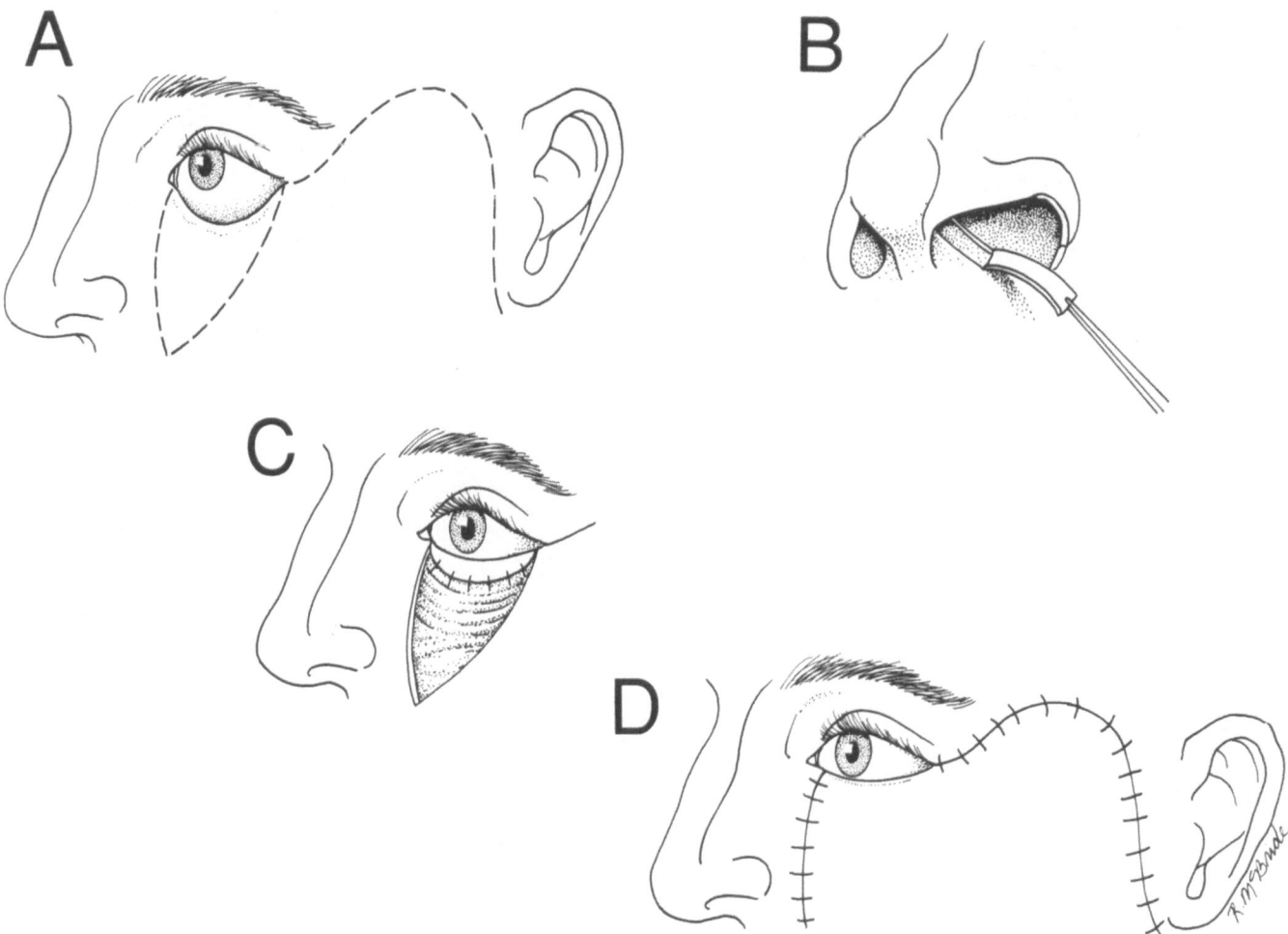

Plate 8-16. (*A*) Lower lid is reconstructed with (*B*) chondral mucosal graft from nasal cavity (may also be harvested with its long axis parallel to the floor of nose). (*C, D*) Skin muscle layer is formed from Mustardé flap. We do not prefer this technique.

flap as possible to include the greatest amount of skin muscle flap in the reconstructed defect in order to give the upper lid a greater vertical dimension.

Composite Grafts in Reconstructing Upper Lid Defects

Composite upper eyelid grafts are free full-thickness sections from the upper lid (Plate 8-18). This technique is helpful in reconstructing large defects in the upper lid when there is not enough adjacent lower eyelid tissue to fill the upper lid defect. To enhance the survival of the composite graft, the composite is denuded of its skin muscle layer; the lid margin and cilia are not removed. The composite graft is obtained from the opposite upper lid and sutured into the recipient upper lid. A skin flap from the recipient upper lid is undermined and

brought over the composite graft. The skin from the composite graft is utilized as a graft to fill the skin defect in the recipient donor lid medially. The muscle layer is discarded.[176]

Reconstruction of the Canaliculus

The lower canaliculus may be reconstructed with as little as one-fourth of the canalicular remnant (Plate 8-19). The distal end of the canaliculus is identified, and the tissue surrounding the canaliculus is undermined so the canaliculus can be stretched. A Johnson wire or Quickert Dryden silicone tube is used to intubate the lacrimal system. The lid is now secured as described above. A notch on the posterior tarsal plate is created in order to reattach the new punctum. The residual canaliculus is then stetched along its axis and sutured to

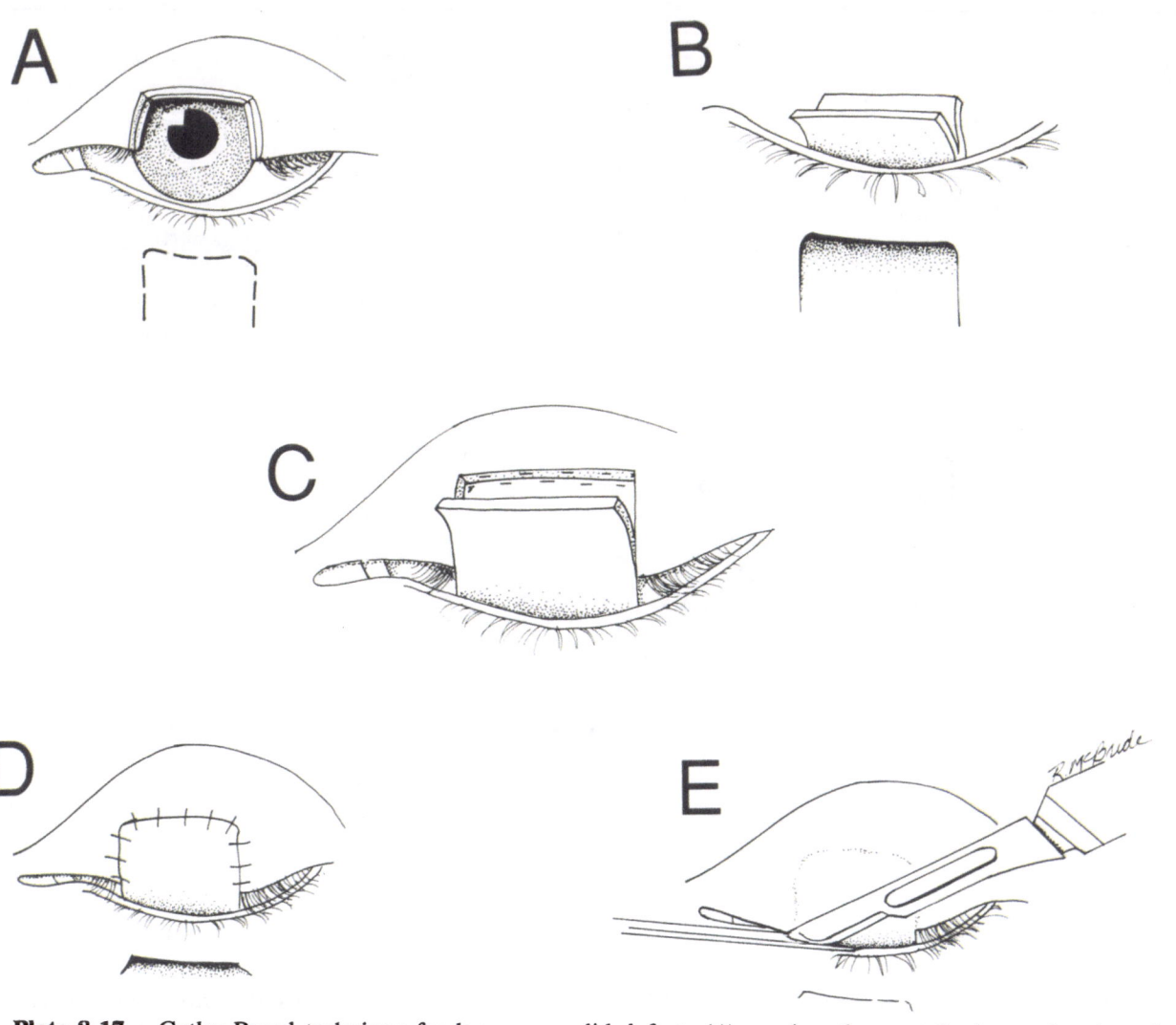

Plate 8-17. Cutler Beard technique for large upper lid defects (*A*) requires the use of a bone plate in order to harvest a full-thickness donor flap (*B*). The flap is advanced into the upper lid defect and orbicular muscle is sutured to levator aponeurosis with a 5–0 chromic running suture; the skin layers are closed (*C,D*). 6–8 weeks later, the flap is severed and the freed flap retracts and after its edges are freshened, it is sutured into the lower lid (*E*).

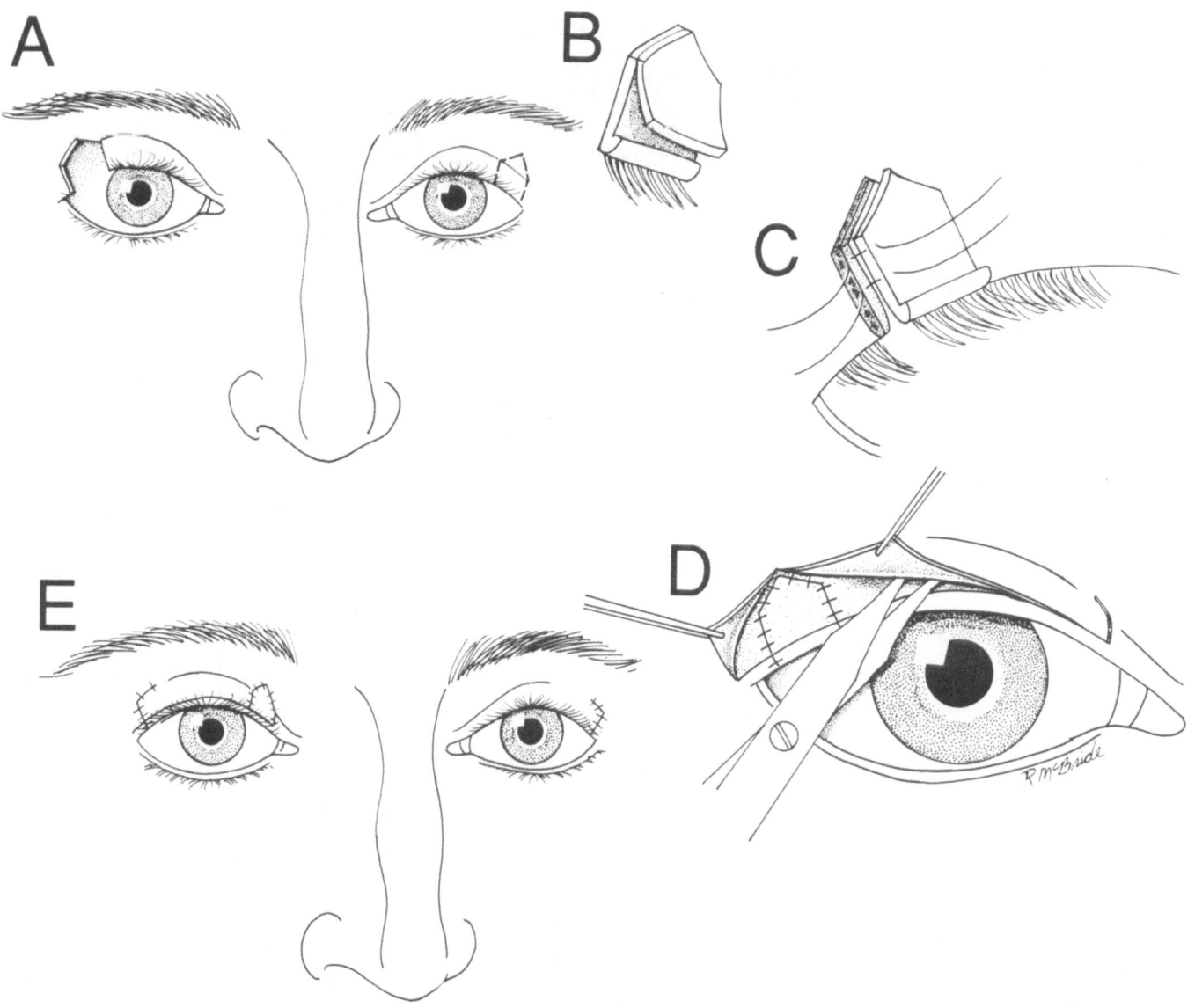

Plate 8-18.   (*A*) Composite graft is harvested from corresponding portion of opposite donor lid. Skin muscle layer is removed and may be utilized for a skin graft; the lid margin including the cilia is undisturbed. (*B,C*) Composite graft is sutured into with 7–0 or 8–0 sutures that are delicate enough to preserve blood supply. (*D*) A skin muscle flap from

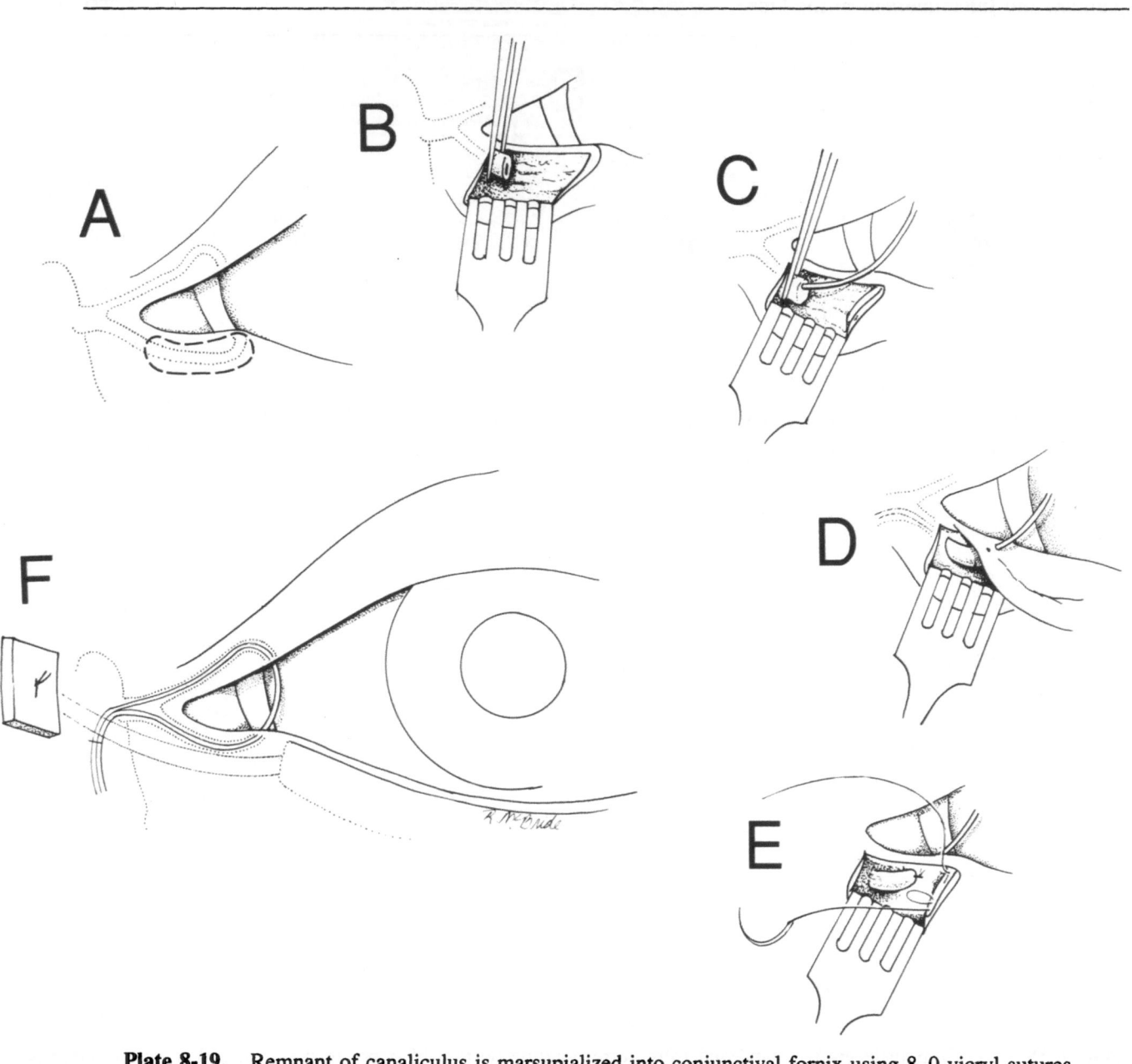

Plate 8-19.   Remnant of canaliculus is marsupialized into conjunctival fornix using 8–0 vicryl sutures.

the posterior border of the tarsal plate with 8–0 silk sutures. The lacrimal stent is left in place for 4–6 weeks.

SUMMARY OF AVAILABLE RECONSTRUCTIVE TECHNIQUES FOR VARIOUS SIZED DEFECTS INVOLVING SPECIFIC AREAS OF THE LIDS AND CANTHI

McCord provides as excellent a summary of this topic as is presently available. Tables 8-14–8-18 have been adapted from his book.[177]

Table 8-14
Upper Lid Defects

Central
  Small
    direct closure
  Moderate
    inverted semicircular flap of Tenzel
    tarsal conjunctival advancement flap from lower lid
      with skin graft
    Cutler Beard bridge flap
  Large
    tarsal conjunctival advancement flap from lower lid
      with skin graft
    Cutler Beard Bridge flap
    nasal chondromucosal graft or tarsal graft with skin
      muscle advancement
  Total
    tarsal conjunctival advancement flap from lower lid
      with skin graft
    Cutler Beard Bridge flap
    nasal chondromucosal graft or tarsal graft with skin
      muscle advancement

Table 8-15
Nasal or Temporal Defects of Upper Lid

Small
  Direct closure
Moderate
  Inverted semicircular flap
  Tarsal conjunctival advancement flaps from lower lid
    with skin graft
  Sliding tarsoconjunctival flap from upper lid with skin
    graft
Large
  Tarsal conjunctival advancement from lower lid and
    skin graft
  Cutler-Beart Bridge Flap

Table 8-16
Central Defects of Lower Lid

Small
  Direct closure
Moderate
  Semicircular flap
Large or total
  Hughes
    Free graft (tarsal, or nasal chondromucosal) with
      skin pedicle flap and skin graft
  Mustarde

Table 8-17
Nasal and Temporal Defects of Lower Lid

Small
  Direct closure
Moderate
  Semicircular flap
Large
  Hughes
  Mustarde
  Free Graft (tarsal, nasal chondromucosal) with skin
    pedicle flap (upper lid) and skin graft

Table 8-18
Medial Canthal Defects

Laissez-faire*
Skin graft, upper lid donor site
Rotation flap from upper lid
Median forehead flap

* with canthal fixation

REFERENCES

1. Jones LT, Reeh MJ, Wirtschafter JD: *Ophthalmic Anatomy.* Rochester. American Academy of Ophthalmology and Otolaryngology, 1970.
2. Hawes MF, Dortzbach RK: The microscopic anatomy of the lower eyelid retractors. *Arch Ophthalmol* 100:1313–1318, 1982.
3. Lever WF, Schaumburg-Lever G: *Histopathology of the Skin,* ed 5. Philadelphia. JB Lipponcott, 1975.
4. Reese A, Wilber J: The eye manifestations of xeroderma pigmentosum. *Am J Ophthalmol* 26:901, 1943.
5. Bellows R, Lahav M, Lepreau R, et al: Ocular manifestations of xeroderma pigmentosum in a black family. *Arch Ophthalmol* 92:113, 1974.
6. El-Hefnaw H, Mortada A: Ocular manifestations of xeroderma pigmentosum. *Br J Dermatol* 77:261, 1965.
7. Gorlin RJ, Goltz RW: Multiple nevoid basal cell epithelioma, jaw cysts, and bifid rib: A syndrome. *N Engl J Med* 262:908–912, 1960.
8. Hammani H, Faggioni R, Streiff EB, et al: Le syndrome d'epitheliomatose naevobasocellulaire multiple. *Ophthalmologica* 172:382–399, 1976.

9. Southwick GJ, Schwart RA: The basal cell nevus syndrome. Disasters occurring among a series of 36 patients. *Cancer* 44:2294–2305, 1979.

10. Clendenning WE, Block JB, Raddle IC: Basal cell nevus syndrome. *Arch Dermatol* 90:38–53, 1964.

11. De Jong PT, Bistervels B, Cosgrove J, et al: Medullated nerve fibers: A sign of multiple basal cell nevi (Gorlin's) syndrome. *Arch Ophthalmol* 103:1833–1836, 1985.

12. Clark WH, Reimer RR, Greene M, et al: Origin of familial malignant melanoma from heritable melanocytic lesions: 'The B-K mole syndrome.' *Arch Dermatol* 114:732–738, 1978.

13. Albert DM, Chang MA, Lamping K, et al: The dysplastic nevus syndrome: A pedigree with primary malignant melanomas of the choroid and skin. *Ophthalmology* 92:1728–1734, 1985.

14. Rodriquez-Sains R: Ocular findings in patients with dysplastic nevus syndrome. *Ophthalmology* 93:661–665, 1986.

15. Wolken SH, Spivey BE, Blodi F: Hereditary adenoid cystic epithelioma (Brooke's tumor). *Am J Ophthalmol* 68:26–34, 1968.

16. Kincaid MC, Green WR, Hoover RE, Farmer ER: Iododerma of the conjunctiva and skin. *Ophthalmology* 88:1216–1220, 1981.

17. Welch RB, Duke JR: Lesions of the lids: A statistical note. *Am J Ophthalmol* 45:415–416, 1958.

18. Aurora AL, Blodi FC: Lesions of the eyelids: A clinicopathological study. *Surv Ophthalmol* 15:94–104, 1970.

19. Kwitko ML, Boniuk M, Zimmerman LE: Eyelid tumors with reference to lesions confused with squamous cell carcinoma I. *Arch Ophthalmol* 69:693–697, 1963.

20. Tesluk G: Eyelid lesions: Incidence and comparison of benign and malignant lesions. *Ann Ophthalmol* 17:704–707, 1985.

21. Lamping K, Fischer MJ, Vareska G, et al: A Merkel cell tumor of the eyelid. *Ophthalmology* 90:1399–1402, 1983.

22. Fett DR, Putterman AM: Primary localized amyloidosis presenting as an eyelid margin tumor. *Arch Ophthalmol* 104:584–585, 1986.

23. Mauriello JA: Trichoepithelioma of the lid margin with loss of lashes. Paper presented at the Biennial AFIP Alumni Meeting, Washington, DC, June, 1985.

24. Herschorn BJ, Jakobiec FA, Hornblass A, et al: Mucoepidermoid carcinoma of the palpebral mucocutaneous junction. *Ophthalmology* 90:1437–1446, 1983.

25. Torre D: Multiple sebaceous tumors. *Arch Dermatol* 98:549–551, 1968.

26. Sacks E, Jakobiec FA, Dodick J: Canaliculops. *Ophthalmology* 94:78–81, 1987.

27. Sacks E, Jakobiec FA, McMillan R, et al: Multiple bilateral apocrine cystadenomas of the lower eyelids: Light and electron microscopic studies. *Ophthalmology* 94:65–71, 1987.

28. Thall E, Grossniklaus H, Cappaert W, Radivoyetvitch M: Acute monocytic leukemia presenting in the eyelid: An immunohistochemical and electron microscopic study. *Ophthalmology* 93:1628–1631.

29. Rulon DB, Helwig EB: Cutaneous sebaceous neoplasms. *Cancer* 33:82–102, 1974.

30. Gardner EJ: Follow-up study of family group exhibiting dominant inheritance for syndrome including intestinal polyps, osteomas, fibromas and epidermal cysts. *Am J Hum Genet* 14:376–398, 1962.

31. Lloyd KM, Dennis M: Cowden's disease: A possible new symptom complex with multiple systems involvement. *Ann Intern Med* 58:136–142, 1963.

32. Brownstein MH, Mehregan AH, Bikowski JB, et al: The dermatopathology of Cowden' syndrome. *Br J Dermatol* 10:667–673, 1979.

33. Macher AM, Palestine AG, Masur H, et al: Multicentric Kaposi's sarcoma of the conjunctiva in a male homosexual with the acquired immnodeficiency syndrome. *Ophthalmology* 90:879, 1983.

34. Fauci AS, Macher AM, Longo DL, et al: Acquired immunodeficiency syndrome. Epidemiologic, clinical, immunologic and therapeutic considerations. *Ann Intern Med* 100:92, 1984.

35. Boniuk M, Zimmerman LE: Eyelid tumors with reference to lesions confused with squamous cell carcinoma. II. Inverted follicular keratosis. *Arch Ophthalmol* 69:698–707, 1963.

36. Boniuk M, Zimmerman LE: Eyelid tumors with reference to lesions confused with squamous cell carcinoma. III. Keratoacanthoma. *Arch Ophthalmol* 77:29–40, 1967.

37. Maize JC: Skin cancer in immunosuppressed patienst. *JAMA* 237:1857, 1977.

38. Peen I: The incidence of malignancies in transplant recipients. *Transplant Proc* 7:323, 1975.

39. Rao NA, Dunn SA, Romero JL, Stout W: Bilateral carcinomas of the eyelid. *Am J Ophthalmol* 101:480–482, 1986.

40. Lins ME, Wirtschafter JD: Polymorphic B-cell lymphoma of the eyelid. *Am J Ophthalmol* 98:634–635, 1984.

41. Gardner TW, O'Grady RB: Mucinous adenocarcinoma of the eyelid: A case report. *Arch Ophthalmol* 102:912, 1984.

42. Lapins NA, Helwig EB: Perineural invasion by keratoacanthoma. *Arch Dermatol* 116:791–793, 1980.

43. Reed RJ: Actinic keratoacanthoma. *Arch Dermatol* 106:858–864, 1972.

44. Boynton JR, Searl SS, Caldwell EH: Large periocular keratoacanthoma: The case for definitive treatment. *Ophthalmic Surg* 17:567–569, 1986.

45. Font RL: Eyelids and lacrimal drainage system, in Spencer WH (ed): *Ophthalmic Pathology: An Atlas and Textbook*, Vol 3. Philadelphia: WB Saunders, 1986, pp 2141–2336.

46. Petrelli R, Cotlier E, Robins S, et al: Dintrochlorobenzene immunotherapy of recurrent squamous papilloma of the conjunctiva. *Ophthalmology* 88:1221, 1981.

47. Neuhaus RW: Bleomycin treatment for recurrent conjunctival papillomas. Paper presented at the 17th Annual Meeting of the American Society of Ophthalmic Plastic and REconstructive Surgery, New Orleans, 1986.

48. Reifler DM, Hornblass A: Squamous cell carcinoma of the eyelid. *Surv Ophthalmol* 30:349–365, 1986.

49. Lund HZ: How often does squamous cell carcinoma of the skin metastasize? *Arch Dermatol* 92:635–637, 1965.

50. Graham JH, Helwig EB: Bowen's disease and its relationship to systemic cancer. *Arch Dermatatol* 80:133–159, 1959.

51. Karp LA, Streeten BW, Cogan DGL: Radiation-induced atrophy of the meibomian glands. *Arch Ophthalmol* 97:303–305, 1979.

52. Martin H, Strong E, Spiro RH: Radiation-induced skin cancer of the head and neck. *Cancer* 25:61–71, 1970.

53. Doxanas MT, Green WR, Iliff CE: Factors in the successful surgical management of basal cell carcinoma of the eyelid. *Am J Ophthalmol* 91:726–736, 1981.

54. Borel DM: Cutaneous basosquamous carcinoma. Review of the literature and report of 35 cases. *Arch Pathol* 95:293–297, 1973.

55. Einaugler RB, Henkind P: Basal cell epithelioma of the eyelid: Apparent incomplete removal. *Am J Ophthalmol* 67:413–417, 1969.

56. Driver JR, Cole HN: Epithelioma of the eyelids and canthi. Report series of 324 cases. *Am J Roentgenol* 41:616–624, 1939.

57. Wiggs EO: Morphea-form basal cell carcinomas of the canthi. *Trans Am Acad Ophthalmol Otolaryngol* 79:649–653, 1975.

58. Gladstein AH: Radiotherapy of eyelid tumors, in Jakobiec FA (ed): *Ocular and Adnexal Tumors*. Birmingham: Aesculapius, 1978, p 484.

59. Forrest AW: Tumors following radiation about the eye. *Trans Am Acad Ophthalmol Otololaryngol* 65:649–771, 1961.

60. Ridenhour CE, Spratt JS: Epidermoid carcinoma of the skin involving the parotid gland. *Am J Surg* 112:504–507, 1966.

61. Shulman J: Treatment of malignant tumors of the eyelids by plastic surgery. *Br J Plast Surg* 15:37–47, 1962.

62. Caya JG, Hidayat AA, Weiner JM: A clinicopathologic study of 21 cases of adenoid squamous cell carcinoma of the eyelid and periorbital region. *Am J Ophthalmol* 99:291–297, 1985.

63. Sternberg I, Buckman G, Levine MR, Sterin W: Trichoepithelioma. *Ophthalmology* 93:531–533, 1986.

64. Mohlenbeck FW: Pilomatrixoma (calcifying epithelioma). *Arch Dermatol* 108:532–534, 1973.

65. Azevedo ML, Milani JA, Souza ED, et al: Pilomatrixoma: An unusual case with secondary corneal ulcer. *Arch Ophthalmol* 103:553–554, 1985.

66. Perez RC, Nicholson DH: Malherbe's calcifying epithelioma (pilomatrixoma) of the eyelid. *Arch Ophthalmol* 97:314, 1979.

67. Hidayat AA, Font RL: Trichilemmoma of eyelid and eyebrow. A clinicopathologic study of 31 cases. *Arch Ophthalmol* 98:844–847, 1980.

68. Rao NA, Hidayat AA, McLean IW, Zimmerman LE: Sebaceous gland carcinoma of the ocular adnexa: A clinicopathologic study of 104 cases with five year follow-up data. *Hum Pathol* 13:113–122, 1982.

69. Condon GP, Brownstein S, Codere F: Sebaceous carcinoma of the eyelid masquerading as superior limbic keratoconjunctivitis. *Arch Ophthalmol* 103:1525–1529, 1985.

70. Tenzel RR, Stewart WB, Boynton JR, Zbar M: Sebaceous adenocarcinoma of the eyelid: Definition of surgical margins. *Arch Ophthalmol* 95:2203–2204, 1977.

71. Ginsberg J: Present status of meibomian gland carcinoma. *Arch Ophthalmol* 73:271–277, 1965.

72. Boniuk M, Zimmerman LE: Sebaceous carcinoma of the eyelid, eyebrows, caruncle, and orbit. *Trans Am Acad Ophthalmol Otolargyngol* 72:619–642, 1968.

73. Putterman AM: Conjunctival map biopsies to determine pagetoid spread. Paper presented at the 17th Annual Meeting of the American Society of Ophthalmic Plastic and Reconstructive Surgery, New Orleans, 1986.

74. Hashimoto K, DiBella RJ, Lever WF: Syringoma: Histochemical and electron microscopic studies. *J Invest Dermatol* 46:150–166, 1966.

75. Glatt HJ, Proia AD, Tsoy ED, et al: Malignant syringoma of the eyelid. *Ophthalmology* 91:987–990, 1984.

76. Ferry AP, Sherman HM: Eccrine acrospiroma (porosyringoma) of the eyelid. *Arch Ophthalmol* 83:591–593, 1970.

77. Headington JT, Niederhuber JE, Beals T: Malignant clear cell acrospiroma. *Cancer* 41:641–647, 1978.

78. Khalil M, Brownstein S, Codere F, et al: Eccrine sweat gland carcinoma of the eyelid with orbital involvement. *Arch Ophthalmol* 98:2210–2214, 1980.

79. Grizzard WS, Torczynski E, Edwards WC: Adenocarcinoma of eccrine sweat gland. *Arch Ophthalmol* 94:2119–2123, 1976.

80. Hood CI, Font RL, Zimmerman LE: Metastatic mammary carcinoma in the eyelid with histiocytoid appearance. *Cancer* 31:793–800, 1073.

81. Jakobiec FA, Austin P, Iwamoto T, et al: Primary infiltrating signet ring carcinoma of the eyelids. *Ophthalmology* 90:291, 1983.

82. Ni C, Wagoner M, Kieval S, Albert DM: Tumours of Moll's glands. *Br J Ophthalmol* 68:502–508, 1984.

83. Hirsch P, Helwig EB: Chondroid syringoma: Mixed tumor of the skin, salivary gland type. *Arch Dermatol* 84:835–847, 1961.

84. Wright JD, Font RL: Mucinous sweat gland adenocarcinoma of eyelid. A clinicopathologic study of 21 cases with histochemical and electron microscopic observations. *Cancer* 44:1757–1768, 1979.

85. Tenzel TR, Boynton JR, Miller GR, et al: Surgical treatment of eyelid neurofibromas. *Arch Ophthalmol* 95:479, 1977.

86. Shields JA, Guibor PE: Neurilemmoma of the eyelid resembling a recurrent chalazion. *Arch Ophthalmol* 102:1650, 1984.

87. Jones IS: Lymphangioma of the ocular adnexa. An analysis of 62 cases. *Trans Am Ophthalmol Soc* 57:602–665, 1959.

88. Pang P, Jakobiec FA, Iwamoto T, et al: Small lymphangiomas of the eyelids. *Ophthalmology* 91:1278, 1984.

89. Charles NC: Multiple glomus tumors of the face and eyelids. *Arch Ophthalmol* 94:1283–1285, 1976.

90. Hidayat AA, Cameron JD, Font RL, Zimmerman LE: Angiolymphoid hyperplasia with eosinophilia (Kimura's disease) of the orbit and ocular adnexa. *Am J Ophthalmol* 96:176–189, 1983.

91. Kalinske M, Leone CR: Kaposi's sarcoma involving eyelid and conjunctiva. *Ann Ophthalmol* 14:497–499, 1982.

92. Rosai J, Sumner HW, Kostianovsky M, Perez-Mesac: Angiosarcoma of the skin. A clinicopathologic and fine structural study. *Hum Pathol* 7:83–109, 1976.

93. Salyer WR, Salyer DC: Intravascular angiomatosis: Development and distinction from angiosarcoma. *Cancer* 36:996–1001, 1975.

94. Kuo T, Sayer P, Rosai J: Masson's "Vegetant intravascular hemangioendothelioma:" A lesion often mistaken for angiosarcoma. Study of seventeen cases located in the skin and soft tissues. *Cancer* 38:1227–1236, 1976.

95. Font RI, Wheeler TM, Boniuk M: Intravascular papillary endothelial hyperplasia of the orbit and ocular adnexa. *Arch Ophthalmol* 101:1731–1736, 1983.

96. Stout AP: Fibrosarcoma: The malignant tumor of fibroblasts. *Cancer* 41:30–63, 1958.

97. Hidayat AA, Font RL: Juvenile fibromatosis of the periorbital region and eyelid. A clinicopathologic study of six cases. *Arch Ophthalmol* 98:280–285, 1980.

98. Fretzin DR, Helwig EB: Atypical fibroxanthoma of the skin. A clinicopathologic study of 140 cases. *Cancer* 31:1541–1552, 1973.

99. Font RL, Zimmerman LE: Nodular fasciitis of the eye and adnexa. *Arch Ophthalmol* 75:475–481, 1966.

100. Stout AP: Fibrosarcoma in infants and children. *Cancer* 15:1028–1040, 1962.

101. Weiner JM, Hidayat AA: Juvenile fibrosarcoma of the orbit and eyelid. A study of five cases. *Arch Ophthalmol* 101:253–259, 1983.

102. Depot MJ, Jakobiec FA, Dodick JM: Bilateral and extensive xanthelasma palpebarum in a young patient. *Ophthalmology* 91:522, 1984.

103. Bullock JD, Bartley GB, Campbell RJ, et al: Necrobiotic xanthogranuloma with paraproteinemia. *Ophthalmology* 93:1233–1236, 1986.

104. Codere F, Lee RD, Anderson RL: Necrobiotic xanthogranuloma of the eyelid. *Arch ophthalmol* 101:60, 1983.

105. Robertson DM, Winkelmann RK: Ophthalmic features of necrobiotic xanthogranuloma with paraproteinemia. *Am J Ophthalmol* 97:173, 1984.

106. Char DH, LeBoil PE, Ljung BM, Wara W: Radiation therapy for ocular necrobiotic xanthogranuloma. *Arch Ophthalmol* 105:174–175, 1987.

107. Reo NA, Font RL: Pseudorheumatoid nodules of the ocular adnexa. *Am J Ophthalmol* 79:471–478, 1975.

108. Carter BT, Sanborn GE, Humphries MK: rheumatoid nodes of the upper lid. *Arch Ophthalmol* 94:2127, 1976.

109. Newell GB, Stone OJ, Mullins JF: Juvenile xanthogranuloma and neurofibromatosis. *Arch Dermatol* 107:262, 1973.

110. Zimmerman LE: Ocular lesions of juvenile xanthogranuloma. Nevoxanthoendothelioma. *Trans Am Acad Ophthalmol Otolaryngol* 69:412–439, 1965.

111. Jaffe HL: Lipid (cholesterol) granulomatosis, in Jaffe HL (ed): *Metabolic, Degenerative and Inflammatory Diseases of Bones and Joints*. Philadelphia: Lea & Febiger, 1972, pp 535–541.

112. Alper MG, Zimmerman LE, LaPiana FG: Orbital manifestations of Erdheim-Chester disease. *Trans Am Ophthalmol Soc* 81:64–85, 1983.

113. Carney JA, Gordon H, Carpenter PC, et al: The complex of myxomas, spotty pigmentation, and endocrine overactivity. *Medicine* 64:270–283, 1985.

114. Pe'er J, Hidayat AA: Myxomas of the conjunctiva. *Am J Ophthalmol* 102:80–86, 1986.

115. Addison DJ: Malakoplakia of the eyelid. *Ophthalmology* 93:1964–1967, 1986.

116. Eagle RC, Brooks JS, Katowitz JA, et al: Fibrin as a major component of ligneous conjunctivitis. *Am J Ophthalmol* 101:493–494, 1986.

117. Kint A: A comparative electron microscopic study of the perivascular hyaline from porphyria cutanea tarda and from lipoid-proteinosis. *Arch Klin Exp Dermatol* 239:203–212, 1970.

118. Weiner JM, Henderson PN, Roche J: Metastatic eyelid carcinoma. *Am J Ophthalmol* 101:252–254, 1986.

119. Mansour AM, Hidayat AA, McLean IW: Metastatic lid disease. *Ophthalmology* 93:101, 1986.

120. Arnold AC, Bullock JD, Foos RY: Metastatic eyelid carcinoma. *Ophthalmology* 92:114, 1985.

121. Zimmerman LE: Phakomatous choristoma of the eyelid, a tumor of lenticular anlage. *Am J Ophthalmol* 71:169–177, 1971.

122. Allen AC: Juvenile melanoma of children and adults and melanocarcinomas of children. *Arch Dermatol* 82:325, 1960.

123. Naidoff MA, Bernardino VB, Clark WH: Melanocytic lesions of the eyelid skin. *Am J Ophthalmol* 82:371, 1976.

124. McGovern VJ, Mihm MC, Bailly C, et al: The classification of malignant melanoma and its histologic reporting. *Cancer* 32:1446, 1973.

125. Folberg RF, MaLean IW, Zimmerman LE: Conjunctival melanosis and melanoma. *Ophthalmology* 91:673–678, 1984.

126. Sutula FC, Dortzbach RK, Bolles JC: Desmoplastic malignant melanoma of the upper eyelid. *Ann Ophthalmol* 14:141, 1982.

127. Searl SS, Boynton JR, Markowitch W, diSant'Agnese PA: Malignant Merkel cell neoplasms of the eyelid. *Arch Ophthalmol* 102:907–911, 1984.

128. Beyer CK, Goodman M, Dickerson R, Doughtery M: Merkel cell tumor of the eyelid: A clinicopathologic case report. *Arch Ophthalmol* 101:1098–1101, 1983.

129. Luthra CI, Doxanas MT, Green WR: Lesions of the caruncle: A clinicohistopathology study. *Surv Ophthalmol* 23:183–195, 1978.

130. Shields CL, Shields JA, White D, Augsburger JJ: Types and frequency of lesions of the caruncle. *Am J Ophthalmol* 102:771–778, 1986.

131. Meekins B, Proia AD, Klintworth GK: Cutaneous T-cell lymphoma presenting as rapidly enlarging ocular adnexal tumor. *Ophthalmology* 92:1288–1293, 1985.

132. Mathew M, D'Souza P, Mehta DK: A new treatment of pthiriasis palpebrarum. *Ann Ophthalmol* 14:439, 1982.

133. Wilhellmus KR: Myiasis palpebrarum. *Am J Ophthalmol* 101:496–498, 1986.

134. Davino D, Margop CE, McCoy, Friedl FE: Dermal myiasis of the eyelid. *Ophthalmology* 93:1225–1227, 1986.

135. Kersten RC, Shoukrey NM, Tabbara KF: Orbital myiasis. *Ophthalmology* 93:1228–1232, 1986.

136. Font RL, Neafie RC, Perry HD: Subcutaneous dirofilariasis of the eyelid and ocular adnexa. Report of six cases. *Arch Ophthalmol* 98:1089–1082, 1980.

137. Perry HD, Font RL: Cysticercosis of the eyelid. *Arch Ophthalmol* 96:1255–1257, 1978.

138. Barr CC, Gamel JW: Blastomycosis of the eyelid. *Arch Ophthalmol* 104:96–97, 1986.

139. Perry DM, Kirby WM: Acute disseminated coccidioidomycosis. Two cases treated with amphotericin B. *Arch Intern Med* 105:929–934, 1960.

140. Chu FC, Rodrigues MM, Cogan DG, Fauci AS: The pathology of idiopathic midline destructive disease (IMDD) in the eyelid. *Ophthalmology* 90:11385–1388, 1983.

141. Huey C, Jakobiec FA, Iwamoto T, et al: Discoid lupus erythematosus of the eyelids. Ophthalmology 90:1389–1398, 1983.

142. Wood TO, Johnson C: Factitious ulceration of the upper eyelid. *Arch Ophthalmol* 93:388–389, 1975.

143. Wesley RE, Close LW, Ballinger WH, et al: Dapsone in the treatment of presumed brown recluse spider bite of the eyelid. *Ophthalmic Surg* 16:116–120, 1985.

144. Browning DJ, Proia AD, Sanfilippo FP: Pyoderma gangrenosum involving the eyelid. *Arch Ophthalmol* 103:551–552, 1985.

145. Rakofksy SI: The adequacy of surgical excision of basal cell carcinoma. *Ann Ophthalmol* 5:596–600, 1973.

146. Payne JW, Duke JR, Butner R, et al: Basal cell carcinoma of the eyelids. *Arch Ophthalmol* 81:553–558, 1969.

147. Older JJ, Quickert MM, Bear C: Surgical removal of basal cell carcinoma of the eyelids using frozen section control. *Trans Am Acad Ophthalmol* 79:658, 1975.

148. Chalfin J, Putterman AM: Frozen section control in the surgery of basal cell carcinoma of the eyelid. *Am J Ophthalmol* 87:802–809, 1979.

149. Anderson RL, Ceilley RI: A multispecialty approach to the excision and reconstruction of eyelid tumors. *Ophthalmology* 85:1150, 1978.

150. Nunnery WR, Welsh MG, McCord CD: Recurrence of sebaceous carcinoma of the eyelid after radiation therapy. *Am J Ophthalmol* 96:10–15, 1983.

151. Hendley RL, Rieser JC, Cavanagh HD, et al: Primary radiation therapy for meibomian gland carcinoma. *Am J Ophthalmol* 87:206–209, 1979.

152. O'Dair RB: The diagnosis and treatment of malignant tumors of the eyelid. *Ophthalmic Forum* 1:44–49, 1983.

153. Zacarian SA: The cryogenic approach to the treatment of lid tumors. *Ann Ophthalmol* 2:706–713, 1970.

154. Beard C: Observations on the treatment of basal cell carcinoma of the eyelids. *Trans Am Acad Ophthalmol Otolaryngol* 70:664–670, 1975.

155. Wojno T, Tenzel RR: Actinic comedonal plaque of the eyelid. *Am J Ophthalmol* 96:687–688, 1983.

156. Liu D, Natielloa J, Schaefer A, Gage A: Cryosurgical treatment of the eyelids and lacrimal drainage ducts of the rhesus monkey. *Arch Ophthalmol* 102:934–939, 1984.

157. Fraunfelder FT, Farris HE, Wallace TR: Cryosurgery for ocular and periocular lesions. *J Dermatol Surg Oncol* 3:841–847, 1977.

158. Tse DT, Kersten RC, Anderson RL: Hematoporphyrin derivative photoradiation therapy in managing nevoid basal-cell carcinoma syndrome. A preliminary report. *Arch Ophthalmol* 102:990–994, 1984.

159. Pizzarell LD, Jakobiec FA, Hofeldt AJ, et al: Intralesional corticosteroid therapy of chalazion. *Am J Ophthalmol* 87:582–583, 1979.

160. Bersani TA, Nichols CW: Intralesional triamcinolone for cutaneous palpebral sarcoidosis. *Am J Ophthalmol* 99:561–562, 1985.

161. Thomas EL, Laborde RP: Retinal and choroidal vascular occlusion following intralesional corticosteroid injection of a chalazion. *Ophthalmology* 93:405–407, 1986.

162. Putterman AM: Semicircular skin flap in reconstruction of nonmarginal eyelid skin defects. *Am J Ophthalmol* 84:708–710, 1984.

163. Fox S, Beard C: Spontaneous lid repair. *Am J Ophthalmol* 58:947–952, 1964.

164. Tenzel RR, Stewart WB: Eyelid reconstruction by the semi-circle flap technique. *Ophthalmology* 85:1164–1169, 1978.

165. Levine MR, Buckman G: Semicircular flap revisited. *Arch Ophthalmol* 104:915–917, 1986.

166. Kersten RC, Anderson RL, Tse DT, Weinstein GL: Tarsal rotational flap for upper eyelid reconstruction. *Arch Ophthalmol* 104:918–922, 1986.

167. Leone CR: Tarsal pedicle flap for lower eyelid reconstruction. *Arch Ophthalmol* 95:1423–1424, 1977.

168. Leone CR, Hand SI: Reconstruction of the medial eyelid. *Am J Ophthalmol* 87:797–801, 1979.

169. Cies WA, Bartlett RE: Modification of the Mustarde and Hughes methods of reconstruction of the lower lid. *Ann Ophthalmol* 7:1497–1501, 1967.

170. Flanagan JC: Eyelid reconstruction. A. Lower eyelid reconstruction, in Stewart WB(ed): *Ophthalmic Plastic and Reconstructive Surgery*. San Francisco: American Academy of Ophthalmology, 1984, pp 247–257.

171. McCord CD, Nunery WR: Reconstructive procedures of the lower eyelid and outer canthus, in McCord CD (ed): *Oculoplastic Surgery* New York: Raven, 1981, pp 198–209.

172. Doxanas MT: Orbicularis muscle mobilization in eyelid reconstruction. Arch Ophthalmol 104:910–914, 1986.

173. Leone CR: Tarsal-conjunctival advancement flaps for upper eyelid reconstruction. *Arch Ophthalmol* 101:945–948, 1983.

174. Mustarde JC: Repair and reconstruction in the orbital region. Edinburg: Churchill/Livingson,

175. McCord CD, Wesley R: Reconstruction of the upper eyelid and medial canthus, in McCord CD(ed): *Oculoplastic Surgery*. New York: Raven Press, 1981, pp 175–187.

176. Putterman AM: Viable composite grafting in eyelid reconstruction. *Am J Ophthalmol* 85:237–241, 1978.

177. McCord CD: System of repair of full thickness eyelid defects, in McCord CD (ed): *Ocuplastic Surgery*. New York: Raven Press, 1981, pp 211–221.

Index